Medical Management of Wildlife Species

Medical Management of Wildlife Species

A Guide for Practitioners

Edited by

Sonia M. Hernandez
DVM, DACZM, PhD
Professor-Wildlife
D.B. Warnell School of Forestry and Natural Resources
and the Southeastern Cooperative Wildlife Disease
Study, Department of Population Health, College of
Veterinary Medicine
University of Georgia
Athens, GA, USA

Heather W. Barron
DVM, DABVP (Avian)
Medical & Research Director
Clinic for the Rehabilitation of Wildlife (CROW)
Sanibel, FL, USA

Erica A. Miller
DVM, CWR
Adjunct Associate Professor of Wildlife Medicine
Department of Clinic Studies
University of Pennsylvania School of Veterinary
Medicine
Philadelphia, PA, USA

Roberto F. Aguilar
DVM, Dip. ECZM (Zoo Health Management)
European Recognized Veterinary Specialist in
Zoological Medicine (Zoo Health Management)
Veterinarian
Tucson Wildlife Center
Tucson, AZ, USA

Michael J. Yabsley
MS, PhD, FRES
Professor-Wildlife
D.B. Warnell School of Forestry and Natural
Resources and the Southeastern Cooperative
Wildlife Disease Study, Department of
Population Health, College of Veterinary
Medicine
University of Georgia
Athens, GA, USA

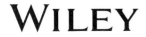

Registered Office
John Wiley & Sons, Inc., 111 River Street, Hoboken, NJ 07030, USA

Editorial Office
111 River Street, Hoboken, NJ 07030, USA

For details of our global editorial offices, customer services, and more information about Wiley products visit us at www.wiley.com.

Wiley also publishes its books in a variety of electronic formats and by print-on-demand. Some content that appears in standard print versions of this book may not be available in other formats.

Library of Congress Cataloging-in-Publication Data

Names: Hernandez, Sonia M., 1969– editor. | Barron, Heather W., 1967– editor.
| Miller, Erica A., editor. | Aguilar, Roberto F., editor. | Yabsley, Michael J., editor.
Title: Medical management of wildlife species : a guide for practitioners /
edited by Sonia M. Hernandez, Heather W. Barron, Erica A. Miller,
Roberto F. Aguilar, Michael J. Yabsley.
Description: Hoboken, NJ : Wiley-Blackwell, 2020. | Includes bibliographical
references and index. |
Identifiers: LCCN 2019017439 (print) | LCCN 2019018358 (ebook) | ISBN
9781119036364 (Adobe PDF) | ISBN 9781119036715 (ePub) | ISBN 9781119036586
(hardback)
Subjects: | MESH: Animals, Wild | Animal Diseases | Communicable
Diseases–veterinary | Veterinary Medicine–methods
Classification: LCC SF996.4 (ebook) | LCC SF996.4 (print) | NLM SF 996.4 |
DDC 636.089/6–dc23
LC record available at https://lccn.loc.gov/2019017439

Cover Design: Wiley
Cover Image: © Alexander Karpikov/Shutterstock
© Roberto F. Aguilar, © Heather W. Barron, © Kim Steininger

Set in 10/12pt Warnock by SPi Global, Pondicherry, India

SKY10091211_111924

Contents

List of Contributors

Noha Abou-Madi, DVM, MSc, DACZM
Associate Clinical Professor
Section of Zoological Medicine
Cornell University
Ithaca, NY
USA

Matthew C. Allender, DVM, PhD
Assistant Professor, Veterinary Clinical
Medicine
Director, Wildlife Epidemiology Lab
Research Affiliate, Prairie Research Institute
Department of Veterinary Clinical Medicine
University of Illinois
Urbana, IL
USA

Heather W. Barron, DVM, DABVP (Avian)
Medical & Research Director
Clinic for the Rehabilitation of Wildlife (CROW)
Sanibel, FL, USA

R. Avery Bennett, DVM, MS, DACVS
Professor of Department of Veterinary Clinical
Sciences
School of Veterinary Medicine
Louisiana State University
Baton Rouge, LA
USA

Linda E. Bowen
Wildlife Rehabilitator
Bats101.info
Falls Village, CT
USA

Allan Casey
WildAgain Wildlife Rehabilitation, Inc.
Evergreen, CO
USA

Edward E. Clark Jr, BA
Director/Founder
Wildlife Center of Virginia
Waynesboro, VA
USA

Leigh Ann Clayton, DVM, DABVP (Avian), DABVP (Reptilian/Amphibian)
Vice President of Animal Care and Welfare
National Aquarium
Baltimore, MD
USA

Kristen Dubé, DVM
Veterinarian
Phillip and Patricia Frost Museum of Science
Miami, FL
USA

Rebecca S. Duerr, DVM, MPVM, PhD
Veterinarian and Research Director
International Bird Rescue
Fairfield, CA
USA

Scott Ford, DVM, DABVP (Avian)
Avian Specialty Veterinary Services
Milwaukee, WI
USA

Laurie J. Gage, DVM, Dipl ACZM
Big Cat and Marine Mammal Specialist
USDA APHIS Animal Care
Napa, CA
USA

Antonia Gardner, DVM
Medical Director
South Florida Wildlife Center (SFWC)
Fort Lauderdale, FL
USA

Michele Goodman, MHS, VMD
Director of Veterinary Services
Elmwood Park Zoo
Norristown, PA
USA

Bethany Groves, DVM
Wildlife Veterinarian
PAWS Wildlife Center
Lynnwood, WA
USA

David Sanchez-Migallon Guzman, DVM, MS, ACZM, ECZM
Associate Professor of Clinical Medicine and
Epidemiology
Companion Exotic Animal Medicine and Surgery Service
Department of Medicine and Epidemiology
School of Veterinary Medicine
University of California Davis
Davis, CA
USA

Michelle G. Hawkins, VMD DABVP (Avian)
Director, California Raptor Center
Professor, Companion Exotic Animal Medicine and
Surgery Service
Department of Medicine and Epidemiology
School of Veterinary Medicine
University of California
Davis, CA
USA

Sonia M. Hernandez, DVM, DACZM, PhD
Professor, D.B. Warnell School of Forestry and Natural
Resources and the Southeastern Cooperative Wildlife
Study at the College of Veterinary Medicine
University of Georgia
Athens, GA
USA

John R. Huckabee, DVM
Veterinary Program Manager
PAWS Wildlife Center
Lynnwood, WA
USA

Helen Ingraham, DVM
Associate Veterinarian
Veterinary Emergency & Critical Care
Las Vegas, NV
USA

Kelli Knight, DVM, CWR
Staff Veterinarian
Southwest Virginia Wildlife Center of Roanoke
Roanoke, VA
USA

Jeannie Lord, PhD
Executive Director/Founder, Pine View Wildlife
Rehabilitation and Education Center
Fredonia, WI
USA

Elizabeth A. Maxwell, DVM, MS
Surgical Oncology Fellow
Department of Small Animal Clinical Sciences
College of Veterinary Medicine
University of Florida
Gainesville, FL
USA

Dave McRuer, MSc, DVM, DACVPM
Wildlife Health Specialist
Parks Canada Agency
Charlottetown, PEI
Canada

Erica A. Miller, DVM, CWR
Adjunct Associate Professor of Wildlife
Medicine
Department of Clinic Studies
University of Pennsylvania School of Veterinary
Medicine
Philadelphia, PA
USA

Terry M. Norton, DVM, DACZM
Director/Veterinarian
Georgia Sea Turtle Center/Jekyll Island Authority
Jekyll Island, GA
USA

Joanne Paul-Murphy, DVM, DACZM, DACAW
Director, The Richard M. Schubot Parrot
Wellness & Welfare Program
Professor, Companion Exotic Animal
Medicine and Surgery Service
Department of Medicine and Epidemiology
School of Veterinary Medicine
University of California
Davis, CA
USA

Nicole Rosenhagen, DVM
Wildlife Veterinarian
PAWS Wildlife Center
Lynwood, WA
USA

Renée Schott, DVM, CWR
Medical Director and Senior Veterinarian
Wildlife Rehabilitation Center of Minnesota
Roseville, MN
USA

David Scott, DVM
Staff Veterinarian
Carolina Raptor Center
Huntersville, NC
USA

Marcy J. Souza, DVM, MPH, DABVP (Avian), DACVPM
Associate Professor
College of Veterinary Medicine
University of Tennessee
Knoxville, TN
USA

Florina S. Tseng, BS, DVM
Director, Wildlife Clinic
Cummings School of Veterinary Medicine
Tufts University
North Grafton, MA
USA

Peach van Wick, MS, DVM
Research Fellow
Wildlife Center of Virginia
Waynesboro, VA
USA

Sallie C. Welte, MA, VMD
Clinic Director Emeritus
Tri-State Bird Rescue and Research, Inc.
Newark, DE
USA; and
Adjunct Associate Professor of Wildlife Medicine
Department of Clinic Studies
University of Pennsylvania School of Veterinary Medicine
Philadelphia, PA
USA

Julia K. Whittington, DVM
Clinical Professor of Zoological Medicine
Veterinary Teaching Hospital Director
College of Veterinary Medicine
University of Illinois at Urbana-Champaign
Urbana, IL
USA

Michael J. Yabsley, MS, PhD, FRES
Professor-Wildlife
D.B. Warnell School of Forestry and Natural Resources and the Southeastern Cooperative Wildlife Disease Study, Department of Population Health, College of Veterinary Medicine
University of Georgia
Athens, GA
USA

Michael Ziccardi, DVM, MS, PhD
Director for Oiled Wildlife Care Network
Associate Director of the Karen C. Drayer Wildlife Health Center
School of Veterinary Medicine
University of California
Davis, CA
USA

Preface

There have always been caring and idealistic people who wanted to help wildlife. Think of tales like Aesop's story about the lion with the thorn in his paw. I wouldn't be surprised if the origins of the domestic dog might have arisen from an early hominid child "rescuing" an "orphan" wolf pup.

This book represents an amazing example of how far wildlife rehabilitation has come. It combines the expertise of some of the top wildlife rehabilitators and goes a long way toward defining the current state of the art. Although much of the focus is clinical, there are also important chapters on aspects of population health and research.

I first got involved in rehab in 1971. Back then, rehab was almost prehistoric by today's standards. There were pitifully few organized centers and even fewer resources. There were no textbooks, no journals, and no state or national organizations holding meetings. Most rehab was carried out in the homes of well-meaning people who had little training and no veterinary support. The internet was a science fiction dream and desktop computers were not yet practical for most of us. In retrospect, it's amazing how rapidly all that changed.

It may have been the combination of several social trends in the 1960s and early 1970s that fostered the emergence of wildlife rehabilitation as an organized discipline. Rachel Carson's 1962 publication of *Silent Spring* heralded a new era of social and environmental concern and consciousness. The succeeding years brought fundamental changes in how people think of our relationships with nonhuman species and the natural world.

Society was in upheaval in the US and abroad. Women's liberation, the civil rights movement, and antiwar sentiment were galvanizing people into action. The first Earth Day in 1970 made popular the philosophical approach "think globally, act locally" (René Dubos). At about the same time the animal rights movement was gaining momentum.

Such energy and activism propelled passage of landmark legislation including the Animal Welfare Act (1966), Clean Air Act (1970), Clean Water Act (1972),

and Endangered Species Act (1973), as well as the establishment of the USEPA (1970) and passage of the Toxic Substances Control Act (1976).

Biologists and veterinarians had been involved in wildlife disease investigation for many years. The Wildlife Disease Association was founded in 1951 but it wasn't until the 1970s that some veterinary schools in the US began to introduce wildlife medicine into their curricula. The American Association of Wildlife Veterinarians was founded in 1979.

The 1970s was also the decade that saw wildlife rehabilitation evolve and begin to develop into state and national organizations. In 1972, rehabilitators in California joined to form the Wildlife Rehabilitation Council – this became the International WRC in 1986. In the midwest and east, the National Wildlife Rehabilitators Association was incorporated in 1982. And overseas the British Wildlife Rehabilitation Council was formed in 1987.

As a rehabilitator, it was encouraging to see all these advances taking place. It was especially exciting to see authors and organizations begin to publish more and more books and journals to assist rehabilitators, veterinarians, and researchers (a partial list of some early books is appended).

And that's where this book comes in. It is an encyclopedic resource that many of us will be using for years to come. In looking at the list of authors for this volume, you will see contributions from an interesting and diverse group of rehabilitators and veterinarians. Some of the vets were rehabilitators first and were drawn to veterinary medicine by their desire to do more for their wildlife patients and their passion for science. Others were environmental educators or wildlife biologists whose commitment to conservation issues introduced them to the need for wildlife care. Still others got their start in rehab through small animal medicine, zoo medicine or training in the military.

One of the lessons that most of us have learned is that academic training alone is not sufficient to make a good rehabilitator. Anyone who is serious about their wildlife interests needs to get as much hands-on experience as they can. This can include formal coursework, internships, participating in professional meetings, and constantly picking the brains of knowledgeable, experienced rehabbers. And we've got to keep reading. The science is always advancing, so if you're still doing things the way you were 10 years ago, you're almost certainly out of date. Rehabilitators need to take advantage of a broad spectrum of literature including taxonomy and wildlife biology, zoological medicine, rehabilitation, exotic pets, and even laboratory animal medicine.

Wildlife rehabilitation is a fascinating hybrid of priorities and activities. Its origins and core values are primarily humane, with caring people rescuing animals that have no owners, providing the best possible care, and releasing these animals back to the wild. In some modest way, this helps many of us feel as though we're making up for the immense damage that our species continues to do to the natural world. One of the most important related goals of wildlife rehab is environmental education. Encouraging people to live more gently on the Earth – a topic that is the focus of many publications other than the present volume.

As the current book amply demonstrates, rehab has also grown to encompass a range of goals that focus on the health and well-being of populations of animals and their environments. Little biomedical information has been gathered and published on many of the species that rehabilitators handle. Rehab can serve an important role in filling in these gaps. If we're speaking of toxins, emerging infectious diseases, or interactions with domestic animals, wildlife rehabilitation can be an important tool for basic research and environmental health monitoring.

One important role of wildlife rehabilitation can be to advance the development of techniques for captive management. How can we improve nutrition, reduce stress, avoid the transmission of disease, and prevent the development of antibiotic-resistant microbes? We must continually challenge ourselves to do better and to come up with improved metrics for how we define "success" in rehabilitation.

Readers should appreciate this book as a marvelous resource that will improve the tools we have to help wildlife. But this book also serves two other important functions. It challenges us all to learn more and to do better. Where is more knowledge needed and how can our efforts contribute to further advances? And finally, I hope that this book inspires us all. It's wonderfully energizing to know that there are other people who share our love, energy and dedication to helping wildlife.

Mark A. Pokras, BS, DVM
Associate Professor Emeritus
Wildlife Clinic & Center for Conservation Medicine
Cummings School of Veterinary Medicine
Tufts University
North Grafton, MA, USA

Carson, R. 1962. Silent Spring. Houghton Mifflin

Collette, R. 1974. My Orphans of the Wild. J B Lippincott

Cooper, J. 1979. First Aid and Care of Wild Birds. David & Charles

Cooper, J.1972. Veterinary Aspects of Captive Birds of Prey. The Hawk Trust

Davis, J. et al. 1971. Infectious and Parasitic Diseases of Wild Birds. Iowa State University Press

Fowler, M. 1978. Zoo and Wild Animal Medicine. W.B. Saunders

Garcelon, D. and Bogue, G.L. 1977. Raptor Care and Rehabilitation. Alexander Lindsay Junior Museum

Hamerstrom, F. 1971. An Eagle to the Sky. Iowa State University Press

Hickman, M. and Guy, M. 1973. Care of the Wild, Feathered and Furred. Unity Press

Keymer, L. and Arnall, I. 1976. Bird Diseases. TFH Publications

McKeever, K. 1979. Care and Rehabilitation of Injured Owls. Owl Rehabilitation Research Foundation

Petrak, M. 1969. Diseases of Cage and Aviary Birds. Lea & Febiger.

Singer, P. 1975. Animal Liberation: A New Ethics for our Treatment of Animals. New York Review/Random House

Thrune, E. 1995. Wildlife Rehabilitation: A History and Perspective. National Wildlife Rehabilitators Association

Yglesias, D. 1962. The Cry of a Bird. E. P. Dutton & Co.

Acknowledgment

Our purpose for this book was to finally compile as much evidence-based information possible, and to capitalize on the experience of so many who work day-in and day-out in the field of wildlife medicine. We also wanted to highlight the importance of the "big picture" of wildlife rehabilitation. As humankind's unprecedented impact on our natural world continues, what we do with every single creature will matter, but in the meantime, we hope the concepts of how this work – the rehabilitation of wildlife – impacts wildlife populations will permeate these chapters.

We owe a huge debt of gratitude to the authors who indulged our mission and shared their expertise.

A project of this scope cannot be completed without the support of family members, as everyone knows that most of the work associated with producing a textbook is squeezed in "here or there." My husband, Michael Yabsley, deserves a lot of thanks, not only because he spent endless days with the other editors and me editing and organizing, but he also held the fort as I disappeared for days to meet with the rest of the group. This project, from conception to reality, went on longer than we expected, in no small part because of the birth of no fewer than four children among us, job changes, promotions, and generally busy lives! I was merely a facilitator, and the other editors (Barron, Yabsley, Miller, and Aguilar) deserve praise for their persistence in aiming for excellence.

The real thanks should go to the thousands of individuals who dedicate their lives to the care of wildlife every day. Most of those people are underpaid and undervalued but are fueled by their passion to help in some way, however small. We hope this book helps them to help wildlife!

Roberto Aguilar is grateful for the time and materials shared by the Tucson Wildlife Center. Their input and generosity were invaluable.

Erica Miller is grateful for parents who nurtured interest in a "nontraditional career," and a wonderfully patient husband who tolerates this continued pursuit. She is also grateful for the many wildlife rehabilitators and wild animals from whom she has learned, and continues to learn every day.

Heather Barron is grateful to the dedicated staff, volunteers, veterinary interns, and students at CROW who care so deeply about the health and welfare of wildlife and who make every day an adventure. She also gives special thanks to her family for their support during the creation of this *magnum opus*.

Finally, we thank those who contributed technical assistance: Henry C. Adams created the cover art and R. Ethan Cooper assisted with formatting.

Sonia M. Hernandez
Spring 2019

Section I

General Topics

1

Regulatory and Legal Considerations in Wildlife Medicine

Allan Casey[1] and Erica A. Miller[2]

[1] *WildAgain Wildlife Rehabilitation, Inc., Evergreen, CO, USA*
[2] *Wildlife Medicine, Department of Clinic Studies, University of Pennsylvania School of Veterinary Medicine, Philadelphia, PA, USA*

Introduction

In virtually all instances, licensed veterinarians can lawfully admit and treat a wild animal that requires medical attention. Except for a few circumstances discussed below, state or federal wildlife regulations do not prohibit such "Good Samaritan" action by a veterinarian. However, once an animal has been medically treated and stabilized, further steps are governed by myriad state, federal, and local regulations, statutes, and ordinances, depending on species and locale. These regulations may be more or less restrictive depending on the government agency imposing them. A veterinarian should not be deterred by this, but should be well informed in advance of administering medical assistance and understand what other actions are allowed regarding wild animals.

Perspective

The information discussed in this chapter is intended for the veterinarian who is licensed to practice veterinary medicine in the United States, but who does not hold any type of license or permit (hereafter referred to simply as "permit") that authorizes possession of wildlife species, such as zoological, alternative livestock, animal sanctuary, falconry, or rehabilitation. It is assumed that holders of those permits are already aware of the requirements granted under those permits regarding the medical treatment of wildlife species that are privately owned or otherwise authorized to be in private possession. In this chapter, wildlife is defined as free-ranging wild animals and migratory birds that prior to admission for medical attention were not under private ownership or otherwise authorized to be in private possession.

Lastly, this chapter is not a definitive source of regulatory requirements or legal advice, but serves as a guide for the types and sources of information a veterinarian should be knowledgeable about if asked to treat any wild animal. Any specific regulation, statute or legislative act discussed or referenced in this chapter is current at the time of publication and is subject to change in the future. It is therefore prudent to stay apprised of any changes that may occur to existing regulations and statutes, and to be alert to newly enacted related regulations or statutes that might affect the rehabilitation of wildlife.

Federal Regulations Pertaining to Wildlife Rehabilitation

The US Fish and Wildlife Service (USFWS) is the federal agency that has responsibility to implement provisions of the Migratory Bird Treaty Act (MBTA), the Bald and Golden Eagle Protection Act (BGEPA) and the Endangered Species Act (ESA) that specifically address authorized activities for these species, including rehabilitation of migratory birds and eagles. Where the BPEGA and ESA are focused on conserving at-risk species, the MBTA protects all migratory birds, regardless of their conservation status. Another federal agency, the National Marine Fisheries Service (NMFS), has promulgated policies, standards, and best practices that govern marine mammal stranding response, rehabilitation, and release.

USFWS – Migratory Birds, Bald Eagles, and Golden Eagles

The federal regulation that addresses criteria for the rehabilitation of migratory birds is 50 CFR §21.31 (Federal Register 2003). The list of migratory birds includes almost all bird species in North America except for invasive species such as European starling (*Sturnus vulgaris*), English sparrow (*Passer domesticus*), Eurasian

Medical Management of Wildlife Species: A Guide for Practitioners, First Edition. Edited by Sonia M. Hernandez,
Heather W. Barron, Erica A. Miller, Roberto F. Aguilar and Michael J. Yabsley.
© 2020 John Wiley & Sons, Inc. Published 2020 by John Wiley & Sons, Inc.

collared dove (*Streptopelia decaocto*), rock pigeon (*Columba livia*), and certain game species governed by state regulations, such as quail (Odontophoridae), pheasant (*Phasianus colchicus*), grouse (Tetraonidae), domestic chicken (*Gallus gallus*), and wild turkey (*Meleagris gallopavo*). The list can be found at https://www.fws.gov/migratorybirds/pdf/policies-and-regulations/MBTA ListofBirdsFinalRule.pdf. However, under §21.12(c), permit exemptions, licensed veterinarians are not required to obtain a federal migratory bird permit to temporarily possess, stabilize, or euthanize sick and injured migratory birds. According to federal regulations, "a veterinarian without a migratory bird rehabilitation permit must transfer any such bird to a federally permitted migratory bird rehabilitator within 24 hours after the bird's condition is stabilized, unless the bird is euthanized" (50 CFR 21.12(c)). "Stabilize" is not legally defined since each medical case presents differently. The veterinarian and the rehabilitator should work together to determine when a bird's condition no longer requires direct veterinary care and it can be moved to the rehabilitator's facility. If a veterinarian is unable to locate a permitted rehabilitator within that time, they must contact the Regional Migratory Bird Permit Office for assistance in locating a permitted migratory bird rehabilitator and/or to obtain authorization to continue to possess the bird.

In addition, veterinarians must: (i) notify the local USFWS immediately upon receiving a threatened or endangered migratory bird species, or bald eagle or golden eagle; (ii) euthanize migratory birds whose injuries are as described in §21.31(e)(4)(iii) and §21.31(e)(4)(iv) (Figure 1.1), although the regulation also establishes criteria for exceptions; (iii) dispose of dead migratory birds in accordance with §21.31(e)(4)(vi)(A–D); and (iv) keep records for five years of all migratory birds that die while in care, including those that are euthanized. The records must include the species of bird, type of injury, date of acquisition, date of death, and whether the bird was euthanized or transferred to a rehabilitator. Euthanasia of any eagle should be coordinated with USFWS permission.

Nonreleasable migratory birds may be placed in educational programs or used for foster parenting, research projects, or other permitted activities with persons licensed, permitted or otherwise authorized to possess such birds, with prior approval from the issuing Regional Migratory Bird Permit Office.

Veterinarians may conduct necropsies on certain species but, prior to conducting the necropsy, they should check first with USFWS because some species may need to be sent to regional or federal diagnostic laboratories. If factors such as oil or chemical contamination, electrocution, shooting, or pesticides are suspected, USFWS law enforcement officials must be contacted immediately.

Other situations that may be helpful to know where the "take" of migratory birds is authorized by regulation, and

---

Federal Regulation Excerpts

Euthanasia

You must euthanize any bird that cannot feed itself, perch upright, or ambulate without inflicting additional injuries to itself where medical and/or rehabilitative care will not reverse such conditions. You must euthanize any bird that is completely blind, and any bird that has sustained injuries that would require amputation of a leg, a foot, or a wing at the elbow or above (humero-ulnar joint) rather than performing such surgery. §21.31(e)(4)(iii)

You must obtain authorization from your issuing Migratory Bird Permit Office before euthanizing endangered and threatened migratory bird species. In rare cases, the Service may designate a disposition other than euthanasia for those birds. If Service personnel are not available, you may euthanize endangered and threatened migratory birds without Service authorization when prompt euthanasia is warranted by humane consideration for the welfare of the bird. §21.31(e)(4)(iv)

Dead birds, parts and feathers

You may donate dead birds and parts thereof, except threatened and endangered species, and bald and golden eagles, to persons authorized by permit (under §21.12) to possess migratory bird specimens or exempted from permit requirements. §21.31(e)(4)(vi)(A)

Rescue by the Public

Any person may remove a migratory bird from the interior of a building or structure under certain conditions (§21.12(d)). Good Samaritan clause–any person who finds a sick, injured, or orphaned migratory bird may, without a permit, take possession of the bird in order to immediately transport it to a permitted rehabilitator. (§21.31)

Education –Specimens /Live Birds Possession

State, federal, and municipal agencies as well as AZA accredited zoos may possess lawfully acquired migratory bird specimens and live birds for educational purposes without a permit. (§21.12(b)) All others must have a Special Purpose Possession permit for education (§21.27)

Figure 1.1 Excerpts from the Code of Federal Regulations §21 pertaining to veterinarians treating native wild animals.

thus exempt from needing a permit, include rescue of birds by the public ("Good Samaritans") and the use of specimens or live birds for educational purposes by certain public and private institutions (Figure 1.1). "Take" has been broadly defined and may include harass, harm, pursue, hunt, shoot, wound, kill, trap, capture or collect, or attempts to do so.

USFWS & NMFS – Threatened and Endangered Species, Including Sea Turtles and Marine Mammals

Aside from rendering immediate medical attention to any federally listed threatened and endangered (T&E) species, sea turtle or marine mammal, it is advisable to immediately contact the state wildlife agency or USFWS or NMFS for further instructions, especially for endangered species.

In the case of sea turtles, the USFWS has issued *Standard Permit Conditions for the Care and Maintenance of Captive Sea Turtles* (USDI/USFWS 2013) in accordance with §10(a)(1)(A) of the ESA, which includes requirements for rehabilitation. For veterinarians who will rehabilitate sea turtles, these conditions include experience requirements, keeping complete health records on each animal, a USFWS- or state-issued permit for euthanasia, submission of a gross necropsy report on each deceased animal, etc. Euthanasia of any sea turtle requires USFWS approval.

NMFS – Marine Mammals (Cetaceans and Pinnipeds)

The NMFS has issued *Policies and Best Practices, Marine Mammal Stranding Response, Rehabilitation and Release, Standards for Rehabilitation Facilities* (NOAA, NMFS 2009) in accordance with Title IV §402(a) of the Marine Mammal Protection Act that includes requirements for rehabilitation of marine mammals. Portions of this document are based on the US Department of Agriculture Animal and Plant Health Inspection Service Animal Welfare Act. To qualify as an attending veterinarian for a marine mammal rehabilitation facility, extensive training and experience are required. For the occasional case presented at a veterinary clinic, it is advisable to contact a local stranding network, facility or veterinarian who is permitted to provide rehabilitative care for consultation on diagnosis, treatment, and medical clearance for release or transport.

State Wildlife Regulations Pertaining to Wildlife Rehabilitation

Every state has its own set of regulations that govern the wildlife native to that state, but all contain a general provision that prohibits the temporary or permanent possession of almost all species of native wild animals (Musgrave and Stein 1993). Exceptions to this rule include activities such as scientific research, bird banding, translocation, animal control, falconry egg harvest, rehabilitation, and, in some states, educational animals that recover from rehabilitation but are deemed nonreleasable. These few exceptions usually require issuance of a permit, which may also include one or more state or federal permits, as discussed later.

Where most veterinarians become involved in the temporary possession of a wild animal is in participating in wildlife rehabilitation, broadly defined as providing assistance to a wild animal that is injured, diseased or distressed, for the purpose of release back to its wild habitat. Most often, this involvement occurs as a direct contact with a rescuer from the public or in assisting a local permitted wildlife rehabilitator.

As mentioned earlier, most state wildlife rehabilitation regulations are silent on any prohibition of a veterinarian rendering immediate, emergency medical assistance to a wild animal in need (Casey and Casey 1994, 1995, 2000, 2005). Thus, it is generally accepted as being allowed. Most states have a clear requirement that the animal, once stabilized and not requiring continuing veterinary care, be transferred to a local permitted rehabilitator as soon as possible for further rehabilitation and release. If such transfer is not possible, either due to a lack of a local rehabilitator authorized for that species or if the rehabilitator's facility is at capacity, the veterinarian should contact the local state wildlife officer or state wildlife agency for guidance and authorization on any next steps, including further care and disposition for that animal.

If a veterinarian finds that wildlife is being delivered by the public on some frequent basis, especially in more urban areas and generally seasonally, and circumstances are such that frequently the local rehabilitator is unable to accept more cases, the veterinarian may consider obtaining a state wildlife rehabilitation permit. The requirements and application forms for a state-issued wildlife rehabilitation permit are available through the state wildlife agency, with many available on the agency's website.

Lastly, many states require that the veterinarian notify the state agency if the animal is a species listed as having some level of protected status, such as a state-sensitive or state T&E species, or a federally listed T&E species.

Another circumstance where veterinarians provide medical assistance on a more regular basis is through a working relationship with a local rehabilitator. States that issue wildlife rehabilitation permits require that the rehabilitator have a veterinarian of record who has agreed to provide medical assistance to wild animals undergoing rehabilitation. Rehabilitation permits do not authorize the practice of veterinary medicine, so a consulting veterinarian is a critical requirement in any successful rehabilitation process.

This partnership may take the form of an informal arrangement between the veterinarian and rehabilitator, or it may be more formal, such as using a written agreement. If a veterinarian agrees to be the veterinarian of record for the rehabilitator, some form of agreement should be clearly discussed and understood, whether formal or informal, written or oral, that articulates the roles, responsibilities, and expectations of both parties. While some states require the rehabilitator to list the name of the consulting veterinarian on the rehabilitation permit, other states require the veterinarian to complete and sign a form specifying and agreeing to the type of services that will be provided for wildlife.

Such discussions of services should clarify if the veterinarian will provide professional services and out-of-pocket costs free of charge, or what portion, if any, are expected to be paid or reimbursed by the rehabilitator, most of whom are volunteers. They also should clarify what initial and continuing medical treatment procedures or supportive care the rehabilitator is authorized to perform under the training and supervision of the veterinarian, such as basic first aid, routine wound management, fluid therapy, and administering prescribed medications. Further details on the communication between the wildlife rehabilitator and the veterinarian can be found in Chapter 8.

Most medical procedures should be performed by the veterinarian and not delegated to the rehabilitator. These would include surgeries, radiography/imaging, stabilization of fractures, and administration of controlled substances such as strong analgesics or euthanasia agents. Correspondingly, the trained and experienced rehabilitator, because of permit requirements, is likely to better understand the captive care and husbandry requirements of a specific species, including diets, enclosure requirements, and pre-release conditioning and considerations. Even when working frequently with a rehabilitator who seems to know and understand all the rules and regulations that may apply, it is good practice for the veterinarian to obtain a copy of regulations to personally understand the rules and arrive at independent interpretations. It is also important to obtain copies of the rehabilitator's state and federal permits.

A few other provisions that often appear in state wildlife rehabilitation regulations that are sound practices for veterinarians to follow include separation of wildlife from domestic animals, prohibition from public display, including social media, and release restrictions. Any wild animal admitted for treatment should be confined and housed separate from all other domestic species in the clinic. This reduces captivity stress on juvenile and adult animals, provides for quarantine against possible transmission of pathogens and parasites, and helps prevent habituation of young animals. Any form of public display of the animal should be prevented, including from curious clinic staff not involved in direct treatment, members of the public, and the media.

The regulations of some states have strict requirements as to when and where animals can be released. Rehabilitators are responsible for preparing and assessing the wild animals for release, and conducting the release. On rare occasions, a brief period of quiet recuperation may be sufficient for the animal to recover and be ready for immediate release. In these cases, the veterinarian may want to consult with a rehabilitator to confirm the appropriateness of the release.

Some states require that the animal be released as close as possible to or within a specified distance from the point of original capture. Other states may require the release location to be chosen in consultation with a wildlife officer, especially involving any state or federal T&E species. States may also outright prohibit the release back to the wild of certain animals, such as those considered to be invasive or nonnative.

Some states may have departments (other than the wildlife agency) that have some level of involvement, jurisdiction, or oversight involving the state's wildlife. For example, some state health departments have reporting requirements for any type of wild animal bites (e.g., rabies vectors) or known or suspected exposure to a zoonotic disease. If involving a rescuer from the public, this notification requirement is most likely the responsibility of the rescuer, if they know to do so. There may be a requirement or strong expectation from the state that the veterinarian who has knowledge of any such occurrence also should report the incident, including the names of any members of the public known to have been exposed.

Additionally, some states have active commercial alternative livestock operations, often governed by a department of agriculture. They may involve wildlife species such as deer and elk, and may have reporting requirements for any of those species that may arrive for rehabilitation, especially if unusual circumstances are suspected or if the state is concerned about the spread and transfer of communicable diseases such as chronic wasting disease.

Local Municipal and County Considerations

Some state wildlife rehabilitation regulations require that rehabilitation must not be in conflict or violation with any local rule or ordinance. While this requirement applies directly to the facility of the rehabilitator, it may create restrictions or a prohibition for wild animals to be housed, even temporarily, within a veterinary facility. Planning and zoning codes and ordinances of some counties and municipalities may prohibit any wild animal species or any species they define as "dangerous" (e.g., venomous snakes) from being kept onsite. Others may allow certain species of wildlife that are not defined as "dangerous" but only if certain conditions are satisfied (e.g., possession of a current state wildlife rehabilitation permit). These restrictions at the local level, if they exist, most likely pose a very low risk to a veterinary clinic for the infrequent squirrel, rabbit or songbird that may be admitted. However, they could pose more significant risks if the veterinarian is admitting wildlife on a more regular basis, or admitting larger carnivore species or those species considered to be disease vectors, especially if any adverse incident should occur involving the public or clinic staff.

Surveillance Reporting

Some public health or wildlife agencies have reporting and surveillance requirements for cases of various diseases observed or suspected. Those of public health importance may include rabies, plague, tularemia, or hantavirus and state wildlife agencies may request information on cases of parvovirus, white-nose syndrome, West Nile virus, highly pathogenic influenza virus, Newcastle's disease virus, etc. Those agencies should be contacted in advance for their reporting and surveillance requirements and that information should be maintained in a readily accessible location. It is almost better to err on the side of more frequent communication, particularly with pathogens that affect public health.

Carcass Disposal and Submission

There are few specific instructions in state-level rehabilitation regulations regarding carcass or animal parts disposal. As a result, it may be reasonable to assume that any form of carcass disposal conforming to local ordinances used on a regular basis by the veterinarian is likely acceptable. A few states do have specific requirements (e.g., incinerate) if poisoning is suspected or euthanasia has involved chemical agents. At times, when the veterinarian is reasonably sure that harmful chemicals, pathogens, disease agents, or drug residues are not present, a carcass may be used as feedstock for wildlife being rehabilitated.

At the federal level, there are certain species for which carcasses and parts are required to be submitted to federal facilities. Carcasses and feathers of bald eagles and golden eagles must be submitted to the National Eagle Repository located in Commerce City, Colorado. Certain marine mammals and sea turtles may need to be submitted to the offices of the NMFS. To assist in the legal acquisition of federally regulated migratory bird feathers, two programs, listed at the end of this chapter, have been established for the distribution of noneagle feathers and carcasses for tribal religious, medical, and ceremonial purposes.

Lastly, it is always good practice to contact the state or local USFWS office to inquire if there are requirements to submit species that are either state or federally listed as T&E.

Law Enforcement

On rare occasions, a veterinarian may be asked to assist in a law enforcement action, at a local, state, or federal level. Examples of this include unlawful take and possession of wildlife, intentional injury to wildlife not covered by legal hunting regulations, unlawful transport or sale of wildlife, and if the nature of the wildlife injury is related to gunshot, poisoning, electrocution, or oil or chemical exposure. The veterinarian's involvement may include a medical assessment of any confiscated wild animals, providing medical assistance or euthanasia, and temporary possession pending transfer to a rehabilitator or other final destination. There are often evidentiary and chain of custody procedures that require strict adherence (Byrd and Sutton 2012). Complete medical records, radiographs, photographs, and other types of evidence, including gunshot or other objects removed from the affected wildlife species, may be required in a form that is later admissible and defendable in a deposition or court of law. The various law enforcement officers involved in any legal action should provide specific and clear guidance to the veterinarian as to any evidentiary requirements and procedures to be followed.

USFWS regional law enforcement offices can be found at https://www.fws.gov/le/regional-law-enforcement-offices.html. A list of state and territorial fish and wildlife offices can be found at www.fws.gov/offices/statelinks.html.

Legal Liability Exposure

Situations that involve physical contact between a human and a wild animal can end badly. A study of rescuers revealed that because of the very strong emotional response that humans demonstrate for animals experiencing pain and suffering, especially young animals, rescues were regularly attempted despite risk of serious injury or disease exposure to the rescuer (Siemer and Brown 1992). When a well-meaning member of the public who is untrained in wild animal capture, restraint, and transport attempts rescue of a wild animal that appears to need help, a plethora of adverse outcomes are very possible, including death or further injury to the wild animal or rescuer.

In the case where clinic staff have advised or coached a rescuer over the phone on capture, restraint or transport, the veterinarian's potential liability exposure begins even before the animal arrives at the clinic. As such, some clinics have chosen to provide no guidance and simply state that the animal will be seen if brought to the clinic. Other clinics simply refer the rescuer to a local experienced rehabilitator or animal control agency to determine if rescue is needed, and if so, to provide for safe methods of capture and transport. This option generally gives the rescuer a more informed source of guidance and instruction, transfers liability away from the clinic, and may result in the rehabilitator offering to perform the tasks for the rescuer in difficult situations. If the veterinarian should decide to provide this type of advice over the phone, very specific training should be given to those clinic staff assigned to speak with rescuers, such as advising the rescuer that particular situations may be unsafe and could result in personal injury and in these cases a rescue should not be attempted.

Once the animal arrives at the clinic, other potential liability exposures are created with clients and clinic staff. To minimize risks to clients, many clinics receive rescued wildlife through an alternative entrance, thus preventing contact with clients or their companion animals. A more real and pronounced set of risks of injury involve clinic staff that assist in the medical treatment of injured or diseased wild animals. Only staff who understand the differences between the behaviors of domestic and wild animals, are trained in safe restraint of wild animals, and in some cases have preexposure rabies vaccinations, should be involved in assisting the veterinarian in any examination, diagnostic or medical procedures.

A thoughtful approach to risk management for the veterinarian and the clinic can mitigate the effects of most of these risks in reducing the likelihood of creating a cause for legal action. Components of a sound defense might include proof that documented policies, procedures, and training were followed to insure the safety of all parties.

The American Veterinary Medical Association (AVMA) suggests that a clinic should have a stated wildlife policy that stipulates whether or not the clinic will accept various wild animal species for treatment. If the clinic does accept wildlife, then clear roles and responsibilities of all staff should be documented and communicated, as well as a list of contacts for referrals and regulatory agencies that may need to be notified (Figure 1.2). The veterinarian should verify that a professional liability insurance policy provides coverage for wildlife treatment, handling, and confinement. If the policy does cover wildlife and classifies them as "small animals" (as opposed to equine or food animal categories), the policy needs to be reviewed to understand if

---

Contact Information Checklist

Governing Authorities:

State Wildlife Agency #_____

Local Wildlife Officer #_____

Local USFWS Agent #_____

Local Animal Control #_____

State Veterinarian #_____

USDA APHIS Area Vet. #_____

Local Public Health Dept. #_____

Regional CDC office #_____

Local Wildlife Rehabilitators:

Name _____ #_____

Name _____ #_____

Name _____ #_____

Wildlife Referrals to other Veterinary Clinics:

Clinic _____ #_____

Clinic _____ #_____

Clinic _____ #_____

(Adapted from "Managing Wildlife Emergencies" prepared by the AVMA –www.avma.org/wildlife)

Figure 1.2 Sample format for a list of helpful contact numbers for veterinarians treating native wildlife. US Fish and Wildlife Service (USFWS) regional law enforcement offices can be found at https://www.fws.gov/le/regional-law-enforcement-offices.html and a list of state and territorial fish and wildlife offices can be found at www.fws.gov/offices/statelinks.html.

certain species or groups of species may be excluded from coverage, such as carnivores, ungulates, raptors, venomous snakes or rabies vector species.

Summary

The successful practice of wildlife rehabilitation has been made possible by the generous support of time, effort, and expertise of countless veterinarians over many decades. This chapter could be interpreted as all the reasons, regulatory hurdles, and legal risks why a veterinarian might hesitate to become involved and volunteer their services, and some will choose to not work with wildlife. However, experience has shown that far more veterinarians will willingly involve themselves, but hopefully do so equipped with knowledge of the rules, regulations, and laws that govern the activity. Just as it is prudent to understand the licensing requirements, laws, and skills needed to operate, for example, a mobile veterinary practice, the same holds true for working with wild animals. Every locale is different, so the veterinarian will need to become familiar with the general set of rules that apply federally, and in their state and local area.

This chapter is a brief discussion to alert the veterinarian to the major considerations to be aware of, and ends with a listing of several helpful resources to further that knowledge. One or more local wildlife rehabilitators also may serve as an excellent source for this information, as they are usually required to fully understand the state and federal regulations that govern wildlife rehabilitation as a primary condition of obtaining and maintaining their permit. Lastly, when in doubt, contact the appropriate governing agency or seek legal counsel.

Resources

1) State wildlife agencies in all 50 states, often within the Department of Natural Resources
2) USFWS offices in all 50 states (www.fws.gov/offices)
3) USFWS Regional Migratory Bird Permit Offices (eight regional offices) (https://www.fws.gov/birds/policies-and-regulations/permits/regional-permit-contacts.php)
4) State and local health departments in all 50 states
5) List of licensed/permitted wildlife rehabilitators – usually available from the state wildlife agency
6) USDA Wildlife Services 1-866-487-3297 (www.aphis.usda.gov/aphis/ourfocus/wildlifedamage/SA_Program_Overview)
7) AVMA website – *Managing Wildlife Emergencies* (www.avma.org/KB/Resources/Reference/wildlife/Pages/default.aspx)
8) USFWS National Eagle Repository (www.fws.gov/eaglerepository)
9) Sia Essential Species Repository (for noneagle feathers), Comanche Nation, OK (www.comancheeagle.org)
10) Liberty Non-Eagle Repository (for noneagle feathers), AZ (http://libertywildlife.org/conservation/non-eagle-feather-repository/)
11) Sea Turtle Stranding and Salvage Network (www.seaturtle.org)
12) USFWS National Sea Turtle Coordinator, Jacksonville, FL (https://www.fws.gov/northflorida/SeaTurtles/seaturtle-info.htm)

References

Byrd, J.H. and Sutton, L.K. (2012). Defining a crime scene and physical evidence collection. In: *Wildlife Forensics: Methods and Applications* (ed. J.E. Huffman and J.R. Wallace). Hoboken, NJ: Wiley.

Casey, A. and Casey, S. (1994). Survey of state regulations governing wildlife rehabilitation. *Journal of Wildlife Rehabilitation* 17 (4): 6–10.

Casey, A. and Casey, S. (1995). State regulations governing wildlife rehabilitation: a summary of best practices. *Journal of Wildlife Rehabilitation* 18 (1): 3–11.

Casey, A. and Casey, S. (2000). A study of state regulations governing wildlife rehabilitation during 1999. In: *Wildlife Rehabilitation*, vol. 18 (ed. D. Ludwig), 173–192. St Cloud, MN: National Wildlife Rehabilitators Association.

Casey, A. and Casey, S. (2005). Survey of state wildlife rehabilitation regulations – 2004. In: *Wildlife Rehabilitation*, vol. 23 (ed. E.A. Miller and D. Nickerson), 175–185. St Cloud, MN: National Wildlife Rehabilitators Association.

Musgrave, R. and Stein, M. (1993). *State Wildlife Laws Handbook*. Rockville, MD: Government Institutes, Inc.

National Oceanic and Atmospheric Administration, National Marine Fisheries Service (2009). *Policies and Best Practices, Marine Mammal Stranding Response, Rehabilitation and Release, Standards for Rehabilitation Facilities*. Silver Spring, MD: National Oceanic and Atmospheric Administration.

Siemer, W. and Brown, T. (1992). *Characteristics, Activities, and Attitudes of Licensed Wildlife Rehabilitators in New York*. Human Dimensions Research Unit Publication 92-1. Ithaca, NY: Cornell University.

US Government Printing Office (2003). Rules and Regulations: Migratory Bird Permits; Regulations Governing Rehabilitation Activities and Permit Exceptions. *Federal Register* 68 (207): 61135.

US Department of the Interior, USFWS. (2013) Standard Permit Conditions for Care and Maintenance of Captive Sea Turtles. Available at: www.fws.gov/northflorida/seaturtles/Captive_Forms/20130213_revised%20_standard_permit_conditions_for_captive_sea_turtles.pdf

2

Human Safety and Zoonoses

Marcy J. Souza

College of Veterinary Medicine, University of Tennessee, Knoxville, TN, USA

Introduction

Working with wildlife can be a rewarding endeavor, but precautions must be taken to ensure the safety and health of the humans who care for these animals. Wild animals are often fractious and, when handled or kept in captivity, can injure themselves or the people caring for them. Additionally, wild animals can be a source of numerous zoonotic diseases, some of which may have not yet been discovered. This chapter provides information on how to reduce the probability of injury or transmission of zoonotic diseases to humans working with wildlife in a rehabilitation setting. In addition to the information found in this chapter, the National Association of State Public Health Veterinarians periodically publishes a compendium on the prevention of zoonoses in veterinary personnel; the latest version can be found on their website (www.nasphv.org/documentsCompendia.html).

Prevention of Traumatic Injury

Limited information is available on the incidence of human trauma inflicted by wildlife, and there is even less focus on wildlife rehabilitation settings (Conover et al. 1995; Bovard 2000; Saito and Shreve 2005). People who work with animals as an occupation are more likely to suffer trauma from animals than people with little animal contact. One report found that 47.6% of surveyed raptor rehabilitators had suffered wounds associated with handling wildlife (Saito and Shreve 2005). In contrast, reports in the literature consistently identify domestic dogs as the most common species that bite members of the general public (Sinclair and Zhou 1995; Moore et al. 2000); bites from other domestic animals are less commonly reported, but are still more frequent

offenders than wildlife. Certainly some species, such as carnivores and raptors, are better equipped to inflict damage to people during handling and procedures and their injuries are therefore more likely to be reported.

Specific precautions to be considered with particular types of animals are covered in other species-specific chapters in this book. For example, carnivores bite, wading birds can inflict painful stabs with their beaks, birds of prey can cause significant trauma with their talons, wild rodents and snakes are quick to bite and scratches from armadillos and other burrowing animals can be very painful. However, there are a few steps that all people working with wildlife can follow to reduce the incidence of injury.

1) *Clear communication*: when two or more people are examining or handling animals together, they should always communicate aloud their respective tasks. For example, when one person is taking control of a raptor foot for examination, both parties involved (the initial holder and the one about to examine) should communicate the transfer of the foot.
2) *Safe, species-specific handling techniques*: animals have a variety of methods to inflict injury on a handler or examiner. Handlers must be aware of the proper restraint technique for the specific animal being examined; in fact, any person working directly with wildlife should have proper training prior to handling any animal (Figure 2.1). For example, if a handler is unfamiliar with birds such as cranes or herons, he or she might not properly restrain the head and neck, increasing the risk of trauma from the bird's beak.
3) *Protective equipment*: to aid in the handling of different species, protective equipment such as nets, towels, gloves, or goggles may be required. The equipment needed will vary with each species.

Medical Management of Wildlife Species: A Guide for Practitioners, First Edition. Edited by Sonia M. Hernandez,
Heather W. Barron, Erica A. Miller, Roberto F. Aguilar and Michael J. Yabsley.
© 2020 John Wiley & Sons, Inc. Published 2020 by John Wiley & Sons, Inc.

(a)

(b)

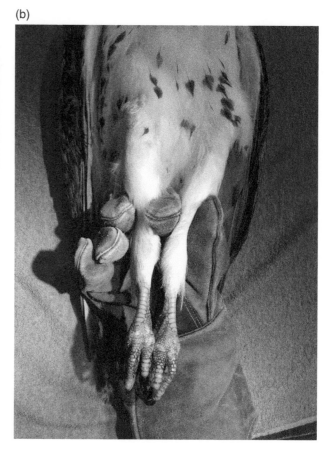

Figure 2.1 Thick gloves should be worn when handling raptors. The raptor's feet should be restrained to prevent talons from causing trauma to individuals working with the bird. When inexperienced individuals are working with raptors, an overhand hold (a) of the feet is recommended to reduce the likelihood of accidental trauma. An underhand hold (b) can be used with experienced individuals or when examining the feet.

4) *Chemical immobilization*: sedation or immobilization with various drug protocols might be the only way to safely handle some animals. Additionally, chemical immobilization of most wild animals will likely be required for diagnostics and other clinical procedures. Sedation or immobilization of animals can not only reduce the likelihood of injury to humans, but also reduce the stress inflicted on the animal.

Routes of Zoonotic Disease Transmission and Steps for Prevention

With the ever-increasing number of emerging infectious diseases identified in wildlife, it is impossible to know every potential pathogen carried by wildlife that could be zoonotic (Taylor et al. 2001). Additionally, collection of biological samples and case data from rehabilitation centers can be time- and cost-prohibitive, although involvement of universities and public health departments, and

the use of electronic record keeping, may improve data collection and review (Stitt et al. 2007).

One of the best disease risk reduction methods for wildlife rehabilitators is knowledge about the routes of exposure to infectious agents and general methods of prevention. One report found that while 88% of rehabilitators wore gloves to prevent injury from raptors, only 45% always or sometimes washed their hands after handling or treatment (Saito and Shreve 2005). Thorough hand washing is a necessary step in disease prevention in both human and veterinary medicine and should always be performed after handling an animal or its waste. Recommendations for prevention of exposure to pathogens vary depending on the typical route of transmission and the animal, but basic precautions like hand washing are always warranted.

Fecal–Oral Transmission

The transmission of infectious agents through the fecal–oral route is one of the most common and easily prevented. People can become infected after handling an animal (dead or alive) that has fecal material on it, cleaning an enclosure, or eating and drinking in areas where animals are housed or examined. Highlighting the importance of the risk of fecal–oral transmission, one study found that 31% of animals in a rehabilitation hospital sampled were shedding at least one zoonotic pathogen, such as *Salmonella* or *Escherichia coli*, in their feces (Siembieda et al. 2011); other zoonotic bacteria, some resistant to common antibiotics, were also isolated from the feces of various animals in rehabilitation centers (Steele et al. 2005; Jijon et al. 2007). In a recent report, raccoons were identified as the source of an outbreak of *Campylobacter* spp. in rehabilitation facility staff in Minnesota (Saunders et al. 2014); a case was characterized as someone who experienced fever and diarrhea or diarrhea lasting three or more days. In addition to zoonotic bacteria, many parasites are also shed in the feces. The recent expansion of the range for the raccoon roundworm (*Baylisascaris procyonis*) warrants extra precaution when working with raccoons, even in areas outside its historical range (Blizzard et al. 2010).

Fortunately, there are a number of simple steps that can be followed to reduce risk of contracting an infectious organism through the fecal–oral route.

1) Enforce a strict hand-washing regimen after handling any animal or samples from animals, or after cleaning animal enclosures. The Centers for Disease Control and Prevention (CDC) recommend using running water and soap to lather and scrub for at least 20 seconds followed by rinsing and drying. Antibacterial soap is not needed. Additional information and free educational posters for printing at the clinic or rehab center are available on the CDC's website: www.cdc.gov/handwashing.

2) Wear appropriate protective equipment such as disposable gloves to reduce contamination of the hands with fecal or other contaminated material. Even when wearing disposable gloves, hand washing is still a necessary step in disease prevention.

3) Designate areas for staff to eat and drink away from animals and prohibit eating/drinking in areas where animal care occurs to reduce the likelihood of food becoming contaminated with fecal material. Although space in some facilities may be limited, this is a crucial step to reduce consumption of contaminated food or drink.

Transmission through Bites and Scratches

Bites and scratches can lead to tissue damage, but infectious organisms can also be transmitted into the tissues through breaks in the skin. Rabies is one of the most common agents associated with bites, but other organisms such as bacteria (*Pasteurella*, *Staphylococcus*) found in the oral cavity or on the nails/talons can also be transmitted (Kunimoto et al. 2004; Carrasco et al. 2011; Hansen et al. 2012; Goldstein et al. 2013). A review of the animal bite literature was recently published by Goldstein and Abrahamian (2015). Much of this review focused on bites associated with keeping animals as pets, and increased pet ownership of traditional animals (dogs, cats) and less traditional pets (exotic species) will likely lead to increases in the number of bites overall. This review also discussed encounters with various wildlife that resulted in bites or other trauma, but the encounters were not specific to individuals who work with animals as an occupation.

Depending on the severity of the trauma and the organism transmitted, infection resulting from a bite or scratch can range from mild and local to systemic and possibly fatal. When a bite or scratch occurs, the area should be immediately and thoroughly washed with soap and water; if there is a concern about rabies exposure, the wound should also be flushed with a povidine-iodine solution (CDC 2015c). Additional information on a useful protocol for thorough wound flushing that has been found to decrease the probability of infection with rabies can be found at www.cdc.gov/rabies/index.html. A mild bite wound that only damages the skin with no deeper tissue affected can often be flushed as described; systemic antibiotics are likely not needed. If the wounds are more severe and include significant tissue damage and/or deep puncture wounds, the individual should seek medical advice from a professional, which may lead to surgical intervention and/or systemic antibiotics.

Additionally, if working in a rabies-endemic area, all staff who handle animals should receive preexposure prophylaxis. If an injury leads to exposure, the animal should be tested to determine its rabies status and the individual injured should be referred to a medical professional immediately for further evaluation and, if deemed necessary, postexposure vaccination. Although wildlife, specifically bats, account for a few human cases of rabies annually in the United States (CDC 2015c), bites from domestic animals, especially dogs, make up the majority of cases in which humans receive postexposure prophylaxis in Tennessee and likely nationwide (H. Henderson personal communication, 2015). Postexposure prophylaxis is not reportable in most states, so exact numbers of people treated, particularly after exposure to wildlife, are difficult to obtain. No reports of rabies specifically in a person who works with wildlife can be found. Recommendations for pre- and postexposure prophylaxis can be found in more detail on the CDC's website (CDC 2011).

Transmission Through Inhalation

Inhalation of infectious agents typically leads to respiratory disease and ranges in severity from mild flu-like symptoms to respiratory failure and death. Infectious organisms are typically shed in the feces, urine, and respiratory secretions of live animals and can be found throughout many tissues in dead animals. These organisms become aerosolized once the biological vehicle has dried and becomes disturbed, often through cleaning of the environment or an enclosure. For example, individuals with hantavirus pulmonary syndrome often become infected after cleaning/dusting/sweeping or camping in buildings that have been infested with mice. The mice shed virus in their urine, which dries in the environment; once disturbed through cleaning or other activities, humans can inhale the virus and become ill. One report found that several wildlife rehabilitation staff became infected with *Chlamydia* (*Chlamydophila*) *psittaci* after handling infected birds (Kalmar et al. 2014). Other organisms such as avian influenza virus, *Yersinia pestis*, and *Francisella tularensis* can also be transmitted by aerosol and lead to grave consequences in infected humans.

When cleaning enclosures or performing a necropsy, the use of a fit-tested mask will reduce the likelihood of inhalation of infectious agents. Surgical masks that are typically used in veterinary medicine are not adequate to prevent inhalation of infectious agents. Masks such as N95 or N99 specifically fitted for the individual should be used (Figure 2.2). Additionally, an enclosure or carcass can be misted with water or a liquid disinfectant prior to cleaning or handling to reduce aerosolization of infectious particles.

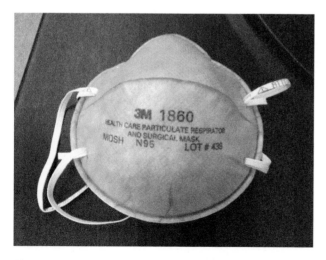

Figure 2.2 Masks with N95 or N99 specifications should be worn to reduce the risk of contracting airborne zoonoses.

Cutaneous Transmission

In veterinary medicine, transmission of infectious organisms directly from contact with the skin is less common than some other routes, although ringworm (dermatophytes) and *Sarcoptes scabei* are common examples. No reports of cutaneous transmission of disease from wildlife are available, and one recent study found that adult white-tailed deer were unlikely to be a source of cutaneous fungal infection for humans (Hall et al. 2011). To prevent cutaneous transmission, exposed skin that comes into contact with animals should be washed with soap and water. Gloves, lab coats, overalls, or other clothing with long sleeves can also be worn to reduce exposure.

Transmission by Biological or Mechanical Vectors

Arthropods, such as mosquitos and ticks, are common biological vectors for many zoonotic diseases, including West Nile virus (WNV), Rocky Mountain spotted fever, and Lyme disease. Fleas may also play a role in the transmission of certain zoonoses including *Y. pestis* and some species of *Bartonella* (Chomell and Kasten 2010). Wildlife may act as reservoirs for a number of these diseases and as hosts for the arthropod vectors responsible for transmission, but typically do not directly transmit the pathogens to humans. One study found that 21% of surveyed raptor rehabilitators experienced symptoms of WNV infection at the same time that a large number of raptors at their facility were diagnosed with WNV infection; however, confirmation of the diagnosis was not made in any of the humans (Saito and Shreve 2005). No risk factors evaluated in this study were found to be significant for illness in people, and the small sample size makes it difficult to determine if there was an increased risk for these individuals compared to the general public. Prevention of these infections is through control of the arthropod vectors. Arthropods, including cockroaches and house flies, can also act as mechanical vectors by transporting an infectious agent on their mouth parts, feet, or other body part to another site.

Reducing arthropod populations in areas where people work and live can reduce exposure to a number of zoonotic organisms. Tick exposure can be reduced by (i) wearing light-colored clothes, including long sleeves and pants, (ii) applying appropriate tick repellants, such as DEET or permethrin, (iii) performing tick checks regularly, and (iv) having landscaping features that discourage ticks and wildlife that carry ticks. For more information, visit the "Stop Ticks" webpage on the CDC web page (2015a).

Similarly, mosquito exposure can be reduced through appropriate clothing, repellants, and enclosure material such as screening of windows. Removal of standing water in flowerpot bottoms, tires, or other objects can also reduce mosquito breeding habitat. Additional information on mosquito bite prevention can be found at "Stop Mosquitoes" on the CDC web page (2015b).

Disinfection Methods

Inanimate objects, or fomites, can act as "reservoirs" of infectious organisms. Fomites can include nondisposable handling gloves, boots, vehicles, instruments used for procedures, and other objects associated with caging.

To most efficiently disinfect any fomite, and allow penetration of disinfectants, all organic material must first be thoroughly removed (NASPHV 2010). Hard, impermeable objects can be cleaned with a scrub brush and soapy water; it is not necessary or recommended to use antibacterial soap. After removal of organic material, these objects can be soaked in or sprayed with an appropriate disinfectant and then rinsed with water or wiped down with a wet towel. Soft objects, such as nondisposable handling gloves or towels, should be washed in hot water with detergent and then dried with heat; it is not advised to place these items into disinfectant baths.

Numerous disinfectants are available for use in rehabilitation facilities. Diluted bleach (1:10 bleach:water) is an effective, inexpensive option that destroys most infectious organisms within a few minutes of contact. Other disinfectants such as alcohols, quaternary ammonium compounds, and biguanides can be used, but they generally offer little to no advantage in terms of disinfection over bleach and are more expensive. The disadvantage of using bleach is its caustic properties and potential for injury to people working with it, the need to dilute it properly to avoid damage to equipment, and the need to both rinse it well and use it in a well-ventilated area. Detailed information on numerous disinfectants summarized by the Center for Food Security and Public Health can be found at www.cfsph.iastate.edu/Disinfection/index.php.

Zoonoses of Particular Concern

To understand the risk for exposure to a zoonotic organism, one must consider not only the animal species involved but also geography and season. For example, plague, caused by *Y. pestis*, occurs in the United States but the risk of exposure varies greatly with location such that it is only a major concern for people working in the western half of the USA.

This section will cover a few zoonoses of concern, but information on additional zoonoses can be found in Table 2.1.

Rabies

Rabies is caused by a lyssavirus and leads to an average of 60 000 human deaths globally each year (WHO 2016). Once symptoms occur, rabies infection is fatal in 99% of cases. Human cases of rabies in the US are rare but when they do occur, are usually caused by exposure to wildlife, bats in particular. Rabies is not present in Hawaii. Since 1980, the overwhelming majority of animals found to be infected with rabies in the US have been wildlife (Monroe et al. 2016). Through vaccination campaigns in dogs and cats, the canine variant of the rabies virus has been eradicated from the US, but numerous variants associated with wildlife are still present (Monroe et al. 2016).

All variants of rabies can cause disease in any mammal; disease caused by rabies has only been reported in mammalian species. Rabies in animals is reportable and cases are compiled by the CDC; surveillance data are published annually in the *Journal of the American Veterinary Medical Association* and are available free to the public (Monroe et al. 2016). Additional valuable information can be found in the Compendium of Animal Rabies Prevention and Control, 2016 which is published periodically and available for free online (NASPHV 2016).

Rabies is most commonly transmitted by a bite from an infected animal. The virus is shed in the saliva of an infected animal, so exposure to infected saliva through open wounds or mucous membranes can also lead to infection, although this route is much less common (Monroe et al. 2016). The virus can also be transmitted through organ or corneal transplants, but this route is rare.

Prevention of infection with rabies can be achieved through wound care and pre- and postexposure prophylaxis steps. Regardless of vaccination status, a person potentially exposed to rabies virus should perform adequate wound cleaning with soap and water (CDC 2016). Individuals who work with animals, particularly wildlife, should receive preexposure prophylaxis. At-risk individuals include wildlife rehabilitators, veterinarians, and veterinary technicians who work with animals such as bats, raccoons, skunks, and canids. Preexposure prophylaxis consists of three vaccinations on days 0, 7, and 21 or 28. These individuals should have their rabies titers checked every two years and if an exposure occurs, the individual should receive two booster vaccinations on days 0 and 3 (ACIP 2010).

Individuals potentially exposed to rabies who have not received preexposure prophylaxis should receive four rabies vaccines on days 0, 3, 7, and 14. If an individual is immunosuppressed, they should receive a fifth dose on day 28. Additionally, human rabies immunoglobulin should be administered around the wound. Additional information on pre- and postexposure prophylaxis can

Table 2.1 Select zoonoses associated with wildlife in rehabilitation settings in the United States.

Disease	Agent	Means of transmission to humans	Most common species associated with transmission to humans	Geographic distribution	Other
Acariasis (mange)	*Sarcoptes scabiei*	Direct contact	Red foxes, coyotes, wolves, bears	Widespread	Human disease is often self-limiting and does not require treatment
Avian influenza	Avian influenza viruses, typically H5 and H7	Inhalation; ingestion less common	Various avian species; Anseriformes and Charadriiformes are often reservoirs	Considered a transboundary disease	Human disease may or may not occur depending on the strain of the virus; wild birds are often asymptomatic reservoirs
Baylisascaris larval migrans	*Baylisascaris procyonis*	Ingestion	Raccoons	Historically northeastern, upper Midwest and West Coast, but increasing prevalence documented in southern and southeastern states	Eggs are extremely resistant in the environment; humans cases have occurred in children or developmentally delayed individuals
Campylobacteriosis	*Campylobacter* spp.	Ingestion	Various avian species, which are typically asymptomatic reservoirs	Widespread	Gastrointestinal disease in humans often associated with poultry consumption, but other birds can also carry
Cryptococcosis	*Cryptococcus neoformans*	Inhalation	Pigeons, other avian species	Widespread	Disease can be severe and life-threatening in immune-suppressed individuals
Cryptosporidiosis	*Cryptosporidium parvum*	Ingestion	Fawns	Widespread	Gastrointestinal disease in humans that often resolves without antibiotic therapy
Colibacillosis	*Escherichia coli* O157:H7	Ingestion	Ruminants, including deer	Widespread	Typically mild and self-limited in humans, but may require topical treatment
Dermatophytosis (ringworm)	*Microsporum* spp., *Trichophyton* spp., *Epidermophyton* spp.	Direct contact	Rabbits, rodents, raccoons, otters	Widespread	Locally acquired cases in humans are rare in the United States
Echinococcosis	*Echinococcus granulosus*, *Echinococcus multilocularis*	Ingestion	Wild canids	Found in wildlife in western and Midwestern states	Prevention of tick attachment is the best prevention
Ehrlichiosis or anaplasmosis	*Ehrlichia* or *Anaplasma* spp.	Vector transmitted (tick)	Deer, rodents are reservoirs	Most cases occur in the eastern half of the United States but some Midwestern and western states also affected	Prevention of mosquito colonies and bites is the best prevention
Encephalitis due to arboviral infection	Eastern equine encephalitis virus (EEEV), Western equine encephalitis virus (WEEV), West Nile virus (WNV)	Vector transmitted (mosquito)	Various avian species are reservoirs	EEEV occurs in east; WEEV occurs in western half of United States; WNV occurs everywhere except Hawaii	

Disease	Organism	Transmission	Reservoir/Host	Geography	Comments
Hantaviral pulmonary syndrome	Hantavirus	Inhalation	Rodents are reservoirs and shed virus in urine and feces	Most human cases occur west of the Mississippi river, although sporadic cases occur in the east	Highest number of cases in New Mexico, Colorado, Arizona, and California; hantavirus pulmonary syndrome (HPS) is severe with approximately 40% mortality
Leptospirosis	*Leptospira* spp.	Direct contact; ingestion	Bacteria are shed in the urine of infected animals	None specific	Human infection often associated with exposure to infected water sources
Lyme disease	*Borrelia burgdorferi*	Vector transmitted (tick)	Small mammals and deer are involved in life cycle in nature	Upper Midwest and New England states; lower prevalence on West Coast	Prevention of tick attachment is the best prevention; tick must be attached 48–72 hours to transmit organism
Mycobacteriosis	*Mycobacterium* spp.	Direct contact, ingestion, inhalation	All animals can potentially be infected; *Mycobacterium* spp. are somewhat species specific with which animal is affected	None specific	*Mycobacterium* spp. are stable organisms in the environment and infection can occur with environmental exposure; *Mycobacterium leprae* associated with armadillos
Plague	*Yersinia pestis*	Vector transmitted (flea); ingestion or inhalation	Rodents and their fleas are the common reservoirs and vectors of disease transmission	Western states	Inhalation of organism leads to most serious disease in humans
Psittacosis/ornithosis	*Chlamydia (Chlamydophila) psittaci*	Inhalation	Various avian species; shed in respiratory secretions and feces	Widespread	Human disease is more commonly associated with pet birds
Rabies	Rabies virus	Inoculation through a bite	Any mammal can become infected	Entire United States except Hawaii; virus variant varies with geography	Although preventable, once clinical symptoms appear in humans, infection leads to death
Rocky Mountain spotted fever	*Rickettsia rickettsii*	Vector transmitted (tick)	Various wildlife (rodents) act as reservoirs but ticks must transmit the organism to people	Entire United States but higher prevalence in southern and southeastern states	Prevention of tick attachment is the best prevention; tick must be attached 6–20 hours to transmit organism
Salmonellosis	*Salmonella* spp.	Ingestion	Commensal gastrointestinal flora in many animals especially birds, reptiles and amphibians	Widespread	Human illness is typically self-resolving but more severe disease can occur
Tularemia	*Francisella tularensis*	Vector transmitted (ticks, deer fly); ingestion; direct contact, inhalation	Rabbits, hares, rodents	Cases occur in all states except Hawaii, but are most common in the south central United States	As few as 50 organisms can cause severe disease in humans

Source: Adapted from National Association of State Public Health Veterinarians (2010).

be found in the recommendations from the Advisory Committee on Immunization Practices (2010).

Neural and Ocular Larval Migrans

Historically, the "raccoon roundworm" (*Baylisascaris procyonis*) has been found in the upper Midwest, Northeast, and selected western portions of the United States, but recent surveys have found an increasing prevalence and increased recognition of it in raccoons in the southern and southeastern United States (Eberhard et al. 2003; Gavin et al. 2005; Souza et al. 2009; Blizzard et al. 2010; Hernandez et al. 2013). Although the number of human cases is limited (less than 50 confirmed in the United States), it is possible that cases are either misdiagnosed or not reported (CDC 2012; Kazacos 2016; Sapp et al. 2016). The larvae of this large ascarid and other related species (*Baylisascaris transfuga* and *B. columnaris*) can cause significant damage to the central nervous system and eyes of infected animals, causing neural and/or ocular larval migrans, but infections in humans have not been confirmed. The incubation period in humans is usually 1–4 weeks. Symptoms vary based on the number of larvated eggs ingested and the tissues in which larvae are migrating, and symptoms may include nausea, lethargy, hepatomegaly, loss of vision and in severe cases neurological disease. Asymptomatic infections, either considered incidental findings at autopsy or by detection of antibodies, have also been reported in people and animals (Hung et al. 2012; Shoieb and Radi 2014; Sapp et al. 2016). Prevention is the best measure because there is no cure once an individual has developed clinical signs due to the parasite, although prolonged treatment with high doses of albendazole in humans has been associated with a decrease in clinical signs.

Eggs of *B. procyonis* are shed in the feces of raccoons and other procyonids and *B. columnaris* and *B. transfuga* are shed by skunks and bears, respectively. The eggs are not infectious immediately and require at least 10–14 days to mature. Prompt removal of fresh raccoon feces in cages and enclosures is paramount to avoid further development of eggs. However, the eggs have a thick outer membrane that allows them to remain viable in the environment for months to years and this covering makes the eggs very "sticky" and more difficult to remove with routine cleaning Gavin et al. 2005) (Figure 2.3).

Humans and other animals become infected through ingestion of infectious eggs. Steps outlined previously to prevent exposure to infectious agents through the fecal–oral route are appropriate (Sapp et al. 2016). However, once cages or enclosures are contaminated, the destruction of eggs is only achieved with boiling water or an open flame. Exposure to undiluted bleach will not kill the eggs, but for items that cannot be immersed in boiling

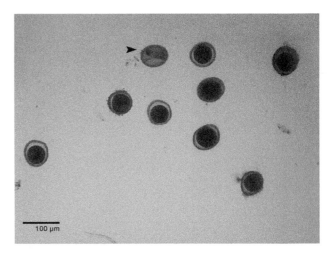

Figure 2.3 *Baylisascaris procyonis* eggs are large (70×60 μm), round, and have a golden-colored mammilated coat.

water or burned, bleach can remove the outer layer of the egg, making removal of eggs easier. Raccoon enclosures in endemic areas in the USA, Europe, Japan, and Central/South America should only be used for housing raccoons and should always be considered contaminated.

Hantavirus

Hantaviruses belong to the Bunyaviridae genus and at least 22 distinct viruses have been found to be pathogenic to humans (Bi et al. 2008). Hantaviruses generally cause one of two types of disease in humans: hemorrhagic fever with renal syndrome (HFRS) or hantavirus pulmonary syndrome (HPS). In North and South America, hantaviruses cause approximately 200 cases of HPS annually with a case fatality rate as high as 40%. In Europe and Asia, hantaviruses cause approximately 150 000–200 000 cases of HFRS; the case fatality rate of HFRS is typically lower than that of HPS but can reach approximately 37% in some outbreaks (Bi et al. 2008). Individuals affected with HPS typically show symptoms approximately two weeks after exposure to the virus. Symptoms include fever, coughing, and pulmonary edema which can lead to death.

Hantavirus is typically found in the western portions of the United States. In the fall of 2012, 10 cases of HPS were confirmed in people who had visited and stayed in campsites/housing in Yosemite National Park (Nunez et al. 2014); of these 10 patients, three died. Several rodent species (deer mouse, cotton rats, rice rats, white-footed mouse) are reservoirs and shed the virus in their urine. Once dried, the infected urine can become aerosolized and inhaled by a person. Handling a live rodent poses little risk of contracting hantavirus, but cleaning rodent enclosures or working in facilities that have pest rodents increases risk. Disease is caused by inhalation of the organism, thus wearing an appropriate mask and wetting an area to prevent aerosolization of rodent urine will reduce risk of exposure.

Mycobacterium leprae

Mycobacterium leprae is an acid-fast, gram-positive bacteria that is very resistant to disinfection. This organism causes leprosy, also known as Hansen's disease, which leads to a variety of symptoms including skin lesions, pain, numbness of affected areas, and muscle weakness.

In recent years in the southern United States, armadillos have been identified as a probable reservoir for *M. leprae* (Truman et al. 2011). Leprosy is relatively uncommon in the United States, with only about 150 cases reported annually. For approximately a third of these cases, armadillos were considered the most likely source of infection (Truman et al. 2011). Direct contact with the blood or fresh tissues of an armadillo increases risk of exposure, and consumption of armadillos is discouraged (Balamayooran et al. 2015). Leprosy can be transmitted between people through respiratory secretions, but it is undetermined whether the bacterium is shed in nasal secretions of armadillos. When handling armadillos in a rehabilitation setting, disposable gloves and protection of the skin to avoid scratches is recommended to prevent transmission; any scratches should be washed thoroughly.

Avian Influenza Virus

Low pathogenic avian influenza strains continually cycle in birds in North America, and water birds, particularly Anseriformes and Charadriiformes, are the most common reservoirs of influenza viruses. Since 2003, numerous highly pathogenic avian influenza (HPAI) strains have been identified in various parts of Asia but had not been found in North American birds. In the fall of 2014, two avian influenza strains, H5N8 and H5N2, were identified in wild birds on the western coast of the United States and Canada; a smaller number of wild birds have also been identified with H5N1 (USGS 2015; WHO 2015). The birds infected with influenza were predominately Anseriformes, but numerous raptor species were also infected. Although similar to the strain that has led to over 800 confirmed cases in humans and approximately 450 deaths in Asia, Africa, and the Middle East, the H5N1 strain in North America is novel and likely a mixed-origin virus of both Asian and North American parts.

Initially, HPAI strains were found in backyard poultry flocks and commercial turkey farms on the western US coast, but commercial farms in the West and Midwest, especially Minnesota and Iowa, have since been adversely affected. Currently, over 48 million birds (poultry) have been affected in 15 states. As of June 2019, a reemergence of influenza virus outbreaks in domestic poultry across North America has not occurred. For the latest information on prevalence and distribution, visit the website of the USDA Animal Plant Health Inspection Service. Fortunately, there has been no human illness associated with any avian influenza strains in the United States or Canada to date. Because wild birds can serve as asymptomatic reservoirs, and some HPAI strains can lead to a case fatality rate of 60% in humans, precautions should be taken, including prevention of inhalation or ingestion of fecal matter or respiratory secretions.

Influenza viruses are shed in the respiratory secretions and feces of infected birds and can become aerosolized. Wearing an appropriate mask and wetting down the feathers of dead birds before necropsy or the caging before cleaning will reduce the risk of inhaling aerosolized viral particles. If a bird is admitted to a rehabilitation facility during an influenza outbreak, that animal should immediately be placed in isolation and the local USDA veterinarian and/or state veterinarian should be contacted. Frequent communication with the appropriate natural resource agency water bird biologist, the state wildlife veterinarian or the state veterinarian (in states where there is no wildlife veterinarian) is highly recommended to keep up to date with recent outbreaks and recommendations.

Conclusion

Although working with wildlife can be fulfilling, precautions must be taken to prevent injury and illness in people. As diseases are constantly emerging onto the global scene, it may sometimes seem impossible to get in front of the next outbreak. But with careful planning and following standard disease prevention steps, veterinarians and others who work with wildlife can protect themselves from most threats. The steps for disease prevention outlined in this chapter do not require large amounts of effort, time, or money. However, they must be performed diligently in order to prevent the transmission of a known or unknown zoonotic agent from the animal patient to the caregiver.

Acknowledgments

Special thanks to Dr Richard Gerhold for scientific review and Misty Bailey for technical editing.

References

Advisory Council on Immunization Practices (2010). Use of a reduced (4-dose) vaccine schedule for postexposure prophylaxis to prevent human rabies. *Morbidity and Mortality Weekly Report* 59 (RR-2): 1–9.

Balamayooran, G., Pena, M., Sharma, H. et al. (2015). The armadillo as animal model and reservoir host for *Mycobacterium leprae. Clinics in Dermatology* 33: 108–115.

Bi, Z., Formenty, P.B.H., and Roth, C.E. (2008). Hantavirus infection: a review and global update. *Journal of Infection in Developing Countries* 2 (1): 3–23.

Blizzard, E.L., Yabsley, M.J., Beck, M.F. et al. (2010). Geographic expansion of *Baylisascaris procyonis* roundworms, Florida, USA. *Emerging Infectious Diseases* 16 (11): 1803–1804.

Bovard, R.S. (2000). Injuries to avian researchers at Palmer Station, Antarctica from penguins, giant petrels, and skuas. *Wilderness and Environmental Medicine* 11 (2): 94–98.

Carrasco, S.E., Burek, K.A., Beckman, K.B. et al. (2011). Aerobic oral and rectal bacteria of free-ranging stellar sea lion pups and juveniles (*Eumetopias jubatus*) in Alaska. *Journal of Wildlife Diseases* 47 (4): 807–820.

Centers for Disease Control and Prevention. (2011). Rabies: What Care will I Receive? www.cdc.gov/rabies/medical_care

Centers for Disease Control and Prevention. (2012) *Baylisascaris* Infection – Epidemiology & Risk Factors. www.cdc.gov/parasites/baylisascaris/epi.html

Centers for Disease Control and Prevention. (2015a). *Stop Ticks.* www.cdc.gov/Features/StopTicks

Centers for Disease Control and Prevention. (2015b). *Stop Mosquitoes.* www.cdc.gov/Features/StopMosquitoes

Centers for Disease Control and Prevention. (2015c). *Human Rabies.* www.cdc.gov/rabies/location/usa/surveillance/human_rabies.html

Centers for Disease Control and Prevention (CDC). (2016). *When Should I Seek Medical Attention?* www.cdc.gov/rabies/exposure/index.html

Chomell, B.B. and Kasten, R.W. (2010). Bartonellosis, an increasingly recognized zoonosis. *Journal of Applied Microbiology* 109 (3): 743–750.

Conover, M.R., Pitt, W.C., Kessler, K.K. et al. (1995). Review of human injuries, illnesses, and economic losses caused by wildlife in the United States. *Wildlife Society Bulletin* 23 (3): 407–411.

Eberhard, M.L., Nace, E.K., Won, K.Y. et al. (2003). *Baylisascaris procyonis* in the metropolitan Atlanta area. *Emerging Infectious Diseases* 9 (12): 1636–1637.

Gavin, P.J., Kazacos, K.R., and Shulman, S.T. (2005). *Baylisascaris. Clinical Microbiology Reviews* 18 (4): 703–718.

Goldstein, E.J.C. and Abrahamian, F.M. (2015). Animal bites and zoonoses: from A to Z: alligators to zebras. In: *Zoonoses – Infections Affecting Humans and Animals, Focus on Public Health Aspects* (ed. A. Sing), 659–679. New York: Springer.

Goldstein, E.J.C., Tyrrell, K.L., Citron, D.M. et al. (2013). Anaerobic and aerobic bacteriology of the saliva and gingiva of 16 captive Komodo dragons (*Varanus komodoensis*): new implications for the "bacteria as venom" model. *Journal of Zoo and Wildlife Medicine* 44 (2): 262–272.

Hall, N.H., Swinford, A., McRuer, D. et al. (2011). Survey of haircoat flora for the presence of dermatophytes in a population of white-tailed deer (*Odocoileus virginianus*) in Virginia. *Journal of Wildlife Diseases* 47 (3): 713–716.

Hansen, M.J., Bertelsen, M.F., Christensen, H. et al. (2012). Occurrence of *Pasteurellaceae* bacteria in the oral cavity of selected marine mammal species. *Journal of Zoo and Wildlife Medicine* 43 (4): 828–835.

Hernandez, S.M., Galbreath, B., Riddle, D.F. et al. (2013). *Baylisascaris procyonis* in raccoons (*Procyon lotor*) from North Carolina and current status of the parasite in the USA. *Parasitology Research* 112 (2): 693–698.

Hung, T., Neafie, R.C., and Mackenzie, I.R.A. (2012). *Baylisascaris procyonis* infection in elderly person, British Columbia, Canada. *Emerging Infectious Diseases* 18 (2): 341–342.

Jijon, S., Wetzel, A., and LeJeune, J. (2007). *Salmonella enterica* isolated from wildlife at two Ohio rehabilitation centers. *Journal of Zoo and Wildlife Medicine* 38 (3): 409–413.

Kalmar, I.D., Dicxk, V., Dossche, L. et al. (2014). Zoonotic infection with *Chlamydia psittaci* as an avian refuge center. *Veterinary Journal* 199: 300–302.

Kazacos, K.R. (2016). *Baylisascaris* Larva Migrans: U.S. Geological Survey Circular 1412. doi:10.3133/cir1412.

Kunimoto, D., Rennie, R., Citron, D.M. et al. (2004). Bacteriology of a bear bite wound to a human: case report. *Journal of Clinical Microbiology* 42 (7): 3374–3376.

Monroe, B.P., Yager, P., Blanton, J. et al. (2016). Rabies surveillance in the United States during 2014. *Journal of the American Veterinary Medical Association* 248 (7): 777–801.

Moore, D.A., Sischo, W.M., Hunter, A. et al. (2000). Animal bite epidemiology and surveillance for rabies post exposure prophylaxis. *Journal of the American Veterinary Medical Association* 217 (2): 190–194.

National Association of State Public Health Veterinarians (2010). Compendium of veterinary standard precautions for zoonotic disease prevention in veterinary professionals. *Journal of the American Veterinary Medical Association* 237 (12): 1403–1421.

National Association of State Public Health Veterinarians (NASPHV) (2016). Compendium of animal rabies prevention and control, 2016. *Journal of the American Veterinary Medical Association* 248 (5): 505–517.

Nunez, J.J., Fritz, C.L., Knust, B. et al. (2014). Hantavirus infections among overnight visitors to Yosemite National Park, California, USA, 2012. *Emerging Infectious Diseases* 20 (3): 386–393.

Saito, E.K. and Shreve, A.A. (2005). Survey of wildlife rehabilitators on infections control and personal protective behaviors. *Wildlife Rehabilitation Bulletin* 23 (2): 42–46.

Sapp, S.G., Rascoe, L.N., Wilkins, P.P. et al. (2016). Baylisascaris procyonis Roundworm Seroprevalence among Wildlife Rehabilitators, United States and Canada, 2012–2015. *Emerging Infectious Diseases* 22 (12): 2128–2131.

Saunders, S., Smith, K., Schott, R., et al. (2014). *Campylobacter jejuni* infections associated with raccoon contact at a wildlife rehabilitation center. Proceedings of 2014 CTSE Annual Conference, Nashville, Tennessee (22–26 June).

Shoieb, A. and Radi, Z.A. (2014). Cerebral *Baylisascaris* larva migrans in a cynomolgus macaque (*Macaca fascicularis*). *Experimental and Toxicological Pathology* 66 (5–6): 263–265.

Siembieda, J.L., Miller, W.A., Byrne, F.A. et al. (2011). Zoonotic pathogens isolated from wild animals and environmental samples at two California wildlife hospitals. *Journal of the American Veterinary Medical Association* 238 (6): 773–783.

Sinclair, C.L. and Zhou, C. (1995). Descriptive epidemiology of animal bites in Indiana, 1990–92: a rationale for intervention. *Public Health Reports* 110 (1): 64–67.

Souza, M.J., Ramsay, E.C., Patton, S. et al. (2009). *Baylisascaris procyonis* in raccoons (*Procyon lotor*) in eastern Tennessee. *Journal of Wildlife Diseases* 45 (4): 1231–1234.

Steele, C.M., Brown, R.N., and Botzler, R.G. (2005). Prevalences of zoonotic bacteria among seabirds in rehabilitation centers along the pacific coast of California and Washington, USA. *Journal of Wildlife Diseases* 41 (4): 735–744.

Stitt, T., Mountifield, J., and Stephen, C. (2007). Opportunities and obstacles to collecting wildlife disease data for public health purposes: results of a pilot study on Vancouver Island, British Columbia. *Canadian Veterinary Journal* 48: 83–90.

Taylor, L.H., Latham, S.M., and Woolhouse, M.E. (2001). Risk factors for human disease emergence. *Philosophical Transactions of the Royal Society B: Biological Sciences* 356 (1411): 983–989.

Truman, R.W., Singh, P., Sharma, R. et al. (2011). Probable zoonotic leprosy in the southern United States. *New England Journal of Medicine* 364: 1626–1633.

United States Geological Survey. (2015) Wild Bird Highly Pathogenic Avian Influenza Cases in the United States. www.aphis.usda.gov/wildlife_damage/downloads/WILD%20BIRD%20POSITIVE%20HIGHLY%20PATHOGENIC%20AVIAN%20INFLUENZA%20CASES%20IN%20THE%20UNITED%20STATES.pdf

World Health Organization. (2015). Cumulative Number of Confirmed Human Cases for Avian Influenza A (H5N1) Reported to WHO, 2003–2015. www.who.int/influenza/human_animal_interface/EN_GIP_20150623cumulativeNumberH5N1cases.pdf?ua=1

World Health Organization (WHO) (2016). Human Rabies. www.who.int/rabies/en

3

Specialized Equipment for Wildlife Care
Florina S. Tseng

Wildlife Clinic, Cummings School of Veterinary Medicine, Tufts University, North Grafton, MA, USA

Introduction

Many practices have general equipment for use on their typical clients. However, for many wildlife species, special equipment or supplies will be needed to safely handle and examine the animals and to provide quality care. Specific tools for handling and restraint will depend on the wildlife species that are most likely to be encountered in the practitioner's geographic location. The supplies needed to raise orphaned young will depend, to a large extent, on whether or not there are local wildlife rehabilitators available who can provide this care. It is strongly encouraged that the veterinary staff work closely with permitted wildlife rehabilitators who have the expertise to care for orphaned young until release and can also provide proper husbandry for adult animals recovering from any medical or surgical procedures. If there are no local wildlife rehabilitators, these animals may be cared for by veterinary staff with proper permits for wildlife rehabilitation but consideration should then be given to caging and other needs that must be available for all stages of growth or recovery from injury and illness. In addition to specific caging needs, proper nutrition for wildlife patients must be available at all times. Knowledge of species natural history will help to inform substitute diets used in captivity as well as the techniques necessary to encourage self-feeding while in care.

The veterinarian and veterinary staff should always be realistic about their level of expertise in working with a particular species as well as availability of proper equipment and supplies to facilitate a successful outcome.

Handling and Restraint Equipment

There is a wide variety of equipment available to assist with safe and successful capture and restraint of different wildlife species. While specific methods of capture for specific groups of animals will be discussed in the appropriate chapters in this book, this section will outline some of the more widely used capture equipment for a variety of different wildlife patients as well as tools necessary for human and animal safety.

The simplest method of restraint for many wildlife patients is to have an appropriately sized towel available that can be used to cover the animal's head and body while simultaneously restraining the body and extremities. This simple method of capture and restraint also serves to decrease the animal's ability to see where the handler is and, once in place, lowers visual stress. For raptors, falconry hoods are also valuable and greatly reduce the bird's visual stress.

Various tools are available that can act as an extension of the handler's arms, thus enabling safe and effective restraint of the animal until it can be more closely handled or sedated. Tools in this category include nets of different lengths and mesh sizes, nets made of different strength materials and those that can cinch together at the opening in order to trap the animal inside. Different snares can be used to capture an animal, usually around a lower extremity or around the neck and one upper extremity. A common example of the latter type of snare is the rabies catchpole. Graspers are also utilized, usually to pin the animal's head to the floor – these can be used on a number of different species but are often used on smaller carnivores and snakes. Cushioned graspers are available, potentially providing a safer means of restraint with certain species. All these tools require practice in order to be used safely and effectively.

Specialized traps and cages are also utilized in order to safely handle and restrain certain wildlife species. For instance, live traps are not only used for animals such as feral cats but can be used to capture wild mammals. Once in a live trap, wild mammals can be safely sedated via injection (Figure 3.1). Squeeze cages are designed so that

Medical Management of Wildlife Species: A Guide for Practitioners, First Edition. Edited by Sonia M. Hernandez, Heather W. Barron, Erica A. Miller, Roberto F. Aguilar and Michael J. Yabsley.

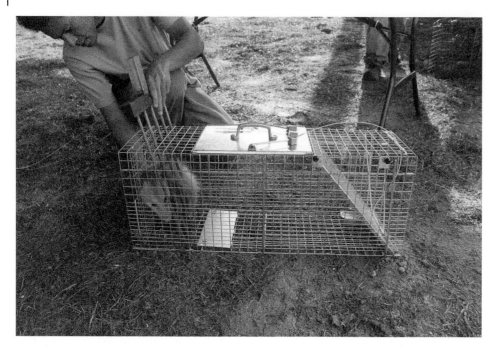

Figure 3.1 Live box traps are often used to capture medium-sized mammals. Custom-made "forks" allow the user to squeeze the animal into a corner to safely and effectively inject it with anesthetics. *Source:* Photo credit Sonia Hernandez.

the animal, generally a mammal, is held between two moveable cage sides, thus allowing the handler to more easily accomplish a procedure, such as an injection. Plastic tubes of varying diameters are available in order to provide safe restraint for different snake species, especially those that are venomous. The snake is encouraged to enter the open end of the tube and, as it moves forward, eventually reaches the closed end. If the proper tube diameter is used, the snake will be unable to double back in the tube and, at this point, the snake's body can be grasped along with the tube and procedures in the caudal half of the animal can be safely administered.

Different methods for safely giving injectable sedatives are sometimes necessary when working with wildlife patients such as carnivores, ungulates. and porcupines. These methods include jab sticks and thumb trigger pole syringes, blow darts, and CO_2-powered pistols and rifles (Figure 3.2).

Jab sticks require the handler to press the needle into the animal and then apply forward pressure in order to complete the injection. When using a thumb trigger pole syringe, the handler gently pushes the needle into the animal and then uses the trigger to give the drug, so there is no additional pressure on the animal. Blow darts utilize different lengths and diameters of piping through which a pressurized dart is introduced. The injectable medication is introduced into the top chamber (Figure 3.3), a needle with a side port blocked by a plastic sleeve is locked onto the syringe and the bottom half of the dart is pressurized with air.

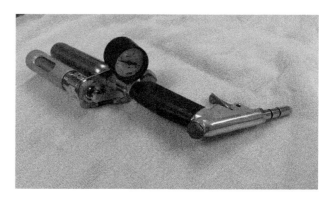

Figure 3.2 A CO_2-powered pistol (DanInject) is a versatile tool to deliver darts in the wildlife medicine setting.

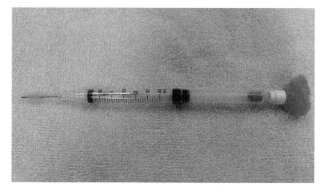

Figure 3.3 Reusable plastic darts are pressurized with air and come in a variety of sizes.

When the dart is blown through the piping and the needle enters the animal, the plastic sleeve is pushed back by the force of the injection and the sedative is quickly injected by the release of the pressurized air. This same dart set-up is utilized in the CO_2-powered pistol and rifle but the use of these firearms allows the handler to fire the dart over longer distances.

Safety equipment is also vital to effective handling and restraint of wild animals. Heavy gloves help to protect the hands of the person who is capturing and restraining the animal. These gloves are of varying lengths and thicknesses and are available in various materials (e.g., synthetic or leather material). Some are lined with Kevlar for additional protection. While these gloves are very useful in protecting the hands and arms, they can compromise the dexterity of the handler. Face shields are recommended for working with certain types of birds (e.g., herons and egrets) which can use their sharp beaks to stab at the handler's face. Physical barriers, such as a board, can be used to herd animals from one space to another as well as for protection, such as may be needed when working with a skunk that might spray as it is being approached.

In general, it is best for the veterinarian and staff to determine which species they are most likely to encounter, acquire the appropriate handling and restraint equipment to work with those species, and then get as much training as possible in safe procedures from more experienced professionals. Written protocols as well as regular refresher training are highly encouraged.

Accurate Measuring Tools

Some of the most important and frequently utilized pieces of equipment to have on hand are accurate weight scales. Animals admitted for rehabilitation can weigh from a few grams (tiny neonatal opossums or small birds) to many kilograms (larger carnivores or large raptors). Thus, it is recommended that different weight scales be available to accommodate the large variety of wildlife species that might be admitted. A small gram scale, capable of weighing to at least 1/10 of a gram, will be very useful for tiny juvenile mammals, small passerines, most amphibians, and smaller reptiles. A human pediatric infant scale is helpful for most medium-sized wildlife species – the most useful size is one that weighs up to 12 lb (~6 kg) and has a resolution up to 1 oz (~2 g). For larger mammals, exam table scales or walk-on scales can be utilized.

Other measuring tools that may be used with wildlife species include goniometers, for measuring range of motion in extremities, and calipers designed to accurately measure various morphological aspects of different birds. Some species of birds are fairly similar in appearance, especially in juvenile plumage, and weight ranges of the males and females may overlap. Accurate morphological measurements of aspects such as culmen and tarsal lengths or wing chord can provide accurate species and, in some cases, differentiate sex of some species of birds.

Heating and Lighting Sources

While heat sources are certainly utilized in small animal practice, their use in wildlife may be different for a number of reasons. For instance, heating pads that are safe to use with mammals may burn much thinner avian skin if set too high or without a protective layer between the pad and the animal. Circulating warm water heating pads or circulating warm air devices are safer and recommended for most species of birds although their use must be closely supervised since some birds, such as raptors, may easily puncture these heat sources. Heat lamps are useful when rehabilitating species, such as turtles, that need to be housed in a preferred optimal temperature zone in order to quickly recover from illness or injury. There are many types of bulbs that can provide heat, some provide light whereas others do not and some produce more heat than others so research is needed in order to determine the species' requirements. Incubators of varying sizes are very useful when working with critically ill wildlife or small neonates that are not yet able to regulate their body temperature. Always ensure that the proper humidity is also provided in these incubators as they can lead to dehydration if used incorrectly. Many incubators have small water chambers that should be used in order to deliver appropriate humidity levels.

Lighting sources can be of equal importance for proper rehabilitation of many wildlife species. Many diurnal animals will not eat well or exhibit appropriate behavior if kept in inappropriately lighted cages during rehabilitation. While natural sunlight is preferred as a light source, this is not always available and various artificial light sources may need to be provided. For example, there are different fluorescent lights that are specifically designed for use with reptiles in captivity. While these are not critical if the animal will only spend a short length of time in captivity, the use of proper lighting in reptiles may enhance their appetite and general activity levels. Make sure to obtain lighting with the proper UVA and UVB output as well as color temperature (color expressed in degrees Kelvin) and color rendering index (degree to which the light sources shows the true colors of the illuminated objects). It is recommended that appropriate light sources are placed between 10 and 12 in. above, and no more than 18 in. above, where the reptile tends to spend most of its time (generally near the heat source). Fluorescent lights can also be used for avian species although the phenomenon of "fluorescent flicker" may be problematic, particularly for birds housed in captivity for longer periods of time. Because most birds process visual stimuli at a higher temporal resolution than their mammalian counterparts, they are susceptible to more stress when exposed to lights with higher flicker frequency rates (Evans et al. 2011). Similarly, crepuscular or nocturnal mammals should be housed in areas that allow the animal to "den" and escape the artificial lighting of the hospital environment.

Caging Requirements

Details concerning caging recommendations are provided in the appropriate species-specific sections. General considerations for captive caging will be discussed in this section and suggestions for a range of different caging options will be presented.

Because being housed in captivity is extremely stressful for wild animals, it is very important that everything possible be done to decrease additional sources of stress that might result from improper caging. General requirements include caging that is safe for both human handlers and the animals, provides visual barriers so that the animals are not able to see outside the cage, and is located in areas that are quiet, where wildlife are not exposed to the sights and sounds of people and domestic animals. In addition, caging should be easily cleaned, allow access to proper temperature and lighting conditions, and provide adequate air exchanges. The current recommendation for laboratory animals is 10–15 full air exchanges/hour (National Research Council 2012).

Most states in the US utilize the "Minimum Standards for Wildlife Rehabilitation" as a guideline for determining appropriate caging for wildlife in captivity (Miller 2012). This publication outlines minimum standards for rehabilitation, disease control, group- and species-specific housing requirements (broken down into restricted activity, limited activity, and unlimited activity categories), and final disposition. Caging recommendations are made taking into consideration the natural history of the animal, the need to allow timely recovery from illness or injury and requirements for enrichment in cage design and furnishings.

Indoor Caging

Many of the wildlife patients will need intensive care housing, whether due to illness or injury. In addition to the general caging requirements outlined above, intensive care housing should be set up so that supplemental heat and oxygen are available if needed. Ideally, these cages should be located in a separate, quiet area from the main hospital but offer easy access for staff to monitor the patient's condition until it is stable enough to be transferred to other indoor caging.

Neonatal and young wild birds, mammals, and reptiles should be housed in incubators or similar caging that allows control of temperature, lighting, and humidity. These parameters must be closely monitored in order to provide optimal conditions for recovery from illness or injury. Older passerines, small mammals, and adult reptiles will also benefit from indoor caging that offers controlled conditions; however, these animals may not be easily housed in incubators. Older passerines that can fly will often escape from incubators so it may be best to house them indoors in caging that allows staff to clean and feed without opening the enclosure, such as cages with bottom trays that slide out for this purpose or soft mesh cages that open from the top. Mesh cages decrease the potential for feather damage and a top opening allows easier capture. Small mammals, such as chipmunks and squirrels, can move very quickly and are also likely to escape from cages with front openings. These animals are also likely to chew through plastic caging so metal or glass caging is preferred (e.g., aquariums with secure tops). Some terrestrial reptiles can also be temporarily housed in aquariums or terrariums although the clear glass sides should be covered in order to reduce stress. Aquatic turtle species will need to be housed in an environment that provides water at a depth that allows complete submersion, proper filtration, and a large, stable basking area.

If waterfowl or other aquatic birds are going to be held for rehabilitation, the ultimate goal is to get them into a pool as quickly as possible. When held out of a pool while indoors, waterfowl should be provided with as large an area as possible that allows them to drink, feed, and move around. These birds are very messy in captivity and the sooner they can have pool access, the better. Pools for waterfowl can be as small as plastic children's pools with an appropriately designed ramp to provide easy access. However, if there are more than two to three individuals, or if larger waterfowl species are being housed, larger wading pools will be necessary. The correct housing is essential when working with seabirds in order to maintain waterproofing and prevent secondary complications, such as pressure sores, that can develop in captivity if incorrectly housed. If these birds have to be held out of pools, they should be housed in net-bottom pens (Miller 2012) to decrease pressure sore development and fecal contamination of their feathers.

Raptors and other wildlife can also be housed while indoors in shift cages that allow staff to easily clean and feed without having to handle the animal excessively (Figure 3.4). A divider is inserted between the two sides of the cage, the empty side is cleaned and the divider is then partially opened. At this point, the animal can be

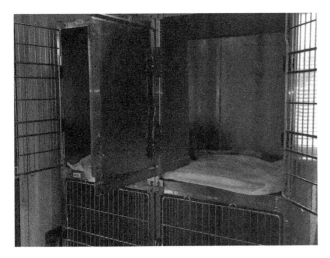

Figure 3.4 Shift cages allow staff to easily clean and feed raptors without having to handle the animal excessively.

gently encouraged to move to the clean side of the enclosure, the divider is closed and the second side is cleaned. Shift cages are also essential if working with larger carnivores that need indoor housing.

An isolation facility is also recommended when working with wildlife since they may be admitted with an infectious and potentially zoonotic disease. Isolation protocols should be prominently displayed and strictly adhered to in order to minimize or eliminate the potential for pathogen transmission.

Outdoor Caging

Since the goal of rehabilitation is release, wildlife should be moved into outdoor caging as quickly as possible. This allows animals to acclimatize to ambient outdoor temperatures and return to normal behavioral and physical conditioning. Every outdoor enclosure must provide some degree of protection from the elements while still allowing the animal to prepare for survival in the wild. It is essential that outdoor caging be constructed so as to be predator proof. Examples of outdoor caging include pools for waterfowl and other aquatic birds and different sizes and types of aviaries for songbirds, raptors, and other bird species. Appropriate mammal housing may be necessary for groups such as rodents, marsupials, lagomorphs, mustelids, hoofed animals, carnivores, and others. Again, detailed information on housing requirements for these diverse groups can be found in the species-specific chapters in this book or in Miller (2012).

Feeding Requirements

The diversity of wildlife that may be presented for care leads to an equally diverse array of dietary needs. Details concerning appropriate diets and feeding techniques are presented in the species-specific chapters. A few general facility requirements to accommodate the need to provide appropriate diets are outlined in this section.

Ideally, dedicated kitchen space for feeding wildlife patients should be available. The kitchen must include freezer space for whole prey as well as other food items. Refrigerator space for thawed whole prey, vegetables and fruit, milk formulas, and other dietary needs should also be provided. In addition, a heat source for making up milk formulas and for warming these formulas prior to feeding is recommended. Dry storage space is also needed for pelleted diets, grains, seed, canned foods, dry milk formulas, and other food. Storage containers should have tight-fitting lids and be made of material that will prevent infestation with pests. If feeding invertebrates to any wildlife patients is necessary, food items such as mealworms and earthworms must be stored in an appropriate environment that allows proper housing and gut loading.

Establishing strict protocols for species-specific diets, adhering to high standards of cleanliness, and labeling all food with expiry dates will help to ensure that wildlife in captivity receive the best possible nutrition.

Conclusion

While most veterinary hospitals are well equipped to work with domestic animals, providing care for wildlife patients can be both challenging and extremely rewarding. Having the appropriate equipment and supplies is a vital component in ensuring safe and successful outcomes for captive wildlife and their caregivers.

References

Evans, J.E., Smith, E.L., Bennett, A.T.D. et al. (2011). Short-term physiological and behavioural effects of high- versus low-frequency fluorescent light on captive birds. *Animal Behaviour* 83: 25–33.

Miller, E. (ed.) (2012). *Minimum Standards for Wildlife Rehabilitation*, 4e. St Cloud, MN.: National Wildlife Rehabilitators Association and International Wildlife Rehabilitation Council.

National Research Council of the National Academies. (2012). *Guide for the Care and Use of Laboratory Animals*, 8e. Washington, DC: National Academies Press.

4

General Principles of Emergency Care

Julia K. Whittington[1] and Nicole Rosenhagen[2]

[1] College of Veterinary Medicine, University of Illinois at Urbana-Champaign, Urbana, IL, USA
[2] PAWS Wildlife Center, Lynwood, WA, USA

The principles of emergency and critical care of veterinary patients are universal, and are globally applicable to all species. Despite differences in anatomy and physiology of nondomestic species, practitioners providing triage and stabilization measures for these patients have significant potential to provide life-saving care. These techniques may also be used when triaging and caring for wildlife, with a few modifications that are highlighted here. Despite the similarities in care, a hospital that cares for wild animals should have a separate area dedicated to these patients, where wildlife and companion animals cannot interact or see one another. This is important for disease control as well as stress management.

Triage

Wild animals present to veterinary practitioners with a wide array of ailments and injuries. The first step to caring for these patients is proper triage. Triage involves sorting cases based on their severity and need. This should initially be done with a thorough history and visual assessment.

Due to the free-living nature of wildlife, the reported history is often minimal or absent. When possible, the person presenting the animal, or "finder," should be asked a series of important questions to determine when and where the animal was found, in what condition it was found, what food or medication the animal has received, if there has been any direct human contact with the animal, including bites or scratches, and if the animal's condition has changed since initial capture. A brief visual assessment will allow for evaluation of respiratory rate and effort, neurological status and mentation, gastrointestinal output, and posture, as well as any urgent conditions such as hemorrhage or seizures.

Patients in critical condition may decompensate quickly, even from undergoing a simple physical examination, and decisions must be made as to how much the animal can tolerate at any given time during diagnostic testing and treatment. Animals exhibiting signs of stress should be given time to rest in a quiet, dark enclosure with supplemental heat and oxygen as needed prior to handling. Brief handling may be appropriate to administer emergency medications or treatments and when evaluating the need for humane euthanasia.

Accurate species identification is critical to the effective triage and management of wildlife patients. Understanding the species' natural history elucidates the survival skills it must possess to be considered for release and may provide information about age, sex, social habits, and migratory status. Additionally, an animal's natural history will dictate necessary daily care, including food and water type and presentation, as well as caging considerations. Field guides, online resources, or specialists may be utilized for species identification.

The survivability of any wild animal is dependent upon its ability to find and apprehend food, avoid predation, interact with conspecifics, and reproduce. Any animal that will not be able to perform these natural behaviors post recovery should not be released. A list of release criteria adopted by the National Wildlife Rehabilitators Association and the International Wildlife Rehabilitation Council is the standard for wildlife triage and includes the following (Miller 2012).

- No animal with vision impairment in both eyes should be released.
- No bird with any portion of its wing missing should be released.
- Birds with fractures close to or involving the joint of a wing that will prevent normal flight when healed should not be released.

Medical Management of Wildlife Species: A Guide for Practitioners, First Edition. Edited by Sonia M. Hernandez,
Heather W. Barron, Erica A. Miller, Roberto F. Aguilar and Michael J. Yabsley.
© 2020 John Wiley & Sons, Inc. Published 2020 by John Wiley & Sons, Inc.

- Mammals with impairment in two or more limbs should not be released.
- Human-imprinted animals should not be released.
- Open fractures with large portions of necrotic bone are generally irreparable.
- Raptors without full function of either leg should not be released.
- Waterfowl with full amputations should not be released; partial foot amputees may be releasable if weight bearing is possible on the leg. Songbirds can be released with one leg in some cases.
- No animal with a high likelihood of shedding a transmissible disease should be released.

In addition to these criteria, traits and behaviors necessary for survival of individual species (such as tail function in an arboreal animal) must be taken into account with any patient.

Patient Assessment

Environmental stress and the physiological stress associated with injury or illness have known detrimental effects on patient healing. Wild animals beyond the age of neonate can be assumed to be experiencing stress from their injury/illness as well as from their captive situation. Minimal handling, decreased auditory stimuli, anxiolytic drugs (Gaskins et al. 2008), and subtle lighting will help reduce this stress.

Visual Examination

The importance of the visual examination cannot be overemphasized. A wild animal's natural instinct is to mask any disability to the extent that it can, especially in the face of perceived danger. Quietly observing an animal from a distance can offer important insight into the true nature of the animal's condition. Take note of respiratory rate and effort, mentation, body posture and position, and use of legs/wings. After a thorough visual examination has been performed, it is prudent to assess the animal's response to visual stimuli as vision can be difficult to interpret during handling. The animal's natural history will again be important to recognizing normal responses for the species and patient's age.

Physical Examination

Following the visual examination, a physical examination is performed when the animal is deemed stable enough for handling. The handler should not begin a hands-on exam without a thorough understanding of the animal's natural defenses. This is critical for the safety of the handler as well as that of the animal. The handler must be aware that responses typical of companion animals during handling and manipulation should not be expected of wildlife under the same circumstances. All anticipated supplies and assistance necessary to complete the assessment should be ready to streamline the exam.

For critical patients, the physical exam begins with a primary survey that follows the "ABC" approach. The patient's airway (A) is assessed first and any compromise or occlusion addressed immediately. Avoid restricting keel movement in birds which may hinder their ability to breathe and mimic airway compromise. Next, the patient's breathing (B) is observed. Take note of the rate and depth of breaths as well as the effort. After breathing, assess circulation (C). Address any external hemorrhage and evaluate perfusion parameters, including pulse quality, extremity temperature, mucous membrane color, capillary refill time, and heart rate. The survey can continue down the alphabet with assessment of disability (D) (is the animal alert, responsive to sounds, responsive to pain or unresponsive?) and finally external assessment (E) to examine for hemorrhage, swelling, fractures, deformities, or other injuries (Crowe 2009).

Following the primary survey, and once the patient is stable, a thorough and complete exam of the entire animal is undertaken. As in companion animals, the exam should be systematic and performed in a routine manner. It may be wise to review normal anatomy for unique or unfamiliar species. During handling, keep the animal's head covered if possible to minimize visual stimuli. The exam should be performed quietly and efficiently. It may be necessary to perform the examination in a stepwise fashion, allowing the patient to recuperate between handling periods as needed. Avoid addressing the most obvious injury first except to rule out the need for euthanasia. Many of the techniques and standard instruments used in companion animal medicine are utilized when assessing wildlife, although patient size and lack of established parameters for many species may limit their use and interpretation of subsequent data.

Always weigh the patient during the initial exam to allow for accurate drug and fluid calculations. Body condition should also be evaluated. For birds, body condition is based on pectoral muscle mass and furcular (interclavicular) and coelomic fat. The pectoral muscle should meet the keel in a "V" shape in most species of good body condition. If the muscle is concave and the keel protruding, the bird is likely in poor body condition; however, young birds or those unable to fly may have decreased muscle mass without losing body condition. Furcular and coelomic fat stores are assessed by gently palpating the thoracic inlet cranial to the clavicles and coelom distal to the keel. Due to the thin nature of avian skin, subcutaneous fat can also sometimes be visualized by parting the overlying feathers. Body condition scoring of amphibians and reptiles, with the exception of chelonians, is based on epaxial muscle mass as well as the presence of coelomic fat. The coelom of a chelonian is palpated by placing the forefingers in the inguinal fossae and applying gentle pressure.

Reptiles and amphibians are ectotherms; therefore, the heart rate, respiratory rate, and blood pressure of these patients will vary with their environmental temperature. In snakes, the heart is located in the cranial third of the body and may be visualized beating through the ventral scutes to determine rate; alternatively, a Doppler probe can be placed over the heart until the blood flow becomes audible. In lizards and turtles, the heart is located between the shoulders and dorsal to the sternum. A Doppler unit with the probe placed between the neck and forelimb is necessary to acquire an audible heartbeat in turtles. In amphibians, Doppler or direct visualization can be used for measuring heart rate.

Of note during the physical exam of amphibians is the unique anatomy and physiology of the integument which is nonkeratinized and semipermeable. The skin acts as a means for fluid and electrolyte balance as well as respiration. Amphibians should never be handled without gloves and the skin should always be kept moist. The color and condition of amphibian skin should be noted during the exam. Often, transillumination of the coelom through the skin can provide direct visualization of internal organs.

Handling

Techniques for restraint are species and animal specific but can be divided into two general categories: manual restraint and chemical restraint. Examination gloves should be worn, in addition to other personal protective equipment deemed appropriate, whenever a wild animal is handled. Protective goggles should be worn by all persons handling wading or seabirds as these animals may use their beaks to stab toward the face in defense.

Manual Restraint

Smaller animals can generally be handled with gentle manual restraint and a towel or sheet. Larger animals may require use of leather gloves and a towel or sheet.

For birds, keep the escape route of the enclosure blocked while gently lowering a sheet or towel over the entire animal, taking care to cover the head. Using gentle pressure, pin the bird's wings against its body in a natural position and maintain this position until the bird's body and legs are secure and controlled. Do not inhibit movement of the keel and secure the head of birds likely to inflict a bite. Small birds can be held in this manner throughout the exam or held in the hand with back and wings pressed against the handler's palm and the handler's thumb and forefinger placed on either side of the bird's head below the mandible. Larger birds can be restrained with hands placed on the sides of the body, each restraining a wing and leg in a flexed, folded position. Additional details specific to raptor, waterfowl, and waterbird restraint are provided in Chapters 17–19.

Small rodents and infant mammals can be held by the scruff or restrained in the hand with thumb and forefinger on either side of the mandible to secure the head. A towel can be used to keep the head covered. Rodents have powerful bites and sharp teeth and may be able to penetrate even thick leather gloves. Very large rodents, such as beavers, may require multiple handlers for secure restraint. Care should be taken to always support the legs of rabbits and hares as these animals have powerful hindlimbs and can fracture their vertebrae with a kick. Neonatal cervids can be cradled to the chest with the legs supported.

Turtles will often attempt to bite. Most can be safely restrained around the bridge between the plastron and carapace, and the head can be gently exteriorized and restrained using a forefinger and thumb below the mandible. Avoid excessive force as this can cause cervical injury. Snapping and soft-shell turtles have an impressive reach and should be held by the base of the tail with one hand beneath the caudal plastron for support. Because box turtles can completely hinge their shells closed, heavy sedation or anesthesia may be required for a thorough exam. Snakes and lizards are best restrained with a thumb and forefinger on either side of the mandible with the body supported. Lizards can be additionally restrained by extending and pinning the rear legs against the tail. Large or venomous snakes may require multiple handlers and specialized equipment (hook, pinning sticks, clear tubes) for safe restraint. Amphibians should be gently restrained with wet, clean, powder-free, nonlatex gloves.

Chemical Restraint

Chemical restraint in the form of sedation or anesthesia is necessary at times to ensure the safety of the handler and animal. Juvenile or adult cervids, large or adult carnivores and omnivores, or any animal that is overly aggressive, requires prolonged handling, has a severe injury, or is highly stressed should be chemically immobilized. Implementation of chemical restraint protocols may require the use of a net, rabies pole, pole syringe, dart gun, squeeze cage, or induction chamber. See species-specific chapters for immobilization protocols.

Exertional Rhabdomyolysis (Capture Myopathy)

When preparing for capture and restraint of a wildlife patient, the handler should be aware of a condition called capture myopathy. Capture myopathy occurs in circumstances of prolonged pursuit, capture, restraint, or transportation of a susceptible animal. The condition manifests as a result of exhaustion of muscular adenosine triphosphate (ATP), decreased oxygen delivery to tissues and increased lactic acid with subsequent metabolic acidosis and muscle necrosis. Clinical signs become apparent acutely or several days after handling and include ataxia, myoglubinuria, hyperthermia, tetany, and acute death. Many species are predisposed to the condition, particularly ungulates, but it has also been reported in birds and various carnivores. Treatment is often unrewarding and management is aimed at prevention, including careful and limited restraint or pursuit, minimizing auditory and visual stimuli, and the use of sedation or anesthesia during restraint in especially high-stress animals. Treatment modalities that have been anecdotally reported include aggressive fluid therapy, vitamin E and selenium injections, muscle relaxants, and analgesics. Readers are directed to a review of this topic (Paterson 2007).

Wildlife Patient Monitoring

Parameters

As with any veterinary patient, a variety of physiological parameters should be monitored during the animal's care to assess progress or decline. In general, these are extrapolated from companion animal medicine. See species-specific chapters for normal parameters.

Equipment

Most equipment required to manage wildlife emergencies will already be available in a veterinary hospital environment. In addition to standard equipment, small-gauge needles and catheters, small-volume blood collection tubes, magnifying loupes, a digital gram scale, noncuffed endotracheal tubes, leather gloves, and eye protection will be beneficial. The small size and unique anatomy of many wild animals often require innovative solutions to common problems, and a variety of nontraditional splinting materials (including paper clips, coat hangers, and foam tubing) will also serve the practitioner well.

Sampling and Timing of Sampling

The principles of diagnostic sample collection are the same in all fields of veterinary medicine. Any sampling should be done prior to initiating treatment that would affect the sample.

Hematological parameters provide valuable insight into patient status and allow for rapid assessment of biochemical and cytological changes. A blood volume equaling 1% of the body weight in kilograms is safe to collect from healthy birds and mammals; in reptiles and amphibians, the volume collected should not exceed 0.5% of body weight. The volume collected must take into account additional loss from hemorrhage or hematoma formation. Animals that are severely debilitated may not tolerate the same volume of loss, and each case should be individually evaluated. It is also necessary to consider the volume of blood needed for testing. In-house diagnostics often require a smaller volume of blood than outside laboratories, and the practitioner should be aware of requirements before collection begins.

Blood collection sites in mammals are similar to domestic species, including the cranial vena cava in sedated or anesthetized small mammals. In birds, phlebotomy of the right jugular vein, the medial metatarsal vein, or the basilic vein coursing over the ventral aspect of the elbow is well tolerated. Chelonian venipuncture sites include the jugular and ventral tail veins and the subcarapacial sinus (lymph contamination is possible from the sinus). In snakes, the ventral tail vein or the cardiac ventricle are used for blood collection, and in amphibians, the ventral tail, abdominal or femoral veins can be used. Anatomy and species-specific venipuncture techniques should be reviewed prior to collection.

Hospitalization of Wildlife Patients

Caging Considerations

A hospital that cares for wild animals should have a separate area where wildlife and companion animals cannot interact or see one another. This is important for disease control as well as stress management. See Chapter 3 and species-specific chapters for more details on housing.

Heat

Supplemental heat is critical for patients that are hypothermic or do not have the ability to thermoregulate. Providing an external heat source reduces the physiological stress on an animal during hospitalization and facilitates healing, particularly in reptiles.

Most wild mammals maintain a core temperature of 37.8–40 °C (100–104 °F), with Virginia opossums being a notable exception having body temperatures of 33.3–35.6 °C (92–96 °F). The normal body temperature of a bird is warmer than most mammals and typically ranges from 40 to 42.2 °C (104–108 °F). Birds in need of thermal

Table 4.1 Preferred optimal temperature and humidity ranges for maintaining reptile and amphibian species.

Species	Temperature in C (F)	% Humidity
Desert reptiles	35–40.6 (95–105)	30–50
Temperate reptiles	23.9–29.4 (75–85)	60–80
Tropical reptiles	26.7–32.2 (80–90)	80–90
Amphibians	23.9–26.7 (75–80)	70–90

Source: Clayton and Gore (2007) and Mitchell (2009).

support may fluff their feathers in an effort to retain heat. These animals should be housed in an enclosure with an ambient temperature of 25–30 °C (77–86 °F) with 50–80% humidity (Dorrestein 2009).

Reptiles and amphibians cannot thermoregulate and each species has a preferred optimum temperature zone (POTZ) for normal physiological function. See Table 4.1 for temperature and humidity ranges.

Cold ectotherms should be warmed to their preferred body temperature (PBT) over 4–6 hours, and should not be fed or medicated until within this range. Full-spectrum ultraviolet light (UVB and UVA) should also be made available (Martinez-Jimenez and Hernandez-Divers 2007).

Pediatric or veterinary incubators are extremely useful in caring for small critical patients. Radiant heat lamps (ideally infrared or ceramic) may be attached to cage doors or placed over aquariums to provide ambient heat when an incubator is not available or suitable. Do not allow the patient or flammable materials to come into contact with the lamp as burns are possible. Forced-air heating blankets, heating pads, discs, bottles, or warm rice socks are good alternatives for patients that are ambulatory and not in need of constant thermoregulation. Heating pads should be used cautiously because animals may chew on the power cord, leading to electric shock. A nonambulatory animal should never be left on a focal heat source without constant monitoring as the animal may become hyperthermic or sustain burn injuries. Heated fluids are also a good source of thermal support.

Whenever possible, a thermal gradient should be created within the enclosure. Animals receiving thermal support should be monitored for signs of hyperthermia, including open-mouth breathing, panting, or distress.

Oxygen Therapy

Oxygen therapy is recommended in many circumstances. Any dyspneic or overly stressed animal should receive supplemental oxygen immediately. An oxygen cage or chamber is ideal for low-stress therapy with the fractional inspired oxygen (FiO_2) >40%. Other options for oxygen support include nasal cannulas, flow-by oxygen,

and direct ventilation via endotracheal tube. However, the stress and additional handling required for these methods are significant and would not be tolerated by many wild patients.

Fluid Therapy

The principles of fluid therapy are universal for all species. The fluid type, dose, and rate of administration depend on patient assessment as well as a basic understanding of fluid pharmacology and the forces governing water movement between body compartments.

Assessment

Assessment of hydration primarily relies on subjective measures of skin tenting, character of mucous membranes, and patient mentation. Generally accepted parameters for assessing percent dehydration are listed in Table 4.2.

It is generally safe to assume at least 5% dehydration for all wild animals that present for care. Animals with relatively good perfusion parameters, strong pulses, and normal mentation will benefit from oral or subcutaneous fluids. The most effective route of fluid administration in patients that are in shock or with very poor perfusion is intravenous (IV) or intraosseous (IO). Intraperitoneal (IP) or intracoelomic (ICe) fluids may be administered to reptiles and mammals but absorption of these boluses may be limited in debilitated animals. Additionally, care must be taken to avoid fluid overload in these patients (Schumacher 2008).

Catheter Placement

Intravenous or IO catheterization should be performed in an aseptic manner. Venous access for catheter placement in mammals is often identical to that for dogs and cats.

Table 4.2 Clinical parameters associated with dehydration in wildlife patients.

Percent (%) dehydration	Clinical signs
4–6%	Slightly dry mucous membranes, skin tent normal or slightly prolonged, normal mentation, CRT <2 s
6–8%	Tacky mucous membranes, 2–5 second skin tent, ropy mucus, slightly depressed mentation, CRT 2–3 s
8–10%	Dry, tacky mucous membranes, >5 s skin tent, ropy mucus, depressed and weak, eyes appear sunken, weak and rapid pulses, CRT >3 s
>10%	Signs of hypovolemic shock or death

CRT, capillary refill time.

The medial metatarsal vein is the preferred location in many avian species although the basilic vein may also be used. Catheterization is possible using the jugular vein and the ventral tail vein in reptiles. Additionally, the cephalic and ventral abdominal veins of lizards may be used for catheter placement but likely will require the use of a cut-down technique to visualize the vessel (Schumacher and Mans 2014). When IV catheterization is not possible due to vascular collapse, limited venous access, or patient size, IO catheterization offers an alternative means for providing effective vascular fluid support.

For IO catheter placement, a short spinal needle or a standard hypodermic needle of appropriate gauge is used. In avian patients, the distal ulna is the most common site for IO catheter placement (Figure 4.1). Local or general anesthesia may be utilized to minimize movement and reduce stress in patients during catheter placement. A local block should be performed to decrease pain associated with catheter placement. Inject 2% lidocaine diluted with sterile saline to achieve a 2 mg/kg dose (Bowles et al. 2007). Fluids infused into the medullary cavity drain directly into the vasculature. However, some resistance to fluid flow is expected due to the rigidity of the cavity and fluid should be administered in a slow, steady fashion. If a hypodermic needle is used for the IO catheter and fluid does not flow through the needle after placement, a bone core may be present. Sterile cerclage wire can be passed through the needle to clear the obstruction or the needle may be withdrawn and replaced with a new one, following the same path. Confirmation of correct placement is challenging in some species, but in birds the basilic vein will "flush" with fluid administered through an IO catheter placed in the ulna. Alternatively, turbulence can be heard when a Doppler probe is placed over the outflow vein. Once the catheter is placed, it is capped with an injection cap or T-port and secured with porous white tape ± suture and a figure-of-eight wrap applied (see Wounds section for bandaging technique) (Figure 4.1).

The proximal tibiotarsus in birds, the tibia in mammals and some reptiles, and the tibio-fibula in amphibians are other common locations for IO catheter placement. For this technique, locate the cnemial crest cranially at the proximal end of the tibia, flex the stifle, and prepare the site. Place the needle at the junction of the cnemial crest and tibial plateau and advance it into the bone in the same manner as described above. In this location, there is no vein available to check for placement, so the clinician will have to monitor the leg for swelling or take orthogonal radiographs to confirm placement.

The femur can also be used in some animals, particularly the proximal femur in small mammals and the distal femur in lizards. Birds have pneumatic bones with air sac communication into the proximal long bones of the legs and wings, so an IO catheter should never be placed in the femur or humerus.

Fluid Selection

Commercially available crystalloid solutions are commonly used for fluid therapy in wildlife species and dextrose or B vitamins may be added as needed. Colloidal solutions are indicated for shock, hypovolemia, or hypoproteinemia. Other fluid solutions (hypertonic saline, 5% dextrose in water) may be indicated in specific circumstances and should be reviewed carefully before use.

Fluid Administration

Fluids should generally be warmed prior to administration and may be given as a bolus or by constant rate infusion using an IV drip set, fluid or syringe pump. The rate and volume will be dependent on the species, presenting problem, percent dehydration, and ongoing losses.

Determining the fluid deficit of an animal is based on the following equation:

$$\text{Percent dehydration (in decimal form)} \times \text{patient weight (g)} = \text{total volume (mL)}$$

This volume is generally administered over a 2–3-day period as follows:

- Day 1 – maintenance volume + 50–75% of deficit volume
- Day 2 – maintenance +25% of deficit
- Day 3 – maintenance ± 25% of deficit
  Daily fluid requirement (maintenance volume) varies by species and physiological stage of life (e.g., neonate/juvenile, lactating adults, etc.) and is directly related to the metabolic rate of the individual. Progress and endpoint of fluid therapy should be based on clinical markers and constant reevaluation, understanding that overhydration is possible and may be indicated by tachycardia or dyspnea.

Maintenance fluid volume:

- Birds – 50–150 mL/kg/day
- Nonherbivorous mammals – 60–120 mL/kg/day
- Herbivorous mammals – 80–150 mL/kg/day
- Reptiles 10–30 mL/kg/day (Mitchell 2009)
- Amphibians – 10–20 mL/kg/day (Clayton and Gore 2007)

Due to the semipermeable nature of amphibian skin, soaking is the most effective route for fluid therapy in these animals. The patient should be placed in an iso- or hypotonic solution for adequate fluid uptake. The bath

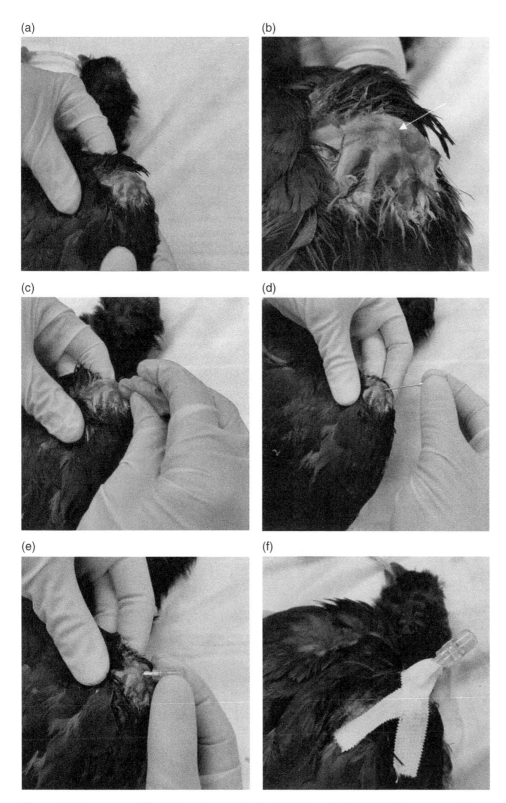

Figure 4.1 Intraosseous (IO) catheter placement in the distal ulna of a bird. IO catheters are used to provide immediate access to the systemic vasculature for administration of fluids and medications when intravenous (IV) access is not practical. To begin, pluck the feathers covering the dorsocranial surface of the carpus (a). Identify the dorsal condyle of the distal ulna (indicated by white arrow in (b)), and aseptically prepare the site (c). Grasp the ulna just proximal to the carpus with the thumb and forefinger of the nondominant hand. With the dominant hand, seat the needle just ventral to the dorsal condyle of the distal ulna, allowing the bevel to drop into the natural "notch" at that location (d). Keep the needle parallel to the longitudinal plane of the ulna and apply steady pressure while rotating the needle to drive it through the cortex of the distal ulna. Once the cortex has been penetrated, the needle should advance easily into the medullary cavity (e). Once properly seated in the bone, the catheter is capped and secured to the wing (f).

solution may be water that is free of chlorine, chloramines, ammonia, nitrites, and nitrates (Hadfield and Whitaker 2005) or an amphibian Ringer's solution can be made using the following formula:

> 6.6 g NaCl, 0.15 g CaCl2, 0.15 g KCl, 0.2 g
> NaHCO3 per liter of fresh dechlorinated water

Fluid Resuscitation for Shock

Shock is a life-threatening condition of cellular dysfunction and death secondary to poor tissue perfusion. Several causes of shock have been documented and include hypovolemia, sepsis, neuropathy, heart failure, and anaphylaxis. In wildlife, shock most commonly manifests from significant loss of intravascular fluid volume as a result of hemorrhage or chronic fluid deprivation (Crowe 2009). Shock in domestic animals is categorized into compensatory, early decompensatory or late decompensatory based on patient heart rate, blood pressure, and a variety of subjective measurements (Lichtenberger 2007). Wild animals will have altered physiological parameters due to stress, so it is difficult to divide these patients into distinct categories. Instead, if shock is suspected based on history and clinical parameters, aggressive therapy should be instituted immediately.

Management of shock is based on early recognition and rapid restoration of circulating blood volume, and the cornerstone of effective treatment is aggressive fluid therapy. It is imperative that fluids be administered directly into the vascular system via IV or IO catheter as subcutaneous or oral fluids will not be properly absorbed into the circulation. Crystalloids are generally considered the mainstay of shock treatment. However, 60–80% of crystalloid volume is redistributed out of the intravascular space and into the interstitium within 30–60 minutes of administration, and aggressive therapy with crystalloids alone can lead to a net positive fluid balance and increased morbidity and mortality (Cazzolli and Prittie 2015).

When high volumes of fluids are warranted, colloids may be indicated for their volume-sparing effect since the region of distribution is theoretically limited to the intravascular space. Treatment with a combination of crystalloid and colloid fluids can allow for resuscitation of a patient with circulatory failure without causing fluid overload. There are many reported adverse effects of synthetic colloid use in humans, and although reports are few in veterinary medicine, judicious use is warranted. Hypertonic saline is another option for treatment of hypovolemic patients; it allows for rapid IV fluid expansion and can decrease the total volume of fluid required for resuscitation. Due to the osmotic effect of colloids and hypertonic saline, both solutions should always be administered slowly and with crystalloids to prevent interstitial fluid depletion.

Determining the etiology of shock is often difficult, especially without an accurate history. Patients suspected to be suffering from septic or anaphylactic shock should be treated with appropriate pharmaceuticals in addition to fluids. Animals with cardiogenic or neurogenic shock have a grave prognosis for prolonged survival and euthanasia should be considered.

Shock doses for mammals are those familiar to the veterinary practitioner. Reported doses for nonmammalian species are provided in Table 4.3. These volumes are administered as a bolus over 10–15 minutes, then the crystalloid repeated as needed for stabilization.

Animals receiving aggressive fluid therapy should be monitored closely for evidence of fluid overload, and therapy adjusted based on clinical signs and changes in parameters.

Transfusion Therapy

In the event of severe anemia or hemorrhage exceeding 25% of the total blood volume, a whole-blood transfusion may provide life-saving support (Morrisey 2013). The decision to transfuse a patient should be based on clinical signs, chronicity, and etiology of blood loss or anemia, packed cell volume, overall prognosis, and availability of a donor.

Blood groups in wild animals are largely unknown, and at least a major cross-match (testing the donor's cells with the recipient's plasma) should ideally be performed before initiating a transfusion. The ideal donor is of the same species, but numerous cases involving donors and

Table 4.3 Reported resuscitation fluid doses for nonmammalian species.

	Crystalloid	Crystalloid + colloid	Crystalloid + hypertonic saline
Avian	NR	10 mL/kg + 5 mL/kg	10 mL/kg + 5 mL/kg
Reptile	NR	5–10 mL/kg + 3–5 mL/kg	5–10 mL/kg + 5 mL/kg
Amphibian	5–10 mL/kg	NR	NR

Volumes are administered as a slow bolus, then the crystalloid dose repeated as needed for patient stabilization. NR, doses have not been reported for treatment of shock in these animals. *Source:* Clayton and Gore (2007), Lichtenberger (2007), Martinez-Jimenez and Hernandez-Divers (2007).

recipients of different species and even genera have been managed successfully. The reported half-life of blood from a homologous species is 6–11 days in birds while the reported half-life of heterologous blood is only 12 hours to three days (Morrisey 2013). However, this can be enough time to stabilize the patient until cell regeneration occurs.

To perform a transfusion, collect blood from the healthy donor in a syringe with added anticoagulant (0.25 mL of sodium heparin for every 10 mL of blood collected). The blood can be transferred to a sterile IV bag for administration or left in the syringe. The blood should be administered to the recipient through a blood filter intravenously or intraosseously as a constant-rate infusion over 2–4 hours (Morrisey 2013). Monitor the patient for reactions including fever, urticaria, or changes in respiration. Any animal requiring multiple transfusions has a poor prognosis for recovery and euthanasia should be considered.

Pharmaceuticals

Antimicrobial and analgesic medications are often incorporated into the emergency and critical care of veterinary patients. Since wild animals will attempt to mask outward signs of pain, conditions that would be painful to a human may be assumed to be painful to the patient. Pain sensation and perception is a complex process that involves many regions and messengers in the body, and a multimodal approach to therapy should be employed whenever possible. Prophylactic antimicrobial use is controversial and careful consideration should be given to the circumstances and likelihood of infection before initiating treatment. Refer to relevant chapters in this text for specific information regarding pharmaceutical selection for the different species.

Nutrition

Nutritional management is vital for patient recovery; wild animals should always be stable and warm before providing any food source. Fluid, thermal, and oxygen support are far more essential than nutritional support in an emergent situation, and feeding an animal that is not physiologically ready for digestion can have grave results. For stable animals, an appropriate diet (based on age and species) should be offered. Animals with evidence of crop stasis, ileus, or impaction should not be fed until the problem is resolved.

Animals that would be self-feeding in the wild will often be anorexic in captivity for a variety of reasons. Degree of debilitation, inability to recognize food (when the animal's natural food is unavailable), abnormal food presentation, and stress can all contribute to apparent lack of interest in eating. These patients will need to be hand or gavage fed, and the route, composition, and frequency of feeding are determined by patient needs. Many neonatal animals must be fed a dozen or more times per day (every 15 minutes for some bird species), requiring careful consideration to the allocation of time and manpower for successful treatment.

The animal's caloric requirements should be estimated with the formula below to provide a baseline for a feeding protocol. Patients should be weighed daily, prior to feeding and after stimulation to defecate/urinate in orphaned mammals, to ensure that nutritional needs are being met.

- Basal metabolic requirements$(\text{kcal}) = k * \text{wt in kg}^{0.75}$
- Metabolic energy requirements$(\text{kcal}) = 1.5 * \text{basic metabolic rate}$
- K values:
  - nonpasserines = 78
  - passerines = 129
  - placental mammals = 70
  - marsupials = 49
  - reptiles at 37 °C = 10 (Dorrestein 2009)

Basal metabolic rate represents the number of kilocalories required for basic physiological functions while metabolic energy requirements determine the kilocalories necessary for an active animal. The metabolic energy requirement can be further adjusted for the animal's specific condition.

Common Conditions

Trauma, malnourishment, toxicosis, and infectious disease are common conditions affecting wildlife species. Rescue efforts employed in domestic animal emergencies may be applicable for wild mammals, but feasibility of follow-up care should be carefully considered for the individual before proceeding with treatment.

Cachexia and Refeeding Syndrome

Severely malnourished animals may be at risk of refeeding syndrome. Refeeding syndrome is broadly defined as the electrolyte disturbances and complications that occur during nutrition rehabilitation of malnourished patients (Skipper 2012). Abnormal levels of phosphorus, potassium, magnesium, and sodium have all been implicated in the manifestation of this syndrome, although hypophosphatemia appears to be the most important determinant of disease (Solomon and Kirby 1990).

During starvation, catabolism of muscle and fat leads to an overall loss of electrolytes; despite this loss, serum electrolyte levels may be within normal limits prior to feeding (Solomon and Kirby 1990). When animals are fed diets containing carbohydrates, the subsequent insulin release enhances the cellular uptake of phosphorus and other electrolytes. In patients with depleted electrolyte stores, the intracellular movement of phosphorus may lead to acute drops in serum levels.

Clinical signs of refeeding syndrome are most often associated with critically low levels of cellular energy in the form of ATP and include cardiac arrhythmias, hemolysis, seizures, and ventilatory failure (Solomon and Kirby 1990). Signs usually become apparent within 2–5 days of feeding, although some animals may die without warning (Skipper 2012). The period of starvation that puts a patient at risk varies by species, age, and presence of concurrent disease and can range from hours to months (Blem 2000). Refeeding syndrome is best avoided with complete rehydration of the patient followed by slow reintroduction of easily digestible food at increasing concentrations until the animal is deemed stable enough for whole foods. Additionally, it is recommended that the practitioner monitor serum chemistry values and supplement electrolytes as needed during the first few days of treatment.

There are currently no published studies documenting the occurrence of refeeding syndrome in avian species. In birds, the pancreatic beta cells that secrete insulin are more sensitive to glucagon, cholecystokinin (CCK), and absorbed amino acids than they are to glucose (Hazelwood 2000). However, the sensitivity of beta cells to glucose varies with species; thus, the condition should not be disregarded and the above precautions should be taken for identified at-risk avian patients.

Respiratory Disease

Respiratory emergencies warrant immediate attention and dyspneic animals should receive supplemental oxygen. See Oxygen Therapy above for details. Animals that do not improve with supplemental oxygen and time alone will require additional treatment. There is a vast array of causes of dyspnea and appropriate management varies so the etiology of the distress should be determined whenever possible. Trauma, infection (especially *Aspergillus* spp.), and toxins are among the most common causes of respiratory difficulty, but other etiologies, such as mechanical obstruction and neurological disease, should also be ruled out. Handling of these patients needs to be planned and efficient. Administering therapeutics targeting the specific etiology and providing nebulization therapy may afford the animal some relief.

Air Sac Cannulation in Birds

Obstructive airway disease is difficult to treat due to the severe respiratory compromise experienced by these patients. The respiratory tract of birds is unique among vertebrates, with air sacs throughout the body communicating with the lungs, trachea, and some bones to facilitate highly efficient, unidirectional airflow during respiration. Air sac cannulation allows for respiration that bypasses the trachea and is indicated for those patients with upper respiratory occlusion or severe facial trauma and swelling. General anesthesia and positive pressure ventilation of the bird can also be administered through an air sac cannula. A variety of readily accessible supplies may be modified into an air sac cannula including teat cannulas, small-diameter endotracheal tubes or red rubber catheters. The tube should be firm so as not to collapse from the pressure of the body wall but pliable enough to not damage internal organs while in place. A cuff is useful to form a seal and stabilize the tube but is not necessary.

The cannula is placed in the caudal thoracic or abdominal air sac on either side of the body, although the air sacs are larger on the left side. Externally, the landmark is caudal to the last rib (for the caudal thoracic air sac) or caudal to the thigh muscles (for the abdominal air sac). In all but emergency situations, the patient is anesthetized for cannula placement. With the bird in lateral recumbency, the leg is extended either caudally or cranially to expose the chosen landmark. The feathers over the site are plucked and the skin aseptically prepared.

A scalpel blade is used to make a small stab incision through the skin. Curved mosquito hemostats are positioned with a finger stop through the incision and directed cranial-to-dorsal with firm pressure to penetrate the body wall. Care must be taken to avoid deep penetration into the coelomic cavity which may cause iatrogenic injury to internal structures. With the hemostats in the air sac, open the tips and introduce the tube so that the end of the tube rests just inside the coelomic cavity. The tube should be tested for patency by administering a breath and watching for keel excursion. A downy feather can also be held over the tube opening to watch for airflow. Secure the tube with a tape butterfly and suture or with a purse-string suture and interlocking pattern (finger trap). To the extent possible, the cannula should be positioned for minimal leg interference. Cannulas can be safely maintained for up to a week (Brown and Pilny 2006; Clippinger and Bennett 1998); however, wild birds in need of long-term respiratory support often have a poor prognosis and euthanasia should be considered.

Respiratory Disease in Reptiles and Amphibians

Chelonians with carapacial fractures may present with signs of respiratory distress if there is damage to the underlying lungs. Clinical signs of respiratory pathology in reptiles include oral and nasal discharge, extension of the neck, and increased respiratory sounds. In severe cases, oxygen should be provided via endotracheal or tracheostomy tube. In reptiles, the glottis is easily visualized at the base of the tongue. Breaths should be administered 2–6 times per minute while the patient is warmed and stabilized. Additional treatment will be indicated based on the nature of the animal's injury or disease (Martinez-Jimenez and Hernandez-Divers 2007).

Amphibians in respiratory distress should be placed in an oxygen chamber or have forced oxygen pumped into the water during soaking (Hadfield and Whitaker 2005). Amphibians can also be intubated and ventilated, although the small size of most North American species makes this procedure technically difficult.

Trauma

Many of the injuries sustained by wildlife are the direct result of human activity or attacks by predators, domestic animals, or conspecifics. Anthropogenic causes of trauma include vehicular trauma, gunshot wounds, power line injuries, and window collisions. Often, the traumatic event is not directly observed but is suspected based on the circumstances of capture and clinical signs. Traumatic events frequently result in life-threatening conditions and patients should be stabilized prior to care for non-life-threatening injuries. The basic tenants of triage for trauma cases are respiratory support, analgesia, and/or fracture management.

Blunt Trauma

Blunt trauma without outward signs of injury is easily missed during initial patient assessment. Signs such as cavity swellings, changes in mentation, lameness, or bruising may indicate internal damage and radiographs or ultrasound may be necessary for directing care and determining overall prognosis.

Wounds

Information on wound management is provided in Chapter 11 and Whittington (2007).

Fractures

Fractures and luxations are commonly sustained by wildlife secondary to trauma. Luxations generally have a poor prognosis; management should include reduction and immobilization as soon as possible for the best chance of success. Open fractures require management of both the fracture and the resulting wound. As the patient is handled, the fracture must be supported to prevent further damage to the surrounding tissue. If a bone end is protruding beyond the skin, measures must be taken to prevent desiccation of the bone. Avoid removing fragments of bone unless the blood supply is obviously compromised as every attempt must be made to preserve vascularity.

Fracture assessment includes determining the nature of the fracture as well as identifying any complications which will affect fracture healing. Nonviable bone, large regions of compromised blood supply, improperly healed fractures or fractures in close proximity to or involving joints will significantly impact a wild animal's return to function and release potential.

Fractures frequently become open in birds due to the minimal amount of soft tissue over the long bones and the potential for sharp bone fragments to lacerate the thin skin. Osteomyelitis and wound infection are potential sequelae of open fractures in any species. The fracture site should be cultured and irrigated with warm saline. Fractures involving the avian humerus or femur should be lavaged carefully to avoid infusing fluid into the pneumatic bones and associated air sacs.

In birds, fractures distal to the elbow can be stabilized with a figure-of-eight wrap (Figure 4.2) and those above the elbow, including bones of the shoulder girdle, should be further managed with a body wrap (Figure 4.3), until healed or until surgical repair is performed. A tape splint can be used (Figure 4.4) for distal leg fractures in small birds and mammals (<300 g). Larger animals require more standard limb immobilization, including modified Robert Jones bandages, Ehmer, or Thomas Schroeder splints until surgical repair.

The size and nature of the patient may necessitate creativity when making splints; modified syringe cases, paper clips, red rubber feeding tubes, coat hangers, and thermal plastic, among others, are options for splinting material. The practitioner should adhere to the principles of domestic animal splinting to prevent venous occlusion and pressure sores.

Confine birds or mammals suffering fractures of the femur, pelvis or spine to a small enclosure until surgical fixation, if indicated, can be pursued. Reptile appendicular fractures can be immobilized by taping the affected limb to the body or tail. Triage of chelonians with shell fractures includes assessment for lung and spine involvement, followed by open wound management until additional stabilization can be performed. Fractures of the pelvis or spine and all fractures in snakes and amphibians are managed with analgesia and cage rest unless euthanasia is warranted.

Traumatic Brain Injury

Traumatic brain injury (TBI) occurs most often as a result of motor vehicle and window collisions. The pathophysiology, clinical signs, and treatment modalities are identical in all animals. If TBI is suspected, the practitioner is advised to evaluate and monitor the patient's mentation, posture, pupil size and symmetry, and cranial nerve reflexes. The modified Glasgow Coma Scale has

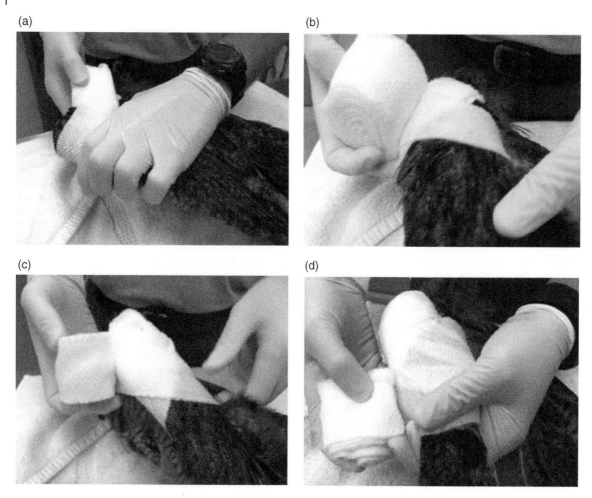

Figure 4.2 Figure-of-eight wing wrap, used to provide external coaptation of fractures of the radius, ulna, major and minor metacarpals and other bones distal to carpus; stabilize elbow or carpal luxations; secure distal ulnar intraosseous (IO) catheter in place; protect soft tissue wounds on the wing distal to the elbow. With the wing held in a naturally flexed position, encircle the carpus with cast padding (a). Ensure that the bandage will be directed ventrally and medially as you continue to wrap the wing. This will avoid placing unnatural torsion on the wing while secured in the wrap. Extend the cast padding from the carpus, over the dorsal wing at a diagonal and under the ventral wing to the axilla. Include the secondary and tertiary covert feathers on the dorsum as the cast padding is placed high in the axillary region and brought back to the dorsal surface of the wing to complete the figure of eight (b). Extend the cast padding to the carpus and encircle the joint as before (c). As the cast padding is applied, it can be placed more distally on the elbow with each subsequent pass to give support to large wings (d,e). The cast padding is covered with conforming gauze (f). The bandage is covered with protective material (g). A properly positioned figure-of-eight wing wrap on a mallard duck (h).

not been adapted for wildlife patients but can be loosely interpreted to provide a general prognosis. When managing these cases, it is prudent to consider both the intracranial and extracranial aspects of the injury. Extracranial damage includes hemorrhage, penetrating wounds, and airway obstruction. As always, life-threatening conditions need to be attended to first. Due to a high correlation between TBI and ocular injury, a complete ophthalmic exam should be performed as soon as possible. Ocular injuries may jeopardize the animal's future release potential and influence treatment.

Current standard of care involves the use of hyperosmotic agents in conjunction with isotonic fluids to maintain intravascular volume and sustain normal mean arterial pressure (MAP). Mannitol and hypertonic saline have been used with reported success in birds and mammals (Rivas et al. 2012). Loop diuretics are not generally recommended due to their potential to cause intravascular volume depletion and subsequent hypotension and decreased cranial perfusion pressure (CPP) (Fletcher and Syring 2009). Doses for mammals are extrapolated from domestic species. In birds, mannitol is dosed at 0.2–2 g/kg IV slowly every 8–24 hours for up to 3 doses (Graham and Heatley 2007) or hypertonic saline may be administered at 5 ml/kg IV slowly every 8 hours and repeated as needed (Lichtenberger 2007).

In addition, animals should receive supportive care, including analgesia and supplemental oxygen to

(e)

(f)

(g)

(h)

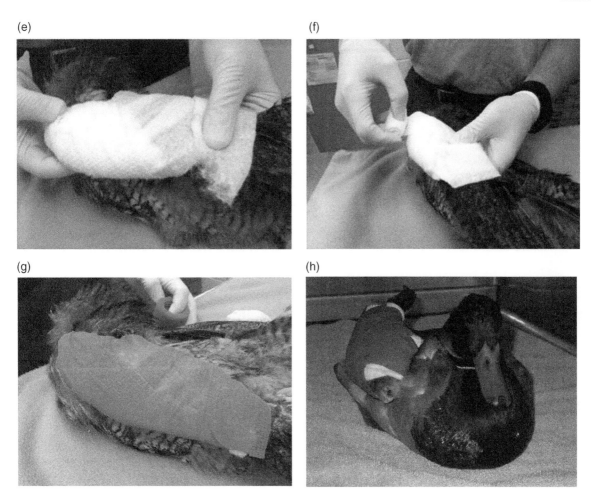

Figure 4.2 (Continued)

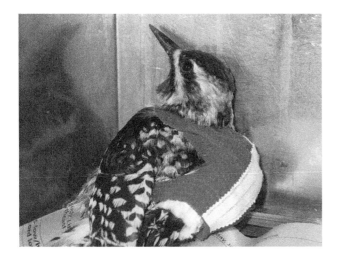

Figure 4.3 The body wrap for birds is used to stabilize the humerus and shoulder. Stretch bandage material or tape (in small birds) is applied to the feathers across the keel, then extended over the figure-of-eight wrap on the affected wing before passing cranial or caudal to the nonaffected wing and secured to the leading edge of the bandage. Take care to avoid impinging on normal excursion of the keel.

encourage normocapnia. Hypoventilation can affect oxygen delivery to the brain, requiring that narcotics be used judiciously and only to effect. The patient's head should be elevated 15–30° to facilitate venous drainage, and jugular compression and hyperthermia should be avoided. Corticosteroids are generally considered to be contraindicated as a treatment for TBI (Fletcher and Syring 2009). When corticosteroids are implemented in the treatment of a wildlife patient, especially avian species, extreme care must be used in order to prevent compromise to the patient's immune system and subsequent susceptibility to secondary infections. If possible, a nonsteroidal antiinflammatory product should be preferentially selected.

Neurological Disease

Signs of neurological disease include ataxia, seizures, paresis or paralysis, changes in posture or mentation, and cranial nerve deficits. A full neurological examination should be performed on any animal exhibiting these

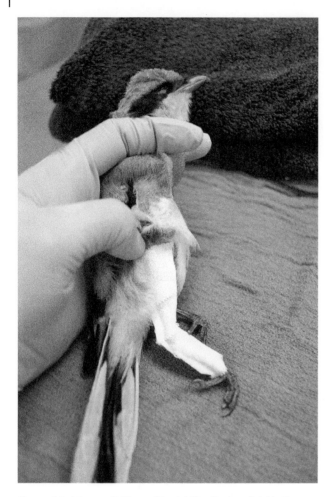

Figure 4.4 A tape splint is used to stabilize the leg, distal to the stifle, in small birds and mammals. Pluck or clip feathers or fur over the area to be splinted. Using white bandage tape, apply a stirrup to the limb to maintain appropriate positioning. Apply white tape over the stirrup in a loose spiral pattern, extending past the joint above and below a fracture if one is present. Use hemostats to crimp the tape against the limb to secure the splint. Cyanoacrylate glue may be added over the tape to increase the stiffness if required.

signs to localize the lesion and determine its severity. The basics of the examination are similar to those of domestic species and should include a fundic exam. In some cases, adjustments need to be made to accommodate differences in anatomy and physiology.

Many of the responses expected in domestic species will not be present. Wildlife patients do not display pain as readily as domestic species, the menace response may not be present in prey animals, and most standard reflexes will be difficult to elicit in reptiles and amphibians. In patients with a chronic injury or illness, the examiner should take care to differentiate musculoskeletal weakness from true paresis.

Birds and reptiles represent a challenge in applying standard neurological assessment techniques. Birds have skeletal muscle in their iris and a complete decussation of the optic nerve, making assessment of ocular reflexes difficult. Postural reactions and gait are good indicators of appendicular limb function, but assessment of reflexes and pain response is difficult to interpret. In stoic wildlife species, pain is best assessed by observing the pupil for change in size to indicate perceived sensation.

Reptiles and amphibians should be examined to the extent possible, but should include assessment of the righting reflex. When placed in dorsal recumbency, a neurologically appropriate patient will return to a normal position immediately. Chelonians may be unable to right themselves without assistance, but the leg and head movement should indicate that the animal perceives its inverted position.

Causes of neurological disease are varied and may not always be determined. The practitioner should be aware of reportable or zoonotic causes of neurological dysfunction and be prepared to handle these animals appropriately. Treatment revolves around supportive care, including bladder or cloacal evacuation as needed, in addition to addressing the underlying cause.

Seizures

Seizures are managed with anticonvulsants, especially diazepam and midazolam. Because midazolam is water soluble and can be administered intramuscularly, it is often the treatment of choice for small patients or those where vascular access is not feasible. See Appendix II: Formulary for more information.

Animals experiencing seizures should also be monitored for hypoglycemia or hyperthermia. Multiple or prolonged seizures carry a poor prognosis for recovery and euthanasia should be considered for these patients.

Toxins and Contaminants

Because many of the patients treated by the wildlife practitioner live in close proximity to humans, the opportunity for toxin exposure is ever-present. Clinical signs are often nonspecific, and exposure can be difficult if not impossible to determine. Common toxicants include heavy metal (lead and zinc), organophosphates, and anticoagulant rodenticides. Naturally occurring toxins, including those associated with red tides and botulism, may also affect wildlife. If there is a definitive treatment for the toxin, it should be implemented promptly. Otherwise, the mainstay of management is supportive care, fluid therapy, and standard measures to prevent further exposure to or absorption of the toxin. Euthanasia may be warranted in severely affected patients.

Animals may also present with oil contamination and management is covered in Chapter 6. Additional information may be found online in this pdf (Welte & Frink 1991).

Infectious Disease

Clinical signs associated with infections may be nonspecific, and any animal suspected of harboring an infectious organism should be segregated, if not quarantined, until a diagnosis is made. Biosecurity is of the utmost importance for the safety of human handlers as well as other animals. Practitioners should be aware of zoonotic diseases and their vectors in the region, and any personnel working with or around wildlife should have protective titers against rabies.

The management of infectious disease often calls for the use of antimicrobials. The antimicrobial choice should be based on a confirmed diagnosis when possible. Animals that will become chronic carriers of a disease despite treatment should not be released.

Cardiopulmonary Cerebral Resuscitation

Animals with respiratory or cardiovascular arrest require cardiopulmonary cerebral resuscitation (CPCR). A stocked and readily available crash cart with trained staff will afford the best chance of success in these efforts. The endgoal of CPCR is restoration of spontaneous circulation and normal neurological function. Standard emergency resuscitation procedures and drugs are used in wildlife patients and the details will not be reviewed here.

The glottis of birds, reptiles, and amphibians is positioned at the base of the tongue and is easily visualized in most species. In general, noncuffed endotracheal tubes should be used as most of these species have complete tracheal rings and compression with an inflated cuff may result in pressure necrosis of the tracheal wall. Once the tube is placed and secure, positive pressure ventilation should begin. Birds that cannot be intubated or that have upper airway obstruction can be ventilated with an air sac cannula. See Air Sac Cannulation in Birds for instructions on cannula placement. For mammals that cannot be intubated due to small size or poor visualization, a tight-fitting mask can be placed over the mouth and nose with forced ventilation using high oxygen flow. While often effective, this technique may lead to air accumulation in the stomach and the patient should be monitored for abdominal distension as this may hinder diaphragm movement (Bowles et al. 2007).

Cardiac compressions in avian, amphibian, and most reptilian species are performed in a manner similar to mammals, and the pressure applied should be adjusted for the animal's size. The plastron of chelonians makes cardiac compressions not feasible in these species. Efficacy of resuscitation efforts can be monitored with endtidal carbon dioxide meters or by monitoring blood gas values, but most often, subjective parameters and degree of normal function are the only indicators of success or failure. Electrocardiogram readings in hypothermic animals should be interpreted with caution because of poor electrical conduction in cold tissue.

Emergency drugs should be administered as life-saving procedures are being performed. See Appendix II: Formulary for drugs and dosages utilized for wildlife emergencies. Clinicians are encouraged to review current formularies and literature for broader options and updated information.

The clinician should be aware that cardiac activity can continue for hours after central nervous system collapse in reptiles and amphibians. As a result, these patients should be left in a cage for 24 hours to assess for signs of life before death can be definitively determined (Martinez-Jimenez and Hernandez-Divers 2007).

Euthanasia

Animals that are nonreleasable can be considered for placement into captive care facilities, but very few wild animals are good candidates for captivity and significant thought should be given to the animal's prospective quality of life.

When euthanasia is deemed appropriate, a lethal injection of sodium pentobarbital is the most commonly used method (see miscellaneous section of Appendix II: Formulary). General anesthesia or heavy sedation prior to administration of a fatal dose may be indicated, especially when using potassium chloride (KCl). All routes of administration utilized in companion animal medicine are viable options for wildlife, including intracardiac and intraperitoneal/intracoelomic injection. Amphibians can be euthanized with IV or ICe pentobarbital or an overdose of the anesthetic MS-222 (tricaine methanesulfonate) (Hadfield and Whitaker 2005).

Importantly, carcasses of animals that have been euthanized by chemical euthanasia should be rendered or incinerated to avoid the potential for relay toxicosis in scavenging wildlife.

References

Blem, C.R. (2000). Energy balance. In: *Sturkie's Avian Physiology*, 5e (ed. G.C. Whittow), 327–341. San Diego, CA: Academic Press.

Bowles, H., Lichtenberger, M., and Lennox, A. (2007). Emergency and critical care of pet birds. *Veterinary Clinics of North America: Exotic Animal Practice* 10 (2): 345–394.

Brown, C. and Pilny, A.A. (2006). Air sac cannula placement in birds. *Lab Animal* 35 (7): 23–24.

Cazzolli, D. and Prittie, J. (2015). The crystalloid-colloid debate: consequences of resuscitation fluid selection in veterinary critical care. *Journal of Veterinary Emergency and Critical Care* 25 (1): 6–19.

Clayton, L.A. and Gore, S.R. (2007). Amphibian emergency medicine. *Veterinary Clinics of North America: Exotic Animal Practice* 10 (2): 587–620.

Clippinger, T.L. and Bennett, R.A. (1998). Successful treatment of a traumatic tracheal stenosis in a goose by surgical resection and anastomosis. *Journal of Avian Medicine and Surgery* 12 (4): 243–247.

Crowe, D.T. (2009). Patient triage. In: *Small Animal Critical Care Medicine* (ed. D.C. Silverstein and K. Hopper), 5–9. St Louis, MO: Saunders Elsevier.

Dorrestein, G.M. (2009). Nursing the sick bird. In: *Handbook of Avian Medicine* (ed. T.N. Tully, G.M. Dorrestein and A.K. Jones), 101–137. Edinburgh: Saunders Elsevier.

Fletcher, D.J. and Syring, R.S. (2009). Traumatic brain injury. In: *Small Animal Critical Care Medicine* (ed. D.C. Silverstein and K. Hopper), 658–662. St Louis, MO: Saunders Elsevier.

Gaskins, L.A., Massey, J.G., and Ziccardi, M.H. (2008). Effect of oral diazepam on feeding behavior and activity of Hawai'i 'amakihi (*Hemignathus virens*). *Applied Animal Behaviour Science* 112: 384–394.

Graham, J.E. and Heatley, J.J. (2007). Emergency care of raptors. *Veterinary Clinics of North America: Exotic Animal Practice* 10 (2): 395–418.

Hadfield, C.A. and Whitaker, B.R. (2005). Amphibian emergency medicine and care. *Seminars in Avian and Exotic Pet Medicine* 14 (2): 79–89.

Hazelwood, R.L. (2000). Pancreas. In: *Sturkie's Avian Physiology*, 5e (ed. G.C. Whittow), 539–555. San Diego, CA: Academic Press.

Lichtenberger, M. (2007). Shock and cardiopulmonary-cerebral resuscitation in small mammals and birds. *Veterinary Clinics of North America: Exotic Animal Practice* 10 (2): 275–291.

Martinez-Jimenez, D. and Hernandez-Divers, S.J. (2007). Emergency care of reptiles. *Veterinary Clinics of North America: Exotic Animal Practice* 10 (2): 557–585.

Miller, E.A. (2012). *Minimum Standards for Wildlife Rehabilitation*, 4e. St Cloud, MN: National Wildlife Rehabilitator Association.

Mitchell, M.A. (2009). Snakes. In: *Manual of Exotic Pet Practice* (ed. M.A. Mitchell and T.N. Tully), 136–163. St Louis, MO: Saunders Elsevier.

Morrisey, J.K. (2013). Practical hematology and transfusion medicine in birds. Proceedings of Western Veterinary Conference, Las Vegas, NV.

Paterson, J. (2007). Capture myopathy. In: *Zoo Animal and Wildlife Immobilization and Anesthesia* (ed. G. West, D. Heard and N. Caulkett), 115–121. Ames, IA: Wiley-Blackwell.

Rivas, A.R., Whittington, J.K., and Emerson, J.A. (2012). The use of hypertonic saline and hetastarch in an American kestrel (*Falco sparverius*) with traumatic brain injury. *Wildlife Rehabilitators Bulletin* 29: 9–12.

Schumacher, J. (2008). Fluid therapy in reptiles. In: *Zoo and Wild Animal Medicine*, 6e (ed. M.E. Fowler and R.E. Miller), 160–164. St Louis, MO: Saunders Elsevier.

Schumacher, J. and Mans, C. (2014). Anesthesia. In: *Current Therapy in Reptile Medicine and Surgery,* (ed. D.R. Mader and S.J. Divers), 134–153. St Louis, MO: Saunders Elsevier.

Skipper, A. (2012). Refeeding syndrome or refeeding hypophosphatemia: a systematic review of cases. *Nutrition in Clinical Practice* 27 (1): 34–40.

Solomon, S. and Kirby, D. (1990). The refeeding syndrome: a review. *Journal of Parenteral and Enteral Nutrition* 14 (1): 90–97.

Welte, S., Frink, L. (1991). Rescue and Rehabilitation of Oiled Birds. Fish and Wildlife Leaflet, 13.2.8. www.nwrc.usgs.gov/wdb/pub/wmh/13_2_8.pdf

Whittington, J.K. (2007). Principles of wound management in wildlife patients. In: *Topics in Wildlife Medicine*, 2e (ed. F. Tseng and M.A. Mitchell), 47–57. St Cloud, MN: National Wildlife Rehabilitator Association.

5

General Principles of Analgesia and Anesthesia in Wildlife

Michelle G. Hawkins[1,2], *David Sanchez-Migallon Guzman*[2] *and Joanne Paul-Murphy*[2]

[1] *California Raptor Center, School of Veterinary Medicine, University of California, Davis, CA, USA*
[2] *Companion Exotic Animal Medicine and Surgery Service and Department of Medicine and Epidemiology, School of Veterinary Medicine, University of California, Davis, CA, USA*

Introduction

The efficacy and safety of anesthetic techniques in wildlife have increased greatly, but complications still exist. Some of these complications are predictable but others, such as hyperthermia, acidosis, and capture myopathy may result from the capture event. It is challenging to perform an examination and determine the health status of many wild animals until they are sedated or anesthetized. In some situations, anesthesia can result in decompensation and emergent situations. With anesthesia of domestic animals, it is often possible to titrate induction drugs to minimize adverse effects, but during anesthesia of wildlife, drugs are often delivered at the higher end of the dose range in an attempt to induce anesthesia rapidly. Anesthesia of wild animals is complicated further by the variety and varied physiology of species. There is a paucity of information concerning anesthetic techniques for many wild species, and thus anesthetists are often forced to extrapolate from closely related species. It is more difficult to obtain preoperative bloodwork, secure an airway or intravenous (IV) access, monitor anesthesia, and prevent hypothermia once the animal is anesthetized, particularly in smaller species.

Balanced Anesthesia/Analgesia

Inhalant anesthetics have the advantage of allowing rapid changes in anesthetic depth, and rapid recoveries due to their low solubility in tissues and elimination via the respiratory tract. But inhalants also induce dose-dependent cardiopulmonary depression. It is important to minimize the concentration used in longer, painful procedures, thereby decreasing their adverse effects. "Balanced anesthesia" uses multiple drugs at lower overall doses, to minimize the adverse effects of each drug while still providing appropriate anesthesia and analgesia. This approach reduces the magnitude of cardiovascular depression and promotes hemodynamic stability.

Even with balanced anesthetic protocols, morbidity and mortality increase with increased duration of anesthesia. Minimize anesthesia time by preparing the patient and all drugs and equipment in advance and provide close patient monitoring so that anesthetic adjustments are identified and corrected immediately. Morbidity and mortality also occur during recovery so it is important to monitor animals until they are fully recovered.

Preanesthetic Considerations

Patient Evaluation

In many cases it is not possible to perform a thorough physical examination without anesthesia or sedation. Place cotton in ears and blindfolds over eyes when possible to help prevent sudden arousal in sedated wild animals. Age should be considered because the margin of safety of anesthesia is generally wider in younger animals. Ideally, obtain an accurate body weight for fluid and drug dose calculations. Evaluate hydration status and correct dehydration prior to anesthesia whenever possible. Severe anemia should be corrected because the patient may not be able to compensate for decreased oxygen delivery. The packed cell volume (PCV) may decrease 3–5% during anesthesia due to vascular hemodynamic changes. Glucose concentration should be monitored and supplemented as necessary. The type of surgery to be performed and potential for blood loss should be assessed for fluid plan preparation.

Medical Management of Wildlife Species: A Guide for Practitioners, First Edition. Edited by Sonia M. Hernandez,
Heather W. Barron, Erica A. Miller, Roberto F. Aguilar and Michael J. Yabsley.
© 2020 John Wiley & Sons, Inc. Published 2020 by John Wiley & Sons, Inc.

Assessment of patency of the nares and nasopharynx is essential in obligate nasal breathers, especially when an inhalant anesthetic mask is used. The thorax of some mammals is very small relative to abdominal volume, the pressure of which can contribute to hypoventilation.

Nutritional Status and Fasting

Prolonged anorexia leads to negative energy balance and hypoglycemia, requiring nutritional support in the perianesthetic period. Nutritional support for the debilitated patient is discussed in species-specific chapters. Schedule procedures early in the day to reduce fasting times. Overnight fasting prior to anesthesia is not performed in many species due to their rapid gastrointestinal (GI) transit times and potential for perioperative ileus. Lagomorphs and some rodents cannot vomit because of their well-developed cardiac sphincter and limiting ridge of the stomach, respectively. Many species store food in their oral cavities; therefore, immediately after induction, syringing water into the oral cavity to remove food materials is recommended. Elevate the neck and turn the nose down during anesthesia if concerned about aspiration. Fasting times vary with species, size, and patient condition and should be determined with prudence, weighing the risks and benefits in the specific patient.

Reptiles
The fasting period is variable, ranging from 2–4 hours in smaller reptiles to 24 hours in large reptiles.

Birds
Species of small birds with crops (>500 g body weight) can be fasted 2–3 hours prior to anesthesia to allow the crop to empty. Raptors and gallinaceous birds should be fasted 8–12 hours to minimize regurgitation. If a bird is in a poor plane of nutrition or has been anorexic, it may be advisable to gavage feed the patient the evening prior to anesthesia.

Mammals
Many medium to larger mammals should be fasted for 12–24 hours. For cervids, remove all concentrates 48 hours before anesthesia, and remove hay for a complete fasting time of 12 hours. Fasting smaller species (e.g., rodents, armadillos, etc.) for 4–6 hours is appropriate.

Clinical Techniques

Vascular Access

Vascular access, sites for IV catheterization and intramuscular (IM) injection, and fluid administration are covered in Chapter 4 and species-specific chapters. Arterial catheterization for evaluation of blood pressure, blood gas tension, and pH can be performed in some species. The most common sites include the pedal arteries in most species, the central auricular artery in lagomorphs, the ventral tail artery in some mammals, and the median ulnar artery in birds. The catheters are usually placed percutaneously, but a cut-down procedure is sometimes used.

Airway Strategy and Intubation

A strategy for keeping an open airway should be developed for each patient. Cuffed tubes are used with caution in species with complete tracheal rings (e.g., birds, chelonians, crocodilians), and the endotracheal tube must be long enough to reach the larynx of species with a long, narrow oropharynx (e.g., cervids). Airway device selection is based upon species, patient size, perceived risk of aspiration, type of procedure, anesthetist experience, whether positive pressure ventilation is required, and whether the surgery is likely to interfere with the airway. Evaluation can be difficult, especially when anesthetizing a new species for the first time. Anatomical variation is considerable across taxonomic groups and thus the anesthetist should gain as much insight into the patient's anatomy as possible prior to induction, and have a wide variety of options available.

Intubation can be simple but when it goes wrong it can be stressful and impact the patient significantly. Poorly assessed anatomy, poor positioning, inadequate induction, abnormalities of the head or peripharyngeal anatomy, foreign bodies, and airway pathology can all cause difficult intubation. It can be extremely useful to have a "difficult airway algorithm" prepared; examples can be found on the American Society of Anesthesiologists (ASA) and Difficult Airway Society (DAS) websites (www.asahq.org; www.das.uk.com). Document the airway strategy in the anesthetic record and medical records, specifically noting anatomical variations, the airway device and size used, and problems or comments associated with airway management during anesthesia. This information is useful for subsequent anesthesias for that individual or the species in general. Disadvantages of intubation include airway mucosal trauma, increased airway resistance, and airway occlusion due to mechanical forces or secretions. Increased airway resistance is of greater importance in very small patients because it is inversely related to the tube radius. Resistance also increases with length of the trachea. Increased resistance can be overcome with positive pressure ventilation.

Specialized endotracheal tubes and light sources are available to aid intubation. The smallest commercial uncuffed tubes have an internal diameter (ID) of 1 mm but tubes <2 mm ID are highly flexible and kink easily. The smallest diameter cuffed tube is 3 mm ID. Uncuffed tubes do not provide a sealed airway, so clean the oral cavity prior to intubation, elevate the head, and monitor the patient for passive regurgitation. When using a cuffed tube, the cuff is carefully inflated with just enough air to prevent leakage when 10–15 cm H_2O pressure is applied. Very small patients can be intubated with Teflon IV, red rubber, or urinary catheters. Care is taken to ensure that the edges on the end are smooth. Application of lidocaine onto the larynx 30–60 seconds prior to intubation should reduce laryngospasm.

Endotracheal tube obstruction is detected by monitoring for a prolonged expiratory phase. Anticholinergics reduce mucus production but increase mucus viscosity, making secretions harder to clear. The use of an endotracheal tube with a Murphy eye decreases the likelihood of mucus occlusion. Humidification of the gases reduces mucus plug formation. Commercial endotracheal tube humidifiers are available (Humidi-vent Mini Agibeck Product, Hudson RCI, Temecula, CA) (Figure 5.1).

Care must be taken to minimize head and neck movement in intubated patients as changes in position may move the tube, causing mucosal trauma. Sublaryngeal tracheal injury, ulceration, and postintubation tracheal strictures have been described in birds and mammals intubated with both cuffed and uncuffed endotracheal tubes (Grint et al. 2006; Phaneuf et al. 2006; Sykes et al. 2013). Other factors that may predispose to mucosal injury include ventilation technique and endotracheal tube disinfection protocols.

Reptiles

Chelonians have a more cranial tracheal bifurcation than some other reptiles. Alligators have an epiglottal flap that needs to be pushed ventrally to intubate. The larynx of the snake is cranial, easy to visualize and directly intubate. In small reptiles, including small snakes, a 16–18 ga IV catheter might be warranted. The catheters have

sharp ends that must be dulled with a file or flamed to smooth the opening before intubation. A piece of sterile tubing such as IV tubing can be glued to the end to provide a soft edge.

Birds

Noncuffed endotracheal tubes are recommended. The endotracheal tube itself will decrease the diameter of the airway and significantly increase resistance to airflow in small birds. Positive pressure ventilation is critical when using anything smaller than a 2 mm diameter endotracheal tube. The avian glottis is easily visualized at the base of the tongue but can be challenging with small birds with fleshy, thick tongues. In gallinaceous birds, the glottis is deep in the oropharynx. A nontraumatic clamp may be necessary to extend the tongue. The crista ventralis is a projection from the ventral aspect of the cricoid cartilage found in a variety of avian species, such as pelicans (*Pelecanus* spp.), that reduces the size of endotracheal tube that can be used (Figure 5.2).

A potential complication of endotracheal intubation in birds is tracheal stricture, as discussed previously. Prevention includes selective intubation, gentle placement of endotracheal tube, minimal head and neck movement after placement, humidification of anesthetic gases, and gentle positive pressure ventilation (Sykes et al. 2013).

Air sac cannulation is a technique for inhalant anesthesia used in birds. It is primarily used with upper airway obstruction or procedures involving the upper airway or cranium and has been used in birds as small as finches (Nilson et al. 2005). Air sac catheters are usually placed in the left caudal thoracic or abdominal air sac to prevent trauma to the larger right liver lobe (Figure 5.3).

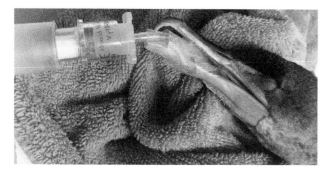

Figure 5.1 Endotracheal tube obstruction occurs often, and especially with smaller diameter tubes. Humidification of the gases can reduce mucus plug formation. Commercial endotracheal tube humidifiers are available that fit into the anesthetic circuit. *Source:* Heather Barron/CROW.

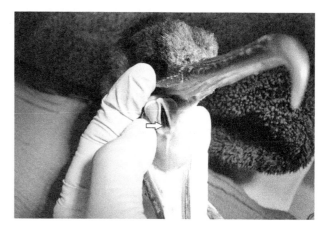

Figure 5.2 The crista ventralis (*arrow*) is a projection from the ventral aspect of the cricoid cartilage found in a variety of avian species, such as this double-crested cormorant, that reduces the size of the endotracheal tube that can be used. *Source:* Heather Barron/CROW.

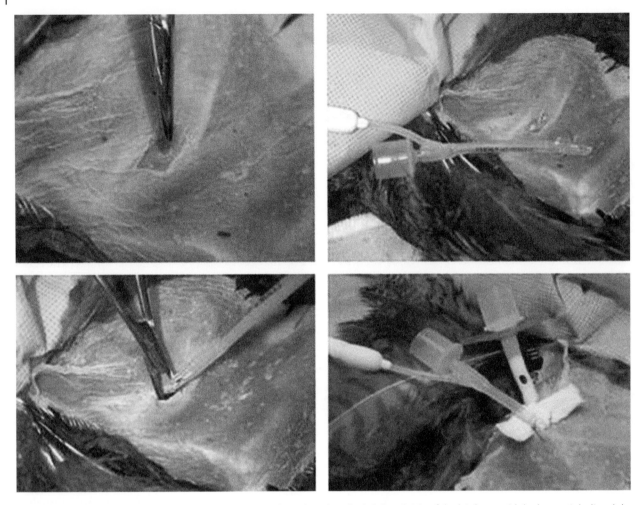

Figure 5.3 Air sac cannula placement in a bird. The cannula is placed on the left-hand side of the bird to avoid the larger right liver lobe. A small incision is made just cranial to the thigh muscles over the last intercostal space. The intercostal muscles are penetrated using a mosquito hemostat to create a hole large enough to insert the tube. The tube is advanced a few millimeters and sutured in place using a finger trap or butterfly tape technique. *Source:* Heather Barron/CROW.

While using air sac cannulas, measured endtidal carbon dioxide (ETCO2) cannot be used in a simple linear fashion to predict $PaCO_2$. Adverse effects include apnea, subcutaneous emphysema, plugging, and contamination of the tube. Following cannula removal, suture the body wall to reduce subcutaneous emphysema and potential contamination.

Mammals

Intubation of most carnivores is straightforward. Intubation of bears requires the patient be in a deep plane of anesthesia. The anatomy is similar to that of canids and intubation is easiest with the bear in sternal recumbency. A long blade laryngoscope facilitates visualization of the glottis. Endotracheal tube size depends on size of the bear, range 8–18 mm ID.

Intubation can be challenging in cervids. Maintain the animal in sternal recumbency with the head and neck extended upwards. Use a laryngoscope with a long flat blade and an endotracheal tube with a stylet. The epiglottis is long and mobile in cervids. The flat blade of the laryngoscope should be carefully placed on the dorsum of the epiglottis, depressing it ventrally. The opening to the glottis can then be visualized and the stylet placed. Animals induced with xylazine and ketamine may swallow or close the glottis during intubation. The "palpation intubation" technique is used in cervids where the anesthetist passes their hand into the oral cavity and pharynx and palpates for the glottis, passing a stylet or the tube alongside their arm.

Lagomorph intubation is challenging with large incisors, long, narrow oral cavities, and thick tongues, making laryngeal visualization difficult. Laryngospasm is easily induced. There are a number of tracheal intubation techniques advocated for use in lagomorphs: direct visualization of the larynx with a laryngoscope; blind intubation with the neck in extension; endoscope-guided intubation; and nasotracheal intubation. Placement of the tube is confirmed by visualizing movement of water vapor ("fog") in the tube, coughing, and auscultation of pulmonary breath sounds; attaching a capnograph and visualizing a characteristic capnographic trace is definitive. Lagomorphs are obligate nasal breathers and the patency of both nares must be carefully assessed post extubation, especially if the animal has been in dorsal recumbency. Reported complications include postextubation obstruction, respiratory arrest, and tracheal mucosal injury (Grint et al. 2006; Phaneuf et al. 2006). Nasotracheal intubation can be used if endotracheal intubation cannot be performed, or for complicated oral procedures. Administer anticholinergics with nasal intubation as vagal-mediated bradycardia can be associated with this procedure. The tube is passed through the ventral meatus with the head held in a normal or slightly extended position.

Supraglottic airway devices (SGAD) are relatively new, considered a bridge between the use of an anesthetic mask and tracheal intubation. SGADs have been used in a number of species, including primates, ungulates, swine, cats, and lagomorphs (Bateman et al. 2005; Cassu et al. 2004; Engbers et al. 2017; Smith et al. 2004). SGADs consist of an inflatable cuff that sits over or above the larynx, joined to a stem that attaches to the anesthetic circuit. It is a reusable device and should undergo evaluation for cuff leakage, eccentric cuff inflation, and failure of the inflation valve prior to use. The SGAD is typically advanced along the hard palate, then the soft palate and guided into place until resistance is felt (Figure 5.4).

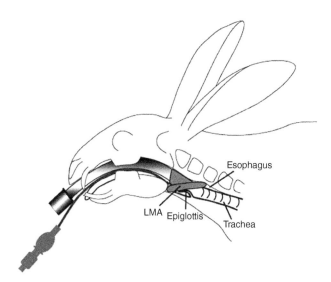

Figure 5.4 Supraglottic airway devices (SGADs) allow an inflatable cuff tube to sit over or above the larynx and are used in species that are difficult to intubate. LMA, laryngeal mask airway. *Source:* Line drawing used with permission from Wiley.

The cuff is then inflated with air. Each has a maximum volume; inflation should be achieved with the lowest optimal volume. Overinflation can increase cuff pressures, reduce the seal, and increase risk of aspiration. Correct placement is confirmed by the mask tip rising 0.5–2 cm on inflation, the neck of the patient seen to slightly fill and the midline of the stem of the tube remains on midline. The SGAD should be refitted if any of these do not occur. With commercial veterinary SGADs, the devices have a shoulder that catches on the palatine arch, confirming correct placement. These lack an inflatable cuff and fit tight locally to affect the seal. SGADs are useful in species that are difficult to intubate, can reduce risk of endotracheal or laryngeal damage, are easy to apply, and are well tolerated by patients, especially during recovery. The primary limitation of the SGAD is the quality of the seal, which is dependent on laryngeal anatomy species variation. SGADs do not guarantee that aspiration will not occur; ventilation is dependent on a tight seal, and gastric insufflation can occur if the seal is not tight or ventilation pressures are high. Complications include failures, displacements, airway obstruction, aspiration, pharyngeal trauma, and nerve injuries from pressure effects.

Squirrels and other rodents have a long, narrow oral cavity, but equipment and techniques for intubating small rodents have been developed (Ordodi et al. 2005; Vergari et al. 2004). Endotracheal tubes of 1–3 mm ID with positive pressure ventilation are often needed. Small rodents may be intubated with IV catheters or IV tubing, but occlusion with mucous plugs occurs frequently. An otoscopic cone, modified pediatric blade, endoscopy, commercially available rodent workstands/ intubation packs and the use of a stylet can help facilitate intubation. Otoscopic cones modified by removing a lateral section can facilitate visualization of the epiglottis and direct placement of the endotracheal tube. Endoscopy provides visualization of the epiglottis and minimizes trauma during tube placement.

Armadillos can hold their breath for long periods of time, so many feel that intubation is necessary. However, their long, narrow snouts make intubation challenging. Utilize lagomorph intubation techniques for armadillos; however, both armadillos and sloths can generally be intubated by visualization with a laryngoscope or endoscope.

Preanesthetic Medications

Parasympatholytics (e.g., atropine, glycopyrrolate) are most commonly used to minimize salivary and bronchial secretions and vagal-induced bradyarrhythmias, but can increase secretion viscosity. For this reason, they are not routinely used in very small patients due to increased risk of endotracheal tube occlusion. Anticholinergics increase heart rate (HR) and because most birds have rapid HRs, it is questionable if increasing the rate and thus the resultant myocardial oxygen demand has adverse effects. Alternatively, glycopyrrolate appears to decrease arrhythmia occurrence, common in birds during induction and recovery with inhalant anesthetics. Preemptive use of parasympatholytics is generally only warranted for surgical procedures with potential to cause vagal effects, such as manipulation of ocular structures, periorbital sinuses, or the GI tract.

Lagomorphs and some rodents have high circulating concentrations of atropine-esterases, reducing efficacy of atropine and prompting use of higher atropine doses, with redosing as often as every 10–15 minutes during bradycardia (Harrison et al. 2006). Large parasympatholytic doses can alter GI motility in hindgut fermenters so the lowest effective doses are recommended (Heard 2014).

Acepromazine has been used extensively in mammals and reported doses vary widely (Heard 2014; Welberg et al. 2006). The peak effect in lagomorphs is often not seen for 30–40 minutes, even when given IV. Vasodilation occurs even at very low doses. Animals that are hypovolemic, anemic, or hypotensive before anesthesia should not receive acepromazine.

Benzodiazepines (e.g., diazepam, midazolam) are increasingly used in all species to provide sedation, hypnosis, anxiolysis, anterograde amnesia, centrally mediated muscle relaxation, and anticonvulsion. Compared with diazepam, midazolam has a faster onset of effect and causes less pain when injected IM. Flumazenil will reverse midazolam, but because its half-life is shorter than midazolam, resedation may occur. Titrate the flumazenil dose to avoid the reversal of the beneficial anxiolysis, sedation, and muscle relaxation. Benzodiazepines coupled with opioid medications provide deeper sedation and preoperative analgesia.

Midazolam in combination with other anesthetic drugs can be administered to birds and some mammals via the intranasal route to provide rapid and effective sedation. The dosage is usually greater than the IM dose and the volume of drug may be challenging for some patients. Reversal agents are also effective when administered via the intranasal route in some species (Mans et al. 2012a; Vesal and Eskandari 2006; Vesal and Zare 2006).

Opioids are administered during the perianesthetic period to provide sedation and preemptive analgesia prior to induction, and are part of balanced anesthesia, reducing minimal anesthetic concentration (MAC) of the inhalant anesthetic. When the anesthetic plan includes the use of a mu opioid agonist constant rate infusion (CRI) then fentanyl, morphine, or hydromorphone is recommended as a premedication.

Other injectable anesthetic agents such as alpha-2 agonists and alfaxolone are used as preanesthetic agents, followed by either other injectable drugs or inhalant anesthetics for induction and maintenance. Combinations of a benzodiazepine, opioid, and an alpha-2 agonist are often used for induction and deep sedation, potentially reducing the dosages of each drug and maximizing the anesthetic effect desired. One disadvantage of using an alpha-2 agonist as a premedication is that it often causes hypotension, making catheter placement more challenging.

Anesthetic Induction and Maintenance

Preoxygenation should be performed routinely, and always when there is potential for hypoxemia. Preoxygenation produces an oxygen reservoir but benefits may take ≥5 minutes in a patient with compromised respiratory function. Preoxygenation is accomplished with an oxygen cage or induction chamber in the unrestrained animal, or a facemask or flow-by nasal insufflation in the physically restrained patient. Ideally, supplemental O_2 should be supplied throughout anesthesia.

Injectable Anesthetics

When working with multiple species, the greatest disadvantage of injectable anesthetics is individual and species variation relative to drug dose and drug response.

Injectable anesthetics are used at low dosages for short procedures where sedation alone is inadequate, or as induction agents and adjuncts to inhalation anesthesia. Most injectable anesthetic agents are associated with pronounced cardiopulmonary depression and prolonged induction and recovery times. Because of this, it is recommended to use balanced anesthetic techniques instead of high dosages of single agents. Additionally, reversible anesthetic agents allow faster recovery. Ultimately, the general dosages published for different protocols are adjusted based on individual factors such as species, gender, age, health status, and others.

Alpha-2 Agonists

Xylazine, medetomidine, and dexmedetomidine are the most commonly used alpha-2 adrenergic receptor agonists in wildlife. Their major advantages are good muscle relaxation and reversal. These drugs are not intended for use as sole agents; combinations with ketamine, opioids, and benzodiazepines are common. Alpha-2 agonists are also being used with local anesthetics in peripheral nerve blocks. Postoperative analgesia should be provided before reversal. These drugs have significant cardio-pulmonary effects including respiratory depression, second-degree heart block, bradyarrhythmias, and increased sensitivity to catecholamine-induced cardiac arrhythmias (xylazine) (Henke et al. 2005), making their use questionable in patients with cardiopulmonary compromise. Supplemental oxygen and assisted ventilation should always be available when using alpha-2 agonists.

Several reversal agents are available for alpha-2 agonists; atipamezole is commonly utilized for detomidine, medetomidine, and dexmedetomidine. Reduce the dose of the reversal agent if the animal is showing signs of recovery, or if anesthestic time has been prolonged. IV administration of atipamezole should be performed very slowly, but IM is generally recommended. Atipamezole (10–20% of calculated dose) may reduce these adverse effects without reversing anesthetic and analgesic effects (P.J. Pascoe, personal communication, 2018). A new peripheral alpha-2 antagonist, MK-467, is being evaluated for coadministration with dexmedetomidine to reduce adverse peripheral effects of the agonist (Honkavaara et al. 2017; Kallio-Kujala et al. 2018).

Reptiles

Medetomidine alone will safely induce sedation in desert tortoises; however, oxygen administration is recommended for procedures longer than two hours (Sleeman and Gaynor 2000). Dexmedetomidine 0.1 mg/kg combined with midazolam 1 mg/kg provided good sedation for physical examination of leopard geckos, and rapid recoveries after both atipamezole and flumazenil antagonists were used (Doss et al. 2017). Dexmedetomidine 0.2 mg/kg IM alone provided antinociception that did not increase when combined with midazolam in Argentine tegu lizards (*Salvator merianae*), but sedation increased when both drugs were combined (Bisetto et al. 2018). A combination of dexmedetomidine 0.2 mg/kg and ketamine 10 mg/kg intranasally induced moderate to heavy sedation for physical examination and minor procedures in yellow-bellied sliders without adverse effects. Anesthesia with ketamine-dexmedetomidine was successful for allowing auditory evoked potential measurements in hatchling leatherback sea turtles (Harms et al. 2014). Respiration in ball pythons (*Python regius*) was reduced 55–70% after IM dexmedetomidine administration, and thermal latencies were increased for approximately two hours post administration (Bunke et al. 2018). Atipamezole IN also appears efficacious for reversal of dexmedetomidine (Schnellbacher et al. 2012). The administration of atipamezole IV was associated with severe hypotension in gopher tortoises, thus IM administration is recommended (Dennis and Heard 2002).

Birds

The use of medetomidine alone or combined with ketamine, ketamine/butorphanol, or a benzodiazepine has been evaluated in pigeons, rock partridges, ducks, and falcons using similar dosages (Atalan et al. 2002; Lumeij and Deenik 2003; Molero et al. 2007; Pollock et al. 2001; Sandmeier 2000; Uzun et al. 2006). Alpha-2 agonists are not recommended for short-term anesthesia in birds because in several studies there was inconsistent immobilization, adverse cardiovascular and respiratory effects, unreliable sedative effects, and excitatory reactions. To date, there are few dexmedetomidine studies alone or in combination with midazolam in raptors and pigeons (Hornak et al. 2015; Santangelo et al. 2009).

Mammals

Xylazine/ketamine given over multiple anesthetic episodes and medetomidine alone or in combination with ketamine and/or diazepam have been associated with myocardial necrosis and fibrosis in lagomorphs (Hurley et al. 1994; Marini et al. 1999). Medetomidine/ketamine allowed rapid intubation, a greater isoflurane-sparing effect, and less esophageal temperature loss than midazolam/ketamine (Grint and Murison 2008) and provided better quality and duration of surgical anesthesia (38.7 ± 30.0 minutes) than medetomidine/midazolam/fentanyl (MMF) (Henke et al. 2005). PaO_2 and pHa were significantly decreased in both groups and apnea occurred post intubation with MMF (Henke et al. 2005).

Sudden recoveries have been encountered with xylazine/ketamine and medetomidine/ketamine in bears, so these combinations are commonly avoided (Caulkett et al. 1999). Induction was smooth and predictable with both medetomidine/tiletamine/zolazepam and dexmedetomidine/tiletamine/zolazepam protocols in free-ranging brown bears (Fandos Esteruelas et al. 2017). Acidemia (pHa < 7.35), hypoxemia (PaO_2 < 80 mmHg), and hypercapnia ($PaCO_2$ > 45 mmHg) were identified with both protocols. African wolves were completely immobilized for physical examination using dexmedetomidine and ketamine, and recoveries were smooth after atipamezole administration (Gutema et al. 2018).

In nine-banded armadillos, xylazine or medetomidine with ketamine provided smooth, rapid induction, good muscle relaxation, and immobilization times of 43.8 ± 27.8 to 66.5 ± 40.0 minutes (Fournier-Chambrillon et al. 2000). Medetomidine combined with butorphanol and ketamine provided good immobilization in Virginia opossums, but did not allow for cardiac puncture for euthanasia (Stoskopf et al. 1999). Dexmedetomidine 25 μg/kg and midazolam 0.2 mg/kg provided adequate sedation for ultrasound examination in pet rabbits, but several individuals required additional doses to lose the righting reflex (Bellini et al. 2014). Dexmedetomidine decreased blood pressure and HR in lagamorphs in a dose-dependent manner, but no effect on myocardial systolic and diastolic function was detected (Ren et al. 2018). Both dexmedetomidine 50 μg/kg with midazolam 0.45 mg/kg and dexmedetomidine 30 μg/kg, midazolam 0.45 mg/kg and butorphanol 0.25 mg/kg provided 30–40 minutes immobilization with excellent muscle relaxation and analgesia adequate for clinical examinations and minor surgical procedures in silver foxes (Diao et al. 2017). The terminal half-life of dexmedetomidine in New Zealand white rabbits after a 20 μg/kg dose was approximately 80 minutes (Bailey et al. 2017). Dexmedetomidine 0.15 mg/kg IM and ketamine 15 mg/kg provided adequate short-term field immobilization with minimal alterations of HR and body temperature and relatively short recovery times in white-eared opossums (*Didelphis albiventris*). The addition of isoflurane to the protocol provided better immobilization but significantly prolonged recovery times (Waxman et al. 2018).

Ketamine

Ketamine is generally well tolerated in stable patients but has sympathomimetic properties that can increase HR, myocardial contractility, and peripheral vascular resistance; therefore, it is not recommend for patients with cardiac or renal disease, or severely stressed patients. Ketamine is a negative inotrope which can cause highly stressed patients to become hypotensive following injection because their sympathetic output is maximized, thus "unmasking" the negative inotropic effect. Renal impairment can markedly prolong recovery. It can be administered subcutaneously (SC), IM, or IV. It increases salivary secretions that can obstruct the airway. It is rarely used alone as it is associated with poor muscle relaxation, muscle tremors, myotonic contractions, opisthotonus, and rough recoveries. Therefore, combination with alpha-2 agonists or benzodiazepines improves relaxation and anesthetic depth (Grint and Murison 2008; Henke et al. 2004, 2005; Ko et al. 1997; Orr et al. 2005; Schernthaner et al. 2008; Welberg et al. 2006). Alpha-2 agonist/ketamine combinations, particularly at higher dosages, produce mild-to-severe dose-dependent hypotension and bradyarrhythmias; ketamine/benzodiazepine combinations produce less cardiopulmonary depression and analgesia with good muscle relaxation (Grint and Murison 2008). Opioids added to ketamine combinations further reduce the dose and each drug's adverse effects. Ketamine may prolong recovery times and reversal of other drugs in ketamine combinations allows its undesirable effects to become apparent.

Reptiles

Medetomidine/ketamine SC or IM can induce general anesthesia in red-eared sliders (Greer et al. 2001; Lahner et al. 2011). A higher dosage combination produced an anesthetic level sufficient for performing a skin incision and suture placement (Greer et al. 2001). Medetomidine/ketamine was also used at high doses for long-term anesthesia necessary for invasive surgical procedures in tegu; anesthesia was maintained up to 16 hours with repeated dosing (Barrillot et al. 2018). Lower dosages resulted in effective short-term immobilization adequate for minor diagnostic procedures in gopher tortoises (Dennis and Heard 2002). Ketamine-diazepam combinations were found to be the most effective of several drug combinations for anesthesia in Caspian pond turtles (*Mauremys caspic*) (Adel et al. 2017).

Birds

Medetomidine/ketamine or xylazine/ketamine combinations have been evaluated in several avian species and often provide a suboptimal plane of anesthesia for painful procedures. Ketamine dosages tend to be higher for smaller birds. When effective, anesthesia occurs within 5–10 minutes of IM injection and may last 5–20 minutes depending on the dose and size of the bird (Atalan et al. 2002; Kamiloglu et al. 2008; Machin and Caulkett 1998; Varner et al. 2004). Ketamine has also been reported to cause salivation, excitation, and convulsions when given to vultures, but these signs are rare in other avian species.

Mammals

Ketamine is one of the most common injectable anesthetic agents used in wild mammals. It can be compounded to 200 mg/mL for use in larger mammals. In small rodents and lagomorphs, hindlimb IM injections have been associated with muscle necrosis and severe sciatic neuritis with self-mutilation. Ketamine has a very short duration of clinical effect in lagomorphs, partly due to redistribution and renal elimination (Avsaroglu et al. 2003). Medetomidine-ketamine was effective shortly after intranasal delivery in lagomorphs, although some rabbits required additional dosing for intubation (Weiland et al. 2017).

Tiletamine-Zolazepam (Telazol®, Zoletil®)

Tiletamine-zolazepam (TZ) produces reliable anesthesia with predictable signs of recovery and is routinely used alone or in combination with ketamine and/or xylazine in Virginia opossums, otters, deer, and skunks. Bears anesthetized with TZ alone with significant head movement generally require a "top-up" of TZ or ketamine for longer procedures, but it will prolong recovery and should only be used if >30 minutes of additional anesthetic time is required (Caulkett and Fahlman 2014). With both xylazine/tiletamine/zolazepam (XTZ) or with medetomidine (MTZ) combinations, head lifting or paw movements should be absent before the bear is approached. Lightly anesthetized bears will begin to breathe deeply, and may sigh. Bears anesthetized with MZT developed hypoxemia, despite lower drug doses used in the captive bears (Fahlman et al. 2011). Telazol/xylazine combinations are used in some rodents as smaller volumes of drug are needed, decreasing potential for muscle and nerve damage if given IM. In rats, duration of telazol anesthesia was dose dependent (59–124 minutes), with minimal cardiorespiratory effects at the higher dosages (Saha et al. 2007). Telazol causes dose-dependent nephrotoxicity in New Zealand white lagomorphs related to the tiletamine (Doerning et al. 1992).

Reptiles

In green iguanas and some chelonian species, telazol 10 mg/kg IM results in good surgical anesthesia for minor procedures, but with some prolonged recoveries of ≥45 minutes. In general, dosages >6 mg/kg IM can cause prolonged recoveries.

Propofol

Propofol has rapid induction and recovery times, few excitatory side effects, and minimal accumulation. Regardless of species, assisted ventilation and oxygen support are strongly encouraged when using this drug. The need for IV access and ventilatory support limits the use of propofol in very small animals. The authors suggest a calculated propofol induction dose given in ¼ increments, each administered over 30–60 seconds, to allow more accurate dosing and minimize apnea and hypotension during induction.

Reptiles

Propofol has been commonly used in wild reptiles, including chelonians (MacLean et al. 2008; Ziolo and Bertelsen 2009) and snakes (Bertelsen et al. 2015; Quesada et al. 2014), with associated apnea and cardiorespiratory depression. Propofol administration in the supravertebral venous sinus was originally considered safe and reliable in red-eared sliders (Ziolo and Bertelsen 2009); however, there have been reports of central nervous system (CNS) complications associated with intrathecal (Quesada et al. 2010) and supravertebral (Innis et al. 2010) administration in chelonians. Current recommendations are to use the jugular or brachial veins in chelonians.

Birds

Propofol has a narrow safety margin in pigeons and chickens (Lukasik et al. 1997; Mehmannavaz et al. 2015); however, low dosages were effective and safe in turkeys and mallard ducks (Machin and Caulkett 1998, 2000; Schumacher et al. 1997). Cardiopulmonary complications of propofol may have contributed to bar-tailed godwit mortality in a field study (Mulcahy et al. 2011). In mute swans, propofol CRI was comparable with multiple boluses for short procedures, but about 50% of the birds from both groups demonstrated short periods of excitement during recovery (Muller et al. 2011). Prolonged recovery, with or without moderate-to-severe CNS excitatory signs, has been reported after use of a CRI in red-tailed hawks and great horned owls (Hawkins et al. 2003).

Mammals

Propofol is commonly used in canids and felids. Propofol as the sole anesthetic demonstrated a narrow therapeutic window in early studies with lagomorphs, but balanced anesthesia provides propofol-sparing effects, reducing its respiratory system disadvantages (Baumgartner et al. 2011; Cruz et al. 2010; Martin-Cancho et al. 2006). Intraosseous (IO) administration of propofol was effective in lagomorphs, suggesting that total IO anesthesia may be performed in lagomorphs with limited vascular access (Mazaheri-Khameneh et al. 2012).

Alfaxalone

Alfaxalone, a schedule IV neuroactive steroid, can be administered IV or IM, which is a major advantage compared to propofol. However, it is costly and large volumes are often needed.

Reptiles

Intravenous use of alfaxalone is a suitable method of induction for inhalation anesthesia in terrapins and tortoises (Knotek 2014). Two dosages of alfaxalone in red-eared sliders provided only 5–10 minutes of light sedation at 35 °C (95 °F), but provided sedation suitable for short noninvasive procedures at lower temperatures (20 °C, 68 °F) (Kischinovsky et al. 2013). Likewise, turtles were more relaxed and easier to handle in cold than warm conditions, whereas warm turtles were more relaxed and easier to handle when administered higher dosages. Cold conditions correlated with lower HR and longer recovery times for each dose category (Shepard et al. 2013). In Horsfield's tortoises (*Agrionemys horsfieldii*), alfaxalone was useful for sedation for nonpainful procedures when combined with medetomidine, provided deeper sedation/

anesthesia; however, some animals developed severe respiratory and cardiovascular depression (Hansen and Bertelsen 2013). Rapid anesthetic induction with a dose-dependent duration of sedation was documented in healthy, yearling loggerhead sea turtles (Phillips et al. 2017).

Alfaxalone 15 mg/kg and midazolam 1 mg/kg SC provided good sedation for physical examination and venipuncture in leopard geckos, but recoveries were prolonged even after flumazenil administration (Doss et al. 2017). In small crocodiles, alfaxalone (3 mg/kg IV) provided adequate induction at temperatures ranging from 17 to 32 °C (62.6–89.6 °F) (Olsson et al. 2013). However, unpredictable results occurred, such as animals recovering without warning and extended recoveries requiring assisted ventilation. Thus, its use in these species should include access to intubation, ventilation, and close monitoring (Olsson et al. 2013). Rapid, smooth anesthetic induction was seen in ball pythons; administration into the cranial third of the body resulted in deeper and longer sedation compared with the caudal third of the body (James et al. 2018; Yaw et al. 2018). Immersion anesthesia with alfaxalone did not provide adequate anesthesia for painful procedures in oriental fire-bellied toads (Adami et al. 2015). Addition of dexmedetomidine provided some antinociception, but failed to potentiate the level of unconsciousness and appeared to lighten the depth of anesthesia (Adami et al. 2016a). A combination of morphine/alfaxalone provided better antinociception than butorphanol/alfaxalone (Adami et al. 2016b).

Birds

To date there is one clinical study using the newly formulated alfaxalone in birds (Villaverde-Morcillo et al. 2014). In flamingos, sedation was rapid and induction quality was smooth, lowering isoflurane concentrations needed for maintenance anesthesia. Alfaxalone produced moderate cardiorespiratory effects not seen in the isoflurane induction group.

Mammals

Alfaxalone has been studied in numerous domestic mammalian species (del Alamo et al. 2015; Santos Gonzalez et al. 2013; Tamura et al. 2015a; Warne et al. 2015) but there is limited literature for wild mammals. Alfaxalone produced dose-dependent, clinically relevant sedation in cats and dogs with relatively mild cardiorespiratory depression in dogs (Tamura et al. 2015a,b). Alfaxalone 10 mg/kg/h used for total intravenous anesthesia (TIVA) in cats provided suitable anesthesia after premedication with no need for ventilatory support. Several studies have been published regarding its use as an induction drug in lagomorphs (Huynh et al. 2015;

Navarrete-Calvo et al. 2014; Tutunaru et al. 2013). Morphine combined with medetomidine and alfaxalone in rabbits produced a suitable level of anesthesia but profound cardiorespiratory depression occurred even in the face of ventilation, so close monitoring is recommended if using this combination (Navarrete-Calvo et al. 2014). Male rats administered alfaxalone intraperitoneally required three times the dose of female rats for the same level of anesthesia; analgesia was enhanced with the addition of dexmedetomidine and fentanyl (Arenillas and Gomez de Segura 2018). Additional work is necessary with this anesthetic to determine efficacy and safety for most species.

Constant Rate Infusions

Intravenous CRIs of anesthetic and analgesic drugs are being evaluated in balanced anesthesia/analgesia protocols and for TIVA (Criado and Gomez de Segura 2003; Hawkins et al. 2003; Mustola et al. 2000; Pavez et al. 2011). Medications administered as CRIs can be titrated to effect. Plasma drug concentrations increase slowly when used as a CRI, so a loading dose of the drug is commonly given prior to CRI initiation. Disadvantages are the need for patient IV access and a syringe pump to accurately deliver low dosages.

In lagomorphs, IO use of a propofol CRI was just as effective as IV, so this route may be effective when vascular access is challenging (Mazaheri-Khameneh et al. 2012). Anesthesia has been maintained with doses of 0.4–0.6 mg/kg/min propofol, but deaths have been reported in lagomorphs following propofol infusions (Kemmochi et al. 2009; Rozanska 2009).

Micro-dose ketamine via CRI can also be an effective analgesic. Ketamine administered at 40 µg/kg/min significantly reduced isoflurane MAC in lagomorphs (Gianotti et al. 2012). Opioid medications can also be used for CRI and because mu receptor agonists can cause respiratory depression, opioids should be used only when a secure airway and ventilation are available (Criado and Gomez de Segura 2003). Opioids have also historically been avoided in small hindgut fermenters for fear of inducing GI stasis, but when used as low-dose IV CRIs, these effects are reduced (Criado and Gomez de Segura 2003). Fentanyl citrate, a mu opioid receptor agonist, is used as a CRI in some birds and mammals (Barter et al. 2015; Criado and Gomez de Segura 2003; Pavez et al. 2011). Administration of fentanyl in isoflurane-anesthetized lagomorphs resulted in improved mean arterial blood pressure and cardiac output, compared with isoflurane alone (Tearney et al. 2015). Anecdotally, butorphanol CRI has been used successfully in the clinical setting for birds.

Inhalant Anesthesia

Inhalant anesthetics offer rapid induction and recovery and the ability to rapidly change anesthetic depth, and their use does not require an accurate body weight. Very little is metabolized, reducing hepatic and renal impact, and recovery is independent of either. But inhalant anesthetics can induce life-threatening cardiovascular and respiratory depression. Inhalants are potent negative inotropes so a dose-related decrease in cardiac output is expected, reflected as a decrease in blood pressure. Thus, the primary goal is to maintain the lightest plane of anesthesia possible allowing for minimal cardiopulmonary depression and completion of the procedure. In some cases, these goals may not be achieved by simply reducing the inhalant; balanced anesthetic/analgesic protocols or the addition of dopamine or dobutamine (only in the volume-loaded patient) may be necessary to offset inhalant-induced hypotension.

Isoflurane, sevoflurane, and desflurane are the currently available inhalants. Their speed of onset and offset is largely determined by their solubility which is isoflurane > sevoflurane > desflurane. Despite these physiochemical differences, the clinical differences overall may be fairly small. All three agents have similar dose-dependent cardiovascular effects. Sevoflurane has a less pungent odor than other inhalants and is generally more tolerated during mask induction. Many practitioners induce using sevoflurane then maintain anesthesia with the more cost-effective isoflurane.

Ventilators appropriate for use in wildlife must cope with the range of tidal volumes in the different species. For some commonly rehabilitated wildlife (e.g., reptiles, birds), ventilators are required if they are to be anesthetized for more than a few minutes. The average tidal volume for many species is 10–15 mL/kg. In very small patients this may be <1 mL but some patients might require several liters. In general, the three things that need to be controlled by a ventilator are tidal volume, rate at which the tidal volume is delivered, and the number of breaths per minute. The way in which each of these is controlled varies from ventilator to ventilator (Hawkins et al. 2014). Commercially available pressure-driven portable ventilators (e.g., Vetronics ventilator, BASi, West Lafayette, IN) used in exotic animal patients are easy to use and reasonably priced (Figure 5.5).

Mask or Chamber Induction

Commercially available masks can be used for induction of anesthesia. A properly sized mask allows the entire head or nostrils to be inserted while minimizing dead space. Masks can be modified to accommodate the widely diverse anatomical variations of species. A proper seal

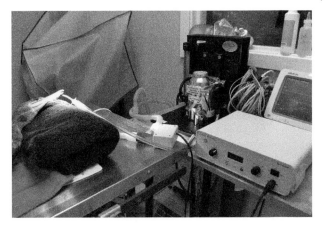

Figure 5.5 Commercially available pressure-driven ventilators are portable, easy to use, and relatively inexpensive. *Source:* Heather Barron/CROW

with a diaphragm or exam glove cut to fit over the end of the mask will create a tight seal. In some mammals, a piece of suture can be placed around the upper incisors and through the breathing circuit for mask security (Figure 5.6).

For animals with long beaks/snouts, a 6–60 mL syringe case or a 1–2 L soft drink bottle can be cut down and used. A custom mask can be made by stretching a latex glove taut over the opening of a plastic syringe case and securing it with tape. A hole is then bored in the narrow end of the case to accommodate an endotracheal adaptor. A slit cut in the latex allows the bird's beak to fit snugly without significant leakage of anesthesia gases.

Depending upon the size of the patient, rebreathing and nonrebreathing circuits are used. The nonrebreathing system uses high gas flow rates to remove CO_2 and provides rapid changes in inhalant concentration with vaporizer setting changes. These circuits have decreased resistance to patient breathing, critical for small patients. Rebreathing systems generally are heavier and bulkier, predisposing to accidental extubation and difficulty working around the head region. These circuits also have a greater resistance to breathing, and are used most commonly for larger patients. Flow rates used for a T-piece or Norman elbow should be 2–3 times the minute ventilation but in the Bain circuit, a flow rate of 150–200 mL/kg/min appears effective.

Induction chambers of various sizes, whether commercially available or home-made, can be useful for very stressed patients that may resist facemask induction (Figure 5.7).

Advantages of appropriately sized chambers are reduced waste gas and shorter induction times. In stressed patients, the chamber can be covered with a towel. Alternatively, for induction of large, intractable, or stressed patients, the front of an animal carrier or hospital cage is sealed with a plastic bag and inhalant anesthetic administered. Disadvantages of induction

(a)

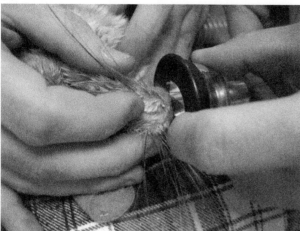

(b)

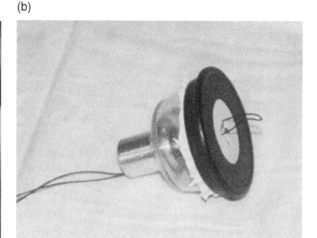

Figure 5.6 (a) An examination glove with a slit in the center can be fitted between the mask and diaphragm to make a seal when the head is positioned inside the mask. (b) In order to keep the head from falling out of the mask during surgery or manipulation, a piece of suture is doubled over and the loop threaded through the slit in the seal, placed around the upper incisors of the patient, and secured by attaching the circuit to the mask.

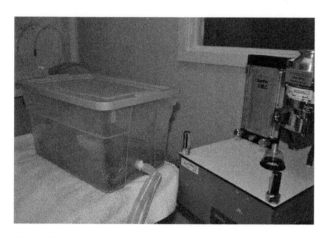

Figure 5.7 Plastic storage bins can easily be converted into inexpensive induction chambers for wildlife patients. *Source:* Courtesy of CROW.

chambers include the inability to assess the patient, gas pollution when opened, and trauma during the excitement phase of anesthesia. Pad the chamber and minimize chamber size to reduce movement and trauma. The patient is promptly removed after the righting reflex is lost. The final phase of induction is accomplished using a mask to facilitate monitoring.

Local and Regional Anesthesia

Local anesthetics block ion channels to prevent pain impulse generation and conduction, and current applications include topical application, tissue infiltration, regional nerve block, intraarticular, or epidural injection. Eutectic Mixture of Local Anesthetic (EMLA) is an emulsion mixture of 25 mg lidocaine and 25 mg prilocaine per gram, used topically to desensitize skin for catheter placement and superficial biopsies and, in combination with heavy sedation, has been used for minor surgical procedures (Keating et al. 2012). Depth of penetration varies by species and skin contact time. Optimal contact time requires application and bandage occlusion for 30–60 minutes in mammals; no data are available on avian or reptile penetration times. Toxicity is associated with improper application to large surface areas, prolonged contact time, and application to damaged skin.

Local line or splash blocks are the most common methods of regional infiltration. To provide appropriate dosages for small patients, dilution of lidocaine with saline may decrease effect so that less concentrated commercial solutions are recommended (e.g., 1% lidocaine or 0.25% bupivacaine).

Reptiles

EMLA was reported to be effective for adjunctive use in chelonians for penile amputation (Spadola et al. 2015). Regional anesthesia for mandibular nerve blocks has been evaluated in crocodilians (Wellehan et al. 2006). Intrathecal administration of lidocaine (4 mg/kg) or bupivacaine (1 mg/kg) in red-eared sliders resulted in motor block of the hindlimbs for approximately one and two hours, respectively (Mans 2014).

Birds

Concerns about avian sensitivity to local anesthetics have been attributed to rapid absorption and delayed metabolism. In birds, toxic effects have been reported to occur at lidocaine doses of 2.7–3.3 mg/kg (Hocking et al. 1997). In contrast, chickens survive higher doses of lidocaine compared to mammals, with the convulsive dose of lidocaine at 30.51 ± 5.15 mg/kg (Imani et al. 2013). High doses of lidocaine, bupivacaine, and ropivacaine were studied for brachial plexus block in chickens and ducks, and adverse effects were not reported (Brenner et al. 2010; Cardozo et al. 2009; de Castro Vilan et al. 2006; Figueiredo et al. 2008). Brachial plexus blocks using palpation, ultrasound, or nerve locator have been used with variable degrees of success in avian species (Brenner et al. 2010; Cardozo et al. 2009; de Castro Vilan et al. 2006; Figueiredo et al. 2008). The safe use of transdermal patches, epidural infusions and spinal blocks has not yet been reported in birds.

Mammals

Topical, intravascular, regional, and intraarticular application is similar for mammalian wildlife and domestic mammals. Recently, a CRI of lidocaine provided better postoperative outcomes with respect to fecal output and food intake in lagomorphs than did buprenorphine (Schnellbacher et al. 2017). Nerve blocks have been successfully used in a number of species (Johnston 2015) but anatomy may differ among species and individuals. Epidural analgesia has been described in rodents, lagomorphs, and mustelids, with the lumbosacral space preferred (Dehkordi et al. 2012; Eshar and Wilson 2010; Johnston 2015). In lagomorphs, and potentially other wildlife mammals, injection into the lumbosacral space may result in subdural injections because the dural sac extends into the sacrum. There appears to be synergism in the epidural space between local analgesics and opioids; drug combinations reduce doses and minimize potential adverse effects of each drug. In general, the total epidural administration volume for all drugs combined should be ≤0.33 mL/kg.

Anesthetic Monitoring and Supportive Care

Effective monitoring requires minute-to-minute patient assessment. The eyes should be well lubricated often to prevent corneal dessication and ulceration. Covering the eyes with damp gauze sponges helps maintain moisture provided by the eye lubrication. Slight corneal and palpebral reflexes are commonly maintained at a surgical plane of anesthesia; absence of these reflexes indicates an excessively deep plane of anesthesia. Withdrawal reflexes include toe pinch, stimulation of the interdigital tissue, tail pinch, and rectal pinch. The toe pinch does not always reliably measure anesthetic depth as involuntary leg movements sometimes occur under anesthesia.

Knowledge of expected HRs for each species is important, but absolute trends in HR during anesthesia are of utmost importance. Decrease the anesthetic concentration with any sudden HR reductions and provide supportive care. Rapid HRs of many wildlife patients can make electrocardiogram (ECG) complexes difficult to assess at standard sweep speeds of 25 mm/s. Needle ECG leads are ideal for small patients to provide excellent conduction without the use of gels. Alternatively, metal alligator clips attached to a hypodermic needle or to a saline-soaked cotton ball or adhesive pads can be used. Peripheral pulse quality is subjectively assessed by changes in pulse loudness using a Doppler probe placed over an artery. This is quite insensitive, but a change in Doppler loudness should alert to reevaluate the patient.

Noninvasive blood pressure monitoring is performed using a Doppler probe, a pressure cuff, and a sphygmomanometer. Oscillometric devices are unreliable in birds and small hypotensive/hypothermic patients with rapid HRs (Zehnder et al. 2009). The size of the blood pressure cuff should be approximately 40% of the limb circumference placed above the Doppler probe. Perfusion is assessed by evaluating the color and capillary refill time of the oral, rectal, or vaginal mucous membranes, femoral pulse quality, HR, blood pressure and venous refill times at the median ulnar vein in birds. Fluid types, uses, and volume calculations are provided in species-specific chapters and Chapter 4.

Respiratory rate and character should be monitored closely, and assisted ventilation provided as needed. Ventilation is monitored by watching the frequency and degree of movement of the thorax/coelom, the movement of the reservoir bag on the anesthesia machine and the endtidal carbon dioxide ($PETCO_2$) via capnography. Respiratory monitors triggered by a thermistor in the airway function well in patients >500 g, but may not respond to small respiratory movements and lower tidal volumes of animals <200 g. Small reservoir bags, such as balloons, can be used to visualize small movements. High respiratory rates are associated with small tidal volumes resulting in more dead space ventilation than pulmonary ventilation. All anesthetics can cause dose-dependent respiratory depression and increased resistance to breathing imposed by the endotracheal tube, providing compelling reasons to ventilate patients. Thoracic/coelomic excursions are assessed and the tidal volume is adjusted to achieve appropriate expansion. Mechanical ventilation can have both positive and negative impacts on blood pressure and blood gases, depending on the frequency and ventilatory pressure used (Bertelsen et al. 2015). If a mechanical ventilator is not available, hand ventilation delivered from the reservoir bag provides assisted ventilation.

Pulse oximetry (SpO_2) is used in many species to evaluate arterial hemoglobin oxygen saturation, but high

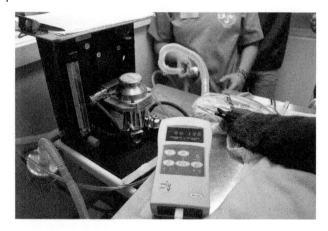

Figure 5.8 A pulse oximeter on the tongue of a North American river otter provides a means of monitoring heart rate (HR) and SpO_2. *Source:* Courtesy of CROW.

normal HRs in many species exceed the upper limits of standard monitors (Figure 5.8). Pulse oximetry has not been validated in birds or reptiles but is commonly used to monitor trends.

Monitoring core body temperature and providing thermal support are mandatory to reduce potential anesthetic-associated morbidity and mortality. Most anesthetics depress thermoregulatory function, and this is exacerbated in small patients prone to heat loss because of high body surface-to-volume ratios. Hypothermia depresses metabolism, cardiopulmonary function, and arrhythmias and disturbances of coagulation occur with deep hypothermia in mammals. Hypothermia decreases anesthetic requirement and prolongs recoveries. Supplemental heat sources should be used regardless of procedure length. Core body temperature is most accurately monitored with an esophageal temperature probe, but rectal/cloacal temperatures can also be used.

Effective techniques to prevent heat loss include minimizing the temperature gradient between the patient and the room by increasing room temperature, insulating the patient with clear plastic drapes, bubble wrap or foil, and wrapping nonsurgical fields. Minimize alcohol/water use for skin preparation, clipping time, surgical time and the time body cavities are open. Latex gloves, empty fluid bags, or plastic bottles can be filled with water, warmed in a hot water bath, wrapped in a towel to prevent burns, and placed next to the patient. Circulating warm water blankets insignificantly diminish the rate of heat loss in small patients. Radiant heat lamps are effective at maintaining core body temperature, but the optimal distance between the heat source and the patient differs with patient size, heat lamp strength and setting. Forced air warmers are more effective at minimizing hypothermia than other methods, and are particularly effective when warm air rises around the patient either

by wrapping the patient in the blanket or by using a perforated table. Lubricate the eyes well to prevent corneal ulceration due to drying from the warm air. Warm replacement fluids prior to administration. Heated, humidified anesthetic gases also help to reduce or prevent development of hypothermia.

One of the most important ways to reduce the potential for complications during anesthesia and recovery is to minimize anesthetic time. Postprocedure recovery should have the patient connected to the circuit or on a facemask with 100% O_2 for as long as possible in a quiet area; however, lower percentages of oxygen are necessary to reduce recovery time in reptiles. Wet animals are gently dried with a loose towel or with warm air. Respiratory depression can continue into the postanesthetic period, so supplemental oxygen should be continued. Use thermal support in the recovery areas, using caution because many animals are susceptible to heat stress. Food and water are provided at a time after recovery appropriate for the species. If IV fluids were not provided during surgery, warm SC fluids should be administered perioperatively.

Analgesic Drugs

Opioid Drugs

Butorphanol
Reptiles
Butorphanol had no analgesic efficacy when evaluated in several species (Fleming and Robertson 2012; Leal et al. 2017; Mosley et al. 2003; Olesen et al. 2008; Sladky et al. 2007, 2008). In red-eared sliders (*Trachemys scripta elegans*), butorphanol did not alter feeding, movement or breathing following unilateral gonadectomy (Kinney et al. 2011). Only in a few studies has butorphanol had any significant effect at increasing tolerance to noxious stimulus (Greenacre et al. 2005, 2006; Sladky et al. 2008). However, with increased availability of suitable alternatives, butorphanol is now rarely used.

Birds
Butorphanol has been considered the drug of choice for pain management in psittacine birds, using dosages of 1–3 mg/kg IM or IV. A major disadvantage is the short (2–3 h) period of effect and the poor oral bioavailability (Guzman et al. 2011; Paul-Murphy et al. 1999). Preoperative butorphanol administration will decrease the inhalation anesthetic concentration needed for general anesthesia with minimal cardiopulmonary changes (Curro et al. 1994; Klaphake et al. 2006). In contrast, 1–6 mg/kg butorphanol did not provide analgesia or sedation for American kestrels; hyperesthesia or hyperalgesia and agitation was seen in males receiving 6 mg/kg (Guzman et al. 2014b).

Mammals

In lagomorphs administered 0.4 mg/kg butorphanol SC, ketamine/medetomidine anesthesia was prolonged, but only minor anesthetic-sparing effects were seen (Hedenqvist et al. 2002) whereas butorphanol 0.4 mg/kg IV significantly reduced the MAC of isoflurane (Turner et al. 2006b). Intranasal butorphanol with dexmedetomidine and midazolam provided 45 minutes of deep sedation and analgesia appropriate for minor procedures in lagomorphs; full recovery was achieved by 90 minutes without any reversal agents (Santangelo et al. 2016). A butorphanol/azaperone/medetomidine combination administered IM provided very good sedation in American black bears, and recovery was quick after reversal with atipamezole and naloxone (Williamson et al. 2018). Adding butorphanol and medetomidine lowered the ketamine dosage necessary for immobilization of bobcats (Rockhill et al. 2011). Butorphanol has also been used as a CRI in the clinical setting, although to date there are no published studies evaluating this in wild mammals.

Buprenorphine

Buprenorphine is a partial mu opioid agonist, while its action on the kappa receptor is less clear.

Reptiles

Buprenorphine had no analgesic efficacy when evaluated using a thermal stimulus in red-eared slider turtles receiving dosages of 0.1, 0.2, and 1 mg/kg SC (Mans et al. 2012b). Similarly, buprenorphine did not alter the response to electrical stimulus in green iguanas administered 0.02 and 0.1 mg/kg IM (Greenacre et al. 2006). Pharmacokinetic studies in red-eared sliders have shown that 0.05 mg/kg SC reaches plasma concentrations similar to those associated with analgesia in humans, thus showing that much higher doses may be necessary to achieve an analgesic effect in this species (Kummrow et al. 2008).

Birds

Buprenorphine (0.1 mg/kg IM) in African gray parrots did not increase withdrawal thresholds to an electrical stimulus, but pharmacokinetic analysis showed that this dose did achieve plasma concentrations considered effective in humans (Paul-Murphy et al. 1999, 2004). In contrast, in American kestrels buprenorphine provided an antinociceptive response at 0.1, 0.3, and 0.6 mg/kg for up to and over six hours, with a mild sedative effect at the higher dosage (Ceulemans et al. 2014). Both concentrated and compounded sustained-release formulations of buprenorphine have been evaluated in raptors (Gleeson et al. 2018; Guzman et al. 2017). It is important to differentiate between these two products as the compounded formulation utilizes a vehicle for sustained release, whereas the concentrated product is a formulation allowing a daily dose to be provided as a single injection. Dosing of the two products may be dramatically different, and published data should not be extrapolated between formulations.

Mammals

Buprenorphine is a preferred opioid in smaller mammals for analgesia because of its longer duration of effect. Analgesic effects at the same dose can be variable among different strains of rodents. GI effects are the most commonly reported adverse effects with buprenorphine. Disparate findings evaluating changes in GI motility in lagomorphs after buprenorphine administration were recently published (Deflers et al. 2018; Martin-Flores et al. 2017). "Pica behavior" may occur when some rodents are housed on certain types of bedding, especially sawdust or wood chips. Buprenorphine is considered safe and effective when administered at 0.01–0.05 mg/kg parenterally, but higher doses are sometimes necessary in smaller mammals. For example, 0.5 mg/kg provided 6–8 hours of analgesia in rats while 2 mg/kg provided 3–5 hours of analgesia in mice (Gades et al. 2000). Buprenorphine administered *per os* (PO) in gelatin to rats was effective only at 8–10 times the parenteral dose (Flecknell 2001). Epidural administration in rats shows consistent, mild to moderate antinociception for at least two hours (Morimoto et al. 2001). Buprenorphine administered as a preanesthetic may not provide timely analgesia for surgical procedures and may prolong recoveries, and so it is most commonly administered postoperatively.

Recently, a compounded, sustained-release formulation of buprenorphine (Bup-SR) and Simbadol™, a commercially available novel combination of dose and concentration for daily dosing in domestic cats, has become available. It is important to differentiate between these two as the compounded formulation utilizes a vehicle for sustained release, whereas Simbadol™ is primarily a formulation that allows a once-daily dose to be provided as a single injection. Therefore, dosing of the two products can be dramatically different and published data should not be extrapolated between formulations. Rats injected with 1.2 mg/kg SC of compounded Bup-SR showed evidence of analgesia for 48 (Healy et al. 2014) to 72 hours (Chum et al. 2014) and plasma concentrations remained over 1 ng/mL for 72 hours after the single dose (Foley et al. 2011). The same dose was only effective for 12 hours in mice (Carbone et al. 2012) but at 2.2 mg/kg achieved 24–48 hours analgesia (Jirkof et al. 2015). Using the same Bup-SR formulation, preoperative administration of 0.12 mg/kg SC in cats or 0.2 mg/kg SC in dogs undergoing ovariohysterectomy appeared to have comparable efficacy and adverse effect profiles to daily administration of buprenorphine HCl (Catbagan et al. 2011;

Nunamaker et al. 2014). Significant injection site abscesses occurred in northern elephant seals with one compounded formulation, and adequate plasma concentrations were not achieved (Molter et al. 2015). Early studies show promising results for the use of a sustained formulation in some wildlife patients, but additional research is needed and extrapolation should be used with caution.

Mu Opioid Agonist Drugs

Morphine, Methadone, Hydromorphone, and Oxymorphone

These mu opioid agonist drugs have similar durations of action.

Reptiles

Morphine had analgesic efficacy when evaluated using a thermal stimulus in red-eared sliders administered 1.5–6.5 mg/kg SC (Sladky et al. 2007), in bearded dragons administered 1–5 mg/kg SC (Sladky et al. 2008), in tegu administered 5 and 10 mg/kg IM (Leal et al. 2017) and in crocodiles (Kanui and Hole 1992). In red-eared sliders, morphine was associated with severe (up to 80%) respiratory depression. Consistent with the previous studies, morphine administered at 1 mg/kg IM to green iguanas (Greenacre et al. 2006) and to bearded dragons (Greenacre et al. 2005) had an analgesic effect when evaluated using an electrical stimulus. Similarly, morphine administered at 5, 7.5, and 20 mg/kg intracoelomically decreased the duration of limb retraction in the formalin test in Speke's hinged tortoise (Wambugu et al. 2010). Ventilatory change data from a study evaluating high morphine dosages in dwarf caimans (*Paleosuchus palpebrosus*) suggested that while these changes would not cause clinical concern during the postoperative period in healthy animals, it was unclear whether they would pose concerns for sick and/or injured caimans (Malte et al. 2018). Hydromorphone had analgesic efficacy when evaluated using a thermal stimulus in red-eared slider turtles receiving dosages of 0.5 mg/kg SC (Mans et al. 2012b).

Birds

Morphine has not been commonly used in avian species because early studies with chickens had conflicting results and it has been shown to have a rapid clearance rate (Singh et al. 2010). Studies in chickens found that increasing doses of morphine at 0.1, 1, and 3 mg/kg lowered isoflurane MAC (Concannon et al. 1995). Hydromorphone administered 0.1–0.6 mg/kg IM to American kestrels has a dose-responsive thermal antinociception effect, suggesting antinociception in this species for up to six hours (Guzman et al. 2013). At the higher dosage, some birds were sedated and when handled they appeared mildly agitated. Methadone at 6 mg/kg IV reduced the MAC of isoflurane by 10–30% in domestic hens (Escobar et al. 2016).

Mammals

Morphine reduced isoflurane MAC by 30% and 50% when administered IM to rats at 3 and 10 mg/kg, respectively (Criado et al. 2000). Both hydromorphone and oxymorphone 0.1–0.3 mg/kg IM have been used by the authors in lagomorphs as primary analgesics for treatment of moderate to severe pain, but they are also useful for preemptive analgesia and postoperative pain. In mustelids, mu agonists can cause profound sedation (Johnston 2005). For many other wild mammals, 0.1–0.3 mg/kg also appears to be effective.

Fentanyl citrate
Reptiles

The application of 12.5 μg/h transdermal fentanyl patches resulted in high plasma concentrations in ball pythons for up to 48 hours, but no response to a thermal stimulus was identified even when achieving these high concentrations (Kharbush et al. 2017). The application of fentanyl patches (10% exposure of total surface area of a 25 μg/h patch for 72 hours) resulted in plasma concentration of 1–4 ng/μL for 72 hours in prehensile-tailed skinks (Gamble 2008), but pharmacodynamic studies have not been published.

Birds

Fentanyl 0.02 mg/kg IM did not affect electrical or thermal nociception of white cockatoos; however, a 10-fold increase in the dosage (0.2 mg/kg SC) produced an analgesic response, but many birds were hyperactive for the first 15–30 minutes after receiving the high dose (Hoppes et al. 2003). In red-tailed hawks, fentanyl as a CRI produces a dose-related decrease of isoflurane MAC with minimal cardiovascular effects (Pavez et al. 2011). Significant differences in the pharmacokinetics of fentanyl were identified between red-tailed hawks and Hispaniolan Amazon parrots; these data strongly discourage dosage extrapolation between species (Pascoe et al. 2018). Transdermal application of a long-acting fentanyl solution in helmeted guineafowl produced plasma concentrations above those analgesic in the dog for five days (Waugh et al. 2016). Plasma concentrations in chickens after a 25 μg/h transdermal patch were similar to humans for up to 48 hours, but significant inter- and intraindividual variability was seen (Delaski et al. 2017). Administration of a single 10 or 30 μg/kg fentanyl bolus in chickens induced a dose-dependent, short-lasting reduction in isoflurane MAC with no significant cardiopulmonary depression during spontaneous ventilation (da Rocha et al. 2017).

Mammals

Fentanyl has an effect for only ~30 minutes after a single IV injection, and is thus most commonly used as a CRI (Criado and Gomez de Segura 2003). As with all mu receptor agonists, fentanyl can cause respiratory depression so a secure airway and ability to ventilate are required when using it as a CRI. Systemic uptake of transdermal fentanyl in lagomorphs with the 25 μg/h patch was highest with the longest duration of activity (3 days) when the hair was clipped at the patch site, but the lagomorphs were more sedated and had a shorter duration of plasma concentrations when the hair was chemically depilated, and no systemic concentrations were identified when hair was present at the patch site (Foley et al. 2001). Although extrapolated effective therapeutic plasma concentrations were obtained, loss of body weight occurred in this study. If this method of analgesia is to be used, appetite and fecal/urine output must be monitored very closely.

Tramadol

Tramadol is a centrally acting mu opioid receptor agonist that also acts at alpha adrenergic and serotonergic receptors. Tramadol is a very weak mu agonist but the O-desmethyl metabolite (M1) is a much more potent agonist in humans.

Reptiles

In red-eared sliders, tramadol 5 mg/kg PO, increased withdrawal latencies for 12–24 hours after drug administration, and at 10 or 25 mg/kg PO increased withdrawal latencies for 6–96 hours (Baker et al. 2011). In the same study, tramadol at the low dosage did not cause respiratory depression, but decreased from 51% to 70% at the higher dosages (Baker et al. 2011). Likewise, in yellow-bellied sliders (*Trachemys scripta scripta*) administered 10 mg/kg IM in the forelimb or hindlimb, withdrawal latencies to a thermal stimulus were increased for 8–48 hours and 0.5–48 hours, respectively (Giorgi et al. 2015a). The pharmacokinetics of tramadol have been evaluated in loggerhead sea turtles, suggesting a dosage of 10 mg/kg PO q72h based on plasma concentrations of tramadol and its metabolite M1 (Norton et al. 2015).

Birds

The pharmacokinetics of tramadol have been evaluated in several avian species, including bald eagles, red-tailed hawks, American kestrels, peafowl, African penguins, and Amazon parrots (Black et al. 2010; Guzman et al. 2014a; Kilburn et al. 2014; Souza et al. 2009, 2011, 2012).

Compared to other avian species, tramadol in Amazon parrots has a low oral bioavailability and rapid clearance and requires a higher oral dose (30 mg/kg), which provides antinociceptive effects up to six hours (Sanchez-Migallon Guzman et al. 2012; Souza et al. 2012). In American kestrels, oral tramadol (5 mg/kg) was antinociceptive for only 1.5 hours (Guzman et al. 2014a).

Mammals

The conversion to the M1 metabolite is variable among species, but it is produced in rats, mice, and lagomorphs (Parasrampuria et al. 2007; Souza et al. 2008; Wu et al. 2006). The pharmacokinetics of tramadol have been evaluated in rats (Parasrampuria et al. 2007; Zhao et al. 2008) and lagomorphs (Souza et al. 2008) but analgesic plasma concentrations have not been studied. Clinically insignificant isoflurane-sparing effects occur in rats and lagomorphs administered 10 and 4.4 mg/kg tramadol PO, respectively (de Wolff et al. 1999; Egger et al. 2009). Significant decreases in HR and transient decreases in systolic arterial pressure were identified in lagomorphs after a single 4.4 mg/kg IV dose (Egger et al. 2009). Results of several studies in rats indicate that it can be an effective analgesic for acute pain (Chandran et al. 2009; Guneli et al. 2007; Hama and Sagen 2007). In rats, tramadol provided analgesia for osteoarthritis (Chandran et al. 2009) but efficacy decreased with increased duration of pain, and its antinociceptive mechanism changed over time, which may partially explain its inconsistent efficacy in chronic pain patients (Hama and Sagen 2007). In one study, there was evidence of tolerance in rats with chronic use, so dosing may need to be readjusted based on individual needs (Valle et al. 2000). Tramadol anecdotally appears to be useful at 5 mg/kg in a number of wild mammals, but does not appear effective in white-tailed deer (H. Barron, personal communication).

Tapentadol

Tapentadol is also a novel atypical opioid medication with mu agonist properties and is a norepinephrine reuptake inhibitor. It is equivalent in analgesic activity in humans to morphine, but has 50-fold lower affinity for mu receptors than morphine (Giorgi et al. 2015b).

Birds

Few studies have assessed the efficacy of tapentadol, but one pharmacokinetic study showed that after a single IV dose (1 mg/kg), plasma concentrations were only higher than the minimum effective concentration for humans for one hour. After a single oral dose of 5 mg/kg, pharmcokinetics parameters could not be calculated, suggesting that further research or higher doses are needed in birds. Twelve days after the last oral dose administered to hens, residues in eggs were undetectable (de Vito et al. 2018).

Reptiles

In both yellow-bellied sliders and red-eared sliders, tapentadol 5 mg/kg IM increased thermal thresholds compared with saline for approximately 10 hours (Giorgi et al. 2014, 2015b).

Nonsteroidal Antiinflammatory Drugs (NSAIDs)

Meloxicam

Meloxicam is a COX-2 selective inhibitor NSAID. It is currently available as oral tablets, suspension, and an injectable form.

Reptiles

In bearded dragons, meloxicam administered at 0.4 mg/kg IM increased tolerance to electrical stimulus (Greenacre et al. 2005). Meloxicam administered at 0.3 mg/kg IM in ball pythons before a surgical placement of an arterial catheter showed effects on physiological parameters when compared to saline (Olesen et al. 2008). The pharmacokinetics of meloxicam have been evaluated in green iguanas, suggesting a dosage of 0.2 mg/kg PO or IV q24h based on plasma concentrations of meloxicam (Divers et al. 2010), and have also been evaluated in red-eared sliders (di Salvo et al. 2016). Regarding safety, meloxicam did not change the hematological or biochemical parameters in green iguanas administered 0.2 mg/kg IM for 10 days (Trkova et al. 2007).

Birds

The pharmacokinetics of meloxicam are published for chickens, ostriches, ducks, turkeys, pigeons, vultures, ring-necked parakeets, Hispaniolan Amazon parrots, African gray parrots, cockatiels, red-tailed hawks, and great-horned owls (Baert and de Backer 2003; Dhondt et al. 2017; Naidoo et al. 2008). There are large differences in meloxicam pharmacokinetics and oral bioavailability between species, underscoring again the challenges of extrapolating drug dosages between species (Baert and de Backer 2003; Dhondt et al. 2017; Lacasse et al. 2013; Molter et al. 2013; Montesinos et al. 2017; Wilson et al. 2004). Pharmacodynamic studies in Amazon parrots and pigeons recommend 1.6 and 2 mg/kg PO every 12 hours, respectively (Cole et al. 2009; Desmarchelier et al. 2012). Safety studies of meloxicam in quail (2 mg/kg IM), Amazon parrots (1.6 mg/kg PO), and gray parrots (0.5 mg/kg IM) found no evidence of significant renal, GI, or hemostatic effects, with the exception of injection site reactions, similar to IM injection of carprofen (Dijkstra et al. 2015; Montesinos et al. 2015; Sinclair et al. 2012; Zollinger et al. 2011). A survey to determine NSAID toxicity in captive birds treated in zoos reported zero fatalities when meloxicam was administered to over 700 birds from 60 species (Cuthbert et al. 2007). Certain vulture species are more sensitive to adverse renal effects of several NSAIDs, with the exception of meloxicam (Swarup et al. 2007).

Despite meloxicam's large therapeutic range and relative safety compared with other NSAIDs, species-specific potential adverse effects should continue to be evaluated. Recently, a compounded sustained-release meloxicam (e.g., ZooPharm, Windsor, CO) has become commercially available, and shows promise for reduced administration frequency.

Mammals

Meloxicam at 1 mg/kg SC dose reduced acute postlaparotomy pain behaviors in rats, but a 0.5 mg/kg SC dose was not effective (Roughan and Flecknell 2003). The pharmacokinetics of single or repeated PO doses (daily for five days) of either 0.3 or 1.5 mg/kg meloxicam in 3-month-old lagomorphs showed that after single oral dosing of either dose, maximal plasma concentrations were achieved at 6–8 hours and were nearly undetectable by 24 hours No drug plasma accumulation was reported at either dose after five days, and meloxicam was rapidly eliminated after drug discontinuation (Turner et al. 2006a). A separate study of the pharmacokinetics of single or repeated PO doses (daily for 10 days) of 0.3 mg/kg meloxicam in 8-month-old lagomorphs identified a slight increase in plasma concentrations over time (Carpenter et al. 2009). However, when administered at 1 mg/kg PO q24h × 29 days, plasma concentrations were similar to those when the same dose was given for five days (Delk et al. 2014). Some rodents and lagomorphs need higher meloxicam doses, but clinical efficacy and safety studies are still necessary to determine appropriate meloxicam analgesic doses and dosing frequency in small mammal patients. Anecdotal data on the new, compounded sustained-release meloxicam suggest it is useful for reduced frequency of administration in bears, raccoons, and deer.

Carprofen

Carprofen is slightly less COX-2 selective than meloxicam. It can be administered parenterally or orally and is well absorbed through the GI tract in mammals.

Reptiles

In bearded dragons, carprofen administered at 2 mg/kg IM increased the tolerance to electrical stimulus (Greenacre et al. 2005). Regarding safety, green iguanas administered carprofen at 0.2 mg/kg IM for 10 days increased alanine aminotransferase (ALT) and aspartate aminotransferase (AST) when compared to saline or meloxicam (Trkova et al. 2007).

Birds

In chickens, carprofen improved lameness in a dose-dependent manner (McGeown et al. 1999). Amazon parrots with experimental arthritis treated with 3 mg/kg IM q12h showed improvement six hours after treatment but not at 12 hours, therefore it may need to be given at a higher dose or more frequently (Paul-Murphy et al. 2009). A safety study with pigeons reported increased AST and ALT concentrations and lesions in the liver and at muscle injection sites (Zollinger et al. 2011).

Mammals

The half-life of carprofen varies considerably among mammalian species, which affects dosing intervals. Very little work has been done evaluating this drug in nondomestic species (Flecknell et al. 1999; Hawkins et al. 2008; Roughan and Flecknell 2003). Carprofen administered at 5 mg/kg SC provided postlaparotomy analgesia in rats for at least five hours, but equivalent effect was found using 2.5 mg/kg (Roughan and Flecknell 2003). Postoperative food and water consumption were improved when rats were administered 5 mg/kg SC but not PO, suggesting higher doses may be necessary with PO dosing (Flecknell et al. 1999). Unlike most species studied, the S(+)-carprofen enantiomer predominates in lagomorph plasma, which may have significant therapeutic and safety implications (see Appendix II: Formulary) (Hawkins et al. 2008). The authors have used 1–4 mg/kg PO, SC, and IM q12–24h short-term (<7 days) in many small mammal species.

Ketoprofen

Ketoprefen is a nonselective COX inhibitor NSAID.

Reptiles

In bearded dragons, ketoprofen administered at 2 mg/kg IM increased tolerance to an electrical stimulus (Greenacre et al. 2005). The pharmacokinetics of ketoprofen have been evaluated in green iguanas (Tuttle et al. 2006).

Birds

Ketoprofen is most commonly used parenterally in birds because of limited oral pharmacokinetic (PK) data and difficulty in accurately dosing the oral formulation in small species. PK studies evaluating a single dose of 2 mg/kg ketoprofen given PO, IM, and IV in Japanese quail showed very low oral and IM bioavailability with a very short half-life (Graham et al. 2005). Studies in mallard ducks found a decrease in inflammatory mediators for 12 hours following ketoprofen administration (Machin et al. 2001). Field use of ketoprofen in two eider species was associated with significant mortalities (Mulcahy et al. 2003).

Mammals

Ketoprofen administered 5 mg/kg SC preoperatively in rats undergoing exploratory laparotomy showed an effect for at least five hours, but this dose was not effective PO, suggesting higher doses may be needed for PO dosing (Flecknell et al. 1999). Ketoprofen is available as a 2.5% topical gel in some countries, but systemic uptake may occur if ingested.

Anesthetic Emergencies

Emergencies during anesthesia should be anticipated and planned for in advance. Most are averted by careful monitoring of HR, respiratory rate, blood pressure, and body temperature. Endotracheal tubes, oxygen, IV catheters and materials for securing them, ventilatory support, and emergency drugs should be close by and ready for use. It is critical that emergency drug doses are calculated and predrawn before induction. Treat respiratory depression and arrest by turning off the anesthetic machine and controlling ventilation. The standard approach of airway, breathing, and circulation (ABC) should be followed. Cardiac massage can be performed and in many small species, the heart is palpable through the thoracic wall. In birds, thoracic compressions should be done digitally with fingers placed along lateral thoracic wall, not over the sternum. If cardiac compressions are unsuccessful, administration of epinephrine IV, transpulmonary, or intracardiac is recommended (in that order of preference). Treat severe bradycardia with atropine, assuming it is due to increased parasympathetic tone.

References

Adami, C., Spadavecchia, C., Angeli, G. et al. (2015). Alfaxalone anesthesia by immersion in oriental fire-bellied toads (Bombina orientalis). *Vet. Anaesth. Analg.* 42: 547–551.

Adami, C., d'Ovidio, D., and Casoni, D. (2016a). Alfaxalone versus alfaxalone-dexmedetomidine anaesthesia by immersion in oriental fire-bellied toads (Bombina orientalis). *Vet. Anaesth. Analg.* 43: 326–332.

Adami, C., d'Ovidio, D., and Casoni, D. (2016b). Alfaxalone-butorphanol versus alfaxalone-morphine combination for immersion anaesthesia in oriental fire-bellied toads (Bombina orientalis). *Lab. Anim.* 50: 204–211.

Adel, M., Sadegh, A.B., Arizza, V. et al. (2017). Anesthetic efficacy of ketamine-diazepam, ketamine-xylazine, and ketamine-acepromazine in Caspian Pond turtles (Mauremys caspica). *Indian J. Pharmacol.* 49: 93–97.

Arenillas, M. and Gomez de Segura, I.A. (2018). Anaesthetic effects of alfaxalone administered intraperitoneally alone or combined with dexmedetomidine and fentanyl in the rat. *Lab. Anim.* 52: 588–598.

Atalan, G., Uzun, M., Demirkan, I. et al. (2002). Effect of medetomidine-butorphanol-ketamine anaesthesia and atipamezole on heart and respiratory rate and cloacal temperature of domestic pigeons. *J. Vet. Med. A Physiol. Pathol. Clin. Med.* 49: 281–285.

Avsaroglu, H., Versluis, A., Hellebrekers, L.J. et al. (2003). Strain differences in response to propofol, ketamine and medetomidine in rabbits. *Vet. Rec.* 152: 300.

Baert, K. and de Backer, P. (2003). Comparative pharmacokinetics of three non-steroidal anti-inflammatory drugs in five bird species. *Comp. Biochem. Physiol. C Toxicol. Pharmacol.* 134: 25–33.

Bailey, R.S., Barter, L.S., and Pypendop, B.H. (2017). Pharmacokinetics of dexmedetomidine in isoflurane-anesthetized New Zealand White rabbits. *Vet. Anaesth. Analg.* 44: 876–882.

Baker, B.B., Sladky, K.K., and Johnson, S.M. (2011). Evaluation of the analgesic effects of oral and subcutaneous tramadol administration in red-eared slider turtles. *J. Am. Vet. Med. Assoc.* 238: 220–227.

Barrillot, B., Roux, J., Arthaud, S. et al. (2018). Intramuscular administration of ketamine-medetomidine assures stable anaesthesia needed for long-term surgery in the Argentine tegu (Salvator merianae). *J. Zoo Wildl. Med.* 49: 291–296.

Barter, L.S., Hawkins, M.G., and Pypendop, B.H. (2015). Effects of fentanyl on isoflurane minimum alveolar concentration in New Zealand White rabbits (Oryctolagus cuniculus). *Am. J. Vet. Res.* 76: 111–115.

Bateman, L., Ludders, J.W., Gleed, R.D. et al. (2005). Comparison between facemask and laryngeal mask airway in rabbits during isoflurane anesthesia. *Vet. Anaesth. Analg.* 32: 280–288.

Baumgartner, C., Koenighaus, H., Ebner, J. et al. (2011). Comparison of dipyrone/propofol versus fentanyl/propofol anaesthesia during surgery in rabbits. *Lab. Anim.* 45: 38–44.

Bellini, L., Banzato, T., Contiero, B. et al. (2014). Evaluation of sedation and clinical effect of midazolam with ketamine or dexmedetomidine in pet rabbits. *Vet. Rec.* 175: 372.

Bertelsen, M.F., Buchanan, R., Jensen, H.M. et al. (2015). Assessing the influence of mechanical ventilation on blood gases and blood pressure in rattlesnakes. *Vet. Anaesth. Analg.* 42: 386–393.

Bisetto, S.P., Melo, C.F., and Carregaro, A.B. (2018). Evaluation of sedative and antinociceptive effects of dexmedetomidine, midazolam and dexmedetomidine-midazolam in tegus (Salvator merianae). *Vet. Anaesth. Analg.* 45: 320–328.

Black, P.A., Cox, S.K., Macek, M. et al. (2010). Pharmacokinetics of tramadol hydrochloride and its metabolite O-desmethyltramadol in peafowl (Pavo cristatus). *J. Zoo Wildl. Med.* 41: 671–676.

Brenner, D.J., Larsen, R.S., Dickinson, P.J. et al. (2010). Development of an avian brachial plexus nerve block technique for perioperative analgesia in mallard ducks (Anas platyrhynchos). *J. Avian Med. Surg.* 24: 24–34.

Bunke, L.G., Sladky, K.K., and Johnson, S.M. (2018). Antinociceptive efficacy and respiratory effects of dexmedetomidine in ball pythons (Python regius). *Am. J. Vet. Res.* 79: 718–726.

Carbone, E.T., Lindstrom, K.E., Diep, S. et al. (2012). Duration of action of sustained-release buprenorphine in 2 strains of mice. *J. Am. Assoc. Lab. Anim. Sci.* 51: 815–819.

Cardozo, L.B., Almeida, R.M., Fiuza, L.C. et al. (2009). Brachial plexus blockade in chickens with 0.75% ropivacaine. *Vet. Anaesth. Analg.* 36: 396–400.

Carpenter, J.W., Pollock, C.G., Koch, D.E. et al. (2009). Single and multiple-dose pharmacokinetics of meloxicam after oral administration to the rabbit (Oryctolagus cuniculus). *J. Zoo Wildl. Med.* 40: 601–606.

Cassu, R.N., Luna, S.P., Teixeira Neto, F.J. et al. (2004). Evaluation of laryngeal mask as an alternative to endotracheal intubation in cats anesthetized under spontaneous or controlled ventilation. *Vet. Anaesth. Analg.* 31: 213–221.

Catbagan, D.L., Quimby, J.M., Mama, K.R. et al. (2011). Comparison of the efficacy and adverse effects of sustained-release buprenorphine hydrochloride following subcutaneous administration and buprenorphine hydrochloride following oral transmucosal administration in cats undergoing ovariohysterectomy. *Am. J. Vet. Res.* 72: 461–466.

Caulkett, N. and Fahlman, A. (2014). Ursids (Bears). In: *Zoo Animal and Wildlife Immobilization and Anesthesia* (ed. G. West, D. Heard and N. Caulkett), 599–607. Ames, IA: Blackwell Publishing.

Caulkett, N.A., Cattet, M.R., Caulkett, J.M. et al. (1999). Comparative physiologic effects of telazol, medetomidine-ketamine, and medetomidine-telazol in captive polar bears (Ursus maritimus). *J. Zoo Wildl. Med.* 30: 504–509.

Ceulemans, S.M., Guzman, D.S., Olsen, G.H. et al. (2014). Evaluation of thermal antinociceptive effects after intramuscular administration of buprenorphine hydrochloride to American kestrels (Falco sparverius). *Am. J. Vet. Res.* 75: 705–710.

Chandran, P., Pai, M., Blomme, E.A. et al. (2009). Pharmacological modulation of movement-evoked pain in a rat model of osteoarthritis. *Eur. J. Pharmacol.* 613: 39–45.

Chum, H.H., Jampachairsri, K., McKeon, G.P. et al. (2014). Antinociceptive effects of sustained-release buprenorphine in a model of incisional pain in rats (Rattus norvegicus). *J. Am. Assoc. Lab. Anim. Sci.* 53: 193–197.

Cole, G.A., Paul-Murphy, J., Krugner-Higby, L. et al. (2009). Analgesic effects of intramuscular administration of meloxicam in Hispaniolan parrots (Amazona ventralis) with experimentally induced arthritis. *Am. J. Vet. Res.* 70: 1471–1476.

Concannon, K.T., Dodam, J.R., and Hellyer, P.W. (1995). Influence of a mu- and kappa-opioid agonist on isoflurane minimal anesthetic concentration in chickens. *Am. J. Vet. Res.* 56: 806–811.

Criado, A.B. and Gomez de Segura, I.A. (2003). Reduction of isoflurane MAC by fentanyl or remifentanil in rats. *Vet. Anaesth. Analg.* 30: 250–256.

Criado, A.B., Gomez de Segura, I.A., Tendillo, F.J. et al. (2000). Reduction of isoflurane MAC with buprenorphine and morphine in rats. *Lab. Anim.* 34: 252–259.

Cruz, F.S., Carregaro, A.B., Raiser, A.G. et al. (2010). Total intravenous anesthesia with propofol and S(+)-ketamine in rabbits. *Vet. Anaesth. Analg.* 37: 116–122.

Curro, T.G., Brunson, D.B., and Paul-Murphy, J. (1994). Determination of the ED50 of isoflurane and evaluation of the isoflurane-sparing effect of butorphanol in cockatoos (Cacatua spp.). *Vet. Surg.* 23: 429–433.

Cuthbert, R., Parry-Jones, J., Green, R.E. et al. (2007). NSAIDs and scavenging birds: potential impacts beyond Asia's critically endangered vultures. *Biol. Lett.* 3: 90–93.

da Rocha, R.W., Escobar, A., Pypendop, B.H. et al. (2017). Effects of a single intravenous bolus of fentanyl on the minimum anesthetic concentration of isoflurane in chickens (Gallus gallus domesticus). *Vet. Anaesth. Analg.* 44: 546–554.

del Alamo, A.M., Mandsager, R.E., Riebold, T.W. et al. (2015). Evaluation of intravenous administration of alfaxalone, propofol, and ketamine-diazepam for anesthesia in alpacas. *Vet. Anaesth. Analg.* 42: 72–82.

de Castro Vilani, R.G.D., Montiani-Ferreirra, F., Lange, R.R. et al. (2006). Brachial plexus block in birds. *Exotic DVM* 8: 86–91.

De Vito, V., Owen, H., Marzoni, M. et al. (2018). Pharmacokinetics of tapentadol in laying hens and its residues in eggs after multiple oral dose administration. *Br. Poult. Sci.* 59: 128–133.

de Wolff, M.H., Leather, H.A., and Wouters, P.F. (1999). Effects of tramadol on minimum alveolar concentration (MAC) of isoflurane in rats. *Br. J. Anaesth.* 83: 780–783.

Deflers, H., Gandar, F., Bolen, G. et al. (2018). Influence of a single dose of buprenorphine on rabbit (Oryctolagus cuniculus) gastrointestinal motility. *Vet. Anaesth. Analg.* 45: 510–519.

Dehkordi, S.H., Bigham-Sadegh, A., and Gerami, R. (2012). Evaluation of anti-nociceptive effect of epidural tramadol, tramadol-lidocaine and lidocaine in goats. *Vet. Anaesth. Analg.* 39: 106–110.

Delaski, K.M., Gehring, R., Heffron, B.T. et al. (2017). Plasma concentrations of fentanyl achieved with transdermal application in chickens. *J. Avian Med. Surg.* 31: 6–15.

Delk, K.W., Carpenter, J.W., Kukanich, B. et al. (2014). Pharmacokinetics of meloxicam administered orally to rabbits (Oryctolagus cuniculus) for 29 days. *Am. J. Vet. Res.* 75: 195–199.

Dennis, P.M. and Heard, D.J. (2002). Cardiopulmonary effects of a medetomidine-ketamine combination administered intravenously in gopher tortoises. *J. Am. Vet. Med. Assoc.* 220: 1516–1519.

Desmarchelier, M., Troncy, E., Fitzgerald, G. et al. (2012). Analgesic effects of meloxicam administration on postoperative orthopedic pain in domestic pigeons (Columba livia). *Am. J. Vet. Res.* 73: 361–367.

Dhondt, L., Devreese, M., Croubels, S. et al. (2017). Comparative population pharmacokinetics and absolute oral bioavailability of COX-2 selective inhibitors celecoxib, mavacoxib and meloxicam in cockatiels (Nymphicus hollandicus). *Sci. Rep.* 7: 12043.

Diao, H.X., Zhang, S., Hu, X.Y. et al. (2017). Behavioral and cardiopulmonary effects of dexmedetomidine-midazolam and dexmedetomidine-midazolam-butorphanol in the silver fox (Vulpes vulpes). *Vet Anaesth Analg.* 44 (1): 114–120.

Di Salvo, A., Giorgi, M., Catanzaro, A. et al. (2016). Pharmacokinetic profiles of meloxicam in turtles (Trachemys scripta scripta) after single oral, intracoelomic and intramuscular administrations. *J. Vet. Pharmacol. Ther.* 39: 102–105.

Dijkstra, B., Guzman, D.S., Gustavsen, K. et al. (2015). Renal, gastrointestinal, and hemostatic effects of oral administration of meloxicam to Hispaniolan Amazon parrots (Amazona ventralis). *Am. J. Vet. Res.* 76: 308–317.

Divers, S.J., Papich, M., McBride, M. et al. (2010). Pharmacokinetics of meloxicam following intravenous and oral administration in green iguanas (Iguana iguana). *Am. J. Vet. Res.* 71: 1277–1283.

Doerning, B.J., Brammer, D.W., Chrisp, C.E. et al. (1992). Nephrotoxicity of tiletamine in New Zealand white rabbits. *Lab. Anim. Sci.* 42: 267–269.

Doss, G.A., Fink, D.M., Sladky, K.K. et al. (2017). Comparison of subcutaneous dexmedetomidine–midazolam versus alfaxalone midazolam sedation in leopard geckos (Eublepharis macularius). *Vet. Anaesth. Analg.* 44: 1175–1183.

Egger, C.M., Souza, M.J., Greenacre, C.B. et al. (2009). Effect of intravenous administration of tramadol hydrochloride on the minimum alveolar concentration of isoflurane in rabbits. *Am. J. Vet. Res.* 70: 945–949.

Engbers, S., Larkin, A., Rousset, N. et al. (2017). Comparison of a supraglottic airway device (v-gel®) with blind orotracheal intubation in rabbits. *Front. Vet. Sci.* 4: 49.

Escobar, A., da Rocha, R.W., Pypendop, B.H. et al. (2016). Effects of methadone on the minimum anesthetic concentration of isoflurane, and its effects on heart rate, blood pressure and ventilation during isoflurane anesthesia in hens (Gallus gallus domesticus). *PLoS One* 11: e0152546.

Eshar, D. and Wilson, J. (2010). Epidural anesthesia and analgesia in ferrets. *Lab. Anim.* 39: 339–340.

Fahlman, A., Arnemo, J.M., Swenson, J.E. et al. (2011). Physiologic evaluation of capture and anesthesia with medetomidine-zolazepam-tiletamine in brown bears (Ursus arctos). *J. Zoo Wildl. Med.* 42: 1–11.

Fandos Esteruelas, N., Cattet, M., Zedrosser, A. et al. (2017). A double blinded, randomized comparison of medetomidine-tiletamine zolazepam and dexmedetomidine-tiletamine-zolazepam anesthesia in free-ranging brown bears (Ursus arctos). *PLoS One* 12: e0170764.

Figueiredo, J.P., Cruz, M.L., Mendes, G.M. et al. (2008). Assessment of brachial plexus blockade in chickens by an axillary approach. *Vet. Anaesth. Analg.* 35: 511–518.

Flecknell, P.A. (2001). Analgesia of small mammals. *Vet. Clin. North Am. Exot. Anim. Pract.* 4: 47–56.

Flecknell, P.A., Orr, H.E., Roughan, J.V. et al. (1999). Comparison of the effects of oral or subcutaneous carprofen or ketoprofen in rats undergoing laparotomy. *Vet. Rec.* 144: 65–67.

Fleming, G.J. and Robertson, S.A. (2012). Assessments of thermal antinociceptive effects of butorphanol and human observer effect on quantitative evaluation of analgesia in green iguanas (Iguana iguana). *Am. J. Vet. Res.* 73: 1507–1511.

Foley, P.L., Henderson, A.L., Bissonette, E.A. et al. (2001). Evaluation of fentanyl transdermal patches in rabbits: blood concentrations and physiologic response. *Comp. Med.* 51: 239–244.

Foley, P.L., Liang, H., and Crichlow, A.R. (2011). Evaluation of a sustained-release formulation of buprenorphine for analgesia in rats. *J. Am. Assoc. Lab. Anim. Sci.* 50: 198–204.

Fournier-Chambrillon, C., Vogel, I., Fournier, P. et al. (2000). Immobilization of free-ranging nine-banded and great long-nosed armadillos with three anesthetic combinations. *J. Wildlife Dis.* 36: 131–140.

Gades, N.M., Danneman, P.J., Wixson, S.K. et al. (2000). The magnitude and duration of the analgesic effect of morphine, butorphanol, and buprenorphine in rats and mice. *Contemp. Top. Lab. Anim. Sci.* 39: 8–13.

Gamble, K.C. (2008). Plasma fentanyl concentrations achieved after transdermal fentanyl patch application in prehensile-tailed skinks, Corucia zebrata. *J. Herpetol. Med. Surg.* 18: 81–85.

Gianotti, G., Valverde, A., Sinclair, M. et al. (2012). Prior determination of baseline minimum alveolar concentration (MAC) of isoflurane does not influence the effect of ketamine on MAC in rabbits. *Can. J. Vet. Res.* 76: 261–267.

Giorgi, M., de Vito, V., Owen, H. et al. (2014). PK/PD evaluations of the novel atypical opioid tapentadol in red-eared slider turtles. *Med. Weter. Vet. Med. Sci. Pract.* 70: 530–535.

Giorgi, M., Salvadori, M., de Vito, V. et al. (2015a). Pharmacokinetic/pharmacodynamic assessments of 10 mg/kg tramadol intramuscular injection in yellow-bellied slider turtles (Trachemys scripta scripta). *J. Vet. Pharmacol. Ther.* 38: 488–496.

Giorgi, M., Lee, H.-K., Rota, S. et al. (2015b). Pharmacokinetic and pharmacodynamic assessments of tapentadol in yellow-bellied slider turtles (Trachemys scripta scripta) after a single intramuscular injection. *J. Exotic Pet. Med.* 24: 317–325.

Gleeson, M.D., Guzman, D.S., Knych, H.K. et al. (2018). Pharmacokinetics of a concentrated buprenorphine formulation in red-tailed hawks (Buteo jamaicensis). *Am. J. Vet. Res.* 79: 13–20.

Graham, J.E., Kollias-Baker, C., Craigmill, A.L. et al. (2005). Pharmacokinetics of ketoprofen in Japanese quail (Coturnix japonica). *J. Vet. Pharmacol. Ther.* 28: 399–402.

Greenacre, C., Paul-Murphy, J., Sladky, K.K. et al. (2005). Reptile and amphibian analgesia. *J. Herp. Med. Surg.* 15: 24–30.

Greenacre, C., Schumacher, J., and Talke, G. (2006). Comparative antinociception of morphine, butorphanol, and buprenorphine versus saline in green iguanas (Iguana iguana) using electroestimulation. *J. Herp. Med. Surg.* 16: 2006.

Greer, L.L., Jenne, K.J., and Diggs, H.E. (2001). Medetomidine-ketamine anesthesia in red-eared slider turtles (Trachemys scripta elegans). *Contemp. Top. Lab. Anim. Sci.* 40: 9–11.

Grint, N.J. and Murison, P.J. (2008). A comparison of ketamine-midazolam and ketamine-medetomidine combinations for induction of anaesthesia in rabbits. *Vet. Anaesth. Analg.* 35: 113–121.

Grint, N.J., Sayers, I.R., Cecchi, R. et al. (2006). Postanaesthetic tracheal strictures in three rabbits. *Lab. Anim.* 40: 301–308.

Guneli, E., Karabay Yavasoglu, N.U., Apaydin, S. et al. (2007). Analysis of the antinociceptive effect of systemic administration of tramadol and dexmedetomidine combination on rat models of acute and neuropathic pain. *Pharmacol. Biochem. Behav.* 88: 9–17.

Gutema, T.M., Atickem, A., Lemma, A. et al. (2018). Capture and immobilization of African wolves (Canis lupaster) in the Ethiopian highlands. *J. Wildl. Dis.* 54: 175–179.

Guzman, D.S., Flammer, K., Paul-Murphy, J.R. et al. (2011). Pharmacokinetics of butorphanol after intravenous, intramuscular, and oral administration in Hispaniolan Amazon parrots (Amazona ventralis). *J. Avian Med. Surg.* 25: 185–191.

Guzman, D.S., Drazenovich, T.L., Olsen, G.H. et al. (2013). Evaluation of thermal antinociceptive effects after intramuscular administration of hydromorphone hydrochloride to American kestrels (Falco sparverius). *Am. J. Vet. Res.* 74: 817–822.

Guzman, D.S., Drazenovich, T.L., Olsen, G.H. et al. (2014a). Evaluation of thermal antinociceptive effects after oral administration of tramadol hydrochloride to American kestrels (Falco sparverius). *Am. J. Vet. Res.* 75: 117–123.

Guzman, D.S., Drazenovich, T.L., KuKanich, B. et al. (2014b). Evaluation of thermal antinociceptive effects and pharmacokinetics after intramuscular administration of butorphanol tartrate to American kestrels (Falco sparverius). *Am. J. Vet. Res.* 75: 11–18.

Guzman, D.S., Knych, H.K., Olsen, G.H. et al. (2017). Pharmacokinetics of a sustained release formulation of buprenorphine after intramuscular and subcutaneous administration to American kestrels (Falco sparverius). *J. Avian Med. Surg.* 31: 102–107.

Hama, A. and Sagen, J. (2007). Altered antinociceptive efficacy of tramadol over time in rats with painful peripheral neuropathy. *Eur. J. Pharmacol.* 559: 32–37.

Hansen, L.L. and Bertelsen, M.F. (2013). Assessment of the effects of intramuscular administration of alfaxalone with and without medetomidine in Horsfield's tortoises (Agrionemys horsfieldii). *Vet. Anaesth. Analg.* 40: e68–e75.

Harms, C.A., Piniak, W.E., Eckert, S.A. et al. (2014). Sedation and anesthesia of hatchling leatherback sea turtles (Dermochelys coriacea) for auditory evoked potential measurement in air and in water. *J. Zoo Wildl. Med.* 45: 86–92.

Harrison, P.K., Tattersall, J.E., and Gosden, E. (2006). The presence of atropinesterase activity in animal plasma. *Naunyn Schmiedebergs Arch. Pharmacol.* 373: 230–236.

Hawkins, M.G., Wright, B.D., Pascoe, P.J. et al. (2003). Pharmacokinetics and anesthetic and cardiopulmonary effects of propofol in red-tailed hawks (Buteo jamaicensis) and great horned owls (Bubo virginianus). *Am. J. Vet. Res.* 64: 677–683.

Hawkins, M.G., Taylor, I.T., Craigmill, A.L. et al. (2008). Enantioselective pharmacokinetics of racemic carprofen in New Zealand white rabbits. *J. Vet. Pharmacol. Ther* 31: 423–430.

Hawkins, M.G., Zehnder, A.M., and Pascoe, P.J. (2014). Cagebirds. In: *Zoo Animal and Wildlife Immobilization and Anesthesia* (ed. G. West, D.J. Heard and J.M. Caulkett), 399–433. Ames, IA: Blackwell Publishing.

Healy, J.R., Tonkin, J.L., Kamarec, S.R. et al. (2014). Evaluation of an improved sustained-release buprenorphine formulation for use in mice. *Am. J. Vet. Res.* 75: 619–625.

Heard, D. (2014). Lagamorphs (rabbits, hares and pikas). In: *Zoo Animal and Wildlife Immobilization and Anesthesia* (ed. G. West, D. Heard and N. Caulkett), 879–893. Ames, IA: Blackwell Publishing.

Hedenqvist, P., Orr, H.E., Roughan, J.V. et al. (2002). Anaesthesia with ketamine/medetomidine in the rabbit: influence of route of administration and the effect of combination with butorphanol. *Vet. Anaesth. Analg.* 29: 14–19.

Henke, J., Baumgartner, C., Roltgen, I. et al. (2004). Anaesthesia with midazolam/medetomidine/fentanyl in chinchillas (Chinchilla lanigera) compared to anaesthesia with xylazine/ketamine and medetomidine/ketamine. *J. Vet. Med. A Physiol. Pathol. Clin. Med.* 51: 259–264.

Henke, J., Astner, S., Brill, T. et al. (2005). Comparative study of three intramuscular anaesthetic combinations (medetomidine/ketamine, medetomidine/fentanyl/midazolam and xylazine/ketamine) in rabbits. *Vet. Anaesth. Analg.* 32: 261–270.

Hocking, P.M., Gentle, M.J., Bernard, R. et al. (1997). Evaluation of a protocol for determining the effectiveness of pretreatment with local analgesics for reducing experimentally induced articular pain in domestic fowl. *Res. Vet. Sci.* 63: 263–267.

Honkavaara, J., Pypendop, B., Turunen, H. et al. (2017). The effect of MK-467, a peripheral alpha2 adrenoceptor antagonist, on dexmedetomidine-induced sedation and bradycardia after intravenous administration in conscious cats. *Vet. Anaesth. Analg.* 44: 811–822.

Hoppes, S., Flammer, K., Hoersch, K. et al. (2003). Disposition and analgesic effects of fentanyl in white cockatoos (Cacatua alba). *J. Avian Med. Surg.* 17: 124–130.

Hornak, S., Liptak, T., Ledecky, V. et al. (2015). A preliminary trial of the sedation induced by intranasal administration of midazolam alone or in combination with dexmedetomidine and reversal by atipamezole for a short-term immobilization in pigeons. *Vet. Anaesth. Analg.* 42: 192–196.

Hurley, R.J., Marini, R.P., Avison, D.L. et al. (1994). Evaluation of detomidine anesthetic combinations in the rabbit. *Lab. Anim. Sci.* 44: 472–478.

Huynh, M., Poumeyrol, S., Pignon, C. et al. (2015). Intramuscular administration of alfaxalone for sedation in rabbits. *Vet. Rec.* 176: 255.

Imani, H., Vesal, N., and Mohammadi-Samani, S. (2013). Evaluation of intravenous lidocaine overdose in chickens (Gallus domesticus). *Iranian. J. Vet. Surg.* 8: 9–16.

Innis, C., de Voe, R., Myliniczenko, N. et al. (2010). A call for additional studies on the safety of subcarapacial venipuncture in chelonians. *Proc. Assoc. Reptile Amphib. Vet* 8–10.

James, L.E., Williams, C.J., Bertelsen, M.F. et al. (2018). Anaesthetic induction with alfaxalone in the ball python (Python regius): dose response and effect of injection site. *Vet. Anaesth. Analg.* 45: 329–337.

Jirkof, P., Tourvieille, A., Cinelli, P. et al. (2015). Buprenorphine for pain relief in mice: repeated injections vs sustained-release depot formulation. *Lab. Anim.* 49: 177–187.

Johnston, M.S. (2005). Clinical approaches to analgesia in ferrets and rabbits. *Sem. Avian Exotic Pet. Med.* 14: 229–235.

Johnston, M.S. (2015). Rabbit and ferret specific considerations. In: *Handbook of Veterinary Pain Management*, 3e (ed. J. Muir and W. Gaynor), 517–535. St Louis: Mosby.

Kallio-Kujala, I.J., Raekallio, M.R., Honkavaara, J. et al. (2018). Peripheral alpha2-adrenoceptor antagonism affects the absorption of intramuscularly co-administered drugs. *Vet. Anaesth. Analg.* 45: 405–413.

Kamiloglu, A., Atalan, G., and Kamiloglu, N.N. (2008). Comparison of intraosseous and intramuscular drug administration for induction of anaesthesia in domestic pigeons. *Res. Vet. Sci.* 85: 171–175.

Kanui, T.I. and Hole, K. (1992). Morphine and pethidine antinociception in the crocodile. *J. Vet. Pharmacol. Ther.* 15: 101–103.

Keating, S.C., Thomas, A.A., Flecknell, P.A. et al. (2012). Evaluation of EMLA cream for preventing pain during tattooing of rabbits: changes in physiological, behavioural and facial expression responses. *PLoS One* 7: e44437.

Kemmochi, M., Ichinohe, T., and Kaneko, Y. (2009). Remifentanil decreases mandibular bone marrow blood flow during propofol or sevoflurane anesthesia in rabbits. *J. Oral. Maxillofac. Surg.* 67: 1245–1250.

Kharbush, R.J., Gutwillig, A., Hartzler, K.E. et al. (2017). Antinociceptive and respiratory effects following application of transdermal fentanyl patches and assessment of brain μ-opioid receptor mRNA expression in ball pythons. *Am. J. Vet. Res.* 78: 785–795.

Kilburn, J.J., Cox, S.K., Kottyan, J. et al. (2014). Pharmacokinetics of tramadol and its primary metabolite O-desmethyltramadol in African penguins (Spheniscus demersus). *J. Zoo Wildl. Med.* 45: 93–99.

Kinney, M.E., Johnson, S.M., and Sladky, K.K. (2011). Behavioral evaluation of red-eared slider turtles (Trachemys scripta elegans) administered either morphine or butorphanol following unilateral gonadectomy. *J. Herp. Med. Surg.* 21: 54–62.

Kischinovsky, M., Duse, A., Wang, T. et al. (2013). Intramuscular administration of alfaxalone in red-eared sliders (Trachemys scripta elegans) – effects of dose and body temperature. *Vet. Anaesth. Analg.* 40: 13–20.

Klaphake, E., Schumacher, J., Greenacre, C. et al. (2006). Comparative anesthetic and cardiopulmonary effects of pre- versus postoperative butorphanol administration in hispaniolan amazon parrots (Amazona ventralis) anesthetized with sevoflurane. *J. Avian Med. Surg.* 20: 2–7.

Knotek, Z. (2014). Alfaxalone as an induction agent for anaesthesia in terrapins and tortoises. *Vet. Rec.* 175: 327.

Ko, J.C., Heaton-Jones, T.G., and Nicklin, C.F. (1997). Evaluation of the sedative and cardiorespiratory effects of medetomidine, medetomidine-butorphanol, medetomidine-ketamine, and medetomidine-butorphanol-ketamine in ferrets. *J. Am. Anim. Hosp. Assoc.* 33: 438–448.

Kummrow, M.S., Tseng, F., Hesse, L. et al. (2008). Pharmacokinetics of buprenorphine after single-dose subcutaneous administration in red-eared sliders (Trachemys scripta elegans). *J. Zoo Wildl. Med.* 39: 590–595.

Lacasse, C., Gamble, K.C., and Boothe, D.M. (2013). Pharmacokinetics of a single dose of intravenous and oral meloxicam in red-tailed hawks (Buteo jamaicensis) and great horned owls (Bubo virginianus). *J. Avian Med. Surg.* 27: 204–210.

Lahner, L., Mans, C., and Sladky, K. (2011). Comparison of anesthetic induction and recovery times after intramuscular, subcutaneous or intranasal dexmedetomidine-ketamine administration in red-eared slider turtles (Trachemys scripta elegans). *Proc. Annu. Conf. Am. Assoc. Zoo Vet* 27.

Leal, W.P., Carregaro, A.B., Bressan, T.F. et al. (2017). Antinociceptive efficacy of intramuscular administration of morphine sulfate and butorphanol tartrate in tegus (Salvator merianae). *Am. J. Vet. Res.* 78: 1019–1024.

Lukasik, V.M., Gentz, E.J., Erb, H.N. et al. (1997). Cardiopulmonary effects of propofol anesthesia in chickens (Gallus gallus domesticus). *J. Avian Med. Surg.* 11: 93–97.

Lumeij, J.T. and Deenik, J.W. (2003). Medetomidine-ketamine and diazepam-ketamine anesthesia in racing pigeons (Columba livia domestica) – a comparative study. *J. Avian Med. Surg.* 17: 191–196.

Machin, K.L. and Caulkett, N.A. (1998). Cardiopulmonary effects of propofol and a medetomidine-midazolam-ketamine combination in mallard ducks. *Am. J. Vet. Res.* 59: 598–602.

Machin, K.L. and Caulkett, N.A. (2000). Evaluation of isoflurane and propofol anesthesia for intraabdominal transmitter placement in nesting female canvasback ducks. *J. Wildl. Dis.* 36: 324–334.

Machin, K.L., Tellier, L.A., Lair, S. et al. (2001). Pharmacodynamics of flunixin and ketoprofen in mallard ducks (Anas platyrhynchos). *J. Zoo Wildl. Med.* 32: 222–229.

MacLean, R.A., Harms, C.A., and Braun-McNeill, J. (2008). Propofol anesthesia in loggerhead (Caretta caretta) sea turtles. *J. Wildl. Dis.* 44: 143–150.

Malte, C.L., Bundgaard, J., Jensen, M.S. et al. (2018). The effects of morphine on gas exchange, ventilation pattern and ventilatory responses to hypercapnia and hypoxia in dwarf caiman (Paleosuchus palpebrosus). *Comp. Biochem. Physiol. A Mol. Integr. Physiol.* 222: 60–65.

Mans, C. (2014). Clinical technique: intrathecal drug administration in turtles and tortoises. *J. Exotic Pet. Med.* 23: 67–70.

Mans, C., Guzman, D.S., Lahner, L.L. et al. (2012a). Sedation and physiologic response to manual restraint after intranasal administration of midazolam in Hispaniolan Amazon parrots (Amazona ventralis). *J. Avian Med. Surg.* 26: 130–139.

Mans, C., Lahner, L.L., Baker, B.B. et al. (2012b). Antinociceptive efficacy of buprenorphine and hydromorphone in red-eared slider turtles (Trachemys scripta elegans). *J. Zoo Wildl. Med.* 43: 662–665.

Marini, R.P., Li, X., Harpster, N.K. et al. (1999). Cardiovascular pathology possibly associated with ketamine/xylazine anesthesia in Dutch belted rabbits. *Lab. Anim. Sci.* 49: 153–160.

Martin-Cancho, M.F., Lima, J.R., Luis, L. et al. (2006). Relationship of bispectral index values, haemodynamic changes and recovery times during sevoflurane or propofol anaesthesia in rabbits. *Lab. Anim.* 40: 28–42.

Martin-Flores, M., Singh, B., Walsh, C.A. et al. (2017). Effects of buprenorphine, methylnaltrexone, and their combination on gastrointestinal transit in healthy New Zealand White rabbits. *J. Am. Assoc. Lab. Anim. Sci.* 56: 155–159.

Mazaheri-Khameneh, R., Sarrafzadeh-Rezaei, F., Asri-Rezaei, S. et al. (2012). Comparison of time to loss of consciousness and maintenance of anesthesia following intraosseous and intravenous administration of propofol in rabbits. *J. Am. Vet. Med. Assoc.* 241: 73–80.

McGeown, D., Danbury, T.C., Waterman-Pearson, A.E. et al. (1999). Effect of carprofen on lameness in broiler chickens. *Vet. Rec.* 144: 668–671.

Mehmannavaz, H.R., Emami, M.R., Razmyar, J. et al. (2015). A comparative study on some cardiopulmonary effects, anesthesia quality, and recovery time of

isoflurane vs. propofol in domestic pigeons (Columba livia domesticus). *Iranian J. Vet. Med.* 9: 33–40.

Molero, C., Bailey, T.A., and di Somma, A. (2007). Anaesthesia of falcons with a combination of injectable anaesthesia (ketamine-medetomidine) and gas anaesthesia (Isoflurane). *Falco: Newsletter of Middle East Falcon Research Group* 17.

Molter, C.M., Court, M.H., Cole, G.A. et al. (2013). Pharmacokinetics of meloxicam after intravenous, intramuscular, and oral administration of a single dose to Hispaniolan Amazon parrots (Amazona ventralis). *Am. J. Vet. Res.* 74: 375–380.

Molter, C.M., Barbosa, L., Johnson, S. et al. (2015). Pharmacokinetics of a single subcutaneous dose of sustained release buprenorphine in northern elephant seals (Mirounga angustirostris). *J. Zoo Wildl. Med.* 46: 52–61.

Montesinos, A., Ardiaca, M., Juan-Salles, C. et al. (2015). Effects of meloxicam on hematologic and plasma biochemical analyte values and results of histologic examination of kidney biopsy specimens of African grey parrots (Psittacus erithacus). *J. Avian Med. Surg.* 29: 1–8.

Montesinos, A., Ardiaca, M., Gilabert, J.A. et al. (2017). Pharmacokinetics of meloxicam after intravenous, intramuscular and oral administration of a single dose to African grey parrots (Psittacus erithacus). *J. Vet. Pharmacol. Ther.* 40: 279–284.

Morimoto, K., Nishimura, R., Matsunaga, S. et al. (2001). Epidural analgesia with a combination of bupivacaine and buprenorphine in rats. *J. Vet. Med. A Physiol. Pathol Clin. Med.* 48: 303–312.

Mosley, C.A., Dyson, D., and Smith, D.A. (2003). Minimum alveolar concentration of isoflurane in green iguanas and the effect of butorphanol on minimum alveolar concentration. *J. Am. Vet. Med. Assoc.* 222: 1559–1564.

Mulcahy, D.M., Tuomi, P., and Larsen, R.S. (2003). Differential mortality of male spectacled eiders (Somateria fischeri) and king eiders (Somateria spectabilis) subsequent to anesthesia with propofol, bupivacaine, and ketoprofen. *J. Avian Med. Surg.* 17: 117–123.

Mulcahy, D.M., Gartrell, B., Gill, R.E. et al. (2011). Coelomic implantation of satellite transmitters in the bar-tailed godwit (Limosa lapponica) and the bristle-thighed curlew (Numenius tahitiensis) using propofol, bupivacaine, and lidocaine. *J. Zoo Wildl. Med.* 42: 54–64.

Muller, K., Holzapfel, J., and Brunnberg, L. (2011). Total intravenous anaesthesia by boluses or by continuous rate infusion of propofol in mute swans (Cygnus olor). *Vet. Anaesth. Analg.* 38: 286–291.

Mustola, S.T., Rorarius, M.G., Baer, G.A. et al. (2000). Potency of propofol, thiopentone and ketamine at various endpoints in New Zealand White rabbits. *Lab. Anim.* 34: 36–45.

Naidoo, V., Wolter, K., Cromarty, A.D. et al. (2008). The pharmacokinetics of meloxicam in vultures. *J. Vet. Pharmacol. Ther.* 31: 128–134.

Navarrete-Calvo, R., Gomez-Villamandos, R.J., Morgaz, J. et al. (2014). Cardiorespiratory, anaesthetic and recovery effects of morphine combined with medetomidine and alfaxalone in rabbits. *Vet. Rec.* 174: 95.

Nilson, P.C., Teramitsu, I., and White, S.A. (2005). Caudal thoracic air sac cannulation in zebra finches for isoflurane anesthesia. *J. Neurosci. Methods* 143: 107–115.

Norton, T.M., Cox, S., Nelson, S.E. Jr. et al. (2015). Pharmacokinetics of tramadol and O-tesmethyltramadol in loggerhead sea turtles (Caretta Caretta). *J. Zoo Wildl. Med.* 46: 262–265.

Nunamaker, E.A., Stolarik, D.F., Ma, J. et al. (2014). Clinical efficacy of sustained-release buprenorphine with meloxicam for postoperative analgesia in beagle dogs undergoing ovariohysterectomy. *J. Am. Assoc. Lab. Anim. Sci.* 53: 494–501.

Olesen, M.G., Bertelsen, M.F., Perry, S.F. et al. (2008). Effects of preoperative administration of butorphanol or meloxicam on physiologic responses to surgery in ball pythons. *J. Am. Vet. Med. Assoc.* 233: 1883–1888.

Olsson, A., Phalen, D., and Dart, C. (2013). Preliminary studies of alfaxalone for intravenous immobilization of juvenile captive estuarine crocodiles (Crocodylus porosus) and Australian freshwater crocodiles (Crocodylus johnstoni) at optimal and selected sub-optimal thermal zones. *Vet. Anaesth. Analg.* 40: 494–502.

Ordodi, V.L., Mic, F.A., Mic, A.A. et al. (2005). A simple device for intubation of rats. *Lab. Anim.* 34: 37–39.

Orr, H.E., Roughan, J.V., and Flecknell, P.A. (2005). Assessment of ketamine and medetomidine anaesthesia in the domestic rabbit. *Vet. Anaesth. Analg.* 32: 271–279.

Parasrampuria, R., Vuppugalla, R., Elliott, K. et al. (2007). Route-dependent stereoselective pharmacokinetics of tramadol and its active O-demethylated metabolite in rats. *Chirality* 19: 190–196.

Pascoe, P.J., Pypendop, B.H., Pavez Phillips, J.C. et al. (2018). Pharmacokinetics of fentanyl after intravenous administration in isoflurane-anesthetized red-tailed hawks (*Buteo jamaicensis*) and Hispaniolan Amazon parrots (*Amazona ventralis*). *Am. J. Vet. Res.* 79: 606–613.

Paul-Murphy, J., Brunson, D.B., and Miletic, V. (1999). Analgesic effects of butorphanol and buprenorphine in conscious African grey parrots (Psittacus erithacus erithacus and Psittacus erithacus timneh). *Am. J. Vet. Res.* 60: 1218–1221.

Paul-Murphy, J., Hess, J., and Fialkowski, J.P. (2004). Pharmacokinetic properties of a single intramuscular dose of buprenorphine in African GREY PARROTS (Psittacus erithacus erithacus). *J. Avian Med. Surg.* 18: 224–228.

Paul-Murphy, J.R., Sladky, K.K., Krugner-Higby, L.A. et al. (2009). Analgesic effects of carprofen and liposome-encapsulated butorphanol tartrate in Hispaniolan parrots (Amazona ventralis) with experimentally induced arthritis. *Am. J. Vet. Res.* 70: 1201–1210.

Pavez, J.C., Hawkins, M.G., Pascoe, P.J. et al. (2011). Effect of fentanyl target-controlled infusions on isoflurane minimum anaesthetic concentration and cardiovascular function in red-tailed hawks (Buteo jamaicensis). *Vet. Anaesth. Analg.* 38: 344–351.

Phaneuf, L.R., Barker, S., Groleau, M.A. et al. (2006). Tracheal injury after endotracheal intubation and anesthesia in rabbits. *J. Am. Assoc. Lab. Anim. Sci.* 45: 67–72.

Phillips, B.E., Posner, L.P., Lewbart, G.A. et al. (2017). Effects of alfaxalone administered intravenously to healthy yearling loggerhead sea turtles (Caretta caretta) at three different doses. *J. Am. Vet. Med. Assoc.* 250: 909–917.

Pollock, C.G., Schumacher, J., Orosz, S.E. et al. (2001). Sedative effects of medetomidine in pigeons (Columba livia). *J. Avian Med. Surg.* 15: 95–100.

Quesada, R.J., Aitken-Palmer, C., Conley, K. et al. (2010). Accidental submeningeal injection of propofol in gopher tortoises (Gopherus polyphemus). *Vet. Rec.* 167: 494–495.

Quesada, R.J., McCleary, R.J., Heard, D.J. et al. (2014). Non-lethal sampling of liver tissue for toxicologic evaluation of Florida cottonmouths snakes (Agkistrodon piscivorus conanti). *Ecotoxicology* 23: 33–37.

Ren, J., Li, C., Ma, S. et al. (2018). Impact of dexmedetomidine on hemodynamics in rabbits. *Acta Cir. Bras.* 33: 314–323.

Rockhill, A.P., Chinnadurai, S.K., Powell, R.A. et al. (2011). A comparison of two field chemical immobilization techniques for bobcats (Lynx rufus). *J. Zoo Wildl. Med.* 42: 580–585.

Roughan, J.V. and Flecknell, P.A. (2001). Behavioural effects of laparotomy and analgesic effects of ketoprofen and carprofen in rats. *Pain.* 90 (1-2): 65–74.

Roughan, J.V. and Flecknell, P.A. (2003). Evaluation of a short duration behaviour-based post-operative pain scoring system in rats. *Eur. J. Pain* 7: 397–406.

Rozanska, D. (2009). Evaluation of medetomidine-midazolam-atropine (MeMiA) anesthesia maintained with propofol infusion in New Zealand White rabbits. *Pol. J. Vet. Sci.* 12: 209–216.

Saha, D.C., Saha, A.C., Malik, G. et al. (2007). Comparison of cardiovascular effects of tiletamine-zolazepam, pentobarbital, and ketamine-xylazine in male rats. *J. Am. Assoc. Lab. Anim. Sci.* 46: 74–80.

Sanchez-Migallon Guzman, D., Souza, M.J., Braun, J.M. et al. (2012). Antinociceptive effects after oral administration of tramadol hydrochloride in Hispaniolan Amazon parrots (Amazona ventralis). *Am. J. Vet. Res.* 73: 1148–1152.

Sandmeier, P. (2000). Evaluation of medetomidine for short-term immobilization of domestic pigeons (Columba livia) and Amazon parrots (Amazona species). *J. Avian Med. Surg.* 14: 8–14.

Santangelo, B., Ferrari, D., di Martino, I. et al. (2009). Dexmedetomidine chemical restraint in two raptor species undergoing inhalation anaesthesia. *Vet. Res. Commun.* 33: S209–S211.

Santangelo, B., Micieli, F., Marino, F. et al. (2016). Plasma concentrations and sedative effects of a dexmedetomidine, midazolam, and butorphanol combination after transnasal administration in healthy rabbits. *J. Vet. Pharmacol. Ther.* 39: 408–411.

Santos Gonzalez, M., Bertran de Lis, B.T., and Tendillo Cortijo, F.J. (2013). Effects of intramuscular alfaxalone alone or in combination with diazepam in swine. *Vet. Anaesth. Analg.* 40: 399–402.

Schernthaner, A., Lendl, C., Busch, R. et al. (2008). Clinical evaluation of three medetomidine-midazolam-ketamine combinations for neutering of ferrets (Mustela putorius furo). *Berl. Munch. Tierarztl. Wochenschr.* 121: 1–10.

Schnellbacher, R.W., Hernandez, S.M., Tuberville, T.D. et al. (2012). The efficacy of intranasal administration of dexmedetomidine and ketamine to yellow-bellied sliders (Trachemys scripta scripta). *J. Herp. Med. Surg.* 22: 91–98.

Schnellbacher, R.W., Divers, S.J., Comolli, J.R. et al. (2017). Effects of intravenous administration of lidocaine and buprenorphine on gastrointestinal tract motility and signs of pain in New Zealand White rabbits after ovariohysterectomy. *Am. J. Vet. Res.* 78: 1359–1371.

Schumacher, J., Citino, S.B., Hernandez, K. et al. (1997). Cardiopulmonary and anesthetic effects of propofol in wild turkeys. *Am. J. Vet. Res.* 58: 1014–1017.

Shepard, M.K., Divers, S., Braun, C. et al. (2013). Pharmacodynamics of alfaxalone after single-dose intramuscular administration in red-eared sliders (Trachemys scripta elegans): a comparison of two different doses at two different ambient temperatures. *Vet. Anaesth. Analg.* 40: 590–598.

Sinclair, K.M., Church, M.E., Farver, T.B. et al. (2012). Effects of meloxicam on hematologic and plasma biochemical analysis variables and results of histologic examination of tissue specimens of Japanese quail (Coturnix japonica). *Am. J. Vet. Res.* 73: 1720–1727.

Singh, P.M., Johnson, C., Gartrell, B. et al. (2010). Pharmacokinetics of morphine after intravenous administration in broiler chickens. *J. Vet. Pharmacol. Ther.* 33: 515–518.

Sladky, K.K., Miletic, V., Paul-Murphy, J. et al. (2007). Analgesic efficacy and respiratory effects of butorphanol and morphine in turtles. *J. Am. Vet. Med. Assoc.* 230: 1356–1362.

Sladky, K.K., Kinney, M.E., and Johnson, S.M. (2008). Analgesic efficacy of butorphanol and morphine in bearded dragons and corn snakes. *J. Am. Vet. Med. Assoc.* 233: 267–273.

Sleeman, J.M. and Gaynor, J. (2000). Sedative and cardiopulmonary effects of medetomidine and reversal with atipamezole in desert tortoises (Gopherus agassizii). *J. Zoo Wildl. Med.* 31: 28–35.

Smith, J.C., Robertson, L.D., Auhll, A. et al. (2004). Endotracheal tubes versus laryngeal mask airways in rabbit inhalation anesthesia: ease of use and waste gas emissions. *Contemp. Top. Lab. Anim. Sci.* 43: 22–25.

Souza, M.J., Greenacre, C.B., and Cox, S.K. (2008). Pharmacokinetics of orally administered tramadol in domestic rabbits (Oryctolagus cuniculus). *Am. J. Vet. Res.* 69: 979–982.

Souza, M.J., Martin-Jimenez, T., Jones, M.P. et al. (2009). Pharmacokinetics of intravenous and oral tramadol in the bald eagle (Haliaeetus leucocephalus). *J. Avian Med. Surg.* 23: 247–252.

Souza, M.J., Martin-Jimenez, T., Jones, M.P. et al. (2011). Pharmacokinetics of oral tramadol in red-tailed hawks (Buteo jamaicensis). *J. Vet. Pharmacol. Ther.* 34: 86–88.

Souza, M.J., Sanchez-Migallon Guzman, D., Paul-Murphy, J.R. et al. (2012). Pharmacokinetics after oral and intravenous administration of a single dose of tramadol hydrochloride to Hispaniolan Amazon parrots (Amazona ventralis). *Am. J. Vet. Res.* 73: 1142–1147.

Spadola, F., Morici, M., and Knotek, Z. (2015). Combination of lidocaine/prilocaine with tramadol for short time anaesthesia-analgesia in chelonians: 18 cases. *Acta Vet. Brno* 84: 71–75.

Stoskopf, M.K., Meyer, R.E., Jones, M. et al. (1999). Field immobilization and euthanasia of American opossum. *J. Wildl. Dis.* 35: 145–149.

Swarup, D., Patra, R.C., Prakash, V. et al. (2007). Safety of meloxicam to critically endangered Gyps vultures and other scavenging birds in India. *Anim. Conserv.* 10: 192–198.

Sykes, J.M., Neiffer, D., Terrell, S. et al. (2013). Review of 23 cases of postintubation tracheal obstructions in birds. *J. Zoo Wildl. Med.* 44: 700–713.

Tamura, J., Ishizuka, T., Fukui, S. et al. (2015a). Sedative effects of intramuscular alfaxalone administered to cats. *J. Vet. Med. Sci.* 77: 897–904.

Tamura, J., Ishizuka, T., Fukui, S. et al. (2015b). The pharmacological effects of the anesthetic alfaxalone after intramuscular administration to dogs. *J. Vet. Med. Sci.* 77: 289–296.

Tearney, C.C., Barter, L.S., and Pypendop, B.H. (2015). Cardiovascular effects of equipotent doses of isoflurane alone and isoflurane plus fentanyl in New Zealand white rabbits (Oryctolagus cuniculus). *Am. J. Vet. Res.* 76: 591–598.

Trkova, S., Knotkova, Z., Hrda, A. et al. (2007). Effect of non-steroidal anti-inflammatory drugs on the blood profile in the green iguana (Iguana iguana). *Vet. Med.* 11: 507–511.

Turner, P.V., Chen, H.C., and Taylor, W.M. (2006a). Pharmacokinetics of meloxicam in rabbits after single and repeat oral dosing. *Comp. Med.* 56: 63–67.

Turner, P.V., Kerr, C.L., Healy, A.J. et al. (2006b). Effect of meloxicam and butorphanol on minimum alveolar concentration of isoflurane in rabbits. *Am. J. Vet. Res.* 67: 770–774.

Tuttle, A.D., Papich, M., Lewbart, G.A. et al. (2006). Pharmacokinetics of ketoprofen in the green iguana (Iguana iguana) following single intravenous and intramuscular injections. *J. Zoo Wildl. Med.* 37: 567–570.

Tutunaru, A.C., Sonea, A., Drion, P. et al. (2013). Anaesthetic induction with alfaxalone may produce hypoxemia in rabbits premedicated with fentanyl/droperidol. *Vet. Anaesth. Analg.* 40: 657–659.

Uzun, M., Onder, F., Atalan, G. et al. (2006). Effects of xylazine, medetomidine, detomidine, and diazepam on sedation, heart and respiratory rates, and cloacal temperature in rock partridges (Alectoris graeca). *J. Zoo Wildl. Med.* 37: 135–140.

Valle, M., Garrido, M.J., Pavon, J.M. et al. (2000). Pharmacokinetic-pharmacodynamic modeling of the antinociceptive effects of main active metabolites of tramadol, (+)-O-desmethyltramadol and (−)-O-desmethyltramadol, in rats. *J. Pharmacol. Exp. Ther.* 293: 646–653.

Varner, J., Clifton, K.R., Poulos, S. et al. (2004). Lack of efficacy of injectable ketamine with xylazine or diazepam for anesthesia in chickens. *Lab. Anim.* 33: 36–39.

Vergari, A., Gunnella, B., Rodola, F. et al. (2004). A new method of orotracheal intubation in mice. *Eur. Rev. Med. Pharmacol. Sci.* 8: 103–106.

Vesal, N. and Eskandari, M.H. (2006). Sedative effects of midazolam and xylazine with or without ketamine and detomidine alone following intranasal administration in Ring-necked Parakeets. *J. Am. Vet. Med. Assoc.* 228: 383–388.

Vesal, N. and Zare, P. (2006). Clinical evaluation of intranasal benzodiazepines, alpha-agonists and their antagonists in canaries. *Vet. Anaesth. Analg.* 33: 143–148.

Villaverde-Morcillo, S., Benito, J., Garcia-Sanchez, R. et al. (2014). Comparison of isoflurane and alfaxalone (Alfaxan) for the induction of anesthesia in flamingos (Phoenicopterus roseus) undergoing orthopedic surgery. *J. Zoo Wildl. Med.* 45: 361–366.

Wambugu, S.N., Towett, P.K., Kiama, S.G. et al. (2010). Effects of opioids in the formalin test in the Speke's hinged tortoise (Kinixys spekii). *J. Vet. Pharmacol. Ther.* 33: 347–351.

Warne, L.N., Beths, T., Whittem, T. et al. (2015). A review of the pharmacology and clinical application of alfaxalone in cats. *Vet. J.* 203: 141–148.

Waugh, L., Knych, H., Cole, G., and d'Agostino, J. (2016). Pharmacokinetic evaluation of a long-acting fentanyl solution after transdermal administration in helmeted guineafowl (Numida meleagris). *J. Zoo Wildl. Med.* 47: 468–473.

Waxman, S., Orozco, M., and Argibay, H. (2018). Comparison of two protocols for field immobilization of white-eared opossums (Didelphis albiventris). *Eur J Wildlife Res* 64 (4): 49.

Weiland, L.C., Kluge, K., Kutter, A.P.N. et al. (2017). Clinical evaluation of intranasal medetomidine-ketamine and medetomidine-S(+)-ketamine for induction of anaesthesia in rabbits in two centres with two different administration techniques. *Vet. Anaesth. Analg.* 44: 98–105.

Welberg, L.A., Kinkead, B., Thrivikraman, K. et al. (2006). Ketamine-xylazine-acepromazine anesthesia and postoperative recovery in rats. *J. Am. Assoc. Lab. Anim. Sci.* 45: 13–20.

Wellehan, J.F., Gunkel, C.I., Kledzik, D. et al. (2006). Use of a nerve locator to facilitate administration of mandibular nerve blocks in crocodilians. *J. Zoo Wildl. Med.* 37: 405–408.

Williamson, R.H., Muller, L.I., and Blair, C.D. (2018). The use of ketamine-xylazine or butorphanol-azaperone-medetoidine to immobilize American black bears (Ursus americanus). *J. Wildl. Dis.* 54: 503–510.

Wilson, H.G., Hernandez-Divers, S., and Budsberg, S.C. (2004). Pharmacokinetics and use of meloxican in psittacine birds. *Proc. Ann. Conf. Assoc. Avian Vet* 7–9.

Wu, W.N., McKown, L.A., Codd, E.E. et al. (2006). Metabolism of two analgesic agents, tramadol-n-oxide and tramadol, in specific pathogen-free and axenic mice. *Xenobiotica* 36: 551–565.

Yaw, T.J., Mans, C., Johnson, S.M. et al. (2018). Effect of injection site on alfaxalone induced sedation in ball pythons (Python regius). *J. Small Anim. Pract.* 59: 747–751.

Zehnder, A.M., Hawkins, M.G., Pascoe, P.J. et al. (2009). Evaluation of indirect blood pressure monitoring in awake and anesthetized red-tailed hawks (Buteo jamaicensis): effects of cuff size, cuff placement, and monitoring equipment. *Vet. Anaesth. Analg.* 36: 464–479.

Zhao, Y., Tao, T., Wu, J. et al. (2008). Pharmacokinetics of tramadol in rat plasma and cerebrospinal fluid after intranasal administration. *J. Pharm. Pharmacol.* 60: 1149–1154.

Ziolo, M.S. and Bertelsen, M.F. (2009). Effects of propofol administered via the supravertebral sinus in red-eared sliders. *J. Am. Vet. Med. Assoc.* 234: 390–393.

Zollinger, T.J., Hoover, J.P., Payton, M.E. et al. (2011). Clinicopathologic, gross necropsy, and histologic findings after intramuscular injection of carprofen in a pigeon (Columba livia) model. *J. Avian Med. Surg.* 25: 173–184.

6

Care of Oiled Wildlife

Florina S. Tseng[1] and Michael Ziccardi[2]

[1] Wildlife Clinic, Cummings School of Veterinary Medicine, Tufts University, North Grafton, MA, USA
[2] Oiled Wildlife Care Network and Wildlife Health Center, Karen C. Drayer Wildlife Health Center, School of Veterinary Medicine, University of California, Davis, CA, USA

Introduction

Petroleum, either as crude oil or a refined product, is transported worldwide via ships, pipelines, and land-based transport. Wildlife may encounter petroleum in its various forms through a number of different scenarios along the pathway – from extraction to consumer delivery, from tanker spills and platform blowouts to accidents at refineries and pipeline breaks. Whatever the cause, oiling of wildlife can result in external and internal effects as a result of both the physical properties of the petroleum product and the toxic components in oil (such as polycyclic aromatic hydrocarbons, or PAHs). Animals not obviously coated with oil may still be affected through inhalation of petroleum vapors or ingestion of oil while feeding or preening.

The Effects of Oil on Wildlife

Birds

The majority of wildlife observed to be affected by oil spills are birds living in the marine environment – specifically seabirds, waterfowl, and shorebirds. Alcids, loons, grebes, and diving ducks tend to be frequently oiled in large numbers and may survive long enough to be brought in for rehabilitation. However, these obligate aquatic species tend to have poorer survival rates during the rehabilitation process than those species with a semi-terrestrial life style. In general, large and/or hardy species, especially those captured soon after oiling, will have the greatest chance of successful rehabilitation leading to release. These species are able to withstand longer periods of fasting, become hypothermic more slowly, and are more likely to be captured before they succumb to the effects of oiling. Many smaller species rarely reach shore or, if they do, are easily predated upon. Birds that nest, roost or feed in groups, especially those with a more generalized diet, are also more likely to survive the rehabilitation process to eventual release due to experiencing less stress in captivity when housed with others of the same species (Helm et al. 2015).

External Effects

Both crude and refined petroleum products affect birds externally in a similar manner. Oiled feathers quickly lose their waterproofing and insulating properties, resulting in loss of buoyancy and subsequent hypothermia (Jenssen and Ekker 1988; Albers 1995). Thus, affected birds may drown at sea or, if they are able to make it to shore, are vulnerable to starvation and predation. In addition, oiled birds spend more time preening, have difficulty foraging for prey, have decreased flight capacity, and have an increased metabolic rate due to heat loss. These difficulties often lead to dehydration and malnutrition exhibited first through loss of body fat and then, subsequently, muscle wasting (Hartung 1967; Holmes et al. 1978; Leighton 1991). Contact with highly volatile refined fuels can also result in varying degrees of skin and corneal burns (Helm et al. 2015).

Internal Effects

Ingested or inhaled petroleum products can result in a variety of acute and long-term health effects. Ingested oils can result in irritation and erosion of the mucosal lining of the gastrointestinal tract, resulting in bleeding, decreased nutrient uptake, and dehydration from ensuing diarrhea (Fry and Lowenstein 1985; Briggs et al. 1996; Tseng 1999). Biotransformation of toxic compounds by the liver can lead to cellular damage and functional impairment, thus decreasing the ability of the liver to

Medical Management of Wildlife Species: A Guide for Practitioners, First Edition. Edited by Sonia M. Hernandez,
Heather W. Barron, Erica A. Miller, Roberto F. Aguilar and Michael J. Yabsley.
© 2020 John Wiley & Sons, Inc. Published 2020 by John Wiley & Sons, Inc.

further detoxify substances (Fry and Lowenstein 1985; Harvey and Brown 1991). Oxidative damage from exposure to PAH forms metabolites that can lead to hemolytic anemia (Leighton et al. 1985; Troisi et al. 2007) and liver impairment via hemochromatosis (Balseiro et al. 2005). Impaired renal function and dehydration are associated with PAH exposure and can potentially result in elevated blood uric acid levels and visceral gout (Fry 1985). Inhalation of volatile fumes may lead to lesions within the upper or lower portions of the respiratory tract.

Serum chemistry values in birds exposed to oil reflect acute liver and kidney damage with increases in aspartate aminotransferase, lactic dehydrogenase, and gamma-glutamyl transferase (Alonso-Alvarez et al. 2007). Muscle wasting may lead to increases in creatine phosphokinase and lactate dehydrogenase. Serum protein levels reflect various factors such as starvation, impaired liver function, stress, and secondary infectious processes.

Adult seabirds exposed to oil in the breeding season may have reproductive failures due to stress, alterations in reproductive hormone levels, abnormal egg formation, decreased or delayed egg laying, nest abandonment, and decreased chick and/or fledging success (Holmes et al. 1981; Leighton 1993).

Captivity-Related Abnormalities

Wild animals are vulnerable to problems associated with being held in captivity. Stress alone results in immune suppression, which can make these animals more susceptible to secondary infectious diseases such as aspergillosis (Figure 6.1). In addition, captivity-related stress can inhibit normal feeding behavior, thus exacerbating problems with malnutrition and dehydration, delay healing from any injuries, and eventually lead to adrenal failure (Rattner et al. 1984).

Because many seabirds are unable to support themselves upright on solid surfaces, inappropriate housing of these species can lead to pressure sores on areas such as the keel (Figure 6.2), feet, and hock joints. Feathers can become soiled with feces and urates if birds are allowed to rest directly on their droppings, resulting in further problems with waterproofing. Finally, housing large numbers of immunosuppressed birds together increases the likelihood of pathogen transmission.

Marine Mammals

Different classes of marine mammals will experience the external effects of oiling in different ways. Those that are heavily furred, such as sea otters, polar bears, and fur seals, rely on their thick coats in order to maintain normal body temperatures and buoyancy in their aquatic

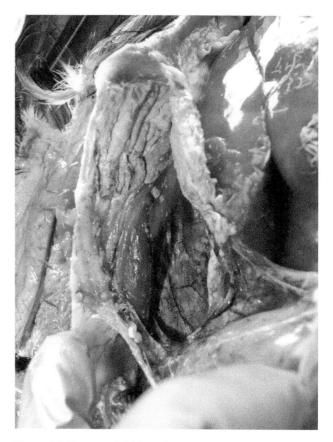

Figure 6.1 Plaque and thickened air sacs on gross necropsy. The lesion is characteristic of avian aspergillosis.

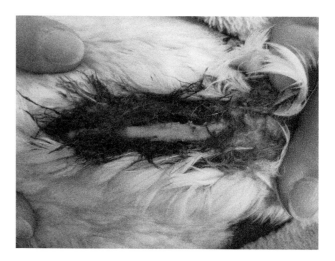

Figure 6.2 Pressure-induced keel lesion on a common mure.

environments. As with oiled seabirds, any disruption in this fur coating allows cold seawater to seep in and can result in hypothermia. Oiled, heavily furred marine mammals will attempt to groom this oil off, resulting in ingestion of the petroleum product. Internal effects of oil exposure are similar to those seen with avian species.

In contrast, those marine mammals that rely on a thick blubber layer (such as true seals, manatees, and cetaceans) are less vulnerable to the external effects of oiling. Ingestion may cause acute and chronic injuries, but the more likely exposure route for this class of animals is through feeding behaviors. Inhaled volatile fumes, however, have been proven to lead to injuries to the respiratory tract, especially in deep-diving mammal species due to their explosive nature of inhalation at the air–water interface (Schwacke et al. 2013; Venn-Watson et al. 2015).

Other Mammalian Species

It is less common for other mammal species to become exposed to oil, but this may occur with mammalian scavengers feeding along shorelines or with mammals exposed in inland spills. For instance, aquatic mammals such as beaver, river otter or muskrat may be exposed in freshwater oil spills and terrestrial mammals may contact oil in their drinking sources.

There is much less specific information available about the effects of oil on nonmarine mammal species, although mink have been studied as a model for the effects of oil on sea otters. Chronic oral exposure to low concentrations of bunker C fuel oil causes development of adrenal hypertrophy in ranch mink (Mohr et al. 2010). Mink that were exposed to bunker C fuel oil in their diets had reduced reproductive success (Mazet et al. 2001). In addition, ingestion of fuel oil was associated with a decrease in erythrocyte numbers, hematocrit, and hemoglobin concentration. Total leukocytes were elevated from increases in neutrophils, lymphocytes, and monocytes (Schwartz et al. 2004).

Reptiles and Amphibians

Most of the information concerning the effects of oil on reptiles is related to exposure in sea turtles. Sea turtles are highly sensitive to oil and, unfortunately, much of their habitat overlaps with areas of oil extraction and transport. Sea turtles are vulnerable to the effects of oil because some of their behaviors, such as indiscriminate feeding choices and large predive inhalations, place them at particular risk for oil exposure. Oil effects on sea turtles include increased egg mortality and developmental defects and direct mortality due to oiling in hatchlings, juveniles, and adults. Morbidity and mortality can result from impacts on skin, gastrointestinal and respiratory tracts, the immune system, and salt glands (Milton et al. 2010).

While less reported in the literature, amphibians are especially vulnerable to environmental contaminants, given the permeability of their skin to water and other substances in their aquatic habitats. A study on the effects of freshwater petroleum contamination on amphibian reproduction demonstrated that, although hatching success was not measurably affected by the presence of oil, no tadpoles successfully metamorphosed from the highest concentrations of oil treatments (Mahaney 1994).

Oiled Wildlife Response: From Recovery to Release

The practice of oiled wildlife response has slowly evolved in the past 50 years from an activity undertaken by small nonprofit organizations with no external support to one that is fully enmeshed into the overall oil spill response effort (Mazet et al. 2002). In the United States, this progress has matched that seen after the *Exxon Valdez* oil spill in 1989, with a more organized and deliberate response effort as dictated by the Oil Pollution Act of 1990 (OPA90). Oil spill responses in the United States now are performed under a structured Incident Command System (ICS). Wildlife response falls under the Wildlife Branch within the Operations Section, while also working closely with other sections under the ICS. An important component of any oil spill response under the ICS is maintaining an awareness of human health and safety throughout the process.

Oiled wildlife responses that involve more than just a few animals necessitate a herd health approach to care. This approach is used in all phases of the response including initial triage, housing, and nutrition guidelines, medical care, and release criteria. The veterinarian plays a critical role in making these decisions in a way that provides consistent, humane care while allowing the rehabilitation process to proceed in an orderly and timely manner.

Because avian species represent the majority of wildlife affected during oil spills, most of this section will be devoted to their care during a spill response. Key differences in approach with other species (particularly marine mammals) will be called out where needed.

Capture and Initial Stabilization

During spill events, most oiled wildlife is captured during search and collection efforts by government agency personnel or by trained and experienced wildlife responders from rehabilitation groups. These personnel must accurately record field data such as date, time, location of capture, species, and name of person responsible for the capture. There may be additional legal requirements for field collection (such as the possibility of starting "chain of custody" procedures immediately), so consult regulatory agency personnel prior to deployment.

Ideally, live oiled animals should either be stabilized *in situ* or quickly taken to a field stabilization site, where initial first aid can be administered. During stabilization, animals should be assessed to determine body temperatures. Normal cloacal temperatures for avian species usually range from 38.9 to 40.6 °C (102–105 °F) (Walraven 1992), while sea otters range between 37.5 and 38.1 °C (99.5–100.6 °F) and pinnipeds from 36.7 to 38.9 °C (98–102 °F) (OWCN 2014). If the animal is hypo- or hyperthermic, methods to restore normal core body temperature should be undertaken. Instant heating or cooling gel packs wrapped in towels may be placed in the transport container. The containers are then placed in a sheltered area with regulated environmental temperatures to encourage heating or cooling. Most birds are gavaged oral electrolyte solutions while at the field stabilization site in order to begin the rehydration process.

Treatment of mammals depends on patient mentation status and the handling capabilities of the staff. If severely debilitated, subcutaneous or intravenous fluids can be started in mammal stabilization, but often wait until reaching the primary care facility due to the need for sedation and/or anesthesia. Large amounts of oil are wiped away from the eyes, nares, or glottis and any other life-threatening conditions are addressed.

Transportation

After initial field stabilization procedures have occurred, oiled wildlife should be transported to the main rehabilitation facility as quickly as possible. Transport containers and vehicles should provide free air exchange and allow temperature regulation to assist in thermoregulation of affected animals. Visual and auditory stimuli should be minimized in order to decrease any captivity-related stress. All animals should be monitored frequently during transport to detect any potential problems, such as overheating.

Intake Procedures

A standardized intake protocol should be in place since, in many circumstances, legal evidence must be obtained. As each oiled animal is brought to the intake station, it is individually identified with a leg band, tag, or other means, and a feather sample or fur swab is taken for proof of oiling. Oftentimes, a photograph of the animal is also taken at intake. These items are collected and stored to maintain appropriate "chain of custody." Threatened and endangered species, or those that require immediate medical care, are prioritized for care. Oiled animals then undergo a thorough physical examination, noting the extent of oiling and signs of hypothermia, dehydration, and malnutrition. For many mammals, this evaluation will require sedation or anesthesia to allow complete exam and sampling to occur. Blood samples are drawn in order to provide, at a minimum, packed cell volume (PCV) and a total protein level but can include complete blood counts and serum/plasma chemistries if medically warranted. All of these data are noted in individual records for each oiled animal.

Oiled animals are triaged at this point into those individuals that should be humanely euthanized, those that require more extensive veterinary care, or those that can be housed with the general population of admitted animals. Some of the considerations that are taken into account during triage include individual animal factors that may predict survival (such as blood values, nutritional status, hydration status, traumatic injuries, and age) and general factors (such as species status and historical success rate of that species in rehabilitation) (OWCN 2014).

Housing

The physical facility should be designed in such a way as to maximize efficient flow of people and animals, while minimizing the possibility of disease spread. Any animals suspected of having an infectious disease of herd or zoonotic importance should be quarantined if at all possible. Treatment of an individual animal with an infectious disease may not be possible in a large spill response, and humane euthanasia may be necessary to protect the population.

Good ventilation is needed to reduce irritating petroleum fumes and the potential for immune-suppressed animals to develop respiratory disease. Of particular concern is the potential for aspergillosis in oiled seabirds. Ten to fifteen air changes per hour have been recommended for indoor animal-holding spaces. Most bird facilities are kept at approximately 26.7 °C (80 °F) in order for them to more easily maintain normothermia, but all facilities should have the ability to adjust and maintain indoor temperatures up to this level while maintaining ventilation status.

Avoiding captivity-related problems prior to cleaning with appropriate housing is important. Certain aquatic bird species, such as loons, grebes, alcids, and sea ducks, should be housed on "net bottomed" caging (Holcomb 1988). These are cages with netting as the flooring surface. They allow for a more even weight distribution for these birds on their ventral surfaces, and for feces and urates to drop through onto easily replaced substrate below the cage. Mammal enclosure requirements may be affected by such factors as the animal's species, age, physical condition, degree of oiling, and nature of the product with which it was oiled. However, all should be constructed using safe materials that can be easily disinfected, and designed to be escape-proof.

In addition to separate housing for oiled and cleaned wildlife, a designated facility should have adequate indoor space and capabilities for intake, veterinary services, quarantine, necropsy, cleaning (washing, rinsing, and drying), food preparation, and storage. It should also have meeting areas for volunteers and staff. Species-appropriate outdoor pens, pools, and aviaries should be set up in order to evaluate waterproofing, diving capability and other behaviors before release.

Nutritional Support

Most oiled animals are dehydrated and malnourished when captured and first admitted into the rehabilitation facility. All oil-exposed birds with normal PCV and total protein levels are typically gavage-fed high-calorie nutritional slurries (such as Emeraid® Exotic Nutritional Care products; LaFeber, Cornell, IL) in combination with crystalloid solutions up to 6–8 times daily, with volumes dependent on species, size, and health status. Particular care must be taken with birds having low total protein values (<2.0 g/dL), with only an easily digestible enteral product being used as the nutritional slurry. Once the total protein levels have risen and the bird shows no signs of regurgitation, it can be gradually moved onto more standard nutritional slurry diet feedings. Debilitated and unweaned marine mammals require specially designed formulas given via gavage feeding, the details of which are beyond the scope of this chapter (Dierauf and Gulland 2001). While these feedings result in much handling and stress, they are necessary procedures until the animals are self-feeding and showing weight gain.

Whole food items can be carefully added to the diet as the patient progresses through rehabilitation. Shallow small pans (sized so that birds cannot climb into them) containing nonoily small fish (whitebait or smelt) may be provided in daylight hours to piscivorous species. Clean, nonoiled birds can be carefully hand-fed fish while housed out of pools but are not left with food in their pens, which might soil their feathers. Sea otters and pinnipeds should be provided whole food items if stable and weaned, the composition of which is specific to the species. After being moved into pools, wildlife should be supplemented with salt and multivitamins following standard rehabilitation guidelines for the species. All animals must be observed for self-feeding and weighed regularly (daily if possible, but definitely whenever handled) during the rehabilitation process.

Medical Considerations

Veterinarians play an important role in oiled wildlife response. Because many of the oiled animals are hypo- or hyperthermic, dehydrated, malnourished, and/or anemic when captured, it is important to address these problems throughout the rehabilitation process. Triage decisions as to whether an individual is too moribund to proceed with any further rehabilitation effort will need to be made and euthanasia should be considered. Examples of conditions that generally warrant euthanasia include animals with irreparable fractures, permanently impaired vision, or inability to fly, dive, or ambulate normally. Only euthanasia procedures approved by the AVMA should be used (AVMA 2013). If legally permissible, it is highly recommended that gross necropsies and full sampling (for both histopathology and petroleum hydrocarbon analyses) of animals that have died or been euthanized take place. These necropsies may assist the veterinarian in determining causes of morbidity and mortality, thus allowing for more refined treatment protocols of the remaining animals.

A common mistake in the rehabilitation of oiled birds and heavily furred mammals is to wash newly admitted animals before they are physiologically stable. Because the washing process is rigorous and stressful, and because these species commonly experience thermoregulatory issues that increase metabolic requirements, stabilization with warmth, fluids, and nutritive support for a period of time is necessary in order for animals to be appropriately stabilized prior to washing (Tseng 1999). Other species, such as pinnipeds (aside from fur seals) and sea turtles, may be able to be immediately cleaned on intake if blood work and initial exam show no abnormalities beyond the physical coating.

Medical problems associated with exposure to highly refined fuels can be difficult to treat directly. Inhalant pneumonia or emphysema has been observed in both birds and mammals, and affected animals will exhibit respiratory difficulty, abnormal lung sounds on auscultation, and characteristic signs of fluid infiltration, lung masses, or bullae on radiography. As an example of this, bottlenose dolphins (*Tursiops truncatus*) in Barataria Bay, Louisiana, in the years following the Deepwater Horizon/Macondo oil spill (2010) were found to have a significantly higher incidence of moderate to severe lung disease, as well as adrenal hormone imbalances and decreased survival (Schwacke et al. 2013). If captured, it is helpful to begin these animals on prophylactic antibiotic and antifungal medications, house them in oxygen cages (if appropriate and available), and provide good supportive care. Skin burns present a special problem in aquatic birds, as the serous exudate from these wounds and feather loss in these areas result in loss of waterproofing. These burns should be thoroughly cleansed with a dilute antiseptic solution and a water-soluble topical antibiotic product can be applied. As is the case with any bird, and especially those involved in oil spill incidents, the use of petroleum-based ointments should be avoided in order to prevent further feather contamination and disruption of waterproofing. Lastly, volatile products can produce significant damage to ocular tissues and sensitive mucous membranes if not removed.

If a product is highly volatile, it may be necessary to give the animal an initial "quick wash" in order to remove the bulk of the oil and reduce inhalant and contact problems. This "quick wash" should take five minutes or less in order to reduce the stress on an already compromised animal. For birds, this wash consists of baths in several tubs of a 1–2% Dawn® (Procter & Gamble, Cincinnati, OH) solution, followed by a rinse to remove most of the soap. The bird must then be completely dried and reenter the standard stabilization process, where a complete cleaning can be done at a later date.

Once an assessment is made of the extent of dehydration, individual animals can be appropriately treated. It is assumed that the average oiled bird that comes into the rehabilitation facility is approximately 8–10% dehydrated, and mammals come in at least 5% dehydrated. See Chapter 4 for fluid therapy protocols.

Gastrointestinal disturbances can further exacerbate dehydration through continued fluid losses from regurgitation and diarrhea. Intestinal protectants, such as bismuth subsalicylate (Peptobismol®, Procter & Gamble, Cincinnati, OH), have been used in spills with some success (Frink and Miller 1993). Similarly, the oral administration of an activated charcoal/kaolin slurry (Toxiban®, Lloyd Inc., Shenandoah, IA) at 6 mL/kg orally has been suggested to adsorb petroleum hydrocarbons, but it is unclear if the effectiveness of this product extends beyond the kaolin protectant aspects. The provision of appropriate rehydration and nutritional slurries will also help to decrease gastrointestinal abnormalities resulting from ingestion of oil.

Anemia and hypoproteinemia, either as a direct effect of crude oil or indirectly from other factors such as stress, malnutrition, and chronic disease, may be a factor in the medical treatment of oiled animals. This may also be a significant complicating factor in the chemical immobilization of marine mammals necessary to safely examine and clean the animal. Treatment of underlying disease states will aid in the resolution of this anemia. In addition, supplementation with appropriate commercial vitamins, such as Mazuri® Auklet vitamins for fish-eating birds (PMI Nutrition International, LLC, St Louis, MO), is recommended. During prewash rehabilitation, oiled birds have blood samples taken for routine checks on PCV and total protein levels approximately every 2–3 days in order to assess their readiness to undergo the next phase in their rehabilitation. Marine mammals and sea turtles typically have complete blood counts (CBCs) and serum chemistry panels conducted and reviewed prior to being approved for cleaning.

Because fungal respiratory diseases are often seen in oil spill responses, prophylactic antifungals may be used (e.g., itraconazole up to 20 mg/kg PO once a day, dependent on the species) (Tell et al. 2005).

Wash/Rinse/Drying Procedures

Birds are usually stabilized for at least 48 hours in captivity prior to the wash, then evaluated by trained personnel to determine if they are physically able to withstand the stressful washing and rinsing procedures. Criteria used to determine if a bird is ready to be washed include an alert attitude, stabilization for at least 48 hours and a normalization of blood parameters. Similarly, marine mammals and sea turtles need to be physiologically stable prior to cleaning but, due to the risks of repeated immobilization and lesser concerns over hypothermia in many species, cleaning can often occur immediately following intake examination.

Oiled animals are always washed by at least two people, a holder and a washer. Large or aggressive animals should be washed by at least three people. Wash personnel should wear appropriate protective clothing, such as waterproof aprons, gloves, boots, and safety goggles. Dawn dishwashing detergent (Procter & Gamble, Cincinnati, OH) has been shown to be the most effective detergent for oil removal (Bryndza et al. 1993). Birds or smaller animals are washed in multiple tubs containing a 1–2% Dawn solution in water heated to and maintained at physiologically normal temperatures. For larger mammals, more concentrated dishwashing liquid solutions (1–4% in otters and fur seals, full strength in other pinnipeds, cetaceans, and sea turtles) are used and poured directly on the pelage/skin for manual agitation. Regular monitoring of rectal or core body temperature in mammals, when logistically feasible, is required to ensure hypothermia does not occur. However, in all instances, handlers should closely observe animals for obvious signs of distress and temperature fluctuations.

Birds/smaller animals are moved from one bath to the next as each tub becomes oily until the animal no longer has any oil on it and the tub water is clean. In birds, the detergent solution is moved through the feathers by lifting the contour feathers away from the body with a gentle against-the-grain stroking (Figure 6.3). The stiff feathers of the wings and tail are gently worked free of oil by manually massaging the feathers in the direction of the feather shafts. In mammals, the detergent solution is manually massaged into the pelage using the fingers until the material coming off the fur/skin is only a white mixture of detergent and water. In all species, the head is carefully cleaned using a soft toothbrush and Waterpik® (Waterpik Inc., Fort Collins, CO) (if available), taking care not to get soap into the eyes, nares/nostrils/blowhole, and ears.

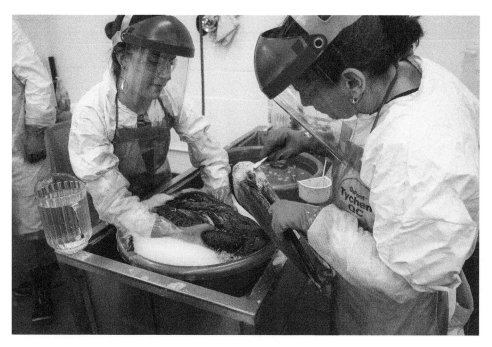

Figure 6.3 A brown pelican being washed.

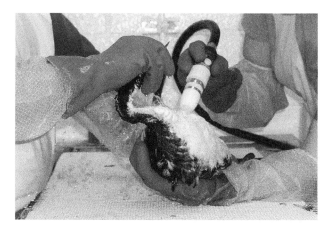

Figure 6.4 A Western grebe on its back, being rinsed, with water beading off.

Safe animal handling should always be practiced. Handlers should work quickly and efficiently, trying to keep the noise level down.

Animals are then rinsed with water heated to physiologically normal temperatures using an adjustable high-pressure nozzle (so that the water pressure can reach 40–60 psi) (Figure 6.4). This water pressure is needed to efficiently rinse the detergent from the feathers or underfur. For birds and heavily furred mammals, it is also recommended that rinse water be 2–5 grains hardness. If the water is softer, it is not effective in rinsing the detergent. If the water is harder, the minerals in the water will bind with microscopic amounts of detergent and can cause calcium carbonate crystals to form in the feathers/fur, which can lead to waterproofing problems (Clumpner 1991). For the same reason, it is recommended that birds/furred mammals be placed into outdoor pools of similar hardness when initially moved outside (at least for the first 24–48 hours). When birds/furred mammals are adequately rinsed, the water will "bead" off the feathers/pelage in small droplets, rather than being absorbed.

After animals are completely clean, birds and furred mammals are then allowed to dry before introducing them into appropriate enclosures or pens. Birds are placed into clean enclosures; larger birds (>500 g body weight) can use a net-bottomed cage while smaller birds can use wall cages or smaller enclosed habitats in which the ambient air temperature has been heated (larger pens with a warm air pet dryer to 32–35 °C [90–95 °F], smaller enclosures with a heat lamp). Heavily furred mammals typically are dried manually using towels and pet groomer dryers if under anesthesia, while other pinnipeds are allowed to dry using ambient conditions in their pen. All animals that are susceptible to hypo- or hyperthermia must be checked frequently for overheating as they dry. The drying time will vary by species, with small birds drying in as little as 30 minutes and larger birds, such as loons, taking as long as three hours.

Waterproofing Considerations

Once animals are thoroughly cleaned and dried, they should be moved into appropriate enclosures (typically outdoor pools, aviaries, or pens) as soon as possible

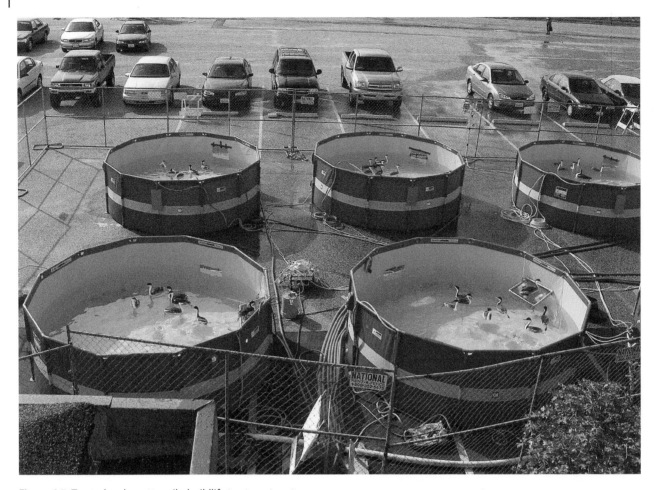

Figure 6.5 Treated grebes at an oiled wildlife treatment center.

(Figure 6.5). For all aquatic animals, it is essential that pools be of sufficient size and depth to allow accurate determination of diving behavior, feeding habits, and waterproofing status. For example, larger pelagic birds should be housed in pools at least 12 ft in diameter and at least 36 in. in depth, while cetaceans require pools of 24 ft or greater in diameter and water depths of one-half body length or 36 in., whichever is greater (Gage 2009). The water quality in pools containing birds and heavily furred mammals must be impeccable in order to prevent further contamination of feathers/fur by oily feces and fish. This is most easily accomplished by having clean water flowing over the pool surface at all times, which serves to skim debris from the surface, in combination with physical filtration means (e.g., sand filters).

When obligate aquatic animals are not waterproof in cold-water pools, water will penetrate to the level of the skin and result in hypothermia and behaviors such as shivering, agitation, excessive preening/grooming, and attempts to haul out of the pool. If any animal exhibits these signs, it must be removed from the pool and

evaluated to determine a cause. Possible causes of inadequate waterproofing include washing-related (inadequate removal of oil, inadequate rinsing of detergent), animal-related (damaged, stripped or missing feathers/fur, or burns and/or wounds that are seeping serous exudate) or pool-related problems (pool water of inappropriate softness or dirty pool water) (OWCN 2014). Steps must be taken to correct any of these underlying problems before animals are again tested for waterproofing.

Release Considerations

Rehabilitated oiled wildlife should be released when their status approximates "normal." Release criteria usually include, at a minimum, normal feeding, swimming, and diving behaviors along with body weights within 10% of normal for the species. In addition, the animal must be waterproof (if warranted), have normal hematology and serum chemistry values and show resolution of any other abnormalities. Certain wildlife species, such as cetaceans, have specific, more rigorous requirements that must be met prior to release, such as auditory assessments (Gage 2009). Physical conditioning may be difficult to assess in captivity, especially in diving animals. Prior to release, animals should ideally be marked with a permanent tag, metal leg band, or other means of identification in order to provide postrelease survival or mortality data. Other means of postrelease monitoring, such as the use of telemetry, are ideal in order to assess the success of rehabilitation efforts.

Caring for the Individual Oiled Bird

In some instances, an individual or a small number of oiled birds may be found and not immediately tied into a known spill event. As these birds may ultimately be tied to a larger event, they should be reported to appropriate state and/or federal wildlife agencies and similar procedures for documenting information as those followed during an organized spill response should be undertaken. The same medical considerations and processes for care that have been described for a larger group of birds should be followed for one or a small number of birds. Under these circumstances, unlike the herd health approach in a larger spill, it may be possible to treat each bird's medical problems on an individual basis.

Conclusions

Excellence in oiled wildlife response requires knowledge of and the expertise to treat the physiological effects of oil exposure on affected animals. The most effective oil spill responses are achieved when plans are put in place prior to the event (e.g., prestocking of supplies, training of volunteers, identification of a facility for the response, and other key readiness steps), and excellent documents providing more details on such plans are readily available (IPIECA 2014). The processes described in this chapter may change based on logistics, available infrastructure, and the number of oiled animals. While an individual or small number of oiled animals may be handled by local veterinarians and wildlife rehabilitation groups, most wildlife affected by oil spills are cared for as part of a larger response organized within an ICS structure. Because this chapter is intended as an overview of the considerations in care for oiled wildlife, veterinarians and wildlife rehabilitators who are interested in working in oil spill response should seek appropriate training through organizations that specialize in this work, such as International Bird Rescue (www.bird-rescue.org), Tristate Bird Rescue & Research (www.tristatebird.org), or the Oiled Wildlife Care Network (www.vetmed.ucdavis.edu/owcn).

References

Albers, J. (1995). Petroleum and individual polycyclic aromatic hydrocarbons. In: *Handbook of Ecotoxicology* (ed. D.J. Hoffman, B.A. Rattner, G.A. Burton Jr. and J. Cairns Jr.), 330–355. Boca Raton, FL: Lewis Publishers/ CRC Press.

Alonso-Alvarez, C., Munilla, I., López-Alonso, M. et al. (2007). Sublethal toxicity of the prestige oil spill on yellow-legged gulls. *Environment International* 33: 773–781.

American Veterinary Medical Association. (2013). *AVMA Guidelines for the Euthanasia of Animals*. Schaumburg, IL: AVMA.

Balseiro, A., Espí, A., Márquez, I. et al. (2005). Pathological features in marine birds affected by the Prestige's oil spill in the north of Spain. *Journal of Wildlife Diseases* 41 (2): 371–378.

Briggs, K.T., Yoshida, S.H., and Gershwin, M.E. (1996). The influence of petrochemicals and stress on the immune system of seabirds. *Regulatory Toxicology and Pharmacology* 23 (2): 145–155.

Bryndza, H.E., Foster, J.P., McCartney, J.H. et al. (1993). Methodology for Determining Surfactant Efficacy in Removal of Petrochemicals from Feathers. In: *Proceedings of the 1993 Conference of the Effects of Oil on Wildlife* (ed. L. Frink). Hanover, PA: Sheridan Press,.

Clumpner, C.J. (1991). Water Hardness and Waterproofing of Oiled Birds: Lessons from the *Nestucca*, *Exxon Valdez* and the *American Trader* Spills. In: *Proceedings of the Second International Effects of Oil on Wildlife Conference* (ed. J. White). Suisun, CA: International Wildlife Rehabilitation Council.

Dierauf, L. and Gulland, F.M. (eds.) (2001). *CRC Handbook of Marine Mammal Medicine: Health, Disease, and Rehabilitation*. Boca Raton, FL: CRC Press.

Frink, L. and Miller, E.A. (1993). Principles of Oiled Bird Rehabilitation. In: *Proceedings of the 1993 Conference of the Effects of Oil on Wildlife* (ed. L. Frink). Hanover, PA: Sheridan Press.

Fry, D.M. and Lowenstein, L.J. (1985). Pathology of common Murres and Cassin's auklets exposed to oil. *Archives of Environmental Contamination and Toxicology* 14: 725–737.

Gage, L. (2009). *Policies and Best Practices Marine Mammal Stranding Response, Rehabilitation, and Release. Standards for Rehabilitation Facilities*. Silver Spring, MD: NOAA Technical Memo. National Oceanic and Atmospheric Administration.

Hartung, R. (1967). Energy metabolism in oil-covered ducks. *Journal of Wildlife Management* 31 (4): 798–804.

Harvey, D.J. and Brown, N.K. (1991). Comparative in vitro metabolism of the cannabinoids. *Pharmacology Biochemistry and Behavior* 40 (3): 533–540.

Helm, R.C., Carter, H.R., Ford, R.G. et al. (2015). Overview of efforts to document and reduce impacts of oil spills on seabirds. In: *Handbook of Oil Spill Science and Technology* (ed. M. Fingas), 431–453. Hoboken, NJ: Wiley.

Holcomb, J.B. (1988). Net-bottom caging for waterfowl. *Wildlife Journal* 11 (1): 3–4.

Holmes, W.N., Cronshaw, J., and Gorsline, J. (1978). Some effects of ingested petroleum on seawater-adapted ducks (Anas platyrhynchos). *Environmental Research* 17 (2): 177–190.

Holmes, W.N., Gorsline, J., and Cavanaugh, K.P. (1981). Some effects of environmental pollutants on endocrine regulatory mechanisms. *Recent Advances of Avian Endocrinology* 33: 1–11.

IPIECA (2014). Wildlife Response Preparedness: Good Practice Guidelines for Incident Management and Emergency Response Personnel. OGP Report Number 516. www.ipieca.org/publication/oiled-wildlife-preparedness-and-response.

Jenssen, B.M. and Ekker, M. (1988). A method for evaluating the cleaning of oiled seabirds. *Wildlife Society Bulletin* 16: 213–215.

Leighton, F.A. (1991). The toxicity of petroleum oils to birds: an overview. In: *The Effects of Oil on Wildlife: Research, Rehabilitation and General Concerns. Proceedings of the 2nd International Effects of Oil on Wildlife Conference* (ed. J. White). Hanover, PA: Sheridan Press.

Leighton, F.A. (1993). The toxicity of petroleum oil to birds. *Environmental Reviews* 1: 92–103.

Leighton, F.A., Lee, Y.Z., Rahimtula, A.D. et al. (1985). Biochemical and functional disturbances in red blood cells of herring gulls ingesting Prudhoe Bay crude oil. *Toxicology and Applied Pharmacology* 81: 25–31.

Mahaney, P.A. (1994). Effects of freshwater petroleum contamination on amphibian hatching and metamorphosis. *Environmental Toxicology and Chemistry* 13 (2): 259–265.

Mazet, J.A.K., Gardner, I.A., Jessup, D.A. et al. (2001). Effects of petroleum on mink applied as a model for reproductive success in sea otters. *Journal of Wildlife Diseases* 37 (4): 286–292.

Mazet, J.A.K., Newman, S.H., Gilardi, K.V.K. et al. (2002). Advances in oiled bird emergency medicine and management. *Journal of Avian Medicine and Surgery* 16 (2): 146–149.

Milton, S., Lutz, P., and Shigenaka, G. (2010). Oil toxicity and impacts on sea turtles. In: *Oil and Sea Turtles: Biology, Planning and Response* (ed. G. Shigenaka), 35–48. Silver Spring, MD: National Oceanic and Atmospheric Administration.

Mohr, F.C., Lasley, B., and Bursian, S. (2010). Fuel-oil induced adrenal hypertrophy in ranch mink (*Mustela vison*): effects of sex, fuel oil weathering, and response to adrenocorticotropic hormone. *Journal of Wildlife Diseases* 46 (1): 103–110.

OWCN (2014). *Protocols for the Care of Oil-Affected Birds*, 3e (ed. C. Fiorello, M. Ziccardi and E. Whitmer). Davis, CA: Oiled Wildlife Care Network.

Rattner, B.A., Eroschenko, V.P., Fox, G.A. et al. (1984). Avian endocrine responses to environmental pollutants. *Journal of Experimental Zoology* 232: 683–689.

Schwacke, L.H., Smith, C.R., Townsend, F.I. et al. (2013). Health of common bottlenose dolphins (*Tursiops truncatus*) in Barataria Bay, Louisiana, following the Deepwater horizon oil spill. *Environmental Science and Technology* 48 (1): 93–103.

Schwartz, J.A., Aldridge, B.M., Lasley, B.L. et al. (2004). Chronic fuel oil toxicity in American mink (*Mustela vison*): systemic and hematological effects of ingestion of a low-concentration of bunker C fuel oil. *Toxicology and Applied Pharmacology* 200: 146–158.

Tell, L.A., Craigmill, A.L., Clemons, K.V. et al. (2005). Studies on itraconazole delivery and pharmacokinetics in mallard ducks (*Anas platyrhynchos*). *Journal of Veterinary Pharmacology and Therapeutics* 28: 267–274.

Troisi, G., Borjesson, L., Bexton, S. et al. (2007). Biomarkers of polycyclic aromatic hydrocarbon (PAH)-associated hemolytic anemia in oiled wildlife. *Environmental Research* 105 (3): 324–329.

Tseng, F.S. (1999). Considerations in care for birds affected by oil spills. *Journal of Exotic Pet Medicine* 8: 21–31.

Venn-Watson, S., Colegrove, K.M., Litz, J. et al. (2015). Adrenal gland and lung lesions in Gulf of Mexico common bottlenose dolphins (Tursiops truncatus) found dead following the Deepwater Horizon oil spill. *PLoS One* 10 (5): e0126538.

Walraven, E. (1992). *Rescue and Rehabilitation of Oiled Birds*. Mosman, Australia: Zoological Parks Board of New South Wales.

7

Vaccination of Wildlife Species

Michael J. Yabsley

D.B. Warnell School of Forestry and Natural Resources and the Southeastern Cooperative Wildlife Disease Study, Department of Population Health, College of Veterinary Medicine, University of Georgia, Athens, GA, USA

Introduction

In domestic animals, vaccines are generally used to protect individual animals against certain pathogens and to create herd immunity. Herd immunity is the development of a high level of protection in a population which makes transmission of a pathogen less likely among those that are not vaccinated or are nonresponders. Vaccines for domestic animals are generally used according to the label, which means that the manufacturer has conducted research into the safety and efficacy of the vaccine and has gained United States Department of Agriculture (USDA) clearance for use of that vaccine in certain species and using specific guidelines. Note that not all vaccines are labeled to prevent disease, as animals may become infected but clinical signs in vaccinated animals tend to be mild.

The only vaccine that is currently approved for use in free-ranging wildlife is the RABORAL V-RG® oral rabies recombinant vaccine (Merial, Lyon, France) which is approved for raccoons and coyotes. This oral bait vaccine is used throughout the eastern US to control rabies in wildlife populations, but it is not commercially available for individual use. Because all other vaccines are not approved for use in wildlife, either in captive or in free-ranging animals, they are used "off-label" or outside of specified label directions. However, some studies have been conducted on the use of domestic animal vaccines in various wildlife species (e.g., Paré et al. 1999) and some have been shown to be efficacious and/or safe, whereas others are known to cause disease.

Why Vaccinate?

Vaccination of wildlife species has become an important conservation tool used to control diseases in endangered or imperiled species or their prey. However, the history of vaccine use in wildlife has been marred by unfortunate instances of well-meaning individuals who vaccinated species with vaccines that ultimately were not safe (i.e., they caused disease). Thus, before using vaccines off-label in wildlife, safety considerations should be reviewed. Knowledge of the efficacy in the species to be vaccinated is also critical, since the use of an ineffective vaccine provides a false sense of security related to protection and is a waste of resources. However, efficacy is rarely evaluated because testing often requires challenge studies of animals with pathogens that can be ethically or logistically challenging.

Some rehabilitators will vaccinate animals to prevent disease after release whereas others vaccinate to produce herd immunity for animals while in care. Animals in rehabilitation equate to a domestic animal shelter environment. They are a random source population of unknown health and pathogen exposure history, high population turnover, may be kept in high density, and are stressed due to being in captivity. All of these factors make it more likely that these animals may suffer from disease. Thus, many clinics who raise orphaned neonates will vaccinate following a standard dog/cat shelter protocol in which animals are vaccinated at intake and then at regular intervals afterwards (see Table 7.2). No vaccine is 100% effective in every animal; therefore, appropriate quarantine, hygiene, and monitoring are essential to minimize disease risks.

Types of Vaccines

Numerous types of vaccines are available, each of which has advantages and disadvantages. In general, vaccines contain dead pathogens, attenuated pathogens, or some natural or synthetic antigen of the pathogen(s). Vaccines can change in composition, even for a similar type of vaccine (e.g., modified live); therefore, when new vaccines enter the market they must be critically evaluated for potential safety and efficacy concerns. Before using any type of vaccine, the risks of using or not using the vaccine for the health of the individual animal or group of animals must be considered. Finally, many commercially available vaccines are now polyvalent, which means that they have components to protect animals against several pathogens. Importantly, the vaccine may contain different types of components (e.g., one pathogen may be modified live whereas another may be a killed component). Thus, some components of a multivalent vaccine may be safe, but other parts may not be, so labels must be examined carefully.

Attenuated or Modified Live Virus Vaccines

Modified live virus (MLV) vaccines are one of the most common types used in veterinary medicine. These vaccines have been developed using viruses that are modified to reduce virulence and thereby cause only mild or no disease in the vaccinated animal. Methods for modification may include serial passage in culture, resulting in natural mutation, or passage through a foreign host, resulting in the pathogen adapting to the new host and thus not being as virulent to the natural host.

These vaccines are useful as rapid onset of immunity is usually provided, fewer doses of vaccine are needed to stimulate response, and they can overcome maternal antibody interference which is an important consideration for neonates (Pratelli et al. 2000). Despite these benefits, there are several very important concerns related to the use of MLV vaccines in wildlife. First, these attenuated viruses may not be attenuated enough for use in certain wildlife species. Thus, they can cause clinical disease and possibly death of the vaccinated animal. Most adverse reactions in wildlife species related to vaccination are due to MLV vaccine use (Table 7.1). Second, not all MLV vaccines are the same; for example, MLV vaccines for canine distemper can be derived from canine cell culture-adapted, avian cell-adapted, or Vero cell-adapted viral strains. In wildlife species, the canine tissue culture-adapted MLV strains have the highest risk of vaccine-induced disease (Halbrooks et al. 1981). However, even avian-adapted strains can potentially represent a risk for highly susceptible species (e.g., black-footed ferrets, gray fox, mink, pandas) (Sutherland-Smith et al. 1997).

Although MLV vaccines contain attenuated pathogen, some vaccinated animal species or individuals may shed the pathogen, particularly in off-label species (Decaro et al. 2014). If the virus reverts to a natural state of virulence, it may be pathogenic to contact animals that are not vaccinated. Although the pathogen is still attenuated, if highly susceptible species are exposed to the shed pathogen, they may become infected and diseased. If an animal is shedding virus, it may test positive by antigen or DNA/RNA detection methods which may complicate the diagnosis of true infections versus shedding of a

Table 7.1 Selected examples of vaccine-induced disease caused by the use of modified live virus vaccines.

Pathogen	Species	References
Canine distemper virus	Black-footed ferrets (*Mustela nigripes*)	Carpenter et al. (1976)
	African wild dogs (*Lycaon pictus*)	Durchfeld et al. (1990)
	Maned wolf (*Chrysocyon brachyurus*)	Thomas-Baker (1983)
	Gray fox (*Urocyon cinereoargenteus*)	Halbrooks et al. (1981)
	Fennec fox (*Fennecus zerda*)	Montali et al. (1987)
	Red/Lesser panda (*Ailurus fulgens*)	McCormick (1983)
	Kinkajous (*Potos favus*)	Bush et al. (1976)
	European mink (*Mustela lutreola*)	Kazacos et al. (1981)
	Long-tailed weasels (*Mustela frenata*)	Sutherland-Smith et al. (1997)
	Ermine (*Mustela erminea*)	Williams (2001)
	South American bush dog (*Speothos venaticus*)[a]	McInnes et al. (1992)
Canine adenovirus-2	Maned wolf	Swenson et al. (2012)
Feline parvovirus	Cheetah (*Acinonyx jubatus*)	Crawshaw et al. (1996)
Parvovirus	Maned wolves	Backues (1994)
Rabies virus	Red fox (*Vulpes Vulpes*) [as part of oral rabies vaccination campaign]	Forró et al. (2019)

[a] Probable case.

vaccine strain of the pathogen (Wilkes et al. 2014). In general, shedding, if it occurs, should be relatively short term (Decaro et al. 2014).

In many rehabilitation clinics, the most commonly admitted group of animals are orphaned neonates. Despite this, studies on the use of vaccines in wildlife neonates are rare (e.g., Paré et al. 1999; Fry et al. 2013), and most studies on the safety and/or efficacy of MLV use in wildlife species are conducted on adult or older juvenile animals (van Heerden et al. 2002). Thus, even if studies show the vaccine may be safe for use in adults of a species, use of a MLV vaccine in neonates or young juveniles may still be a risk (Durchfeld et al. 1990; Truyen et al. 2009). Immunosuppressed individuals may be susceptible to clinical disease even if the vaccine is typically safe for use in that species or age group.

Finally, because MLV vaccines do contain live pathogens, correct storage and handling of the vaccine are important to ensure the vaccine remains potent. This requirement may limit the usefulness of MLV for use in free-ranging wildlife in remote areas.

Inactivated or Killed Virus Vaccine (KV)

These vaccines are made with pathogens that have been killed by either heat or chemical methods. They are generally quite safe because no live pathogen is present; however, they may not stimulate as vigorous an immune response as MLV or recombinant vaccines. Protective titers may take a much longer time to develop and multiple boosters may be required to produce a long-lived response. Even with boosters, for some vaccines or species, a protective response may not develop. For wildlife that are present in stressful, crowded, or mixed-origin groups, this prolonged period of time can result in ineffectiveness.

Most killed vaccines contain adjuvants to boost the immune response. There are hundreds of compounds that have been used as adjuvants and while those in commercially available vaccines are generally safe, local or systemic reactions to the adjuvants can occur. Animals should be watched for swelling, pain, abscesses, or systemic disease following vaccination.

One of the more common killed vaccines used in wildlife is an inactivated rabies vaccine. One study found that intramuscular injection of a single vaccine into raccoons and striped skunks resulted in 98% and 100% seroconversion respectively and that antibodies persisted in most animals beyond a year (Rosatte et al. 1990). Six of the skunks were challenged with rabies virus 90 days post vaccination and five survived, indicating that most vaccinated animals were protected. Another study found that 88% of 29 raccoons similarly vaccinated seroconverted, but challenge of three vaccinated raccoons a year later resulted in the death of two (Brown and Rupprecht 1990). Similarly, another study found that only 31% of vaccinated raccoons maintained a titer beyond one year. However, an anamnestic response was noted in raccoons that were seronegative but given an inactivated rabies booster (Sobey et al. 2010). A trap-vaccinate-release strategy using an inactivated rabies vaccine has been used in several locations to decrease the incidence of rabies in free-ranging carnivores (Rosatte et al. 1992).

Killed parvovirus vaccines are commonly used in wildlife but few studies have investigated their efficacy. One study in coyotes found that only one of 37 8-week-old coyotes vaccinated with a killed feline parvovirus vaccine developed antibodies. However, these pups may have still had maternal antibodies and none received boosters (Green et al. 1984).

A commercial killed West Nile virus vaccine approved for horses has been used in birds. It lowered mortality and the amount of virus present in the blood of vaccinated western scrub-jays (*Aphelocoma californica*) (Wheeler et al. 2011), and so was hypothesized to be a useful strategy to protect highly susceptible wild corvids (Boyce et al. 2011). Several other studies have failed to detect antibodies in vaccinated birds but different studies used variable numbers of vaccines and doses so direct comparison is difficult and probability of protection is difficult to evaluate in any species without a challenge trial (Phalen and Dahlhausen 2004; Okeson et al. 2007). More details are given below in the West Nile virus section.

Subunit or Recombinant Vector Vaccines

Neither subunit nor recombinant vector vaccines have intact pathogen so they are considered much safer than MLV vaccines in highly susceptible species. Unfortunately, animals vaccinated with subunit or recombinant vaccines, compared with MLV, take longer to develop a response. The difference between subunit and recombinant vector vaccines is the way antigens are presented to the vaccinated animals.

Subunit Vector Vaccines

Subunit vaccines include one or many antigen(s) of the pathogen that are known to stimulate an immune response. The source of these antigens may be from the pathogen itself (grow pathogen and then harvest specific antigens) or synthesized using recombinant DNA technology (AKA recombinant subunit vaccines, which clone the protective antigens and propagate them in bacteria or yeast from which they are purified). For these vaccines to be effective, the proteins involved in a protective response must be known, which takes considerable research. Few commercially available subunit vaccines are used in wildlife, but examples used in domestic animals include a *Borrelia burgdorferi* OspA for dogs (Eschner and Mugnai 2015) and a porcine circovirus type 2 for pigs (Shelton et al. 2012). In general, subunit vaccines often require repeated boosters and strong adjuvants. In order to overcome these limitations, protective antigen sequences are genetically engineered into a vector which is then injected into the animal.

Recombinant Vector Vaccines

These vaccines use a vector to introduce the target microbial DNA to cells of the body. "Vector" refers to an attenuated virus or bacterium used as a carrier. After vaccination, the virus or bacterium backbone then produces recombinant proteins that stimulate an immune reaction. An increasing number of recombinant vaccines are becoming available that may be used in wildlife species because they pose no risk of infection with the pathogen.

Two common backbones used to make recombinant vaccines for use in veterinary species are the vaccinia virus and canarypox virus. An advantage of vaccinia virus is that it has a wide host range and replicates well in mammals, so large amounts of protein are produced. Canarypox virus has limited ability to replicate in mammals, but still effectively expresses proteins.

There are numerous examples of recombinant vector vaccines being used in wildlife species. Some have experimental data to support their use whereas others are used without data to support their efficacy. A commercial canarypox recombinant West Nile virus vaccine approved for horses has been tested in various raptors and has been shown to provide partial protection (Angenvoort et al. 2014). Because this virus is extremely pathogenic to raptors, even partial protection is important. Researchers found that giving a series of three vaccines (versus the recommended two for horses) provided better protection (Angenvoort et al. 2014). Minor to moderate side effects have been noted, so vaccinates should be monitored (Wheeler et al. 2011; Angenvoort et al. 2014).

Many vaccinia- and canarypox-vectored vaccines are used in wild mammals (e.g., rabies virus, canine distemper virus [CDV]). One of the most successful wildlife vaccination campaigns was the RABORAL V-RG oral rabies recombinant vaccine (Merial) vaccination of red fox (*Vulpes vulpes*) in Europe that led to the complete or near complete eradication of terrestrial rabies in numerous countries (Freuling et al. 2013). The RABORAL V-RG vaccine is a vaccinia-vectored vaccine expressing the surface glycoprotein (G) responsible for protection against virus-neutralizing antibodies. This same oral rabies recombinant bait vaccine is being used in the eastern United States to control rabies spread.

In the United States, this vaccine is currently labeled for use in raccoons and coyotes but has been evaluated in a wide range of rabies-susceptible species, including red fox (*V. vulpes*), gray fox (*Urocyon cinereoargenteus*), and arctic fox (*Vulpes lagopus*) (Slate et al. 2009; Follmann et al. 2011). This platform appears to be effective in eliciting an immune response in skunks; however, the current format of the oral rabies bait does not result in a high percentage of skunks being exposed to the vaccine contained in the bait sachets (Grosenbaugh et al. 2007). Furthermore, this vaccine is not 100% effective in raccoon kits as 29% of kits failed to respond to this vaccine, highlighting that kits may not respond the same as adult animals (Fry et al. 2013). A recently developed live recombinant human adenovirus rabies virus glycoprotein vaccine (ONRAB) was shown to be safe for use in raccoons and a high percentage of animals developed antibodies (Slate et al. 2014).

Several other types of recombinant vector vaccines commercially available for dogs and cats are used in wildlife (e.g., canarypox-vectored CDV), but they have not been evaluated for efficacy (Larson and Schultz 2006). However, anecdotal evidence suggests that this CDV vaccine is safe for use in raccoons (Yabsley, personal discussions with several wildlife rehabilitators).

Other Vaccine Types

Numerous other types of vaccines exist, but they are not commonly used in wildlife species. For example, DNA vaccines can be used to immunize animals with naked DNA that encodes for protective proteins. These vaccines are desired because there are fewer safety concerns as compared with live or MLV vaccines; however, additional research and optimization are needed before DNA vaccines are readily available for most pathogens of concern in wildlife. This type of vaccine is becoming more common and may be more available in the future.

Another type of vaccine is a gene-deleted vaccine, created by deleting an essential virulence gene. These viruses will replicate like wild-type viruses but lack the virulence genes. However, it is possible for the gene-deleted viruses to recombine with wild-type virus and acquire the necessary virulence genes. Safety of these vaccines can be increased by deleting more than one virulence gene, so two recombination events would be needed to recover a virulent pathogen. Few of these vaccines have been evaluated in wildlife, but one example is the vaccination of raccoons with gene-deleted vaccines for pseudorabies virus (causes "mad itch" in raccoons). Findings were mixed: not all raccoons developed antibodies and not all vaccinated raccoons survived challenge; however, this virus should not be a concern for raccoons in rehabilitation as long as they are not in contact with swine infected with pseudorabies virus (Weigel et al. 2003).

Toxoid vaccines are commonly used in humans, domestic animals, and captive wildlife (e.g., zoo animals, exotic pets) but rarely in free-ranging wildlife species. Some bacteria, such as *Clostridium* spp. and *Corynebacterium diphtheriae*, produce toxins that can cause disease in their host. Toxoid vaccines are made from inactivated toxins that are produced by these bacteria so if animals are exposed to toxins in the future, the immune response can inactivate the toxin.

Administration of Vaccines

In a captive setting, most vaccinations administered to wildlife are injectable. The timing, quantity, and spacing of vaccine administration vary for each individual vaccine. Importantly, nearly all of the vaccines used in wildlife species are used off-label or are experimental. Therefore, adherence to label use as described for domestic species or humans may not result in adequate protection.

Proper administration of vaccines is important to ensure effectiveness. For example, oral administration of a canarypox-vectored CDV vaccine to African wild dogs (*Lycaon pictus*) failed to induce an immune response, although all dogs vaccinated intramuscularly developed presumably protective titers (Connolly et al. 2013). This particular type of vaccine (canarypox vector) was not developed for oral use.

There are oral vaccination formulations for several pathogens of particular zoonotic or domestic animal concern (e.g., rabies virus, *Yersinia pestis*, and *Mycobacterium bovis*). However, these are rarely used in wildlife in rehabilitative care so they will not be discussed in this chapter. Good reviews of oral vaccination strategies have been published (Slate et al. 2009; Buddle et al. 2013; Tripp et al. 2014).

Repeated administration of the same vaccine is called homologous boosting. However, several studies on human and veterinary pathogens have shown that a heterologous prime-boost strategy, where the vaccine type is changed, can achieve a stronger immune response, one that is more appropriate (i.e., Type 1 and Type 2 helper T cells [Th1 vs Th2]), and/or longer-term protection with fewer boosters needed (Kardani et al. 2016). For example, in species that are sensitive to MLV vaccines, it is possible that administering a killed vaccine or canarypox-vectored vaccine first followed by a MLV vaccine after an immune response has developed may be safe. This strategy takes advantage of the MLV vaccine's strengths while offering a safer alternative than using only MLV vaccines. However, this strategy has not been used in native North American wildlife, although it is the suggested strategy for vaccinating maned wolves for parvovirus (Padilla and Hilton 2014).

Concerns Related to Use of Vaccines in Wildlife

A major concern with the use of vaccines in wildlife is adverse reactions; primarily that the animal will develop clinical disease due to vaccination (Table 7.1). Animals should also be watched for signs of anaphylaxis and treated if necessary. Many of these reports occurred when MLV were being used most commonly in new wildlife species. After the list of species that developed severe disease grew, the use of MLV was more limited. The increased use of a recombinant canarypox vectored (RCPV) CDV vaccine with greater safety has decreased the number of reports of adverse reactions.

Most vaccines are given without major reactions, but local inflammation, swelling, or hair loss are possible. Anaphylaxis following use of a MLV vaccine (Fervac D®, United Vaccines Inc., Madison, WI, USA) has been reported for some mustelids and viverrids. As noted before, CDV MLV can result in disease in some wildlife species, but postvaccinal encephalitis has also been reported in dogs for which the vaccine is labeled, highlighting that each animal is unique and may develop a severe reaction despite the vaccine being safe in other individuals (Fairley et al. 2015). Other than these MLV concerns, systemic reactions are rare. Other concerns previously discussed include possible risk due to mixed components in polyvalent vaccines and possible shedding by vaccinates.

Vaccine failure may occur due to maternal antibody interference (e.g., Fry et al. 2013; Niewiesk 2014). When neonates are admitted for care, they are often part of large, mixed-origin groups, so pathogen transmission is a concern. Thus, rehabilitation centers often want to begin vaccination as soon as young animals are admitted. The risk of maternal antibody interference varies by individual, animal species and level of antibodies present. Also, the time period that maternal antibodies persist varies by the number of antibodies transferred from the dam to young, the pathogen, and the individual animal. In general, the period of greatest risk of pathogen transmission and development of disease is when maternal antibodies are waning (6–18 weeks) but are still high enough to interfere with the response to vaccination.

Evaluation of Vaccines for Use in Wildlife

The typical way to evaluate a vaccine's efficacy for domestic animals is to vaccinate groups of animals using appropriate vaccine or contact controls and then challenge animals with a virulent strain of the pathogen to determine the degree of protection. These studies are essential to our understanding of the efficacy of a particular vaccine strategy to prevent disease. However, with wildlife, such studies can be problematic because appropriate naive animals may not be available, housing of larger numbers of wildlife species may be logistically or financially prohibitive, or the animal species may be imperiled and thus induction of disease is not an option. Also, similar to studies in domestic animals, some researchers have ethical concerns with the purposeful induction of disease in animals.

Often, serological response is used as a proxy for protection, but using this simple measure can sometimes be misleading. Some animals that fail to seroconvert or have decreasing antibody titers may still be protected due to effective cell-mediated immune responses, while others that have high antibody titers as a result of vaccination may still become infected or diseased (Paré et al. 1999; Brown et al. 2011). In the absence of available data for a wildlife species, the literature should be investigated for closely related domestic species; however, it is critical to remember that differences between closely related species may occur.

Vaccines Commonly Used against Important Pathogens of Rehabilitated Animals

In general, killed vaccines or canarypox-vectored vaccines should be used in wildlife species because they are less likely to cause problems than MLV vaccines.

Rabies

Rabies is nearly always fatal, so considerable effort is used to control rabies in wildlife and domestic animals. Because of a long history of the use of rabies vaccines in animals, several companies produce safe killed virus vaccines (KV) that may be used in wildlife (Table 7.2). There is also a recombinant oral vaccine (RABORAL V-RG) that is used for control of rabies in free-ranging raccoons. This vaccine is not commercially available, but a recent study found that nearly a third of raccoon kits failed to respond to this vaccine, highlighting that kits may not respond the same as adult animals (Fry et al. 2013).

Table 7.2 Table of vaccines commonly used in selected wildlife species.

Pathogen	Vaccine name (Manufacturer)	Component type*	Used in which species	Reported frequency or protocols	Notes
Canine distemper virus (CDV)	Recombitek® C3 (Merial Inc.)	RCPV	Raccoons Skunks Otter Coyotes Fox Bobcat	At least 2 vaccinations, 2–3 weeks apart (juveniles booster until >16 weeks old)	Also includes canine parvovirus (MLV) and canine adenovirus type 2 (MLV) components.
	Nobivac® Puppy-DPv (Merck Animal Health)	MLV	Raccoon	At least 2 vaccinations, 2–4 weeks apart until 16 weeks old	Although a CDV MLV vaccine (Galaxy D®) was shown to be safe and efficacious in raccoons (Pare et al., 1999), there are reports of disease in raccoons due to use of CDV MLV vaccines; **use is not recommended.** Also includes canine parvovirus (MLV) component.
	Duramune® Max 5/4L (Boehringer Ingelheim)	MLV	Raccoon	At least 2 boosters at 3 and 6 wks (possibly longer)	See comment above
Canine parvovirus	Recombitek® C3 (Merial Inc.)	MLV	Raccoons Skunks Otter Coyotes Fox Bobcat	Follows canine distemper virus schedule	
Feline panleukopenia virus	Fel-O-Vax® PCT (Elanco Animal Health)	KV	Raccoons Bobcat Cougar	at 8 wks, booster 3–4 wks later; if vaccinating at <12 wk, revaccinate at 12–16 wks.	Also contains feline herpesvirus-1 and calicivirus components.

Table 7.2 (Continued)

Pathogen	Vaccine name (Manufacturer)	Component type*	Used in which species	Reported frequency or protocols	Notes
	PureVax® Feline 3/4 (Merial Inc.)	MLV	Raccoons	Neonates: at admission, then every 2–3 wks until 14–16 wks of age Juveniles: at least 2 doses given 2–3 wks apart	PureVax 3 also contains feline herpesvirus-1 and calicivirus, both MLV, components. PureVax 4 contains these as well as MLV *Chlamydia psittaci.*
Rabies virus	Imrab® 3 (Merial Inc.)	KV	Raccoon and possibly other rabies hosts	14–16 wks of age	Check local regulations regarding legality of vaccinating non-domestic animals for rabies virus.
	Rabvac® 1 or Rabvac 3 (Elanco Animal Health)	KV	Raccoon and possibly other rabies hosts	>12 wks of age	Check local regulations regarding legality of vaccinating non-domestic animals for rabies virus.
	Nobivac® 1 or 3 (Merck)	KV	Raccoon and possibly other rabies hosts	>12 wks of age	Check local regulations regarding legality of vaccinating non-domestic animals for rabies virus.
	Defensor® 1 or 3 (Zoetis)	KV	Raccoon and possibly other rabies hosts	>12 wks of age	Check local regulations regarding legality of vaccinating non-domestic animals for rabies virus.
	PureVax® Rabies (Merial Inc.)	RCPV	Potential rabies hosts	At least 12 wks of age (per label for domestic cats)	No known evidence that rehabilitators are using, but other RCPV vaccines are considered safe to use in a variety of wildlife species.
Feline herpesvirus (Feline viral rhinotracheitis)	FVRCP (Ultra™ Hybrid™ or Ultra™ Fel-O-Vax®, Elanco Animal Health) or PureVax Feline 3/4 (Merial Inc.) as used for feline panleukopenia virus	KV	Bobcat	At least 8–10 wks of age with booster 3–4 wks (per label for domestic cats)	
Feline calicivirus	FVRCP (Ultra™ Hybrid™ or Ultra™ Fel-O-Vax®, Elanco Animal Health) or PureVax Feline 3/4 (Merial Inc.) as used for feline panleukopenia virus	KV	Bobcat	At least 8–10 wks of age with booster 3–4 wks (per label for domestic cats)	
West nile virus	Recombitek® rWNV(Merial)	RCPV	Raptors	0.5ml for birds <500 g 1ml for birds >500 g 3 doses spaced 2 weeks apart	Boost annually before mosquito activity if kept overwinter.
	West Nile Innovator (Zoetis)	KV	Raptors	1ml divided between both sides of pectoral muscles with boosters at 3 and 6 wks.	Boost annually before mosquito activity if kept overwinter.

It is important to note that none of these vaccines have been approved for use in wildlife species. Although the vaccines listed in this table have been used by rehabilitators without major adverse effects, there is always the risk of adverse reactions, especially with modified live vaccines. Also, many of these vaccines are polyvalent, so even if one or more components are safe in one species, other components of that vaccine may not be safe. KV, killed virus vaccine; MLV, modified live virus vaccine; RCPV, Recombinant canarypox vectored.

One should always check local statutes before vaccinating wildlife species. One concern related to the vaccination of animals that are released is the need for differentiating infected from vaccinated animals (DIVA). Some areas or states use oral rabies vaccination programs in which they capture animals and test them for antibodies to rabies virus to determine if sufficient numbers of animals are being vaccinated with the oral rabies baits and whether vaccination at rehabilitation centers might interfere with these efforts to understand vaccine uptake in the wild. Finally, it is important to remember that despite being vaccinated against rabies, any wild mammal that bites a human (or a domestic pet) will be recommended for euthanasia and submission for testing.

Canine Distemper Virus

Canine distemper is a major concern for wildlife species in captive situations. Wild raccoons and other carnivores generally have a high rate of exposure to canine distemper virus, as measured by the presence of antibodies; thus, many orphaned neonates will present with maternally derived antibodies (Paré et al. 1999; Bischof & Rogers 2005; Junge et al. 2007; Raizman et al. 2009). One study showed that raccoon kits had detectable maternally derived antibodies at 16–20 weeks of age (Paré et al. 1999).

Historically, many centers vaccinated raccoons using MLV vaccine (Galaxy D®, Solvay Animal Health), which had been shown safe and efficacious in a small challenge study, although there was evidence of maternal antibody interference (Paré et al. 1999). Another MLV vaccine (Duramune® Max 5/4 L, Revival Animal health) was safe when used in raccoon kits and of the 31 raccoons without prevaccination positive titers, all had increases in titers post vaccination. In contrast, only five of 15 animals with prevaccination titers had increases in antibody titers post vaccination and the titers decreased throughout the study for the remaining 10 raccoons (Staudenmaier et al. 2014). Two MLV vaccines (Galaxy D® and Fervac-D® [no longer available] were safe in wild river otters (*Lutra canadensis*) and vaccinated otters developed presumed protective titers (Peper et al. 2014). However, there is variation in response to these vaccines as fishers (*Pekania pennanti*) failed to respond to Fervac D® but did have elevated titers in response to Galaxy D® (Peper et al. 2015). Although there is difficulty in understanding these data because of possible previous exposure, they do suggest that single vaccines probably are not sufficient to produce protective responses. In a rehabilitation setting, this is not usually an issue as an animal is in care for a long enough period to allow multiple vaccinations.

Currently many wildlife rehabilitators still use CDV MLV vaccines in raccoons, apparently safely (Table 7.2). However, sporadic cases of vaccine-induced disease in neonatal raccoons have been noted, so canarypox vaccines are preferred. Also, some strains circulating in free-ranging raccoons originated from MLV vaccine strains, suggesting that vaccination has resulted in sustained transmission (Lednicky et al. 2004). The CDV strain detected in a sick black bear (*Ursus americanus*) from Pennsylvania was similar, but not identical, to the Rockborn-Candur vaccine strain (Cottrell et al. 2013).

Canine cell line-adapted MLV CDV vaccines are not safe for use in foxes (Halbrooks et al. 1981) and this information has resulted in slow acceptance of a canarypox recombinant CDV vaccine (Merial) as a safe alternative for most carnivore species, including fox (Padilla & Hilton 2014) (Table 7.2). Although safe, the efficacy of the canarypox recombinant CDV vaccine has not been shown in native US wildlife species, although a wide range of wildlife species develop presumably protective titers after vaccination (Bronson et al. 2007; AZA Small Carnivore TAG 2010; Padilla & Hilton 2014). However, controlled studies are limited. A recent study on red fox found that although most animals seroconverted and remained healthy after vaccination with Recombitek® C6, not all animals developed titers considered protective (Hidalgo-Hermoso et al. 2019). This vaccine type is generally given subcutaneously, but a study on Siberian polecat (*Mustela eversmanni*) showed that oral administration can create protection; however, as noted earlier, the effectiveness of this vaccine may vary by species, route, and vaccine schedule (Wimsatt et al. 2003). A study on ferrets showed that intranasal administration of a CDV canarypox vaccine did not result in protection, so this route should be avoided (Welter et al. 2000).

Parvovirus

Parvoviruses have been reported from numerous wildlife species; however, clinical disease is most severe in raccoons and possibly bobcats and wild canids (Allison et al. 2012, 2013). Raccoons, and possibly other hosts, can be infected with canine or feline parvoviruses, but the majority of parvoviruses detected in raccoons are canine parvovirus (CPV)-2 variants, although sporadic reports of feline parvovirus (FPV) (panleukopenia) are detected (Allison et al. 2012, 2013). Regardless, it is believed that cross-protection occurs with parvovirus vaccines so most rehabilitators only vaccinate against either canine or feline parvovirus.

As noted earlier, maternally derived antibodies may interfere with MLV parvovirus vaccine efficacy. In a study with kittens, 25% of domestic kittens vaccinated at 12 weeks with three different MLV failed to servoconvert when maternal antibodies were present (Jakel et al. 2012). In a study in which raccoons were vaccinated with inactivated feline panleukopenia vaccine (Fel-O-Vax® FVRCP, Boehringer Ingelheim, St Joseph, MO) on admission to a rehabilitation center, only two of 25 vaccinated raccoons had an elevation in titer levels compared to one of six in the unvaccinated group (Broersma 2013). In a study using a modified live vaccine in raccoon kits, those individuals with prevaccination titers greater than 1:10 had a decrease in antibody titers, with 17/18 (94%) of kits becoming seronegative (<1:10 titer) by eight weeks post-vaccination (Berry & Ludwig 1988). This was in contrast to an increase in titers in all vaccinated raccoons that were initially seronegative, with 18 of these 19 (95%) kits remaining seropositive at 12–13 weeks post vaccination (Berry & Ludwig 1988). Another study in which raccoon kits were vaccinated with a modified live FPV vaccine (Fel-O-guard® Plus3) found that 12 of 14 seronegative raccoons developed titers >1:80 (considered protective in domestic cats) (Staudenmaier et al. 2014). In contrast, the 34 kits with positive titers (<1:20) at vaccination had a decrease in antibody titers and only seven kits had titers considered protective at 11 weeks (Staudenmaier et al. 2014).

Similar results were noted in raccoon kits vaccinated with a killed FPV vaccine as the two litters with prevaccination titers failed to respond to vaccination (Evans et al. 1988). It was also found that frequent boosters were needed to maintain positive titers which is common for killed virus vaccines (Evans et al. 1988).

Because exposure of raccoons to parvoviruses is common (Junge et al. 2007; Allison et al. 2012, 2013; Kamps et al. 2015), maternal antibody interference may be an issue in kits. Although controlled studies to determine efficacy of vaccination are needed, especially in kits with maternal antibodies, success in preventing disease has been reported with the use of MLV Recombitek® or PureVax® Feline 3 or 4 vaccines (Merial) (Yabsley, discussions with several rehabilitators) (see Table 7.2). This could be due to protection against parvovirus in raccoons with low titers, even those <1:10, because currently, it is not known if antibody levels alone are indicative of protection.

Canine Adenovirus (CAV)

There are two species of adenovirus (CAV-1 and -2) that infect canids; however, CAV-1 is the species reported in wildlife (Gerhold et al. 2007; Knowles et al. 2018). CAV-1 causes the disease called infectious canine hepatitis. Although CAV-1 is the virus of concern for wildlife, vaccines containing CAV-2 are used because CAV-1 and CAV-2 are antigenically cross-reactive and vaccines containing CAV-1 cause severe side effects. Although CAV-1 exposure among wild carnivores is common, vaccination specific for CAV-1 appears to be rare, although the Recombitek® C3 or C4 vaccines have a MLV CAV-2 component. Importantly, this vaccine has not been evaluated for efficacy in most wildlife species. A single study focused on CDV and CPV in red wolves (*Canis rufus*) did detect CAV antibodies in wolves of unknown vaccination history, suggesting that previously used polyvalent vaccines prior to the study contained CAV and that these antibodies persisted for at least three years (Anderson et al. 2014).

Feline Herpesvirus and Feline Calicivirus

Vaccination of wild felids is often used to prevent acute and chronic upper respiratory tract disease caused by feline herpesvirus and feline calicivirus. Many wildlife rehabilitation centers use a combination vaccine for parvovirus that also includes protection for these two viruses (Table 7.2). Although experimental data on native wild felids are limited, these vaccines have been used safely in many exotic felid species (e.g., lions, tigers) (Risi et al. 2012).

West Nile Virus

West Nile virus (WNV) can be a significant cause of morbidity and mortality in many bird species, especially corvids and raptors. Many centers vaccinate raptors that are going to be held long term (education/nonreleasable birds). Experimental data are mixed on the efficacy of different types of WNV vaccines (i.e., limited seroconversion or protection to challenge with virus) (Nusbaum et al. 2003; Johnson 2005; Okeson et al. 2007; Redig et al. 2011). However, use of a third dose of either a commercially available recombinant canarypox vector vaccine (Merial) or a formalin inactivated vaccine (Innovator®, Zoetis) reduced/eliminated mortality and alleviated clinical signs in gyrfalcons and hybrid falcons (*Falco rusticolus* × *Falco cherrug* and *F. rusticolus* × *Falco peregrinus*) and sandhill cranes (*Grus canadensis*) (Angenvoort et al. 2014). Regardless, prevention is important, and screens should be used to prevent mosquito bites.

Conclusions

Vaccination is an important management tool for the prevention of disease in a wide range of wildlife species. In the past, there has been considerable concern about adverse reactions or induction of clinical disease with certain vaccines for specific pathogens. These vaccines were MLVs that, when used in highly susceptible species, resulted in the attenuated virus replicating enough to cause disease. Most of these were CDV vaccines, and although CDV MLVs are still commercially available, they are prepared using different protocols that make them generally safer. However, it is critical to remember that even when a MLV has been shown to be safe for a particular species, individuals may still develop disease. Use of these vaccines in new species requires special thought and evaluation.

With proper use, vaccination of wildlife in care can assist rehabilitators in minimizing risk of pathogen transmission within their facility. This protection may also extend beyond their time in care and decrease disease risk during the high stress period after release.

The field of vaccination is constantly evolving, so it is important to stay informed of what has been shown to be safe and efficacious. This could also be important if novel pathogens were to be detected in US wildlife and for which vaccines are available that have not been previously used in wildlife species.

References

Allison, A.B., Harbison, C.E., Pagan, I. et al. (2012). Role of multiple hosts in the cross-species transmission and emergence of a pandemic parvovirus. *Journal of Virology* 86 (2): 865–872.

Allison, A.B., Kohler, D.J., Fox, K.A. et al. (2013). Frequent cross-species transmission of parvoviruses among diverse carnivore hosts. *Journal of Virology* 87 (4): 2342–2347.

Anderson, K., Case, A., Woodie, K. et al. (2014). Duration of immunity in red wolves (*Canis rufus*) following vaccination with a modified live parvovirus and canine distemper vaccine. *Journal of Zoo and Wildlife Medicine* 45 (3): 550–554.

Angevoort, J., Fischer, D., Fast, C. et al. (2014). Limited efficacy of West Nile virus vaccines in large falcons (*Falco* spp.). *Veterinary Research* 45: 41.

AZA Small Carnivore TAG (2010). *Mustelid (Mustelidae) Care Manual*, 136. Silver Spring, MD: Association of Zoos and Aquariums.

Backues, K.A. (1994). Problems with maned wolf puppies and parvovirus immunization. *Zoo Veterinarians News* 10: 6.

Berry, D.R. and Ludwig, D.R. (1988). Antibody response to a modified-live feline panleukopenia vaccine and blood cell values of young raccoons. *Wildlife Rehabilitation* 7: 57–70.

Bischof, R. and Rogers, D.G. (2005). Serologic survey of select infectious diseases in coyotes and raccoons in Nebraska. *Journal of Wildlife Diseases* 41 (4): 787–791.

Boyce, W.M., Vickers, W., Morrison, S.A. et al. (2011). Surveillance for West Nile virus and vaccination of free-ranging island scrub-jays (*Aphelocoma insularis*) on Santa Cruz Island, California. *Vector Borne and Zoonotic Diseases* 11 (8): 1063–1068.

Broersma, M.-L. (2013). Does Vaccination Against Feline Parvovirus Protect Hospitalized Raccoon Kits From Clinical Outbreaks of Parvoviral Disease? Second cycle, A2E. Uppsala: SLU, Department of Clinical Science. http://urn.kb.se/resolve?urn=urn:nbn:se:slu:epsilon-s-2907

Bronson, E., Deem, S.L., Sanchez, C. et al. (2007). Serologic response to a canarypox-vectored canine distemper virus vaccine in the giant panda (*Ailuropoda melanoleuca*). *Journal of Zoo and Wildlife Medicine* 38 (2): 363–366.

Brown, C.L. and Rupprecht, C.E. (1990). Vaccination of free-ranging Pennsylvania raccoons (*Procyon lotor*) with inactivated rabies vaccine. *Journal of Wildlife Diseases* 26 (2): 253–257.

Brown, L.J., Rosatte, R.C., Fehlner-Gardiner, C. et al. (2011). Immunogenicity and efficacy of two rabies vaccines in wild-caught, captive raccoons. *Journal of Wildlife Diseases* 47 (1): 182–194.

Buddle, B.M., Parlane, N.A., Wedlock, D.N. et al. (2013). Overview of vaccination trials for control of tuberculosis in cattle, wildlife and humans. *Transboundary and Emerging Diseases* 60 (Suppl 1): 136–146.

Bush, M., Montali, R.J., Brownstein, D. et al. (1976). Vaccine-induced canine distemper in a lesser panda. *Journal of the American Veterinary Medical Association* 169 (9): 959–960.

Carpenter, J.W., Appel, M.J., Erickson, R.C. et al. (1976). Fatal vaccine-induced canine distemper virus infection in black-footed ferrets. *Journal of the American Veterinary Medical Association* 169 (9): 961–964.

Connolly, M., Thomas, P., Woodroffe, D. et al. (2013). Comparison of oral and intramuscular recombinant canine distemper vaccination in African wild dogs (*Lycaon pictus*). *Journal of Zoo and Wildlife Medicine* 44 (4): 882–888.

Cottrell, W.O., Keel, M.K., Brooks, J.W. et al. (2013). First report of clinical disease associated with canine distemper virus infection in a wild black bear (*Ursus americana*). *Journal of Wildlife Diseases* 49 (4): 1024–1027.

Crawshaw, G.J., Mehren, K.G., Pare, J.A. (1996). Possible Vaccine Induced Viral Disease in Cheetahs. Proceedings of the American Association of Zoo Veterinarians Annual Conference, pp. 557–560.

Decaro, N., Crescenzo, G., Desario, C. et al. (2014). Long-term viremia and fecal shedding in pups after modified-live canine parvovirus vaccination. *Vaccine* 32 (30): 3850–3853.

Durchfeld, B., Baumgärtner, W., Herbst, W. et al. (1990). Vaccine-associated canine distemper infection in a litter of African hunting dogs (*Lycaon pictus*). *Zentralblatt für Veterinarmedizin Reihe B* 37 (3): 203–212.

Eschner, A.K. and Mugnai, K. (2015). Immunization with a recombinant subunit OspA vaccine markedly impacts the rate of newly acquired *Borrelia burgdorferi* infections in client-owned dogs living in a coastal community in Maine, USA. *Parasites and Vectors* 8: 92.

Evans, R.H., Squires, L., and Getson, P. (1988). Vaccination of young raccoons with a killed feline panleukopenia vaccine. *Wildlife Rehabilitation* 7: 71–86.

Fairley, R.A., Knesl, O., Pesavento, P.A. et al. (2015). Post-vaccinal distemper encephalitis in two border collie cross littermates. *New Zealand Veterinary Journal* 63 (2): 117–120.

Follmann, E., Ritter, D., Swor, R. et al. (2011). Preliminary evaluation of Raboral V-RG® oral rabies vaccine in Arctic foxes (*Vulpes lagopus*). *Journal of Wildlife Diseases* 47 (4): 1032–1035.

Forró, B., Marton, S., Kecskeméti, S., Hornyák, Á., and Bányai, K. (2019). Vaccine-associated rabies in red fox, Hungary. *Vaccine* 37 (27): 3535–3538.

Freuling, C.M., Hampson, K., Selhorst, T. et al. (2013). The elimination of fox rabies from Europe: determinants of success and lessons for the future. *Philosophical Transactions of the Royal Society of London. Series B* 368 (1623): 20120142.

Fry, T.L., Vandalen, K.K., Shriner, S.A. et al. (2013). Humoral immune response to oral rabies vaccination in raccoon kits: problems and implications. *Vaccine* 31 (26): 2811–2815.

Gerhold, R.W., Allison, A.B., Temple, D.L. et al. (2007). Infectious canine hepatitis in a gray fox (*Urocyon cinereoargenteus*). *Journal of Wildlife Diseases* 43 (4): 734–736.

Green, J.S., Bruss, M.L., Evermann, J.F. et al. (1984). Serologic response of captive coyotes (*Canis latrans* say) to canine parvovirus and accompanying profiles of canine coronavirus titers. *Journal of Wildlife Diseases* 20 (1): 6–11.

Grosenbaugh, D.A., Maki, J.L., Rupprecht, C.E. et al. (2007). Rabies challenge of captive striped skunks (*Mephitis mephitis*) following oral administration of a live vaccinia-vectored rabies vaccine. *Journal of Wildlife Diseases* 43 (1): 124–128.

Halbrooks, R.D., Swango, L.J., Schnurrenberger, P.R. et al. (1981). Response of gray foxes to modified live-virus canine distemper vaccines. *Journal of the American Veterinary Medical Association* 179 (11): 1170–1174.

Hidalgo-Hèrmoso, E., Mathieu-Benson, C., Celis-Diez, S., et al. (2019). Safety and serological response to multivalent canine distemper virus vaccine in red foxes (vulpes vulpes). *Journal of Zoo and Wildlife Medicine* 50 (2): 337–341.

Jakel, V., Cussler, K., Hanschmann, K.M. et al. (2012). Vaccination against feline panleukopenia: implications from a field study in kittens. *BMC Veterinary Research* 8: 62.

Johnson, S. (2005). Avian titer development against West Nile virus after extralabel use of an equine vaccine. *Journal of Zoo and Wildlife Medicine* 36 (2): 257–264.

Junge, R.E., Bauman, K., King, M. et al. (2007). A serologic assessment of exposure to viral pathogens and *Leptospira* in an urban raccoon (*Procyon lotor*) population inhabiting a large zoological park. *Journal of Zoo and Wildlife Medicine* 38 (1): 18–26.

Kamps, A.J., Dubay, S.A., Langenberg, J. et al. (2015). Evaluation of trapper-collected bobuto filter-paper blood samples for distemper and parvovirus antibody detection in coyotes (*Canis latrans*) and raccoons (*Procyon lotor*). *Journal of Wildlife Diseases* 51 (3): 724–728.

Kardani, K., Bolhassani, A., and Shahbazi, S. (2016). Prime-boost vaccine strategy against viral infections: mechanisms and benefits. *Vaccine* 34 (4): 413–423.

Kazacos, K.R., Thacker, H.L., Shivaprasad, H.L. et al. (1981). Vaccination-induced distemper in kinkajous. *Journal of the American Veterinary Medical Association* 179 (11): 1166–1169.

Knowles, S., Bodenstein, B.L., Hamon, T. et al. (2018). Infectious canine hepatitis in a Brown bear (*Ursus arctos horribilis*) from Alaska, USA. *Journal of Wildlife Diseases* 54 (3): 642–645.

Larson, L.J. and Schultz, R.D. (2006). Effect of vaccination with recombinant canine distemper virus vaccine immediately before exposure under shelter-like conditions. *Veterinary Therapeutics* 7 (2): 113–118.

Lednicky, J.A., Dubach, J., Kinsel, M.J. et al. (2004). Genetically distant American canine distemper virus lineages have recently caused epizootics with somewhat different characteristics in raccoons living around a large suburban zoo in the USA. *Virology Journal* 1: 2.

McCormick, A.E. (1983). Canine distemper in African cape hunting dogs (*Lycaon pictus*) – possibly vaccine induced. *Journal of Zoo and Animal Medicine* 14: 66–71.

McInnes, E.F., Burroughs, R.E., and Duncan, N.M. (1992). Possible vaccine-induced canine distemper in a South American bush dog (*Speothos venaticus*). *Journal of Wildlife Diseases* 28 (4): 614–617.

Montali, R.J., Bartz, C.R., and Bush, M. (1987). Canine distemper virus. In: *Virus Infections of Carnivores* (ed. M. Appel), 437–443. Amsterdam: Elsevier Science.

Niewiesk, S. (2014). Maternal antibodies: clinical significance, mechanism of interference with immune responses, and possible vaccination strategies. *Frontiers in Immunology* 5: 446.

Nusbaum, K.E., Wright, J.C., Johnston, W.B. et al. (2003). Absence of humoral response in flamingos and red-tailed hawks to experimental vaccination with a killed West Nile virus vaccine. *Avian Diseases* 47 (3): 750–752.

Okeson, D.M., Llizo, S.Y., Miller, C.L. et al. (2007). Antibody response of five bird species after vaccination with a killed West Nile virus vaccine. *Journal of Zoo and Wildlife Medicine* 38 (2): 240–244.

Padilla, L.R. and Hilton, C.D. (2014). Canidae. In: *Fowler's Zoo and Wild Animal Medicine*, 8e (ed. R.E. Miller and M.E. Fowler), 457–467. St Louis, MO: Elsevier.

Paré, J.A., Barker, I.K., Crawshaw, G.J. et al. (1999). Humoral response and protection from experimental challenge following vaccination of raccoon pups with a modified-live canine distemper virus vaccine. *Journal of Wildlife Diseases* 35 (3): 430–439.

Peper, S.T., Peper, R.L., Kollias, G.V. et al. (2014). Efficacy of two canine distemper vaccines in wild Nearctic river otters (*Lontra canadensis*). *Journal of Zoo and Wildlife Medicine* 45 (3): 520–526.

Peper, S.J., Peper, R.L., Mitcheltree, D.H. et al. (2015). Utility of two modified-live virus canine distemper vaccines in wild-caught fishers (*Martes pennanti*). *Veterinary Quarterly* 36 (4): 197–202.

Phalen, D.N. and Dahlhausen, B. (2004). West Nile virus. *Seminars in Avian and Exotic Pet Medicine* 13 (2): 67–78.

Pratelli, A., Cavalli, A., Normanno, G. et al. (2000). Immunization of pups with maternally derived antibodies to canine parvovirus (CPV) using a modified-live variant (CPV-2b). *Journal of Veterinary Medicine B Infectious Diseases and Veterinary Public Health* 47 (4): 273–276.

Raizman, E.A., Dharmarajan, G., Beasley, J.C. et al. (2009). Serologic survey for selected infectious diseases in raccoons (*Procyon lotor*) in Indiana, USA. *Journal of Wildlife Diseases* 45 (2): 531–536.

Redig, P.T., Tully, T.N., Ritchie, B.W. et al. (2011). Effect of West Nile virus DNA-plasmid vaccination on response to live virus challenge in red-tailed hawks (*Buteo jamaicensis*). *American Journal of Veterinary Research* 72 (8): 1065–1070.

Risi, E., Agoulon, A., Allaire, F. et al. (2012). Antibody response to vaccines for rhinotracheitis, caliciviral disease, panleukopenia, feline leukemia, and rabies in tigers (*Panthera tigris*) and lions (*Panthera leo*). *Journal of Zoo and Wildlife Medicine* 43 (2): 248–255.

Rosatte, R.C., Howard, D.R., Campbell, J.B. et al. (1990). Intramuscular vaccination of skunks and raccoons against rabies. *Journal of Wildlife Diseases* 26 (2): 225–230.

Rosatte, R.C., Power, M.J., MacInnes, C.D. et al. (1992). Trap-vaccinate-release and oral vaccination for rabies control in urban skunks, raccoons and foxes. *Journal of Wildlife Diseases* 28 (4): 562–571.

Shelton, N.W., Tokach, M.D., Dritz, S.S. et al. (2012). Effects of porcine circovirus type 2 vaccine and increasing standardized ileal digestible lysine: metabolizable energy ratio on growth performance and carcass composition of growing and finishing pigs. *Journal of Animal Science* 90 (1): 361–372.

Slate, D., Algeo, T.P., Nelson, K.M. et al. (2009). Oral rabies vaccination in North America: opportunities, complexities, and challenges. *PLoS Neglected Tropical Diseases* 3 (12): e549.

Slate, D., Chipman, R.B., Algeo, T.P. et al. (2014). Safety and immunogenicity of Ontario rabies vaccine bait (ONRAB) in the first us field trial in raccoons (*Procyon lotor*). *Journal of Wildlife Diseases* 50 (3): 582–595.

Sobey, K.G., Rosatte, R., Bachmann, P. et al. (2010). Field evaluation of an inactivated vaccine to control raccoon rabies in Ontario, Canada. *Journal of Wildlife Diseases* 46 (3): 818–831.

Staudenmaier, A., Miller, E., and Dubovi, J. (2014). Immune response in the common raccoon (*Procyon lotor*) to modified live canine distemper and feline panleukopenia vaccines. *Wildlife Rehabilitation Bulletin* 32 (1): 26–33.

Sutherland-Smith, M.R., Rideout, B.A., Mikolon, A.B. et al. (1997). Vaccine-induced canine distemper in European mink, *Mustela lutreola*. *Journal of Zoo and Wildlife Medicine* 28 (3): 312–318.

Swenson, J., Orr, K., and Bradley, G.A. (2012). Hemorrhagic and necrotizing hepatitis associated with administration of a modified live canine adenovirus-2 vaccine in a maned wolf (*Chrysocyon brachyurus*). *Journal of Zoo and Wildlife Medicine* 43 (2): 375–383.

Thomas-Baker, B. (1983). Vaccination-Induced Distemper in Maned Wolves, Vaccination-Induced Corneal Opacity in a Maned Wolf. In: Silberman MS, Silberman SD, eds. *Proceedings of the American Association of Zoo Veterinarians*, Scottsdale, AZ, p. 53.

Tripp, D.W., Rocke, T.E., Streich, S.P. et al. (2014). Season and application rates affect vaccine bait consumption by prairie dogs in Colorado and Utah, USA. *Journal of Wildlife Diseases* 50 (2): 224–234.

Truyen, U., Addie, D., Belák, S. et al. (2009). Feline panleukopenia. ABCD guidelines on prevention and management. *Journal of Feline Medicine and Surgery* 11 (7): 538–546.

van Heerden, J., Bingham, J., van Vuuren, M. et al. (2002). Clinical and serological response of wild dogs (*Lycaon pictus*) to vaccination against canine distemper, canine parvovirus infection and rabies. *Journal of South African Veterinary Association* 73 (1): 8–12.

Weigel, R.M., Hahn, E.C., and Scherba, G. (2003). Survival and immunization of raccoons after exposure to pseudorabies (Aujeszky's disease) virus gene-deleted vaccines. *Veterinary Microbiology* 92 (1–2): 19–24.

Welter, J., Taylor, J., Tartaglia, J. et al. (2000). Vaccination against canine distemper virus infection in infant ferrets with and without maternal antibody protection, using recombinant attenuated poxvirus vaccines. *Journal of Virology* 74 (14): 6358–6367.

Wheeler, S.S., Langevin, S., Woods, L. et al. (2011). Efficacy of three vaccines in protecting Western scrub-jays (*Aphelocoma californica*) from experimental infection with West Nile virus: implications for vaccination of island scrub-jays (*Aphelocoma insularis*). *Vector Borne and Zoonotic Diseases* 11 (8): 1069–1080.

Wilkes, R.P., Sanchez, E., Riley, M.C. et al. (2014). Real-time reverse transcription polymerase chain reaction method for detection of canine distemper virus modified live vaccine shedding for differentiation from infection with wild-type strains. *Journal of Veterinary Diagnostic Investigation* 26 (1): 27–34.

Williams, E.S. (2001). Canine distemper. In: *Infectious Diseases of Wild Mammals*, 3e (ed. E.S. Williams and I.K. Barker), 50–59. Ames, IA: Iowa State University Press, Ames, IA, pp. 50–59.

Wimsatt, J., Biggins, D., Innes, K. et al. (2003). Evaluation of oral and subcutaneous delivery of an experimental canarypox recombinant canine distemper vaccine in the Siberian polecat (*Mustela eversmanni*). *Journal of Zoo and Wildlife Medicine* 34 (1): 25–35.

8

The Veterinary Practitioner and the Wildlife Rehabilitator

Building the Right Relationship and Touching All the Bases

Edward E. Clark Jr

Wildlife Center of Virginia, Waynesboro, VA, USA

Introduction

The definition of wildlife rehabilitation is *the treatment and temporary care of injured, diseased and displaced indigenous animals, and the subsequent release of healthy animals to appropriate habitats in the wild* (Miller 2012). Appropriate and necessary care for any wild animal generally falls somewhere along a broad spectrum, with highly sophisticated medical intervention, such as surgery and complex drug therapies, at one end and the simple provision of basic nutrition and suitable housing at the other. Similarly, the skills and capabilities of care providers can range from highly specialized training, equipment, and facilities to rudimentary knowledge of simple husbandry techniques and a cardboard box. In wildlife rehabilitation, it is absolutely necessary to be able to determine what kind of care is needed to restore a wild patient to good health, for return to the wild, not just to save its life. It is also critical to realistically assess and understand who has the training and resources to provide what level of care. If a patient requires extensive orthopedic reconstruction but the care provider only has basic first aid skills, the animal needs to be transferred to other, more capable care providers; if other placement options are not available, euthanasia needs to be considered.

An awareness of both the kind of care that is required and the capacity of available care providers is essential in the realistic triage of patients and development of a treatment plan that is workable in a wildlife rehabilitation setting. A good working relationship between the veterinarian and the cooperating wildlife rehabilitators will greatly improve decision making and increase the potential for a successful outcome for wild patients.

The Complementary Roles of Veterinarian and Wildlife Rehabilitator

Across North America and around the world, very few communities have access to full-service veterinary hospitals that deal exclusively with wildlife. Fortunately, many veterinarians in private practice are willing to admit and treat wildlife patients, both as a service to members of the public who might find and present injured and orphaned wildlife and because of their own personal interest in wildlife. While many medical issues are best treated in a clinical setting, it makes little sense, and may actually be counterproductive, for patients that require more than a few days to recover, let alone uninjured wildlife, to remain in a hospital setting for extended periods of time. Ideally, the individual veterinarian or the veterinary practice that admits wildlife will have working relationships with one or more wildlife rehabilitators. These are trained individuals or organizations that hold permits issued by the relevant state, provincial, and/or federal governments, allowing them to care for injured and orphaned native wildlife. A list of licensed wildlife rehabilitators can be obtained by contacting the relevant wildlife agencies. Many state wildlife agencies post a list of current, permitted wildlife rehabilitators on the agency website.

Typically, wildlife rehabilitators provide temporary care for wild patients at their homes or in private, non-profit wildlife rehabilitation centers where there may be more space and more appropriate housing for wild species than is available in a typical veterinary clinic. Most wildlife rehabilitators have some level of specialized

Medical Management of Wildlife Species: A Guide for Practitioners, First Edition. Edited by Sonia M. Hernandez, Heather W. Barron, Erica A. Miller, Roberto F. Aguilar and Michael J. Yabsley.
© 2020 John Wiley & Sons, Inc. Published 2020 by John Wiley & Sons, Inc.

training in wildlife rehabilitation and can provide housing or enclosures specific to the appropriate confinement of wildlife during the rehabilitation process.

Effective working relationships between veterinary practitioners and wildlife rehabilitators significantly increase the likelihood that wild patients will have access to the short-term and long-term care and housing they need to be restored to health and returned to life in the wild. Establishing the right working relationships between the veterinarian and the wildlife rehabilitator is essential to ensuring that the needs of the injured or orphaned wild patient will be met, the interests of the public protected, and the collaboration between the veterinarian and wildlife rehabilitator is both sustainable and fulfilling for both parties.

At some point along the continuum from clinical medicine to rehabilitation and release, primary responsibility for providing care shifts from the veterinarian or veterinary clinic to the wildlife rehabilitator or rehabilitation center. The precise transition point will vary somewhat, and may alternate based on the specifics of a given animal's health issues, the capacity or willingness of the veterinarian to treat or house wild patients, and the training or competence of the wildlife rehabilitator. In an effective partnership, both parties will have a good understanding of the full range of factors influencing where a patient's needs fall along this continuum and how best to sustainably optimize the quality of care. Good communication about both the case and the working relationship is essential.

Success in wildlife rehabilitation means returning the healthy animal to an appropriate habitat in the wild, able to survive on its own and function normally in that habitat. An understanding of the natural history of each species (morphology and physiology, ecology, behaviors, diet, etc.) is vital to make informed decisions about which treatment options are appropriate for each wild patient. Decisions about appropriate care and reasonable outcomes made jointly by the veterinarian and wildlife rehabilitator, with each contributing their expertise and involving the full spectrum of considerations, tend to be most successful.

Setting the Ground Rules and Defining the Relationship

As a first step in building an effective team, the veterinarian and the wildlife rehabilitator need to candidly discuss their respective areas of expertise and experience, as well as their expectations for the relationship and each other. The wildlife rehabilitator's access to the veterinarian for consultation and patient evaluation and treatment will often be one of the most challenging issues to manage.

Veterinarians who work in busy private practices may not be able to simply drop everything in order to deal with a rabbit that has been attacked by a cat or a bird that has flown into a window, even when timely treatment may be essential for an animal's survival. To avoid frustration, disappointment, and conflict, fully exploring and discussing the realities of each partner's personal and professional situation is key. It is critically important for the veterinarian and wildlife rehabilitator to establish ground rules for when and how the veterinarian will be available to see wild patients, the terms under which care will be provided, and who will bear the financial costs. Contingency planning needs to be part of that discussion.

Treating Wildlife in your Clinic

Some veterinarians will allow clients, members of the public, local animal control officers, animal welfare organizations, or the wildlife rehabilitators themselves to drop off wild patients needing care so they can be seen when time permits throughout the day. Allowing this practice is often well received by those presenting the wild patients, but conveys to the veterinarian full responsibility for guaranteeing appropriate care, timely feeding, and segregated housing (away from people and other patients) while wild patients are in the clinic. It is always inappropriate to house wild species in the same room or in close proximity to domestic animals, especially dogs or cats. Noise, smells, and the sight of potential predators can be extremely stressful for wild patients, especially prey species. Such stress can exacerbate medical conditions or become a life-threatening problem in itself. Unnecessary handling, observation, or photography of wild patients by clinic personnel, clients, or visitors should also be prohibited.

Some practitioners prefer to schedule specific days or times when wild patients can be brought to the clinic by the wildlife rehabilitator. This is a common scenario, especially for nonemergency care. Even when such a schedule is established, all parties need to understand what is expected of both the veterinary clinic staff and the wildlife rehabilitators.

If the wildlife rehabilitator has a dedicated facility for the care of injured and orphaned wildlife, some veterinarians prefer to provide general (nonemergency) medical care at that facility, either on an as-needed basis or on a fixed schedule. For this to be effective, the veterinarian and wildlife rehabilitator should discuss what tools, materials, and supplies need to be available, as well as what kind of work space is required. Sanitary standards for the room in which medical procedures will take place may be significantly higher than a room simply used for the housing of patients. When the veterinarian routinely provides care in any setting, he/she is responsible for ensuring that these minimum requirements have been met.

In relationships between veterinarian and wildlife rehabilitator, regardless of where the care is provided, there must be a certain degree of flexibility to accommodate the unexpected or unpredictable. Under any such arrangement, the wildlife rehabilitator will likely need access to the veterinarian or his/her staff outside scheduled appointment times for consultation on appropriate medical care until the veterinarian can actually see a given patient. This is especially true where high-priority cases are received, or where the medical issues involved are outside the normal range of issues typically treated.

Hospitalization of Wildlife – Engagement of the Clinical Team

Any time wild patients are being treated in or admitted to a veterinary clinic or practice, the cooperation, understanding, and assistance of entire clinic staff are necessary to ensure appropriate care. All personnel must understand and accept that what is necessary and appropriate for their domestic patients may be entirely inappropriate for wild animals. It is also essential that any technicians, kennel staff or other personnel having contact with or access to wild patients understand the legal, medical, and ethical standards for providing appropriate care (see Chapter 1). The wildlife rehabilitator can be extremely helpful in training designated clinic personnel to perform necessary tasks such as feeding juveniles, stimulating small mammals to urinate and defecate, or safely handling and restraining wild patients during examinations and treatment. The rehabilitator can often provide specialized diets or formulas required for wild patients, to ensure that their nutritional needs are met during hospitalization. The veterinarian and wildlife rehabilitator should also discuss biosafety, common zoonoses of the species at hand and the risks of pathogen transmission from one species to another.

Emergency Care

Regardless of how available the veterinarian tries to be, there will always be emergency situations in which wild animals are presented needing immediate, time-critical care and treatment. In the human world, these are the treatments a first responder, such as an emergency medical technician or a paramedic, might administer during the short interval before an accident victim arrives at the emergency room. In wildlife rehabilitation, it is the lay rehabilitator who frequently fulfills the role of first responder. However, unlike human medicine, or even companion animal medicine, where higher levels of care are readily available, wildlife rehabilitators must often provide certain emergency treatments that would typically be provided by veterinarians, such as the administration of antibiotics or pain medications. Without such emergency care, many wild patients might not survive the first few hours in captivity.

It is important for veterinarians to evaluate the skills and competence of their cooperating wildlife rehabilitators. Whether it is simple animal handling and examination skills or more advanced bandaging techniques and fluid therapy administration, wildlife rehabilitators should not be allowed to perform any procedures for which they have not been adequately trained and in which they have not demonstrated competence, let alone directed to do so. The veterinarian should assess that the wildlife rehabilitator has the necessary skills to adequately evaluate the condition of patients, calculate the appropriate doses of any emergency medications, and administer the necessary treatments.

Training can be provided by a qualified third-party trainer or the veterinarian. However, it is up to the veterinarian to ensure that the skills of anyone involved in the care of a wild patient are adequate, including the wildlife rehabilitator and the clinic staff. In all veterinary/rehabilitation partnerships, the veterinarian, as a licensed professional, has primary responsibility to ensure that adequate standards of medical care are met, and the permitted rehabilitator has the primary responsibility to ensure all requirements for husbandry needs are met.

Since not all wildlife emergencies occur during regular business hours, the veterinarian and the cooperating wildlife rehabilitator should discuss policies and procedures for after-hours access, consultation, and care. Frequent calls in the middle of the night about situations that may not be actual emergencies have the potential to quickly sour any working relationship. The veterinarian can prevent a great deal of inconvenience by working with the wildlife rehabilitator to establish standard protocols for common wildlife situations such as cat attacks, head traumas, or other common injuries. Protocols for emergency care may also include criteria for providing or withholding food and water, or whether anesthesia may be required for advanced diagnostics or care. If it is allowed by state and federal law, the veterinarian may choose to supply the wildlife rehabilitator, in advance, with the materials and medications needed to provide basic emergency care until the animal can be seen by the veterinarian. Specific guidance can often be obtained by contacting the state boards of pharmacy and/or veterinary medicine.

In some instances, certain scheduled or prescription-only medications may only be possessed by licensed veterinary professionals, except on an animal-specific prescription basis. While a veterinary license authorizes the practitioner to prescribe and dispense medications, it may not authorize a veterinarian to provide medications, in advance, to wildlife rehabilitators. Determining what is allowed, before dispensing medications or establishing protocols, will help avoid many potential problems.

Who Will Provide What?

For any relationship between a veterinarian and a wildlife rehabilitator to be sustainable, both parties must understand what the other is bringing to the partnership, and what limits must be recognized and accepted. When a critically injured wild patient is on the examination table, in need of immediate care, it is not the time discuss budgets, resources, and funding. A question as simple as what fees, if any, the practitioner will charge for medications or services could have profound implications for the degree to which the wildlife rehabilitator will be willing or able to consult the veterinarian, let alone present an animal for diagnosis and treatment. Even though it may be frustrating for all parties to have to give up on an animal because available care is simply too expensive or too time-consuming, such decisions are more easily made and accepted if the limits and reasonable expectations are discussed and understood in advance. Having a candid discussion about the cost of medications and treatments, consumable medical supplies, food, bedding, or other specific services can help quantify fundraising goals and open the door to creative solutions for securing the needed financial or medical resources. Reaching an agreement about who will pay for what *before* the patient is in hand will reduce the potential for misunderstanding and conflict in the veterinarian/rehabilitator relationship, thus benefitting all parties concerned.

While such decisions may not be easy, it is sometimes better to conserve limited resources needed to treat larger numbers of less critical patients than to invest a disproportionate amount of resources on a severely injured individual or one that has little chance of returning to the wild. In the real world of wildlife rehabilitation, especially when the veterinarian is working with an individual rehabilitator or a very small organization, funding is almost always limited. *Economic triage* is sometimes as necessary as the medical evaluation. If the care of a certain patient is found to be too expensive for the reality of a particular veterinarian/rehabilitator relationship, advanced planning will facilitate the timely decision to transfer that patient to another facility where more resources may be available or to quickly recognize that the patient's needs simply cannot be met, so euthanasia is an appropriate and ethical choice.

Legal, Regulatory, and Ethical Issues for the Veterinarian to Consider

In addition to identifying and meeting the medical needs of the wild patient, the veterinarian must successfully navigate what can be a confusing and conflicting labyrinth of laws, regulations, permits, and ethical mandates. Unfortunately, no two states or provinces have precisely the same requirements, so it is up to the veterinarian and the wildlife rehabilitator to determine what rules apply in their location. Legal issues are discussed in Chapter 1.

In most states and provinces, individuals authorized to engage in wildlife rehabilitation are encouraged – if not required – to establish some level of working relationship with a licensed veterinarian as a condition for securing a permit to possess and care for wild animals. In some localities, a licensed veterinarian must actually sign the wildlife rehabilitation permit application form and express a willingness to provide medical expertise, guidance, and assistance to that permit holder.

However, even in jurisdictions where regulations state that such a relationship must exist, the degree to which the veterinarian is involved in patient management decisions, let alone the actual provision of care, is seldom defined. While the level of specificity varies from state to state, it is typically up to the veterinarian and rehabilitator to set the terms of their relationships. In practice, this may range from a close working partnership to a distant and noninteractive acquaintance. In all cases, for the partnership to reach its full potential, a genuine interest in collaboration must be the foundation upon which an effective program for the treatment and rehabilitation of wild patients is built.

Veterinarians who accept wild patients from the public need to recognize that, with few exceptions, the person presenting the wild animal for care is unlikely to be legally authorized to possess captive wild animals. Therefore, returning a wild animal to those individuals may be strictly forbidden. Consequently, even if the veterinarian or veterinary practice does not have a formal relationship with wildlife rehabilitators in the area, it behooves the veterinarian to become acquainted with them and know how to contact them, since they are authorized to provide long-term care for wildlife. The practitioner or clinic should transfer those patients to authorized individuals or organizations as soon as appropriate. Any veterinarian who ignores or fails to comply with regulatory mandates and legal prohibitions does so at his/her own peril, and could be held accountable for the criminal possession of wildlife or the conveyance of protected species to unauthorized personnel.

It is important for the veterinarian to inquire about applicable rules and regulations prior to getting involved in wildlife care. It is typically a matter of simply visiting the website of the state or provincial wildlife agency, or calling their law enforcement or permits offices to secure a copy of applicable laws and regulations related to the possession of wildlife and the provision of veterinary care to wild species. A veterinary license is no protection against prosecution for the violation of wildlife laws or regulations.

Many people seem to labor under the mistaken impression that so-called "Good Samaritan" protections exist for people who are "trying to help" wildlife in need, or that such declarations somehow give them immunity from prosecution for possessing wildlife without a permit, as long as they are "trying to help." This is seldom the case. Where such permission or tolerance has been granted to individuals having wildlife in their possession without a permit, it is generally limited to rescuing an animal in distress or removing it from harm's way, and delivering it directly to duly authorized personnel. Very rarely is this permission specifically articulated in law or regulation; rather, it is simply the policy of some wildlife law enforcement agencies not to prosecute individuals who are genuinely acting in good faith to get help for injured or orphaned wildlife. However, when individuals without authorization take the animal home, try to raise it, feed it, or provide any other form of do-it-yourself care, without attempting to contact authorities, any assumption of good faith evaporates quickly and prosecution is a real possibility.

Authorities often choose to euthanize wildlife that has been in such unauthorized captivity or which has received inappropriate care, especially if the animals have become tame or habituated to humans or domestic animals, or if their captive care has resulted in some physical or behavioral abnormality. Sadly, this scenario is all too common with the young of species like deer and raccoons because they tame quickly and can become dangerous as adults if they have lost their natural fear of humans.

For the veterinarian, an awareness of the policies of the local wildlife authorities can prevent potentially serious legal trouble for both the practitioner and clients or members of the public who seek veterinary help for wildlife in illegal captivity. When contacted by anyone who has captive wildlife without a permit, the veterinarian is well advised to recommend prompt communication with a wildlife rehabilitator, conservation officer or game warden, or animal control agency.

The Broader Context of Wildlife Care and Rehabilitation

In most states and provinces, there are wildlife-specific guidelines, requirements, and prohibitions related to the captive care of wild species, including housing requirements for specific animal groups, prohibition on exposure of wild patients to domestic animals or the public, and certain occupational health and safety requirements, especially related to zoonotic diseases, such as rabies. While these rules and regulations are typically intended for wildlife rehabilitators, all mandates will likely apply to anyone caring for wildlife, even the veterinary practitioner or the staff of a veterinary clinic. To avoid legal complications or other wildlife-specific problems, it pays to inquire about the legal issues that govern the captive care of wildlife.

In addition to the wildlife-specific regulations administered by wildlife management or natural resource agencies, there are other, more general laws and regulations governing the practice of veterinary medicine and the use of prescription-only medications that cannot be overlooked. There may also be local zoning or land use restrictions on the type or numbers of animals that may be maintained in a specific location.

Regardless of who is *willing* to do what aspect of wildlife care, it is essential to be aware of, and comply with, all local, state, provincial, and federal laws and regulations that define or restrict any aspect of animal care, or require that certain procedures must be provided *only* by a licensed veterinarian.

In general terms, the diagnosis of illness/injury, the prescription of drugs, and the performance of surgical procedures are activities restricted to the veterinarian alone, and within the context of the doctor–patient relationship. In some cases, wildlife rehabilitation activities authorized and allowed under the regulations of a state wildlife agency may be interpreted as being in conflict with the prohibitions of the agency charged with regulating the practice of veterinary medicine or the possession and use of controlled substances. Failing to determine the mandates and limits of the regulatory regime of the respective government entities can put both the wildlife rehabilitator and veterinary practitioner at risk.

The message to take away from this situation is that those involved in wildlife care need to be familiar with the full context within which they are working, including wildlife regulations and the laws and regulations governing veterinary medicine and pharmacy. In most cases, compliance is readily achievable, but it is incumbent on the licensed veterinary professional to determine what rules and regulations apply.

Euthanasia: When, Why, and by Whom?

One of the most challenging issues related to the practice of wildlife rehabilitation is the question of euthanasia – to humanely end the life of the patient. Certainly, no one gets involved in the provision of care to injured and orphaned wildlife for the purpose of killing wild animals, but there are many situations in which it is not only ethically allowable but ethically and legally required to end the life of a wild patient that is not eligible for rehabilitation and/or release.

The role of the veterinarian in euthanasia is absolutely critical, both for the determination of which patients need to be euthanized and for its administration.

By definition, the entire purpose of wildlife rehabilitation is to provide care for injured, diseased, or displaced wildlife to enable "the subsequent release of healthy animals to appropriate habitats in the wild" (Miller 2012). This means that any animal unable to return to the wild is not a candidate for wildlife rehabilitation and needs to be considered a candidate for euthanasia.

There are certainly many reasons for an animal to be considered nonreleasable: a bird that is unable to fly; an arboreal mammal unable to climb a tree; a burrowing animal unable to dig a hole; a predator without depth perception or full mobility; or an animal that may be carrying a communicable disease. The choice may be obvious with animals whose injuries are so extensive that there is little chance of recovery. There will be others in such discomfort and pain that euthanasia is actually the most merciful thing to do, thus ending their suffering. For other animals, the decision on euthanasia may not be as easy or clear-cut, and the veterinarian and wildlife rehabilitator may not always agree. It is worth keeping in mind that the wildlife rehabilitator, through experience and specialized training, might have unique insights about the physical and physiological requirements needed for an animal to survive in the wild or tolerate captivity; their input may be invaluable in helping to make an appropriate decision early in the case.

While there are a few situations in which a nonreleasable animal may have a potential role in educational outreach, breeding programs, or foster care of orphaned members of its species, it is often the veterinary professional who must make the difficult decisions of whether or not an animal can really have an adequate quality of life if it remains in captivity. A wildlife rehabilitation permit is for the care of animals that are intended for release; a separate permit may be required to maintain any animal that is not a candidate for release.

Another significant issue related to euthanasia is the means for ending an animal's suffering, and the skills required to administer euthanasia. While the intravenous administration of a commercial euthanasia solution may be the most common method for humanely ending the life of an animal in domestic animal medicine, many rehabilitators do not have the specific training, licensure, or experience to use this method; alternative methods must be available for those with limited formal instruction or facilities. Many of the products used in these procedures are closely regulated by federal, state, and provincial authorities, restricting access to licensed professionals or other designated personnel. The bodies of animals euthanized with certain drugs must also be managed as hazardous material, and disposed of properly. Alternative methods can be obtained from the AVMA Guidelines for the Euthanasia of Animals (www.avma.org).

Record Keeping and Documentation of Cases

One of the aspects of a wildlife care partnership that is often neglected is the question of record keeping and documentation of the case history for each patient seen. It is every bit as important to document all procedures performed on, or medications given to, wild patients as it is for any other animal receiving veterinary care. While the immediate focus of most veterinarians and wildlife rehabilitators is the individual animal, situations or health issues can often be encountered that have potentially profound implications for entire species or ecosystems, or for human health and safety. For this reason, in addition to recording the patient's medical history, it is also extremely important to capture and document all human contact with that patient, especially those which could be carrying an infectious disease. Adequate information must be gathered and available to allow appropriate follow-up investigations or responses.

For example, if a wild patient develops neurological symptoms and is subsequently found to have rabies, the lives of every unvaccinated person or family pet who has had direct contact with that animal could be at risk. If the records for the patient do not included contact information (names, addresses, telephone numbers, email addresses) for the rescuer or transporter of the rabid animal, there may be no way to reach them and provide information about their exposure to this deadly disease. It is arguably negligent for either the veterinarian or the wildlife rehabilitator to fail to gather this information, therefore it is extremely important to ensure that all personnel understand the need to have a complete record for all animals.

Training in, and attention to, record keeping must include veterinary hospital staff and front desk personnel who may be the ones accepting a wild patient dropped off by a client or a member of the public. Even if the patient record is simply handwritten on a piece of paper, the information collected must be complete and accurate.

There are several sophisticated patient record-keeping databases available to wildlife rehabilitators, some of which allow for remote access to patient files by the veterinarian. Three of the more commonly used programs are the Wildlife Center of Virginia's Wildlife Incident Log/Database and Online Network (WILD-ONe) (https://www.wildlifecenter.org/training-opportunities/ WILD-ONe), Wildlife Rehabilitation Medical Database (WRMD) (www.wrmd.org), and Carolina Raptor Center's RaptorMed (www.raptormed.com). Also, there are standard templates available that identify the basic information that should be collected in all wildlife cases.

Another valuable advantage of complete patient records is that it is far easier to comply with restrictions on when certain animals can be released following the administration of medications; specifically, game species which may be hunted and consumed by humans. Complete records will include the dates when those medications were given and should include information on release considerations. While it is standard procedure to consider the necessary withdrawal time period between the administration of an antibiotic or other medication to a food animal and when it is sent to the market, this consideration is often overlooked in wildlife rehabilitation. Many types of wildlife are legally hunted for food (e.g., deer, rabbits, squirrels, waterfowl, and others). These species must be considered "food animals" and the appropriate drug withdrawal periods must be observed before such an animal is released, if the legal hunting season will occur prior to the end of the drug withdrawal period.

Even if the only medications administered are immobilization drugs used to capture an animal or anesthetize it during examination or surgery, adequate time must be allowed for the drugs to dissipate from the animal's body before it can be released, if there is any chance it could legally be harvested and consumed by humans. Withdrawal periods vary with medication and species, and should be carefully researched and considered with all game species used for human consumption. Such medical management is the veterinarian's responsibility, and all such considerations need to be included on the patient record. Ultimately, the veterinarian is responsible for the use of all authorized medications dispensed or prescribed.

Follow-up and Outcomes

Ideally, the veterinarian and the wildlife rehabilitator will remain in communication throughout the duration of care of all wild patients. This will enable the veterinarian to intervene in a timely manner if problems are encountered during recover and rehabilitation. Understanding the outcomes of specific cases and the implications of various decisions made during the course of treatment can deepen the understanding of the medical issue involved and the effectiveness of therapeutic choices made. It is also very satisfying to know that care provided to a wild animal has actually led to its return to the wild, the very goal of wildlife rehabilitation.

Summary – It Can Work, But It Takes Work!

While the complexity of working with a wildlife rehabilitator may seem like a potential quagmire, such relationships can also be highly rewarding for all participants and extremely beneficial for wildlife. The most important admonition is to determine which rules and regulations apply to the care of wildlife, then follow them with the same rigor as for traditional companion animal, exotic, or large animal practice.

Communication is the key to a successful partnership on any level, and especially so with wildlife rehabilitation. The veterinarian must be just as explicit and rigorous in informing the wildlife rehabilitator about the condition and care of the wild patient as would be the case with a pet owner. Since the care of wildlife patients is typically done in multiple locations, all aspects of patient care must be documented, both to ensure the consistency of care in all locations and for the protection of the various partners in the relationship. Whenever decisions or instructions can be captured in writing or electronically, the chances for mistakes, misunderstandings, and conflict are reduced.

Both the veterinarian and wildlife rehabilitator need to be flexible and understanding of each other's needs and capabilities. Above all, all parties need to deal with each other in a respectful, professional manner. Each partner brings specific capabilities and knowledge to the relationship, and neither partner can do as much alone as the team can do together.

Perhaps the best way to care for the relationship is to treat it like a patient. The partnership needs the right kind of nurturing to grow. Potential problems can be anticipated and avoided with the right kind of preventive care and advanced planning. When problems do occur, addressing them quickly and in a focused manner can return the partnership to good health. In the long run, the degree to which a good working relationship between a veterinarian and a wildlife rehabilitator achieves and maintains the right balance and level of collaboration will determine what difference the team will make for its wild patients and for wildlife in general.

Acknowledgments

The author wishes to thank Dr Dave McRuer of the Wildlife Center of Virginia, Waynesboro, VA, and Dr Kelly Gottschalk of Wellesley Animal Hospital, Henrico, VA, for their insightful comments, good suggestions, and positive input.

Reference

Miller, E.A. (ed.) (2012). *Minimum Standards for Wildlife Rehabilitation*, 4the. St Cloud, MN: National Wildlife Rehabilitators Association.

9

Pre-Release Conditioning
Scott Ford¹ and Kristen Dubé²

¹ Avian Specialty Veterinary Services, Milwaukee, WI, USA
² Phillip and Patricia Frost Museum of Science, Miami, FL, USA

Introduction

After successful treatment and convalescence, wildlife patients enter a phase of evaluation and conditioning that will prepare them for release. This is necessary as the exposure to humans, nonnative food sources, inactivity due to disease or injury and confinement can affect the animal's overall fitness and its ability to survive in its natural habitat (Sleeman and Clark 2003; Mullineaux 2014). The evaluation is particularly rigorous at the beginning and end of the conditioning phase, but should also include ongoing checks of progress. The evaluation should consider physical and behavioral health with the goal of ensuring that the animal is prepared to support itself and interact with other animals, people, and the environment in an appropriate manner. Likewise, the activities of conditioning should address physical and behavioral preparedness.

Holistic physical conditioning manages pain, encourages repair and rebuilding of damaged tissues, increases strength and agility, and increases cardiopulmonary stamina. Following injury or surgery, there is a tendency for contracture of tendons and muscle to occur accompanied by formation of adhesions between damaged layers of tissue. The adhesions and contractures, in particular, can be detrimental to limb mobility (Wimsatt et al. 2000). Application of physiotherapy, starting early, diminishes the untoward effects of these processes and has many short- and long-term benefits (Shumway 2007). The inactivity accompanying injury and convalescence results in loss of strength and cardiopulmonary performance, so there must be efforts to rebuild ability and endurance prior to release. Behavioral conditioning includes efforts to assess and, where necessary, "instruct" an animal to forage normally, interact with conspecifics appropriately, and avoid common hazards, particularly anthropogenic dangers.

Adult wildlife patients have, by necessity, acquired a level of skill needed for survival in the wild, including recognition and appropriate avoidance of predators, including humans, social skills with conspecifics, ability to locate or build nests or dens, and hunting or foraging for food and defending territories (Diehl and Stokhaug 2002; Llewellyn 2003; Miller 2012). However, for neonatal patients, this vital skill set will vary depending on the animal's age and time spent with parents, and may be limited or even nonexistent. The onus then falls upon the rehabilitator to ensure the juvenile animals have undergone both physical and behavioral species-appropriate preparation prior to release.

Avian Species

Assessment

Health Evaluations
Principles of examination and behavioral assessment are discussed in other areas of this book. This chapter will discuss the most important components for determining an appropriate conditioning program, evaluating progress, and determining fitness for release.

In the context of a patient already in treatment in a wildlife facility, evaluation starts with observing the bird in its enclosure and take note of its responses to captors and conspecifics, its ability to evade capture, and its general ability to walk and run. If the bird is in a larger chamber, both vertical and horizontal flight modes should be observed, looking for asymmetry in posture, ease of flight and landing, and cardiopulmonary stamina. Digital video at 60 frames per second is commonly available and can be very helpful for review of flight nuances. Special attention should be paid to the symmetry of the wingtips and the direction of the legs and tail during straight flight. Shifts to one side may indicate compensation for a painful or less aerodynamically effective wing (e.g., the legs/tail will point away from the injured wing) (Scott 2014; Ponder 2011).

The physical examination at the start or conclusion of a physical conditioning program should be thorough, from beak to tail. Important points include checking that original injuries are healed, measurement of the range of motion (ROM) of joints, a check for captivity-related injuries such as carpal or cere abrasions, pododermatitis, or broken flight feathers, a check of molt status, and an evaluation of vision. These findings will guide the style and aggressiveness of the physiotherapy program you carry out.

Particularly in the case of injuries to bone, muscle, joints, or tendons, the ROM of the affected limbs should be thoroughly assessed. It is very important that all evaluators perform ROM assessments in a consistent manner to ensure reliability of the results and usefulness for tracking progress. A goniometer is a simple tool for performing joint angle measurements and will lend objectivity. Figure 9.1 demonstrates how to apply a goniometer to the joints of the wing. The maximum angle is the point at which resistance is felt and just before discomfort is expressed. For maximum accuracy, the measurement should be conducted two or three times, with a relaxation phase in between.

There are three portions to examining the ROM of the limbs. First, the wing or leg should be palpated for swelling or obvious injury before being extended. The examiner should also note any hyperesthetic responses (e.g., unusual jerking, writhing, or vocalizing in response to touching the limb) which may indicate pain.

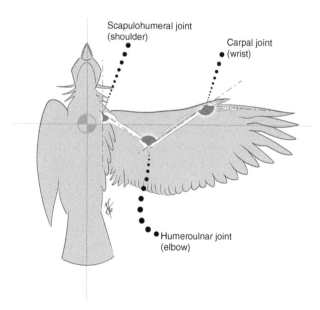

Figure 9.1 Use of a goniometer.

Second, the limb is extended gently to assess passive ROM. In the case of the wing, the quality of the feathers is also assessed and the symmetry of how the feathers spread. The examiner takes note of any crepitus, pain, or deficit in extension. If a deficit is unclear, a comparison with the contralateral limb is recommended for comparison. Next, each joint is individually manipulated. It is critical, particularly for the wings, that extension for measurement be performed in a consistent angle and plane. For example, the wing should be extended straight outward from the body, maintaining it in the same plane as the shoulders. Similarly, when each component, such as the shoulder, is extended, it should be kept in that same plane. With legs, it is most natural to evaluate them in a sagittal plane (Figure 9.1). Goniometer measurements should use consistent reference points. In the case of the shoulder, the angle is measured between an imaginary line drawn through the shoulder joint, parallel to the spine, and an imaginary line drawn down the long axis of the humerus. Other joints are simpler to visualize, such as the long axis of the humerus and the long axis of the fore-wing for measuring the humeroulnar (elbow) joint angle.

Finally, the function of tendons and joints is assessed by manipulation of the reciprocal apparatus of the wings and legs. In the case of the wings, the carpus is depressed caudally while the elbow is depressed cranially. These combined forces should cause the elbow and carpus to pivot open and spread the wing utilizing the tendons primarily.

If more than three flight feathers from any wing or five from the tail are broken or less than half grown, they should be imped or allowed to molt prior to beginning forced exercise regimens (Ponder et al. 2015). Imping is the process of cutting off a damaged grown feather and using glue and dowel to splice in a similar feather, molted or harvested from another bird. The practice is adopted from falconry and is a quick way to restore functional feathers (Lierz and Fischer 2011).

Diagnostics should include a recheck of any tests that previously produced out-of-range results. Orthogonal radiographic views should be repeated in the case of orthopedic injuries, foreign bodies, aspergillosis, or other conditions that produced radiographically detectable lesions. In essence, illness and injuries should be deemed resolved to the point that enduring the stress and demands of a conditioning program will not exacerbate them and delay healing. Also, before initiating strenuous activities such as flight exercise, a minimum laboratory database of packed cell volume and total serum solids is advisable as a simple, albeit incomplete, assessment of oxygen-carrying capacity.

Use of serum lactate, determined from blood samples collected before and after exercise, has been reported in the literature as a means for measuring improvements in cardiopulmonary fitness (Holz et al. 2006; Pollard-Wright et al. 2010; Ponder 2011). The general protocol is to collect blood immediately before exercise sessions and then immediately after and again 20 minutes later. Samples can be rapidly and inexpensively checked utilizing a point-of-care analyzer (e.g., Lactate Plus, Nova Biomedical, Waltham, MA). The testing regimen can be performed weekly during the exercise phase of a patient's conditioning. The results are analyzed for downward trends at all points from session to session, but most especially between the two postexercise samples which should presumably indicate increased ability to clear lactate and deliver oxygen to tissues. Rather than focusing on specific ranges, recovery trends are analyzed (e.g., how much the serum lactate changes post exercise). With repeated measurement, a point of diminishing returns may be noticed, which would prompt evaluation for release.

Managing Pain and Stress

Much of physiotherapy involves rehabilitation of torn tissues and broken bones and it is reasonable to assume pain is present, particularly in the early stages, whether or not a bird expresses discomfort. Pain can interfere with the rehabilitation process by causing muscle tightening and unwillingness to use the affected limb. Also, pain can suppress appetite and induce corticosterone production, thereby suppressing immune function. At all stages of rehabilitation, pain should be judiciously considered and addressed for the welfare of the patient and for optimum progress in treatment. Willingness to fly in the presence of people is not sufficient to assume a lack of pain since fear of humans can be a powerful motivator. Signs of comfort with most birds include good appetite, normal preening and bathing behaviors, resting with wings symmetrically held and, sometimes, one foot tucked up under the feathers (Mazor-Thomas et al. 2014). Also, nonpainful birds will fly in the absence of humans and show a general interest in conspecifics and their surrounding environment. Obviously, nocturnal species will tend to show more resting and hiding behaviors during the daytime. Birds that are painful may be reluctant to fly without human motivation, may sit fluffed up more often, hold limbs asymmetrically, eat less than their counterparts, and may exhibit less upkeep of plumage. Remote camera monitoring or use of motion sensors may help to evaluate the activity levels of patients while not being directly observed.

Preemptive use of multimodal analgesia is recommended (i.e., a nonsteroidal antiinflammatory drug (NSAID), e.g., meloxicam, and opioid, e.g., butorphanol combination – see Chapter 5). During times of direct human involvement, personnel should conduct their activities in a careful, calm manner, recognizing that their actions and body language can have a direct impact on the stress of the bird. Actions should be slow, deliberate, and predictable with no excited shouts, running, or aggressive actions. Eye contact can be a powerful motivator on its own and may obviate the need for raising arms or hands. Used judiciously – that is, only when about to capture or prompt a bird to fly – eye contact can instruct birds on when to expect flushing for exercise versus capture. Similarly, use of consistent visual cues (e.g., a capture blanket, leather handling apparel, or even a prop such as a creance rig) while capturing or exercising birds, which is different from cues present during routine cleaning or feeding activities, can minimize stress to just those times when it is most appropriate. These are examples of operant conditioning and can even be extended into use of rewards such as food, fresh baths, or rest periods to provide positive reinforcement for tolerating periods of physiotherapy.

Evaluation of Progress

It is extremely important to track progress during a conditioning program so that regular, objective assessments can be made. For rehabilitators dealing with multiple cases on a daily basis, it can be difficult to accurately remember the progress of each patient. A written record will accomplish this and even allow others to assist in making decisions regarding the case. Moreover, over time and multiple cases, this documentation becomes evidence to help you systematically evolve your protocols involving conditioning. Figure 9.2 demonstrates a simple log that can be added to a patient's record to provide a means of quickly looking at the progress being made. Note that concerns can also be flagged to direct attention to more detailed notes in the medical record. In cases involving range-of-motion deficits, records should include an assessment of maximum joint angles before and after each session to track progress.

Setting Goals

Although the ultimate goal of pre-release conditioning is to achieve sufficient mobility, agility, and hunting experience for a bird to survive in the wild, this goal by itself can be lofty and intangible when starting from zero in a case involving severe trauma or emaciation. Smaller, realistic performance goals should be set to aid in evaluation of progress. Goals should be specific, such as hitting target joint angles or percentages of performance improvement within a given time period. For example, for a flighted bird that is building muscle, perhaps 100% increase in stamina per week would be sensible. So, if it can only fly three laps in 15 minutes at the start, after a few sessions you might expect it to fly six at the start of the following week, 12 the next week, and so on until it can fly continuously during those sessions. Goals should

Generic Raptor Rehab Center   Patient# 16-449   Species: BAEA

Date/Time	PT Type	Total Distance	Ambient Conditions	Notes	Ini
9-13-16 Start: 09:45 End: 10:00	PROM	5 min. repititions	Indoors	Heat pack 5 min. prior Starting elbow angle: 135° Ending " " : 145°	SF CS
9-14-16 Start: 08:30 End: 09:00	Flight cage	9 lengths (450 m)	20°C, calm, dry	Slow recoveries between flights. Good control & symmetry	SF CS
9-15-16 Start: 08:00 End: 08:30	Creance	900 m	18°C, calm, lt. rain	Strong, symmetric wingbeats. Short recoveries. Became wet & heavy.	SF CS
Start: __:__ End: __:__					

Figure 9.2 Example of a raptor conditioning record.

be stated in the conditioning log so that the target is known. Goals and progress should be reevaluated regularly; weekly is generally an acceptable period of time. This is because there will likely be variations in performance based upon weather, soreness from previous therapy sessions, and physiological changes such as presence or absence of food in the gastrointestinal (GI) tract.

Methods of Physiotherapy

Selecting Methods

Three categories of physiotherapy modalities are discussed here: physical agent modalities (PAMs), exercise, and manual therapy (Hanks et al. 2015). For best results, use of at least one component from each of these categories is recommended. Early in rehabilitation, the emphasis should be upon low-impact methods that encourage anatomically correct soft tissue repair, such as use of PAMs. These include massage, therapeutic ultrasound, low-level laser therapy, and application of cold or heat. At this early stage, exercise may be limited to providing a small enclosure for stretching limbs and walking short distances. Manual therapy would involve passive stretching under general anesthesia. As injuries resolve, typically after the first two weeks, ROM improves, and the risk of adhesions diminishes, a transition is made away from PAMs and manual therapy to self-exercise in larger enclosures and eventually to forced exercise regimens that build muscle and cardiopulmonary performance.

Physical Agent Modalities
Cold Application
Cold therapy is most indicated during the acute stages (48–72 hours) of injury or surgery (Hanks et al. 2015).

Benefits include temporary reduction of blood flow, edema, hemorrhage, histamine release, cellular metabolism, muscle spindle activity, and improvement of nerve conduction velocity. In summary, there is reduction of pain, swelling, and inflammation. Cold compresses are applied to surgical sites for up to 10 minutes. Birds in particular are prone to hypothermia and some species, such as Pelecaniformes, seem particularly prone to frostbite of the extremities. Therefore, it is prudent to monitor the patient and limit application of cold to as focused an area as possible. Means of applying cold include cold packs made of crushed ice and covered in a layer of fabric, use of cold gel, or small amounts of crushed ice applied directly. With direct application of ice, continuous circular motions should be used. Frequency of application could be 1–2 times daily but will need to be balanced with the detriments of the stress of handling and restraint.

Heat Application
Direct application of heat produces vasodilation, improves tissue elasticity, relaxes muscles, and increases the pain threshold (Hanks et al. 2015). It typically does not penetrate more than 2 cm which is more than adequate for many wild birds, particularly around the joints of the wings and legs where muscle coverage is most scant. As with cold packs, heat is applied for up to 10 minutes, 1–2 times per day or at the start of each physical therapy session. Heat can be applied with use of a compress soaked in hot water, chemically activated handwarmers, or small bags of raw rice heated briefly in a microwave. Care must be taken to avoid local thermal injury or hyperthermia. A compress should be no warmer than 43°C (110°F) at its surface (hot to the touch but not painful).

Massage

Gentle manipulation of the soft tissues may be useful for diminishing adhesions, stimulating endorphin release, and increasing blood flow to an area, which in turn improves oxygen delivery, reduction of edema, and easing of muscle tension (Ponder 2011). Massage should start with effleurage, a light superficial stroking. Pressure is gradually increased to gentle kneading or circular massage. Massage is contraindicated around freshly closed surgical wounds or friable tissues.

Therapeutic Ultrasound

Therapeutic ultrasound utilizes high-frequency (>20 kHz) acoustic waves to produce deep physiological heat (Hoppes and Sessum 2008). It has been widely applied to the treatment of soft tissue injuries in humans, domestic animals, and birds. The mode of action includes increasing temperature in specifically targeted tissue and induction of acoustic cell streaming (Wimsatt et al. 2000). The thermal effects encourage blood flow and analgesia (by increasing the pain threshold) (Wimsatt et al. 2000; Hoppes and Sessum 2008; Ponder 2011). Acoustic streaming is presumed to enhance healing through increased cell permeability to calcium ions, increased protein synthesis, and release of growth factors. The result is stimulation of collagen deposition, increased formation of new blood vessels, and fibroblast proliferation (Ponder 2011). This may accelerate fracture and wound healing.

Several parameters should be considered when using therapeutic ultrasound, including frequency, duty cycle, rate of transducer motion, duration of treatment, and frequency of treatment. Most commonly, 1–3 MHz is used in birds and heats to depths of 5–30 mm. As frequency is increased, penetration decreases, such that 3 MHz is ideal for superficial lesions. Ultrasound waves striking bone may cause periosteal pain and damage and so its use over areas of bone covered with thin tissue (common around the joints of the wings and legs) is discouraged. Intensity, measured in watts/cm^2, is the rate of energy delivered. Increasing tissue temperature to 40–45°C (104–113°F) can be accomplished with 1–2 W/cm^2 with a continuous wave duty cycle for 5–10 minutes. The normal recommendation for transducer movement is 4 cm/s or slower. Treatments can be performed daily or every other day, depending upon the needs and relative fractiousness of the patient (Hoppes et al. 2008).

Therapeutic ultrasound is discouraged for use around freshly closed wounds, friable tissues, or infected joints (Hoppes and Sessum 2008). However, it can be initiated sooner than passive/active extension physical therapy (PAEPT) since it does not produce strain on bones and soft tissues. However, there are benefits to its use even in chronic cases of contracture of the wing (Wimsatt et al. 2000).

Phototherapy/Low-Level Laser Therapy (LLLT)

Low-level laser therapy involves the use of focused, coherent light of various intensities and wavelength to penetrate tissues without thermal injury. It is thought to stimulate oxygen penetration, cellular metabolism, and cell division (Ponder 2011). There also appear to be pain management benefits, probably from endorphin release. There are few documented uses of LLLT in avian species but the modality has demonstrated benefits in other animal species. One paper documents use of LLLT as part of a multimodal analgesic program to successfully manage automutilation from neuropathic pain in a prairie falcon (*Falco mexicanus*) (Shaver et al. 2009). This paper also discusses that the dose of LLLT, as well as other components of multimodal analgesia, must be carefully considered to ensure treatment is adequate. There appear to be no side effects to LLLT recognized at this time. Clear benefits in avian species have not yet been documented.

Manual Therapy
Passive Extension Physical Therapy

The terms active and passive, in terms of physical therapy, refer to whether the motion is performed by the animal (active) or by an external force (passive). ROM is the total amount of freedom of movement of a joint (Shumway 2007). ROM exercises increase blood flow, improve synovial fluid production, decrease pain, and reduce potential for adhesions and bony entrapment of tendons at fracture sites. The goals of extension therapy are to assess wing function and, through repetition, to improve ROM (Crook et al. 2007). Massage, heat application, therapeutic ultrasound, or LLLT are good precursors to a passive extension session as they will loosen tight muscles and increase circulation.

Most ROM exercises of wild birds would be considered passive. The clinician applies gentle traction or pressure to manipulate individual joints (Ponder 2011). As discussed in the evaluation section, the reciprocal apparatus of the wing and leg can be utilized to produce simultaneous extension or flexion of multiple joints and assess the function of joints and tendons. Forces should only be sufficient to flex or extend the joint to the point of gentle resistance. After massage, the limb is first stretched and held for 30–60 seconds. This process is repeated 3–5 times. Then each joint is flexed and extended gently for 10–30 cycles. If discomfort is expressed then the manipulations are slowed, decreased in intensity, or discontinued. ROM measurements should be taken before and after each session to track progress.

Active Extension Physical Therapy

Active extension physical therapy can be applied in the form of restraint that encourages flapping. In this exercise, the bird is restrained by the legs in one hand and held upright so that its weight is supported at the hips. The hand is then tilted slowly forward or back to encourage the bird to spread its wings. In the case of raptors, a hood can be applied to diminish stress and encourage more gentle use of the wings or removed to encourage more active use of the wings. With large birds, such as bald eagles, the opposite hand can support the breast and the bird may flap softly in place for several minutes. This should be performed in a quiet and distraction-free environment, perhaps even with lights dimmed for particularly fractious individual birds. Hooded or not, an outdoor breeze or fan can be used to further encourage spreading of the wings. This method is not recommended for use in the first 4–5 days after major orthopedic or tendon repair. The degree of stress response should dictate whether this approach is appropriate. Its primary benefit tends to be close evaluation of the bird's ability to manipulate its wings if neural deficits or other deficits that are difficult to localize are suspected.

Exercise

Creance

Equipment required for creance flying includes a pair of jesses, creance with appropriate weight or reel, water spray bottle, and a large, safe flight area. Jesses are leather straps for securing the legs of a raptor or other strong-legged bird. They are not appropriate for all species. Typical jess styles include traditional jesses or aylmeries. Traditional jesses are easy to make (Figure 9.3). Aylmeries involve the application of anklets with grommets and use of a button jess that slides through the grommet. While requiring more time to apply initially, application of jesses is very quick for each exercise session thereafter. Traditional jesses are recommended for most rehabilitation situations.

Once applied to the legs, jesses are fastened to a swivel which is tied securely to the end of a long cord or reel of high-test fishing line. The swivel should be of high-quality stainless steel, ball-bearing construction, such as is used with falconry or sailing equipment. These are available through online suppliers and commonly referred to as "Sampo swivels" (Sampo Inc., Barneveld, NY, USA). The cord or line should be braided in construction and be capable of withstanding the force of many times the weight of the bird since there can be abrupt loading applied. An 1/8″ braided "parachute cord" is suggested for large birds, 100-pound test braided fishing line for medium-sized and smaller birds. The opposite end of the creance is attached to a weight such as a board or secured to a heavy-duty fishing rod and reel. If using a fishing rod, the rod can be shortened for convenience in operation (or use a rod intended for ice fishing). The advantage to a fishing rod is that it provides less resistance for beginning birds and can be adjusted for more resistance as the bird's performance improves. Moreover, the user can apply increasing tension to the reel using a gloved hand, should the bird begin to stray toward hazards such as trees, people, or traffic, particularly helpful in forested regions of the country or where large athletic fields are not available. In the case of very powerful birds, the rod should also be attached to the person or weighted to ensure that it does not get pulled free of the user's control.

Proximity to hazards such as power lines, traffic, random foot traffic, pets, or even the presence of nesting birds of prey should be avoided when selecting a creance site. A sports field or farm pasture can be excellent choices. Weather should be moderate without unseasonably hot or cold temperatures (e.g., –12–29 °C [10–85 °F]), heavy rain, or gusts of wind. Birds should be housed at outdoor ambient temperatures for 1–2 weeks prior to starting creance sessions (Ponder 2011). The spray bottle is used for applying water mist to the bird's feet and face to assist in heat dissipation.

Before each session, previous comments on performance and a current weight should be taken and compared to recent weight trends. If there has been a weight decline of 10% or more within a week, exercise should not be performed until a more complete health assessment is made. Exercise should also be aborted if the bird

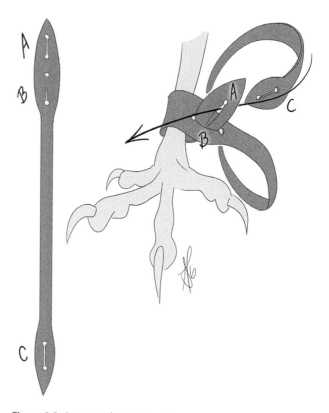

Figure 9.3 Jesses and creance system.

has a full crop or any fresh injuries. Common captive-care injuries, such as abraded carpi or beak or foot lesions, may indicate restlessness. They may prompt increased intensity/frequency of exercise sessions, an evaluation of the safety of the flight enclosure, or a pre-release evaluation.

Sessions are best performed with two persons – one to handle the bird and one to handle the line. In some cases, more people can be placed strategically to assist in driving and guiding the flight of a bird. Flights should be conducted into the wind or, if wind is calm, toward an attractive goal such as open space or perches. If a weight is used instead of a reel, the session starts by laying out line in loose loops on the ground behind the line handler. The line handler uses leather gloves to hold the line in front of these loops. If using a reel, the line handler positions a gloved thumb on the reel and the reel tension is adjusted so as to provide a mild degree resistance (if no resistance is present, backlashes and tangles tend to occur).

The bird is set on the ground, facing into the wind, in front of the line handler and the bird handler urges the bird to fly. As the bird flies, the line handler allows the line to spool out in a controlled fashion. If the bird approaches danger or is nearing the end of the line, the line handler applies a series of braking pulses to the line, just prior to applying harder pressure to slow the bird down and force it to land. With repetition, pulse-braking the line in such a manner can train a bird to make a controlled landing prior to being forced to land. Placement of obvious perches can also provide goals for the bird to attain and make controlled landings.

There are two strategies for setting up for subsequent flights. In some situations, such as a calm day or areas with plenty of space, the bird can be flown along in the same direction or back the opposite direction without retrieval. Personnel approach the bird calmly with the line held in the hands to provide control pressures should it fly again. If a reel is used, the line is reeled in as the line handler approaches. Once within a reasonable distance of the bird, flight is repeated. Birds tend to take off into a breeze so if winds are present and the edge of the field has been reached, the bird must be retrieved and returned to the starting point. The bird is retrieved by the bird handler approaching quietly, treading on the line to prevent further flight. As they approach, they take up the line in their gloved hands, crouch low, and calmly approach. Raptors will usually try to fly away so if the line is immobilized, they will end up on their breast with legs behind them or may try to turn for confrontation. If lying on their breast, the handler can reach forward to the jess swivel and hoist them off the ground. If the bird has turned to face the handler, they can pull up gradually on the line until the bird is dangling. In either of these situations, birds may flap and care should be taken to avoid feather and wing damage. Grass will usually be forgiving and prevent injury. They can be raised momentarily until they cease flapping and then lowered until the shoulders lightly rest on the ground. This position often seems to calm them. The feet and shanks (tarsometatarsi) can be secured in one hand and the bird swiveled gently into a horizontal flying position, facing away from the handler, with the opposite hand bracing the upper breast (Figure 9.4). In this configuration, they can be safely carried back to the starting point for further flights without hampering their ability to breathe and cool themselves. Smaller birds may simply be cupped to the breast with the feet secured for carrying.

Each flight's distance is recorded and the session is stopped when a target total distance is achieved, the bird exhibits significantly shorter flights (or refusal to fly), or develops signs of stress or hyperthermia (panting for longer than 1–2 minutes between flights). During flight, temperature naturally increases as much as 2–4 °C (3.6–7.2 °F) because of muscle activity. Also, lactic acid builds up in muscle tissues as their oxygen-carrying and delivery capacity is exhausted. The University of Minnesota Raptor Center has established guidelines for optimal total distances of flight sessions for a few common species, based upon results of blood lactate studies (Table 9.1). Sessions are usually started at two times per week and build up to 3–5 times per week as the bird demonstrates increased stamina, stability, and strength (Ponder 2011).

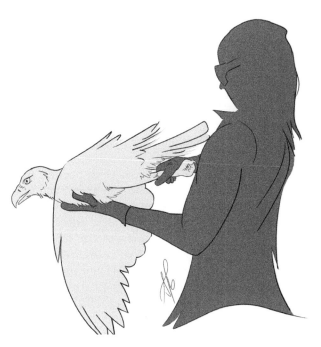

Figure 9.4 Carrying raptors during creance flights.

Table 9.1 Optimal creance flight distances[a].

Species	Total distance flown in meters (feet)
Small raptors (<200 g body weight)	600 (2000)
Barred owl (*Strix varia*)	600 (2000)
Great horned owl (*Bubo virginianus*)	300–450 (1000–1500)
Red-tailed hawk (*Buteo jamaicensis*) (1000 g body weight) (1400 g body weight)	600 (2000) 300–450 (1000–1500)

[a] Adapted from Ponder (2011).

Birds of prey are best suited to the use of creance exercise due to their strong legs for attachment of jesses. This technique can be applied to some other species, provided their legs are strong and they can be encouraged to fly. Modifications are possible using body harnesses that leave the legs and wings free and provide a site for attachment of the creance line. In one paper, a portable tower and bird launcher were used in concert with creance and harness to exercise a mallard (Pollard-Wright et al. 2010).

Flight Enclosures

The rehabilitation process for most species of birds can be broken into several phases: admission/stabilization, treatment, convalescence, and conditioning/rehabilitation. Enclosures utilized for stabilization and treatment phases emphasize minimizing stress, conserving energy, and providing ease of access for monitoring and treatments. Enclosures range from just large enough to allow perching and spreading the wings up to enough room for bathing or housing with a few conspecifics. Convalescence requires a bit more space and may include ramps and low perches that do not require flight for transitioning to the floor. Convalescent spaces typically provide ambient outdoor temperatures, fresh air, and sunlight for enrichment. Use of limbs is encouraged but space for full flight is not provided. Birds in both of these stages of rehabilitation, if they have had limbs bandaged or have undergone surgery, can easily be captured and receive massage, therapeutic ultrasound, phototherapy, or physical therapy on a regular basis (every 2–3 days). These enclosures provide some ability to assess patient mobility, although smaller birds may also benefit from flight assessments in a narrow flight corridor, such as an obstacle-free hallway (Ponder 2011). Once birds are able to attain the highest perches in such an enclosure (or make horizontal flights in a corridor) and fractures and wounds have healed sufficiently, they may be moved to larger flight cages and more aggressive conditioning modalities.

Flight conditioning enclosures should provide sufficient space to attain flight speed and still glide to a controlled landing (Pollock 2002). If enclosures are provided as the only means for flight conditioning then they should demand vertical and horizontal performance. Horizontal performance is easily obtained by placing perches at opposite ends of a long enclosure. Vertical performance is encouraged by placement of high perches that do not have ramps, netting, sequential perches, or other means of assisting ascension. Most bird species will prefer these higher perches and will attempt to get to them as their flight ability improves. However, lower perches should also be provided so that they can gain some elevation from the floor and feel safe until they are able to make it to higher perches. Minimum Standards of Wildlife Rehabilitation contains reference values for the minimum size of enclosures for many North American wild bird species (Miller 2012). This resource is the guide referenced by the US Fish and Wildlife Service for permit regulations. It can be accessed through the International Wildlife Rehabilitation Council or National Wildlife Rehabilitators Association websites (Miller 2012).

Use of flight enclosures for conditioning has several advantages such as requiring less staff time, potentially being less stressful to the birds, and being less prone to weather interference. However, raptors tend to sit quietly when undisturbed in an enclosure so merely being in a flight enclosure is not sufficient to ensure adequate exercise (Ponder 2011). Moreover, it can be difficult to force repeated flights of varying pitch (e.g., the birds tend to fly straight from one perch to another without climbing or descending) and therefore complicate the assessment process. Creance and falconry techniques have been shown to have significant advantages over flight chambers with regard to weight gain post survival, suggesting better physical fitness (Holz et al. 2006). Combining enclosure exercise with a creance flight program may provide the best advantages of both modalities.

To exercise birds in an enclosure, a single person enters and slowly walks around the perimeter of the cage. The bird is watched for cues that it will fly (turning around to face the interior, defecating, leaning forward with wings slightly outward, and head bobbing to gauge distance to a target perch). A slow pace by the exerciser allows the bird time to consider its options and make a flight to a perch. Moving too fast can panic a bird and force it to fly into windows or walls. Often, only eye contact and a steady approach is all that is necessary to prompt a bird to fly. In cases where this is insufficient, hands can be raised and waved calmly or a padded pole or soft "throw" object, such as a towel or glove, can be tossed in the air above the handler (i.e., not at the bird). If the exerciser keeps to a predictable pattern and the bird is comfortable with flying, they may begin to anticipate the movements of the handler and calmly fly from one perch to the other. This "cooperation" can be further encouraged by use of food rewards, mist baths, or a fresh pan of water immediately following the exercise session, depending on the species and individual reactions. The exercise session concludes when the bird begins to demonstrate signs of fatigue, discomfort, or overheating such as panting for longer than 1–2 minutes, or an inability to reach target perches.

Many species of birds have anatomical or flight characteristics that are not compatible with the hands-on techniques widely described for the exercise of birds of prey. However, flight enclosures can be created to cater for flight exercise of almost any species of bird.

Falconry

Falconry's primary goal is the free flying of birds of prey for hunting. This activity demands high performance and good health if it is to be successful. Because a falconry bird may actually encounter several kill opportunities per hunting trip, the experiential gains can be tremendous. Many falconers also practice an exercise known as "jump-ups" or "verticals" where the bird is required to fly vertically to the fist for small food rewards. The distance can be increased by the falconer standing on a chair or ladder. Vertical flight is extremely demanding of all of the joints, tendons, and muscles of the wing so it provides an excellent means of assessing wing function as well as building muscle and stamina. In a study involving the release of rehabilitated peregrine falcons (*Falco peregrinus*) and brown goshawks (*Accipiter fasciatus*), those conditioned with falconry techniques, versus forced exercise in an enclosure, demonstrated superior weight maintenance when recaptured after release (Holz et al. 2006). The falconry-exercised birds also demonstrated lower postexercise lactate levels.

In most jurisdictions, falconry requires separate permits from those required for rehabilitation. In some countries or states, the practice is completely forbidden. However, there may be exceptions possible for the rehabilitation of wildlife so check with your permitting agency and wildlife authorities to investigate the options. In most US, states, federal and state permits are required, which are earned through a series of steps (e.g., finding an experienced falconry sponsor, taking a written test, having facilities inspected). Falconers progress through a series of license ranks based upon experience ("Apprentice," "General," and "Master"). Depending upon their license, they are restricted to acquiring specific numbers, ages, and species of birds. A rehabilitation bird would still be counted as one of those birds, if it is in the falconer's care. Because of all these requirements, it is good to establish a working relationship with local, experienced falconers with General or Master falconer licenses. They can be an excellent resource for the final pre-release conditioning of birds but also for other bird-keeping and training questions.

If it is not practical to work with falconers in your area, you can still perform most of a falconer's activities with a raptor attached to a creance, without being required to possess a falconer's license. This includes use of lures to build and test hunting ability. In some cases, rehabilitation permits may be modified to allow free flight of species not normally permitted for falconry (e.g., bald eagles), particularly where experienced trainers or falconers are involved.

Falconry techniques are suitable, for the most part, only with birds of prey. There can also be hazards to personnel if birds are improperly trained (e.g., attacking personnel for food). For these reasons, if you are considering using falconry, it is best to consult with experienced people and to start the process with relatively "easy" birds such as postfledging red-tailed hawks or kestrels (an apprentice falconer's usual options). As long as a bird of prey is not human imprinted when entering a falconry program, it should not have long-lasting habituation issues post release. Falconry birds develop a good rapport with their caretakers in a cooperative hunting sense but typically return to being wild and aloof when no longer subjected to a regular falconry regimen.

Behavioral Considerations

For successful rehabilitation, physical fitness and flight ability are only part of the equation. A wild bird must also be able to select shelter, forage successfully, avoid hazards such as predators or people, and interact normally with conspecifics. Behavioral assessment starts at admission and carries on throughout all stages of treatment and conditioning. Malimprinting and habituation are two important behavioral aspects of which to be particularly aware.

Imprinting is a process that occurs early in a bird's life, typically around the time they are first able to see parents clearly. For precocial species of birds, such as waterfowl, the phenomenon occurs immediately upon hatching. For many birds of prey, it is around 7–14 days of age and varies by species (Jones 2001). For owls, the process seems to occur much later during fledgling stages, when they are out of the confines of the nest and can see more clearly. Imprinting is not completely genetically dictated and precedes other forms of learning (Park 2003). It has permanent ramifications that may not be obvious until much later in life. These effects include social selection, mate selection, and possibly even food selection. One study found that in at least some songbirds, cross-fostering with other species of birds negatively impacts the ability to form successful pairs later in life (Slagsvold et al. 2002). There is some modification of mate selection later in life, based upon the responses to courtship, but much depends on what species is approached as conspecific (e.g., a mate must recognize and respond appropriately to the bird's advances) (Jones 2001). In young birds, however, malimprinting is recognizable as a lack of fear, display of infantile behaviors directed at people such as food begging, and during the fledging period may manifest as aggression or inordinate curiosity about humans and their activities.

Learned behaviors can be modified throughout the life of a bird (e.g., they are not permanent) (Jones 2001). Some learned behaviors are considered involuntary. These include habituation, operant conditioning, learning by association, and trauma learning. Other learned behaviors are voluntary, defined as behavior modified through insight and experience. Habituation and operant conditioning can be used to great advantage when training birds for exhibition or falconry. The behaviors diminish when not regularly reinforced (Park 2003). A good example of this is when falconry birds are relinquished back to the wild.

In summary, imprinting is typically considered a permanent phenomenon whereas habituation and other learned behaviors are reversible. Because human-imprinted birds can be misunderstood by or even dangerous to humans, and because the condition is permanent, they are not considered releasable. For this reason, it is extremely important to prevent human imprinting from occurring when hand rearing birds.

Preventing human imprinting in nestlings requires obscuration of humans to avoid their recognition as parents, particularly during the phases when imprinting is most likely to occur. After this period, birds should demonstrate apprehensive behaviors toward any caregiver considered novel and not of their species. Anthropogenic sounds such as voices and equipment should also be minimized. Hand puppets can be used for direct feeding of young. Surrogate parents of the same species can also be used to raise fledglings and ensure proper species orientation. Static aids, such as taxidermy mounts, stuffed animals, or feather dusters, can be used to provide some of the most important elements of a parent bird. For example, chicks of precocial species may benefit from periods in contact with a feather duster to simulate a brooding and protective parent. While raising whooping cranes (*Grus americana*) at the Patuxent Wildlife Research Center, crane head props are aimed into food dishes to direct foraging efforts. These examples illustrate that there can be specific cues that are most important to the learning and comfort of a particular species. Rehabilitators should research the biology and rearing techniques of the species they intend to raise.

Young birds may also benefit from training to recognize threats. In a study involving the release of captive-raised red-legged partridges (*Alectoris rufa*), birds that were raised with "tutors" and exposed to simulated threats (wooden raptor silhouettes and humans) were more likely to survive post release (Gaudioso et al. 2011).

Learning proper food selection and how to forage are important developmental steps. Captive diet should contain elements that are identifiable with natural foods that the species would normally consume. Housing with conspecifics and performing captive prey or foraging trials may be beneficial. As previously indicated, falconry also offers an excellent means for raptors to learn to hunt and gain experience. Finally, soft releases or "hacking" is recommended for birds that have been raised in captivity (see below).

Releasing Birds

Release Criteria

Before release, a final health and behavior evaluation should be performed to assess preparedness for the rigors of survival in the wild. The precise criteria vary among species and even individual patients. In other words, a bird released at a time of local abundance of food may not have the same demands upon it as one released during other times of the year such as migration or wintering. In addition, logistics vary from facility to facility, so it is prudent for each facility to formulate its own criteria for release assessment. This protocol should include general criteria as well as species-specific criteria for the most common taxons or species received. Below is an example of general criteria, adapted from Ponder (2011), Miller (2012), and Scott (2014).

1) Anatomical
   a) Original injuries or lesions resolved completely
   b) Wings, legs, beak, talons, eyes fully functional and not requiring assistance to maintain (there are exceptions, see below)
   c) Fully restored plumage (including imping flight feathers if necessary)
   d) Does not demonstrate asymmetry in flight, lands lightly from upward or level flight
   e) Does not demonstrate asymmetry in the wings when perched, particularly after exertion
2) Physiological
   a) Normal baseline bloodwork
      i) Refer to Appendix I for normal values.
      ii) CBC and serum biochemistry recommended. PCV and total plasma solids as a minimum.
      iii) Exceptions: presence of nonpathogenic blood parasites in moderate numbers
   b) Able to maintain body mass appropriate for the species, gender, and season at ambient temperatures
   c) Producing normal droppings
   d) Excellent cardiopulmonary stamina in flight (generally this means that the bird can transit a flight

chamber effortlessly dozens of times without becoming exhausted or demonstrating overheating or shortness of breath)

  e) Able to maintain normal body temperature in ambient temperatures and weather conditions

3) Biological

  a) Appropriate age for life independent of parents

  b) Minimal risk of territory incursion (e.g., some species should not be released into areas of active breeding territories to avoid intraspecific conflict)

4) Behavioral

  a) Makes normal food choices and demonstrates ability to forage naturally. This is particularly critical for raptors admitted during their first year of life

  b) Normal avoidance of humans, not aggressive toward humans (falconry-trained birds will tolerate humans but should not show food-begging behaviors indicative of imprintation)

  c) Able to avoid predation

  d) Responds appropriately to conspecifics

5) Ecological

  a) Suitable habitat available with good carrying capacity (e.g., adequate shelter and food) for the species and time of year

  b) Presence or absence of conspecifics may be important, depending upon time of year and social preferences of the species

  c) Habitat that is subject to minimal disturbance by humans and pets. One study demonstrated that rest disorders are likely common in birds introduced to new areas (Henry et al. 2013)

  d) Access to said habitat in compliance with applicable laws and landowner permission

As noted, there are exceptions made for some cases of loss of vision or toes. Some birds do compensate well for loss of vision in one eye. This seems particularly true when it occurs prior to fledging. A failure to compensate often manifests as a bird that circles or acts more easily surprised. If a unilaterally blind raptor can pass all of the other criteria for release, then release can be considered.

For many species of birds, lack of one or even two toes on one foot may not be life-threatening. For birds that use their feet for powerful swimming, such as loons, the effects may be more dramatic than for surface swimmers, such as mallards. Likewise, loss of toes for raptors can negatively impact their ability to forage whereas a crow or songbird may experience negligible impact. Moreover, which toes are lost can be important; for example, in raptors, the first and second digits are considered the most important for hunting. Functional effects can be tested in swim tanks (for waterfowl) or perching and prey testing (for raptors). One additional consideration is symmetry of weight bearing. If excessive pressure is applied to the contralateral foot, it will likely develop pododermatitis. In general, loss of part of one toe of one foot is probably acceptable. More loss than this should elicit careful case-by-case scrutiny of the health of the feet over time in captivity.

Performing the Release

There are two main categories of release: soft and hard. Soft release gives a bird time to observe the new location, observe and interact with conspecifics, and receive food while it gradually acclimatizes to the wild. Soft release is a particularly attractive option for captive-raised birds. In raptors, this process is referred to as "hacking" and is performed using an elevated box with slatted front that can eventually be opened. Food is delivered through openings in the back of the box to diminish association with humans. With songbirds, portable soft-sided screened cages can be situated close to outdoor feeders to provide observational and social opportunities with conspecifics. With waterfowl, soft release can be conducted utilizing private ponds where owners may or may not provide supplemental food and which can provide feedback to the rehabilitator on how well the birds are adapting.

Hard release is the process of taking a bird to a site and letting it go directly into the wild with minimal opportunity for ongoing observation or assistance. Hard release is most appropriate for birds admitted as adults and being returned to the same locale as their capture, especially when very little time has elapsed.

Selecting a site for release should consider the habitat needs for the species and time of year. There should be adequate shelter from the elements or from predators as well as abundant food resources. There should also be minimal likelihood of human disturbance or anthropogenic hazards (e.g., foot/car traffic, hunting, power lines, and pets). The weather on the day of release should meet similar criteria to those for creance exercising (see above).

Legal issues also should be considered. For instance, release of any animals upon some federal or public lands in the US may be prohibited. Large tracts of private land can be excellent. Landowners may also take pride in monitoring the birds and reporting on their progress. For public releases involving large gatherings, the majority of the public should be kept well back to one side of the release area so that the bird can feel safe to depart in almost any direction. Birds prefer to take off into the wind, so consider this in the final moments before release, leaving the windward path clear and free of people.

Release should minimize stress. Opening the transport box and standing back is recommended, followed by allowing the bird to venture out on its own.

Nonavian Species

Habituation

Some studies have shown that habituation to and loss of fear of humans or domestic animals can affect an animal's survival and can be a negative prognostic indicator of successful rehabilitation (Houser et al. 2011; Beringer et al. 2004). Habituation can influence many aspects of an animal's normal social behavior, including reducing their chance of finding appropriate food and mates, and decreasing skills of predator avoidance. However, age at admittance does not necessarily affect the chance of release, as many wildlife centers have higher release rates for several species of juveniles compared with adults (Molony et al. 2007; Kelly et al. 2010, 2012; Mullineaux 2014). Therefore, reducing and mitigating the effects of habituation becomes a paramount part of the pre-release conditioning protocol in juvenile wildlife.

Due to the human involvement necessary in the rearing process, a certain amount of contact is unavoidable, particularly in the preweaning period. However, once weaned, human contact should be avoided except when absolutely necessary. The sights, smells, and sounds of humans should all be considered when interacting with captive wildlife, and in decisions regarding housing for postweaning juveniles to minimize habituation (Llewellyn 2003; Sleeman 2007; Houser et al. 2011). The following points are particularly important.

1) Visual barriers can be constructed using shade cloth attached to wire surfaces, or nontoxic foliage and branches or towels can be used.
2) At no time should wildlife have a positive association with or be housed in proximity to a domestic species, especially dogs.
3) Many species of wildlife, including most types of carnivores, need to be reared with conspecifics to ensure proper behavioral development. In special circumstances, surrogates can be utilized under the authority of state or federal wildlife agencies.
4) Necessary handling and contact for physical exams or vaccinations should never involve "comforting" the animal, including speaking to or stroking it.
5) Loud voices and human sounds from devices such as televisions and radios should not be used near wildlife.

In addition, food hatches and privacy screens should be utilized in enclosures when possible to allow feeding and observation without direct human contact. Ideally, closed-circuit cameras can be used to observe animals at will without disrupting or influencing behavior, which is crucial in determining fitness for release (Llewellyn 2003). Many cameras utilize smartphone technology to allow the user to view the animal from virtually any remote location.

On occasion individual juvenile animals may be irreversibly habituated and incapable of survival in their native habitat although at a developmental stage suitable for release. These animals may have been reared in a solitary situation if conspecifics were not available, and exhibit behavior that is abnormal. Generally, they will show signs of comfort when in the presence of humans and distress at their absence, and can be seen to beg for food from their caretakers, and may attempt grooming or other intimate or unusual behaviors with humans (Diehl and Stokhaug 2002; Llewellyn 2003). In very specific and rare circumstances, one of these individuals may be found to be suited to life in captivity as an exhibit or education animal. Generally, these animals are sociable with humans and amenable to handling and training. However, there also needs to be the proper housing, state or federal permits, and the creation of protocols and training of staff to properly care for the animal. Often these animals are only desirable if they are a unique or protected species. Euthanasia is the more commonly chosen option in these situations, as release would not be advisable for many reasons (Woodford 2000; Molony et al. 2007; Guy et al. 2013).

Behavioral Training

Animals reared in the predictable surroundings of captivity will not always readily adapt to the dynamic conditions of their natural habitat after release, which can affect their survivability. Behavioral training is essential for many species of juvenile wildlife to become adept at hunting and foraging for food. Generally these animals will not have had the opportunity to practice through observation and repetitive mimicry of these actions by their parents. The ability and interest of prey-driven species to seek and ingest natural food items are innate, but the ability to complete these tasks proficiently is a skill that needs to be developed. This skill may be muted in hand-reared wildlife, depending on the level of human habituation.

In several species, providing native food items prior to release has been shown to increase feeding on them in the wild (Guy et al. 2013; McWilliams and Wilson 2014). Native food items can be placed in hollowed-out logs, underneath substrate such as leaf litter, or presented in small pools for semiaquatic species. In bats, mealworms provided in perforated containers or dispensers stimulated normal foraging activity. O'Connor (2000) and Houser et al. (2011) showed that hunting proficiency in juvenile large felids improved within a month of being introduced to live prey.

Considerations for holding vertebrate live prey items and space allowances for hunting behaviors in the predator's enclosure need to be completed prior to the introduction of live prey. When any live prey is used, it must be monitored closely to ensure it is eaten and does not cause harm to the patient. Live rodents, crickets, and even mealworms have been known to injure mammals and reptiles if left uneaten in the enclosure (Hayes et al. 1998). To improve postrelease survivability in endangered species, specialized taste aversion conditioning has also been successfully undertaken in juvenile marsupials to dissuade them from preying on toxic cane toads (*Bufo marinus*) (O'Donnell et al. 2010), but this technique would only be feasible in specific situations.

Nutrition for Juveniles

The proper nutrition must also be considered in the complete diet offered, as most animals will selectively eat the most appealing foods which may not satisfy developmental needs (Donoghue 2006; Miller 2012; Miller and Fowler 2015). Details on suitable diets for juvenile wildlife species are discussed in other chapters.

Behavioral Conditioning

Captive-reared wildlife have not been exposed to predators, except humans. Rather than consider people a threat, habituated juvenile animals will seek out humans to beg for food and may be considered a nuisance or even dangerous. This is documented in many species, especially carnivores, and can result in euthanasia of the animal (Mazur 2010; Guy et al. 2013; McWilliams and Wilson 2014). Aversive conditioning techniques, including chasing and the use of rubber slugs, could be considered in special situations in large predators (ursids and felids) if any interaction with humans is likely to result in a fatal outcome to the animal, but must be undertaken with the guidance of experienced individuals. Rehabilitators can use a frightening noise (i.e., shaking a can or jar filled with rocks or coins) as a negative conditioning tool when in close contact with an animal if habituation is still a concern prior to release, although it is important to change the stimulus if acclimation is seen. Predator training can also be undertaken to introduce juveniles to threatening species, since for many types of animals, avoidance behavior is learned from parents. Evasive action has also been shown to improve with experience to a predator stimulus. Sound recordings of alarm calls and video of responses by conspecifics to key predators as well as realistic models have been used successfully for training in several species including mustelids, marsupials, and primates (Griffin et al. 2000; Guy et al. 2013; McWilliams and Wilson 2014). This training was effective for several months, after which time exposure to natural predators and reinforcement of the appropriate response is likely to have occurred.

Adults

Mature wildlife admitted due to disease conditions or trauma must be treated with the same precautions to prevent habituation to humans as previously discussed for postweaning juveniles, but their age and generally limited contact with people in the wild confer a significant advantage in preventing habituation. Housing and nutrition must then be carefully planned to ensure their time in captivity does not negatively influence their survivability post release.

Housing and Enrichment

Enclosures should provide the animal with a safe naturalistic area to reduce stress and stereotypical behavior and encourage normal activity and increase fitness prior to release, particularly in mammalian species (Diehl and Stokhaug 2002; Llewellyn 2003; Sleeman 2007; Guy et al. 2013). Unlike in avian species, specific exercise routines are not generally undertaken in mammals or reptiles, as the added exposure to humans can exacerbate stress and possibly habituation, and these programs are generally not needed if the proper environment is created in their pre-release enclosure. Purpose-built flight enclosures incorporating gentle forced air and flying insects have been used to encourage sustained flight and increase endurance in juvenile bats (Routh 2003; Grogan and Kelly 2013), but success has been variable. Scent trails can be created in enclosures for predatory mammals and reptiles by dragging a carcass or even a spice scent (e.g., cinnamon) to encourage foraging (Fleming and Skurski 2014). Vertical space needs to be considered in animals that are semi- or fully arboreal, as well as platforms and hide boxes to allow seclusion.

The life history of the animal should be kept in mind when making enrichment decisions, such as the addition of untreated wood for chewing in rodent species, artificial burrows for lagomorphs and tortoises, and pools for semiaquatic animals. Natural materials must be free of toxins and sharp edges to prevent injury, and ropes and material carefully inspected on a regular basis for loose threads and strings and removed when worn to prevent entanglement or strangulation (Bourne 2010).

Due to space restrictions, housing animals individually in the final stages of rehabilitation may not be possible and sometimes not warranted in social species, but mixing adult animals must be done with caution, as many species are territorial when mature, and will become aggressive when housed with conspecifics. It is best to move animals into a new enclosure at the same time, and provide additional hide space, forage, and cover to minimize negative interactions, and be prepared to quickly separate them if needed. Overcrowding also needs to be avoided, as animals need to have the proper space to move in their enclosure to increase their fitness prior to release. At no time should juvenile animals be mixed with unrelated adults since animals in earlier stages of rehabilitation may possess different pathogens (Hartup 2004). It is best to adhere to an "all in, all out" policy to prevent the spread of pathogens and allow proper disinfection between groups of animals.

Visual barriers need to be used to protect wildlife from the sight of humans, but also to prevent visualization of predator species by prey animals, which can lead to undue stress. Ideally, species such as small marsupials, rodents, and lagomorphs should not be housed in close proximity to predators at all, as their scent can also elicit a stress response in prey species.

Indoor enclosures are often utilized in temperature-sensitive species, particularly reptiles, or when outdoor space is limited. At a minimum, reptiles generally require a photoperiod, an ultraviolet light source, and an external heat source with a setting appropriate to their native environment and allowing them to select a preferred optimum temperature zone. Natural history information needs to be collected to provide optimal housing (Miller 2012). Species-appropriate enrichment needs to be provided indoors as well.

Nutrition in Adults

The base diet in adult animals should be nutritionally complete (Marcum 2002; Llewellyn 2003). Forage or food enrichment with low nutritional value should be offered as no more than 10% of the diet. Insects, arachnids, amphipods, and small fish and shrimp can be captured using nets. Road kill has been used in carnivorous species but the age and condition of the carcass, as well as the presence of parasites, could present a health risk. Obtaining fresh meat from a reliable source, such as through hunters, is a viable and safer alternative. Occasionally, media appeals can also result in donations of fresh native meat or fish from businesses or the public to help support larger predators.

Pre-release Assessment of Fitness for Release

Juvenile Animals

For a wild animal to be successfully released into its native habitat, it must have both physical and behavioral fitness after completing rehabilitation. For juvenile mammals admitted as orphans, development must be advanced enough for them to survive independently. They must be weaned and maintaining body weight while eating native food and possess dentition allowing them to capture prey or masticate food items. Coat quality needs to be substantial enough to provide warmth. Coordination and muscle development must be advanced

enough to allow proper locomotion and evasion from predators or capture of prey. Table 9.2 outlines general guidelines for release in selected species.

Pre-release behavioral assessment should be completed as unobtrusively as possible, which is best achieved by the use of remote viewing via video cameras. In this way, foraging and hunting skills, interactions with conspecifics, and the ability to ambulate effectively in a naturalistic environment can be evaluated. Inactivity can be further assessed to rule out a physical rather than behavioral impediment. However, manifestations of habituation will most likely be obvious while evaluating the animal's responses to humans. Any lack of fear by the animal can be considered significant enough to incorporate some form of aversive conditioning into the pre-release protocol. On occasion, when a juvenile has passed the developmental milestones required for release but still maintains a low level of habituation, a soft-release situation may be the best option to further distance the animal from humans.

Assessment of Deficits

All animals completing rehabilitation must possess the faculties to survive and adapt in the wild, including recovery from admitting injury or illness (Diehl and Stokhaug 2002; Sleeman and Clark 2003). This must be weighed with heavy consideration of the species and normal activity and life history if any deficits are appreciated. A small rodent missing a digit should not be significantly impaired at release, but a tortoise with amputated digits would need to be evaluated for the ability to excavate a burrow and ambulate properly in rocky terrain to be releasable. Any residual lameness from an orthopedic injury needs to be fully evaluated to ensure the animal is not experiencing pain that would affect its ability to evade a predator or capture prey. A minor functional abnormality may not preclude release but if pain is elicited on exam, such as when carrying out a ROM assessment of a limb, then euthanasia should be considered on welfare grounds.

Pre-release Exam

A thorough physical exam is a routine part of admitting a wildlife patient, but is also an essential part of the pre-release assessment. An animal that has undergone an antibiotic course should have completed the treatment 7–14 days prior to the exit exam to ensure the therapy is not masking clinical signs. It is also important to adhere to antibiotic and drug withdrawal times in animals that could potentially be used as a human food source after release. A full recovery benefits the patient by improving survivability after release, but it can also prevent the introduction of an infectious disease to wild populations.

Table 9.2 Minimum release guidelines for selected wildlife (Diehl and Stokhaug 2002; Mullineaux et al. 2003).

Species	Age	Weight	Acclimatization	Additional requirements
Reptiles	Variable		Several days prior to release	Release >2 weeks prior to brumation period
	Hatchlings		Some centers head start	Immediate release if captive born (chelonians)
Virginia opossum (*Didelphis virginiana*)	4–5 months	>250 g	~2 weeks in outdoor enclosure	Should bare teeth/ attempt escape from humans
Raccoon (*Procyon lotor*)	3–5 months (min age 3 months)	>1.2 kg	Outdoor enclosure when >1 kg	Fed ~10% diet foods from native habitat once outside
River otter (*Lutra canadensis*)	>8 months	>2.5–3 kg	Raise outdoors with min human contact after weaning; >2 months water training	
Spotted skunk (*Spilagale putorius*)			Housed outdoors >10 days prior to release	
Striped skunk (*Mephitis mephitis*)	4–5 months	>1.0–1.5 kg	Housed outdoors >10 days prior to release	
American badger (*Taxidea taxus*)	6–8 months	> 5 kg	Fed varied natural diet once weaned	Reared in social groups
Coyote (*Canis latrans*)	4–6 months	Adult weight	N/A	Must be able to hunt live food
Bobcat (*Lynx rufus*)	8–9 months	Adult weight	N/A	Must be able to hunt live food
Gray fox (*Urocyon* spp.) Red fox (*Vulpes vulpes*)	3–4 months		Important to raise with conspecifics; move group to naturalistic enclosure once weaned	Must be able to hunt live food
Black bear (*Ursus americanus*)	Variable		Variable	
Bats	>3 months		Move to flight cage with conspecifics once weaned	Must be capable of sustained flight
Woodchuck (*Marmota monax*)	2.5 months		More than 10 days outside being fed natural foods	
Eastern gray squirrel (*Sciurus carolinensis*)	3 months	>150–200 g	Outside for 2–4 weeks	Thick coat and bushy tail; able to navigate branches well in enclosure
Fox squirrel (*Sciurus niger*)		>350 g	Outside for 2–4 weeks	Eating natural foods; ability to crack whole nuts
Flying squirrels (*Glaucomys* spp.)	3–3.5 months	> 60 g	Outdoors for >2 weeks; eating native foods	Avoid human contact once weaned; particularly susceptible to habituation
Deer mouse (*Peromycus maniculatus*)	~4 weeks		Eating seeds	Fully furred and at 50% adult size
Beaver (*Castor canadensis*)	2 years		They do not reach sexual maturity or learn appropriate skills until 2 years of age	Release to a pond that doesn't have a resident beaver family (highly territorial and aggressive)
Muskrat (*Ondatra zibethicus*)	6–8 weeks		Eating native diet well; outdoors with pool for >1 week	Must be strong swimmer
Eastern cottontail rabbit (*Sylvilagus floridanus*)	1–2 months	100–200 g	Outdoors >1 week	Eating grass/native diet well and weaned >1 week
Hares (*Lepus* spp.)	6–12 weeks		Outdoors >1 week	Enclosure large enough for adequate movement/ exercise
White-tailed deer (*Odocoileus virginianus*)	3.5–4 months		Eating native foods	Vital to minimize exposure to humans pre-release
Nine-banded armadillo (*Dasypus novemcinctus*)	~6 months	1.1–1.4 kg	Eating native foods	

Additional details are provided in species-specific chapters.

This exam allows screening of the patient for nosocomial infections, including parasites and possible zoonoses, emerging diseases, or other important conditions that may have not been apparent earlier. The clinician has an opportunity and a responsibility to ensure the fitness of the individual and to help protect the health of the ecosystem and the public (Woodford 2000; Hartup 2004).

Diagnostic Testing

As a minimum database in an exit exam, a complete blood cell count, packed cell volume, total protein and whole blood and fecal parasite checks can be undertaken with nominal expenditure of resources. In addition, radiographs should be required for a thorough reassessment of a trauma case and a biochemistry profile should be completed when possible (Myers 2006). Diagnostic testing for pathogens may not change a course of treatment during an animal's rehabilitation, but depending on the pathogen, these data may guide decisions regarding housing and potential quarantine, and releasability in a particular area. For example, feline leukemia virus (FeLV) is often asymptomatic in nondomestic felids, but a cat that remains persistently viremic may act as a reservoir for disease in a naive population, where the outcome for another species may not be as favorable (Guimaraes et al. 2009; Blanco et al. 2011.) Where funds are limited, testing and treatment need to be prioritized to maximize resources to benefit the greatest number of animals, whether that is the individual in the clinician's care or the population of the species at large. If possible, archiving samples of frozen whole blood and plasma is advantageous for retrospective studies.

Vaccination

There are concerns with vaccination practicality and effectiveness in rehabilitated wildlife that will eventually be released. See Chapter 7 for more details.

Physical and Seasonal Considerations for Release

Beyond resolution of the inciting cause of admittance and establishment of the animal's disease status, it must possess the physical attributes that will allow it the best chance for reacclimation and success in its native habitat (Myers 2006; McWilliams and Wilson 2014). Assessment of weight and body condition score will help determine fitness for release. In most mammals, palpation of the soft tissue at the vertebrae and along the ribs will give an accurate determination of body condition, while evaluation for reptiles is best done by assessing the hips and tail base. In general, releasing an animal that is slightly overconditioned is preferable as there is usually a trend for weight loss after release, although obesity should be avoided (Myers 2006; Guy et al. 2013). Coat quality in furred animals needs to be assessed for completeness to ensure proper insulation, particularly if fur was missing due to injury or disease, or removed for surgical procedures (Diehl and Stokhaug 2002). Snakes need to have intact skin and should not be undergoing or preparing to shed at release.

In northern climates, an animal needs to be acclimated properly to the season prior to release. Raccoons (*Procyon lotor*) can have a 30% increase in fat stores in the fall and early winter, but most other mammals also need to put on condition in preparation for winter (Whiteside 2009). For species that have a dormant period, such as most bears, release must not be undertaken in the late fall or winter to ensure there is the proper time to increase fat stores and prepare dens. Reptiles must also not be released during this period as many species of turtles, tortoises, and snakes brumate/hibernate. If the animal is ready for release at an inappropriate time then accommodation must be made for overwintering with release in mid-spring after temperatures have stabilized and natural foods are available (Diehl and Stokhaug 2002; Donoghue 2006).

Rehabilitation of wildlife takes considerable time and resources. It is considered a success when the animal has completely recovered from its admitting problem or has matured to be a functional and productive member of its species and is deemed healthy and releasable. The animal must not have any physical or behavioral impediments to prevent it from normal activity in its native habitat; it needs to successfully forage or hunt for food and build or seek out shelter, evade predators, including dogs and humans, not exhibit any stereotypy or other abnormal behavior, and relate socially and react appropriately to conspecifics (Miller 2012; Guy et al. 2013; Mullineaux 2014). In all situations, the animal's welfare and survivability post release must be considered in the final decision on its disposition, whether it be release, euthanasia or, rarely, permanent captivity.

References

Beringer, J., Mabry, P., Meyer, T. et al. (2004). Post-release survival of rehabilitated white-tailed deer fawns in Missouri. *Wildlife Society Bulletin* 32: 732–738.

Blanco, K., Pena, R., Hernandez, C. et al. (2011). Serological detection of viral infections in captive wild cats from Costa Rica. *Veterinary Medicine International* 2011: 1–3.

Bourne, D.C. (2010). Avoiding killing with kindness: risk assessment and mitigation to prevent injury or death associated with environmental enrichment. *British Veterinary Zoological Society Proceedings* 2010: 16–19.

Crook, T., McGowan, C., and Pead, M. (2007). Effect of passive stretching on the range of motion of osteoarthritic joints in 10 labrador retrievers. *Veterinary Record* 160 (16): 545–547.

Diehl, S. and Stokhaug, C. (2002). Release criteria for rehabilitated wild animals. In: *NWRA Principles of Wildlife Rehabilitation*, 2e (ed. A.T. Moore and S. Joosten), 10.9–10.28. St Cloud, MN: National Wildlife Rehabilitators Association.

Donoghue, S. (2006). Nutrition. In: *Reptile Medicine and Surgery*, 2e (ed. D.R. Mader), 251–298. St Louis, MO: Elesvier.

Fleming, G.J. and Skurski, M.L. (2014). Conditioning and behavioral training in reptiles. In: *Current Therapy in Reptile Medicine and Surgery* (ed. D.R. Mader and S.J. Divers), 128–132. St Louis, MO: Elsevier.

Gaudioso, V.R., Sanchez-Garcia, C., Perez, J.A. et al. (2011). Does early antipredator training increase the suitability of captive red-legged partridges (*Alectoris rufa*) for releasing? *Poultry Science* 90 (9): 1900–1908.

Griffin, A.S., Blumstein, D.T., and Evans, C.S. (2000). Training captive-bred or translocated animals to avoid predators. *Conservation Biology* 14 (5): 1317–1326.

Grogan, A. and Kelly, A. (2013). A review of RSPCA research into wildlife rehabilitation. *Veterinary Record* 172: 211.

Guimaraes, A.M.S., Brandao, P.E., Moraes, W. et al. (2009). Survey of feline leukemia virus and feline coronaviruses in captive neotropical wild felids from southern Brazil. *Journal of Zoo and Wildlife Medicine* 40 (2): 360–364.

Guy, A.J., Curnoe, D., and Banks, P.B. (2013). A survey of current mammal rehabilitation and release practices. *Biodiversity Conservation* 22: 825–837.

Hanks, J., Levine, D., and Bockstahler, B. (2015). Physical agent modalities in physical therapy and rehabilitation of small animals. *Veterinary Clinics of North America: Small Animal Practice* 45 (1): 29–44.

Hartup, B.K. (2004) Considerations for Veterinarians Involved in Wildlife Rehabilitation. *North American Veterinary Conference Proceedings*, pp. 1426–1427.

Hayes, M.P., Jennings, M.R., and Mellen, J.D. (1998). Beyond mammals environmental enrichment for amphibians and reptiles. In: *Second Nature* (ed. D.J. Shepherdson, J.D. Mellen and M. Hutchins), 205–235. Washington, DC: Smithsonian Institution Press.

Henry, P., Salgado, C.L., Munoz, F.P. et al. (2013). Birds introduced in new areas show rest disorders. *Biology Letters* 9 (5): 20130463.

Holz, P.H., Naisbitt, R., and Mansell, P. (2006). Fitness level as a determining factor in the survival of rehabilitated

peregrine falcons (*Falco peregrinus*) and brown goshawks (*Accipiter fasciatus*) released back into the wild. *Journal of Avian Medicine and Surgery* 20 (1): 15–20.

Hoppes, S. and Sessum, D. (2008). Therapeutic ultrasound in a blue and gold macaw (*Ara ararauna*). *Proceedings of the Association of Avian Veterinarians* 29: 403–407.

Houser, A., Gusset, M., Bragg, C.J. et al. (2011). Pre-release hunting training and post-release monitoring are key components in the rehabilitation of orphaned large felids. *South African Journal of Wildlife Research* 41 (1): 11–20.

Jones, M.P. (2001). Behavioral aspects of captive birds of prey. *Veterinary Clinics of North America – Exotic Animal Practice* 4 (3): 613–632.

Kelly, A., Scrivens, R., and Grogan, A. (2010). Post-release survival of orphaned wild-born polecats *Mustela putorius* reared in captivity at a wildlife rehabilitation Centre in England. *Endangered Species Research* 12: 107–115.

Kelly, A., Goodwin, S., Grogan, A. et al. (2012). Further evidence for the post-release survival of hand-reared, orphaned bats based on radio-tracking and ring-return data. *Animal Welfare* 21: 27–31.

Lierz, M. and Fischer, D. (2011). Clinical technique: imping in birds. *Journal of Exotic Pet Medicine* 20 (2): 131–137.

Llewellyn, P. (2003). Rehabilitation and release. In: *BSAVA Manual of Wildlife Casualties* (ed. E. Mullineaux, D. Best and J.E. Cooper), 29–36. Gloucester, UK: British Small Animal Veterinary Association.

Marcum, D. (2002). Mammal nutrition: diets part II – post-weaning diets – dietary staples. In: *NWRA Principles of Wildlife Rehabilitation*, 2e (ed. A.T. Moore and S. Joosten), 8.59–8.64. St Cloud, MN: National Wildlife Rehabilitators Association.

Mazor-Thomas, J.E., Mann, P.E., Karas, A.Z. et al. (2014). Pain-suppressed behaviors in the red-tailed hawk 1 (*Buteo jamaicensis*). *Applied Animal and Behavioral Science* 152: 83–91.

Mazur, R.L. (2010). Does aversive conditioning reduce human-black bear conflict? *Journal of Wildlife Management* 74 (1): 48–54.

McWilliams, M. and Wilson, J.A. (2014). Home range, body condition, and survival of rehabilitated raccoons (*Procyon lotor*) during their first winter. *Journal of Applied Animal Welfare Science* 18 (2): 133–152.

Miller, E.A. (2012). *Minimum Standards for Wildlife Rehabilitation*, 4e. St Cloud, MN: National Wildlife Rehabilitators Association.

Miller, R.E. and Fowler, M.E. (2015). *Fowler's Zoo and Wild Animal Medicine*, 8e. St Louis, MO: Elsevier.

Molony, S., Baker, P.J., Garland, L. et al. (2007). Factors that can be used to predict release rates for wildlife casualties. *Animal Welfare* 16: 361–367.

Mullineaux, E. (2014). Veterinary treatment and rehabilitation of indigenous wildlife. *Journal of Small Animal Practice* 55: 293–300.

Mullineaux, E., Best, D., and Cooper, J.E. (2003). *BSAVA Manual of Wildlife Casualties*. Gloucester, UK: British Small Animal Veterinary Association.

Myers, D.A. (2006). Common procedures and concerns with wildlife. *Veterinary Clinics Exotic Animal Practice* 9: 437–460.

O'Connor, K.I. (2000). Mealworm dispensers as environmental enrichment for captive Rodrigues fruit bats (*Pteropus rodricensis*). *Animal Welfare* 9: 123–137.

O'Donnell, S., Webb, J.K., and Shine, R. (2010). Conditioned taste aversion enhances the survival of an endangered predator imperiled by a toxic invader. *Journal of Applied Ecology* 47: 558–565.

Park, F. (2003). Behavior and behavioral problems of Australian raptors in captivity. *Seminars in Avian and Exotic Pet Medicine* 12 (4): 232–241.

Pollard-Wright, H.M., Wright, M.T., and Warren, J.M. (2010). Use of a portable tower and remote-controlled launcher to improve physical conditioning in a rehabilitating wild mallard (*Anas platyrhynchos*). *Journal of Avian Medicine and Surgery* 24 (4): 308–315.

Pollock, C. (2002). Postoperative management of the exotic animal patient. *Veterinary Clinics of North America – Exotic Animal Practice* 5 (1): 183–212.

Ponder, J.B. (2011). Avian physiotherapy and reconditioning in a rehabilitation program. *Proceedings of the Association of Avian Veterinarians* 32: 149–160.

Routh, A. (2003). Bats. In: *BSAVA Manual of Wildlife Casualties* (ed. E. Mullineaux, D. Best and J.E. Cooper), 95–108. Gloucester, UK: British Small Animal Veterinary Association.

Scott, D. (ed.) (2014). *Internal Protocols*. Huntersville, NC: Carolina Raptor Center.

Shaver, S.L., Robinson, N.G., Wright, B.D. et al. (2009). A multimodal approach to management of suspected neuropathic pain in a prairie falcon (*Falco mexicanus*). *Journal of Avian Medicine and Surgery* 23 (3): 209–213.

Shumway, R. (2007). Rehabilitation in the first 48 hours after surgery. *Clinical Techniques in Small Animal Practice* 22 (4): 166–170.

Slagsvold, T., Hansen, B.T., Johannessen, L.E. et al. (2002). Mate choice and imprinting in birds studied by cross-fostering in the wild. *Proceedings of the Royal Society B: Biological Sciences* 269 (1499): 1449–1455.

Sleeman, J.M. (2007) Keeping Wildlife Wild: How to Prevent Habituation and Imprinting in Rehabilitated Wildlife. *North American Veterinary Conference Proceedings*, pp. 1708–1709.

Sleeman, J.M. and Clark, E.E. (2003). Clinical wildlife medicine: a new paradigm for a new century. *Journal of Avian Medicine and Surgery* 17 (1): 33–37.

Whiteside, D.P. (2009). Nutrition and behavior of coatis and raccoons. *Veterinary Clinics of North America: Exotic Animal Practice* 12: 187–195.

Wimsatt, J., Dressen, P., Dennison, C. et al. (2000). Ultrasound therapy for the prevention and correction of contractures and bone mineral loss associated with wing bandaging in the domestic pigeon (*Columba livia*). *Journal of Zoo and Wildlife Medicine* 31 (2): 190–195.

Woodford, M.H. (2000) Quarantine and Health Screening Protocols for Wildlife Prior to Translocation and Release into the Wild. IUCN Species Survival Commission's Veterinary Specialist Group, Gland, Switzerland, the Office International des Epizooties (OIE), Paris, France, Care for the Wild, UK, and the European Association of Zoo and Wildlife Veterinarians, Switzerland.

10

Postrehabilitation Release Monitoring of Wildlife

Sonia M. Hernandez

D.B. Warnell School of Forestry and Natural Resources and the Southeastern Cooperative Wildlife Study at the College of Veterinary Medicine. University of Georgia, Athens, GA, USA

Introduction

The rehabilitation of wildlife continues to gain popularity for many reasons, one being that it is perceived as a way to mitigate the effects of human activities on wildlife. This topic is subject to much debate among biologists and rehabilitators, where biologists and wildlife managers discount rehabilitation activities as having little effect on wildlife populations and disagree with the diversion of resources toward these often high-profile, "feel good" activities in preference to preventive measures such as protection or restoration of habitat. In fact, most state natural resource agencies do not philosophically or financially support rehabilitation centers, with notable exceptions, such as efforts to rescue endangered species (e.g., marine mammals or sea turtles). The philosophy and ethics of wildlife rehabilitation and the controversy about it are beyond the scope of this chapter; however, well-designed postrelease monitoring studies of rehabilitated and released animals can help provide factual information that can guide the discourse.

The International Wildlife Rehabilitation Council defines rehabilitation as "The treatment and temporary care of injured, diseased, and displaced indigenous animals, and the subsequent release of healthy animals to appropriate habitats in the wild" (www.theiwrc.org). This mission statement is similar to that of many wildlife clinics. For example, the University of Georgia's wildlife clinic's mission statement is (paraphrasing) "to provide care to injured wildlife for the purpose of returning them to 100% function and releasing them back into the wild," thereby excluding treatment or care that would result in animals that were not able to fend for themselves once released or rehabilitating animals for a lifetime in captivity, with only very specific and special exceptions (e.g., an animal needed for breeding or educational purposes).

At the center of the debate among rehabilitators and biologists and the mission of rehabilitation activities is the "success" of individual animals after they are released. Specifically, the definition of "success" varies among stakeholders. For example, a wildlife medicine practitioner might be interested in how an individual may function in its environment post release in order to determine if the particular clinical technique applied was successful. In that case, short-term monitoring aimed at evaluating the function of a particular system (e.g., whether the animal can hunt after a particular fracture repair) might be sufficient. A biologist, on the other hand, may have a more comprehensive concern about the ability of an individual rehabilitated animal to, for example, recognize, hunt/forage for food, successfully compete with others, join social groups, defend/maintain territories, withstand weather fluctuations and other environmental extremes, or acquire/maintain a mate and reproduce successfully as measures of that individual's contribution to its population. For endangered animals, even a few individuals contributing to the population could be significant.

Lastly, both groups can likely agree that at the core of this topic is the welfare of both the individual animal being released and the recipient population. It is assumed that an animal that is unprepared or unfit for release will die, perhaps suffering in the process, which is undesirable. Likewise, released animals that are diseased or will attack resident conspecifics can be disruptive to local populations. Regardless, whether one cares about (i) the information needed to modify clinical techniques, (ii) the individual animal's welfare, or (iii) its contribution to the population, monitoring of released individuals is paramount and provides a means to inform whether and how rehabilitation should continue. Unfortunately, postrelease monitoring studies are rarely conducted.

Medical Management of Wildlife Species: A Guide for Practitioners, First Edition. Edited by Sonia M. Hernandez, Heather W. Barron, Erica A. Miller, Roberto F. Aguilar and Michael J. Yabsley.

For further reviews that suggest that survival after release varies greatly both within and between species, please see Ellis et al. (1990), Priddel and Wheeler (1994), Pietsch (1995), Carrick et al. (1996), Reeve (1998), Fajardo et al. (2000), Goldsworthy et al. (2000), Lander et al. (2002), and Guy and Banks (2011).

Postrelease Monitoring Informs the Clinician

At its simplest, postrelease monitoring can inform the clinician and staff whether a particular technique was successful. For example, the abnormal growth of scutes below and surrounding a shell injury repaired with epoxy in radio-tagged aquatic turtles monitored for two years suggested that turtles are best not released prior to removal of epoxy implants, a practice that although once common, has now fallen out of favor (Hernandez, unpublished data). In some cases, postrelease monitoring information can lead to modifications that result in more efficient and less consuming rehabilitation activities. For example, assessment of the success and survival of animals after oil spills and intervention activities has led to changes in the triage and methodology employed during these events (Mazet et al. 2002). Gartrell et al. (2013) found that intensive captive husbandry to convert birds to a captive diet and improve nutritional status was the main factor needed to improve survival of dotterels collected after an oil spill. In fact, the rehabilitation of animals, particularly birds, after oil spills is likely the most systematically assessed rehabilitation activity and its success can be attributed to its adaptive strategy based on scientific studies (Newman et al. 2004; de la Cruz et al. 2013).

Sometimes postrelease studies can help clear up ethical questions about release. For example, 16 screech owls (seven normal, nine vision impaired) were tracked for ~115 days, during which five died (3/5 were vision impaired). The study concluded there was a higher survival in the normal group but there were no wild counterparts used as controls and small sample sizes limit data interpretation (Allbritten and Jackson 2002).

Measuring Postrelease Monitoring

Prior to release, animals must be physically and psychologically fit to resume their life in the wild. Chapter 9 outlines pre-release conditioning in detail. Postrelease monitoring can rely on passive reporting of recovered animals (often after they die; e.g., with tattoos, bands, tags, microchips, etc.) or active monitoring with transmitters (e.g., via radiotelemetry, global positioning systems, geolocators, etc.). The recent and rapid development of battery technology and miniaturization of tracking devices has expanded the range of options available to monitor animals. Text reviews on the use of remote sensing technology to monitor animals are useful for general principles (e.g., Kenward 2000; Millspaugh et al. 2012) but to keep up with the latest technology, the reader should consult species-specific primary literature. Remote sensing technologies allow the monitoring of animal movements and habitat use, but require both trained individuals and, depending on the goal of the study, adjunctive methods.

As a way to examine how rehabilitation or time spent in captivity might impact an animal, we can consider measuring effects in three broad categories: survival, behavior, and reproductive success. Most postrelease monitoring measures survival and requires locating an animal at regular intervals for a predetermined amount of time. Whereby it is understood that rehabilitated individual animals are expected to survive for some period after their release, the extent to which postrelease survival has been monitored is extremely varied, tends to be short term and is often limited by the technology and cost of the monitoring equipment. For example, radiotelemetry requires trained personnel who can spend the time moving in the environment in search of a radio signal with hand-held, truck-mounted, or aerial antennas. Triangulation of the signal is required to determine an exact location. Conversely, GPS systems utilize satellites to determine the location of an animal, and allow for data to either be stored in the device (and later retrieved if the animal dies or the attachment device falls off) or delivered to the researcher via satellite or cell phone networks. Most devices are equipped with "mortality indicators" which turn on when an animal has not moved for a predetermined number of hours/days and can help in measuring survival.

Survival alone is not the only measure of rehabilitation success. In fact, it is imperative that animals released after rehabilitation behave in ways that will allow them to succeed in their environments. Measuring behavior will often require a combination of monitoring techniques, including direct observations or reliance on reports from the public. The most obvious negative effects to animal behavior considered in rehabilitation are imprinting and/or other types of habituation to humans. For example, one study concluded that approximately half of deer fawns released after rehabilitation died within the first month after release and those that survived did so near human-inhabited areas, likely due to some degree of habituation (Beringer et al. 2004). In contrast, much effort has been devoted to avoid imprinting of birds of prey, waterfowl and other imprinting-prone species, but the success of these efforts has not always been measured. A story promoting the role that rehabilitation can have on the conservation of the wombat detailed the success of rehabilitated animals (77%) after eight years of monitoring, but warned that imprinting needed to be avoided (Saran et al. 2011).

A major concern among biologists and rehabilitators alike is that animals admitted to rehabilitation centers, which often present with conditions related to anthropogenic activities, return to situations or behaviors that place them at high risk for the problem to repeat itself. For example, urban coyotes that were struck by vehicles and suffered long bone fractures were radio-collared and monitored for one year post surgical repair and rehabilitation. Despite being released more than 20 miles outside a large city, all the animals returned to scavenging in urban areas with high human density and likely were at high risk of suffering a similar fate in the future (Hernandez, unpublished data). Four out of 10 monitored bats rehabilitated in England survived, but were found trapped in buildings, prompting the authors of the study to recommend that rehabilitation activities "teach" bats how to exit enclosed spaces through small holes (Kelly et al. 2012). All three cheetahs monitored in one study were shot within seven months of their release, illustrating that they returned to situations that resulted in human–wildlife conflicts (Houser et al. 2011).

Lastly, if an individual survives and goes on to reproduce in the wild, it may be considered as having contributed to its population. Few studies have measured the reproductive success of rehabilitated animals, particularly when compared with their free-ranging counterparts, and again, this likely requires a combination of monitoring efforts, including long-term tagging and observations. For example, one study compared the reproductive success of koalas rehabilitated after wild fires to a control population and determined that their reproductive rates did not differ (Lunney et al. 2004).

Comprehensive assessment of the behavior, longevity, and reproductive activities of rehabilitated wildlife is rarely done because it is expensive and time-consuming. In a review of rehabilitation methods in Australia, the most important constraint on postrelease monitoring was lack of funds (87%) (Guy et al. 2013) and consequently monitoring was only undertaken by one third of centers surveyed. In fact, the majority of postrelease studies, because they tend to be poorly financially supported and/or opportunistic, are conflicted by some significant design flaws: (i) they rely on small sample sizes that may not reflect the large variation in behavior (phenotypic plasticity) that individuals can display (e.g., monitoring of three Stellar sealion pups [*Eumetopias jubatusa*]; Lander and Gulland 2003), (ii) monitoring is often only undertaken for short periods of time

(<1 year), (iii) they often lack a control group of free-living animals that were not rehabilitated with which to compare, and (iv) they fail to control for extraneous variables such as differences in habitat, climate, or rehabilitation/release methods (soft vs hard releases), etc. "Researcher bias" (i.e., the inherent desire by animal caretakers for animals to succeed) can complicate such studies. To address these concerns, it is suggested that rehabilitation centers, animal welfare organizations, and other groups collaborate with researchers and wildlife managers trained in conducting scientifically sound wildlife monitoring studies.

Postrelease monitoring is not prioritized, in part perhaps because of the perception that negative results would bring into question the purpose of rehabilitation activities. Yet, there are positive stories, particularly for endangered species (e.g., sea turtles tracked for 688 days which survived and returned to their natural feeding ranges) (Mestre et al. 2014) and information gained from controlled studies contributes to the overall management of wildlife species. The most common and frequently rehabilitated animals (e.g., raccoons, songbirds, etc.) are rarely, if ever, monitored after release. A study of adult raccoons in Canada demonstrated that rehabilitated raccoons survived at a similar rate as nonrehabilitated raccoons (Rosatte et al. 2010). For other species, results are often variable, depending on methodology, study design, and location. European hedgehogs were monitored in the UK and some studies found good postrelease survival (82% survival at six weeks, 77% survival at six weeks, and 75% survival at five weeks post release) while others had less successful rates (33% survival at six weeks, 25% survival at eight weeks) (Mullineaux 2014).

A Different Perspective

Rehabilitation and release of wildlife are akin to, and should be firmly rooted in, two activities that are well studied within the disciplines of conservation biology and ecology: the movement of wildlife and urban wildlife ecology. These disciplines have developed evidence-based principles which can serve to inform rehabilitation activities.

To begin, definitions matter. *Introduction* is defined as the release of a species into an area outside its historical range (IUCN 2013); *reintroduction* aims to establish a species in an area where it used to exist; *supplementation* is the addition of individuals to an existing population; and finally *relocation/translocation* involves moving individuals from an area where they are threatened to where their habitat is secure (Dodd and Seigel 1991). Biologists generally consider these activities to be successful if it leads to the "establishment of a self-sustaining population, obtained by the survival and breeding of the released individuals, and persistence of this new population" (Dodd and Seigel 1991; Seddon 1999). For example, gopher tortoises are one of the most translocated animals in the USA, yet postrelease monitoring has led to significant changes in how these animals are managed in their translocated range. Tuberville et al. monitored gopher tortoises for two years post release using various management treatments and concluded that for the successful establishment of translocated tortoises to occur, the area where tortoises were released had to be fenced for at least one year (Tuberville et al. 2005). In lieu of limiting the movement of tortoises with fences, the animals, confused and devoid of their pretranslocation social hierarchy, dispersed far away and never established a viable population. Gopher tortoise managers have adopted these recommendations and temporary fencing of release areas has become the standard in gopher tortoise translocation.

The urban wildlife ecology literature abounds in studies of animals that are translocated and subsequently monitored because they have become a public nuisance and the practice of wildlife rehabilitation can also benefit

from those studies. For example, nine-banded armadillos were captured, translocated, monitored, and compared to a resident population. Researchers found that translocated individuals dispersed away from their translocation site and made large movements toward to their original site of capture, concluding that their translocation is unlikely to be successful (Gammons et al. 2009). In contrast, reintroduction of bobcats onto a barrier island was considered highly successful (93% of animals survived and reproduced) because the area was protected, there was strong public support for the project, and bobcats rarely cause public conflict (Diefenbach et al. 2009).

Thus, in rehabilitation and release, we should not try to reinvent the wheel and instead, look to factors that have contributed to the success of reintroduction, translocation, and other similar activities, particularly because the majority of these efforts, according to one review, have failed (Fischer and Lindenmayer 2000). Guidelines for reintroduction are outlined by the International Union for Conservation of Nature (IUCN) guidelines (IUCN 2013) and could serve as a baseline for rehabilitation activities.

References

Allbritten, M. and Jackson, D. (2002). A post-release study of rehabilitated western screech owls (Otus kennecotti) in Douglas County, Oregon. *Journal of Wildlife Rehabilitation* 25 (4): 5–10.

Beringer, J., Mabry, P., Meyer, T. et al. (2004). Post-release survival of rehabilitated white-tailed deer fawns in Missouri. *Wildlife Society Bulletin* 32: 732–738.

Carrick, F.N., Beutel, T.S., Ellis, W.A.H., and Howard, N. (1996). Re-establishment of koalas in the wild following successful rehabilitation. In: *Koalas: Research for Management. Proceedings of the Brisbane Koala Symposium* (ed. G. Gordon), 123–128. Brisbane: World Koala Research Inc.

De La Cruz, S., Takekawa, J.Y., Spragens, K.A. et al. (2013). Post-release survival of surf scoters following an oil spill: an experimental approach to evaluating rehabilitation success. *Marine Pollution Bulletin* 67: 100–106.

Diefenbach, D.R., Hansen, L.A., Conroy, M.J., et al. (2009). Restoration of bobcats to Cumberland Island, Georgia, USA: lessons learned and evidence for the role of bobcats as keystone predators. Iberian Lynx Ex-situ Conservation Seminar Series. Sevilla, Spain: Fundación Biodiversidad.

Dodd, C.K. Jr. and Seigel, R.A. (1991). Relocation, repatriation, and translocation of amphibians and reptiles: are they conservation strategies that work? *Herpetologica* 62: 336–350.

Ellis, W.A.H., White, N.A., Kunst, N.D., and Carrick, F.N. (1990). Response of koalas (Phascolarctos cinereus) to re-introduction to the wild after rehabilitation. *Australian Wildlife Research* 17: 421–426.

Fajardo, I., Babiloni, G., and Miranda, Y. (2000). Rehabilitated and wild barn owls (Tyto alba): dispersal, life expectancy and mortality in Spain. *Biological Conservation* 94: 287–295.

Fischer, J. and Lindenmayer, D.B. (2000). An assessment of the published results of animal relocations. *Biological Conservation* 96: 1–11.

Gammons, D.J., Mengak, M.T., and Conner, L.M. (2009). Translocation of nine-banded armadillos. *Human-Wildlife Conflicts* 3 (1): 64–71.

Gartrell, B.D., Collen, R., Dowding, J.E. et al. (2013). Captive husbandry and veterinary care of northern New Zealand dotterels (Charadrius obscurus aquilonius) during the CV Rena oil-spill response. *Wildlife Research* 40: 624–632.

Goldsworthy, S.D., Giese, M., Gales, R.P. et al. (2000). Effects of the Iron Baron oil spill on little penguins (Eudyptula minor). II. Post-release survival of rehabilitated oiled birds. *Wildlife Research* 27: 573–582.

Guy, A.J. and Banks, P. (2011). A survey of current rehabilitation practices for native mammals in eastern Australia. *Australian Mammalogy* 34 (1): 108–118.

Guy, A.J., Curnoe, D., and Banks, P.B. (2013). A survey of current mammal rehabilitation and release practices. *Biodiversity and Conservation* 22: 825.

Houser, A., Gusset, M., Bragg, C.J. et al. (2011). Pre-release hunting training and post-release monitoring are key components in the rehabilitation of orphaned large felids. *African Journal of Wildlife Research* 41: 11–20.

IUCN/SSC Re-introduction Specialist Group (2013). *Guidelines for Reintroductions and Other Conservation Translocations*. Gland, Switzerland: IUCN.

Kelly, A., Goodwin, S., Grogan, A. et al. (2012). Post-release survival of hand-reared pipistrelle bats (Pipistrellus spp). *Animal Welfare* 17 (4): 375–382.

Kenward, R. (2000). *A Manual for Wildlife Radio Tagging*, 2e. Cambridge, MA: Academic Press.

Lander, M.E. and Gulland, F.M. (2003). Rehabilitation and post-release monitoring of Steller Sea lion pups raised in captivity. *Wildlife Society Bulletin* 31: 1047–1053.

Lander, M.E., Havery, J.T., Hanni, K.D., and Morgan, L.E. (2002). Behavior, movements and apparent survival of rehabilitated and free-ranging harbor seal pups. *Journal of Wildlife Management* 66: 19–28.

Lunney, D., Gresser, S.M., Mahon, P.S. et al. (2004). Post-fire survival and reproduction of rehabilitated and unburnt koalas. *Biological Conservation* 120: 567–575.

Mazet, J., Newman, S., Gilardi, K. et al. (2002). Advances in oiled bird emergency medicine and management. *Journal of Avian Medicine and Surgery* 16 (2): 146–150.

Mestre, F., Bragança, M.P., Nunes, A., and dos Santos, M.E. (2014). Satellite tracking of sea turtles released after prolonged captivity periods. *Marine Biology Research* 10 (10): 996–1006.

Millspaugh, J.J., Kesler, D.C., Kays, R.W. et al. (2012). Wildlife radiotelemetry and remote monitoring. *The Wildlife Techniques Manual* 1: 258–283.

Mullineaux, E. (2014). Veterinary treatment and rehabilitation of indigenous wildlife. *Journal of Small Animal Practice* 55 (6): 293–300.

Newman, S.H., Golightly, R.T., Craig, E.N., et al. (2004). The Effects of Petroleum Exposure and Rehabilitation on Post-Release Survival, Behavior, and Blood Health Indices: A Common Murre (Uria aalge) Case Study Following the Stuyvesant Petroleum Spill. Final Report. Oiled Wildlife Care Network, Wildlife Health Center, UC Davis, Davis, CA.

Pietsch, R.S. (1995). The fate of urban common brushtail possums translocated to sclerophyll forest. In: *Reintroduction Biology of Australian and New Zealand Fauna* (ed. M. Serena), 239–246. Chipping Norton, New South Wales: Surrey Beatty & Sons.

Priddel, D. and Wheeler, R. (1994). Mortality of captive raised malleefowl, Leipoa ocellata, released into a mallee remnant within the wheat-belt of New South Wales. *Wildlife Research* 21: 543–552.

Reeve, N.J. (1998). Survival and welfare of hedgehogs (Erinaceus europaeus) after release back into the wild. *Animal Welfare* 7: 189–202.

Rosatte, R., Ryckman, M., Meech, S. et al. (2010). Home range, movements and survival of rehabilitated raccoons (Procyon lotor) in Ontario, Canada. *Journal of Wildlife Rehabilitation* 30: 7–12.

Saran, K.A., Parker, G., Parker, R. et al. (2011). Rehabilitation as a conservation tool: a case study using the common wombat. *Pacific Conservation Biology* 17: 310–319.

Seddon, P.J. (1999). Persistence without intervention: assessing success in wildlife reintroductions. *Trends in Ecology & Evolution* 14 (12): 503.

Tuberville, T.D., Clark, E.E., Buhlmann, K.A. et al. (2005). Translocation as a conservation tool: site fidelity and movement of repatriated gopher tortoises (Gopherus polyphemus). *Animal Conservation* 8 (4): 349–358.

11

Wound Management in Wildlife

Elizabeth A. Maxwell[1] and R. Avery Bennett[2]

[1] *Department of Small Animal Clinical Sciences, College of Veterinary Medicine, University of Florida, Gainesville, FL, USA*
[2] *Department of Veterinary Clinical Sciences, School of Veterinary Medicine, Louisiana State University, Baton Rouge, LA, USA*

Introduction

Wound healing is a complex process. It is important to understand the healing process when managing patients so we are able to assess change over time and select appropriate therapies as healing progresses. Critical assessment of the wound site is important in determining when the treatment protocols should be changed.

It is not feasible to recommend a step-by-step approach when managing specific types of wounds in wildlife. This chapter is a review of the stages of wound healing and the treatment options available for managing wounds in the various stages of the healing process. We review wound irrigation, topical treatments, bandaging techniques, and relatively new therapies such as laser and negative pressure wound therapy. Also described are when different treatments, topical medications and other therapies are indicated during the healing process.

The clinician attending the patient must evaluate the wound on a regular basis, usually during bandage changes, and change therapies as healing progresses. It is very important that the person making decisions about wound therapies and treatment changes be involved as wound healing progresses. It is difficult to make decisions if the clinician has not been following wound progression. After a wound has healed, the scar tissue may be fragile until it has matured. It is best to keep the animal in captivity for a period of time after wound closure to make sure the healed wound can withstand any environmental stressors following release back to the wild.

Wildlife species may present with wounds inflicted from various causes. As a result, wildlife wound management is complex and challenging. The majority of wounds seen in wildlife are over eight hours old and are contaminated by the time of presentation. Consequently, most wounds in wildlife are allowed to heal by second intention or delayed primary closure. Wound management in wildlife that present following trauma may be further complicated by the animal being in shock, dehydrated, malnourished or having suffered polytrauma. Stabilization of the patient is critical before attempting to manage wounds.

Biology of Wounds

The entire wound-healing process is a complex sequence of events that begins from the moment of the initial insult and can continue for months. This section will discuss the phases of second intention healing.

Phases of Healing

Inflammatory and Debridement Phase (Days 1–5)
The inflammatory phase is characterized by redness, swelling, and pain. Vasoconstriction occurs initially, as part of hemostasis, and is followed by vasodilation, which leaks clotting elements into the wound. Platelet aggregation allows for hemostasis and provides a scaffold for cell migration. Neutrophils release enzymes that facilitate the breakdown of bacteria, extracellular debris, and necrotic material. In avian, reptilian, amphibian, and some mammalian species, heterophils are the predominant granulocyte and are equivalent to neutrophils in function. Monocytes migrate into tissues and become macrophages which release cytokines and phagocytize debris. Macrophages also secrete chemotactic and growth factors that initiate, maintain, and coordinate the formation of granulation tissue.

Proliferative/Granulation Phase (Day 4–Week 2)
During this phase, capillary ingrowth, collagen production, wound contraction, and wound coverage take place. Macrophages stimulate fibroblast proliferation.

Medical Management of Wildlife Species: A Guide for Practitioners, First Edition. Edited by Sonia M. Hernandez,
Heather W. Barron, Erica A. Miller, Roberto F. Aguilar and Michael J. Yabsley.

Fibroblasts invade wounds to synthesize and deposit collagen. Wound fibrin disappears as collagen is deposited. The combination of new capillaries, fibroblasts, and fibrous tissue forms bright red, fleshy granulation tissue 3–5 days after injury. The granulation tissue fills defects and protects the wound. It is resistant to infection, provides a surface for epithelial migration, and is a source of special fibroblasts (i.e., myofibroblasts), which are imperative for wound contraction. Unhealthy granulation tissue is pale and has a high fibrous tissue content with few capillaries.

The epithelium serves as a barrier to external infection and internal fluid loss. Epithelial repair involves mobilization, migration, proliferation, and differentiation of epithelial cells. Epithelialization begins in open wounds when an adequate granulation bed has formed. Epithelial migration is guided by collagen fibers. Cells advance until the wound surface is covered, augmented by wound contraction. Contact on all sides with other epithelial cells inhibits further cell migration. Wound contraction can be inhibited by a number of factors such as excessive tension, movement, infection, and exuberant granulation tissue.

Maturation/Remodeling Phase (Week 3 to 18 Months)
Wound maturation begins once collagen has been adequately deposited in the wound. Collagen fibers remodel and the number of capillaries in the fibrous tissue declines. Scars become less cellular, flatten, and soften during maturation.

Reptile and mammalian healing differ in the character of the inflammatory reaction, the pattern of fibroplasia, and epithelial migration, but the temporal sequence, but not duration, of wound healing is the same (Smith and Barker 1988). There are no significant differences in mammalian and avian healing (Katiyar et al. 1992).

Management of Open Wounds

During the initial assessment, a decision must be made whether to close the wound primarily, perform a delayed primary closure, or allow the wound to heal by second intention. If the wound was sustained recently, appears clean and has minimal bruising, it may be closed immediately. If the wound is contaminated, as is often the case with wildlife patients, appears infected or the tissue appears traumatized or necrotic, closure should be delayed until a healthy bed of granulation tissue is formed. Once there is healthy granulation tissue, surgical closure may be performed (delayed primary closure). If there is not sufficient skin for closure, second intention healing should be considered, with possible soft tissue reconstruction at a later date.

Wound Preparation

Sterile water-soluble lubricant should be placed within the wound to help protect it when clipping hair, plucking feathers, or scrubbing the surrounding area with antiseptics. After the surrounding skin has been prepared, the wound should be lavaged to remove dirt and debris, and reduce bacterial load. Tap water is useful for removing gross contaminants but has cytotoxic effects on fibroblasts *in vitro* (Buffa et al. 1997). In the study by Buffa et al., lactated Ringer's solution was shown to be the least damaging to fibroblasts and had a more physiologically acceptable pH. Chlorhexidine (0.05%) has also been shown to be more beneficial to wound healing when compared to saline alone, and has residual antimicrobial activity (Sanchez et al. 1988). Chlorhexidine typically comes in a 2% stock solution, thus 2.5 mL of 2% chlorhexidine solution should be added to 97.5 mL saline to create a 0.05% solution. A close approximation is attained by adding 25 mL chlorhexidine to 1 L of saline solution. A precipitate forms in this solution but does not affect its efficacy.

Various methods have been employed for irrigating wounds. The most commonly recommended pressure for wound irrigation to remove bacteria and foreign material is 7–9 psi. This amount of pressure will not drive bacteria and debris deeper into the tissues. One study showed that a 1 L bag under 300 mmHg of pressure using a fluid bag compression device was the most consistent technique for achieving this ideal wound irrigation pressure (Gall and Monnet 2010). Another less accurate method involves using a 35 mL syringe, an 18 gauge needle or catheter, and a three-way stopcock connected to a 1 L bag of irrigation solution. Wound irrigation using a 1 L 0.9% saline bottle with holes poked through the lid with a 20 gauge needle is also a commonly used technique. Cultures should be obtained after surface contaminants have been removed and before antiseptics have been applied. Bandages reduce dead space, protect the wound from microorganisms, debride the wound surface, and provide an optimal environment for healing.

Dressing the Wound

Primary (Contact) Layer
Choosing the right contact layer is critical to allow for optimal healing. This layer should be sterile and may initially assist in debridement of the wound surface.

Nonadherent Pads or Gauze
Nonadherent pads or gauze may be used for small lacerations and minimally exudative wounds that do not need debridement. They may also be used on healthy granulation

tissue. A nonadherent pad (TELFA nonadherent dressing, Kendall Co., Mansfield, CT, USA) consists of a thin layer of absorbent cotton fibers enclosed in a sleeve of polyethylene terephthalate, which is perforated in a regular pattern and sealed along the edges. The outer film layer prevents the dressing from adhering to the surface of the wound, while its perforated surface allows the passage of exudates from the wound into the body of the pad. Nonadherent pads may be used to cover dry sutured wounds, superficial cuts, or abrasions. They have a low absorbent capacity and are intended for use on lightly exuding wounds and to prevent damage to granulation tissue. Leaving these dressings for several days on an exudative wound may cause adherence to the wound bed, and will damage the healthy tissue when removed.

Petroleum-impregnated mesh (ADAPTIC®, Systagenix, San Antonio, TX, USA) consists of knitted cellulose acetate fabric impregnated with a petrolatum emulsion. It is designed to help protect the wound bed while preventing the dressing from adhering to the wound surface. It also minimizes pain and trauma upon removal. The mesh is indicated for dry to moderately exuding wounds such as surgical incisions, lacerations, abrasions, burns, healthy granulation tissue, and skin grafts.

Semipermeable Adherent

Semipermeable or semiocclusive coverings (Tegaderm™, 3 M Animal Care Products, St Paul, MN, USA; Bioclusive®, Johnson and Johnson Medical, New Brunswick, NJ, USA) allow for transfer of gases, such as air and water vapor, but are impermeable to liquids. They provide an effective barrier to external contamination, maintaining moisture by reducing water vapor loss. This type of dressing can be applied directly over minor lacerations or abrasions. It can also be used to secure other primary dressing layers such as nonadherent pads or moisture-retentive dressings, particularly calcium alginate, hydrocolloids, and hydrogels.

Wet-to-Dry

Wet-to-dry dressings are appropriate for use in early wound management as an aid to debridement. The contact layer is applied wet and allowed to dry on the wound surface. Sterile gauze can be soaked in saline or 0.05% chlorhexidine solution. A secondary layer of dry gauze should be placed over the first to absorb exudate and to allow debris to adhere to the primary layer as it dries. These dressings provide nonselective debridement, removing both healthy and unhealthy tissue when they are removed. As a result, they should not be applied to healthy granulation tissue. Sedation and pain management will help facilitate removal, as there is usually pain associated with the process. Moisture

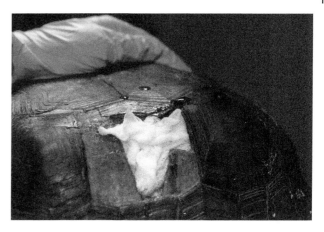

Figure 11.1 The first layer of a wet-to-dry bandage (wet gauze) was applied to the carapacial wound of a gopher tortoise. The dry layer would be added and secured in place with self-adhesive tape.

added to the bandage to facilitate removal defeats the debridement function of the wet-to-dry and should not be done (Figure 11.1).

Hyperosmolar Dressings

Hyperosmolar dressings include sugar, hypertonic saline (20%), and honey. These dressings draw exudate and debris out of the wound and have antimicrobial effects through the dehydration of microorganisms. Plain granulated sugar should be placed at least 1 cm deep. Honey provides antimicrobial effects through the production of hydrogen peroxide (it contains glucose oxidase) and phytochemicals (Mathews and Dinnington 2002a, 2002b). Other properties of honey include the reduction of inflammation and the stimulation of B and T lymphocytes. Studies in mice and rabbits show that honey accelerates wound healing in experimentally created wounds. Medical-grade honey (MEDIHONEY®, Derma Sciences, Princeton, NJ, USA) is manuka honey sterilized by gamma irradiation. This ensures the inactivation of *Clostridium botulinum* spores that may be present in unsterilized honey. Honey found in grocery stores should be used with caution, as it may contain spores. Pasteurization inactivates the glucose oxidase that is responsible for the antibacterial properties of honey, so only unpasteurized honey should be used. Manuka honey is preferred due to additional antimicrobial activity not present in other types of honey. Hyperosmolar dressings are indicated during the inflammatory stage of wound healing and for wounds that are infected. Edematous wounds may also be treated with hyperosmolar dressings. By decreasing edema at the wound bed, there is decreased pressure on capillaries, resulting in an increase in wound perfusion. These dressings should be changed daily or more frequently in heavily exudative wounds.

Hydrophilic (Moisture-Retentive) Dressings

Hydrophilic (moisture-retentive) dressings include calcium alginate, hydrocolloid dressings, and hydrogels. These dressings have varying absorptive capabilities. All of them maintain a moist wound environment, which promotes granulation tissue formation and epithelialization.

Alginates

Heavily exudative wounds may be managed with calcium alginate dressings, since they have high absorptive capacity. Alginates are derived from seaweed and interact with wound exudate to form an odorous gel. The appearance and odor of the gel may seem similar to that of an infection. When the gel is removed by lavage, the wound bed should appear healthy. Release of cations stimulates the inflammatory cascade and allows the release of endogenous growth factors. These stimulate healing and formation of granulation tissue. Calcium alginate is often in the form of a sheet or rope. It must be covered with a semipermeable adhesive dressing (Tegaderm, Bioclusive), or a similar transparent dressing that allows for transfer of gases such as air and water vapor but which is impermeable to liquids. Calcium alginate sheets should be cut to the size and shape of the wound, but the permeable adhesive dressing covers the alginate and surrounding skin to hold the alginate in place.

Exuberant granulation tissue may result from use of this type of dressings. A bandage with hypertonic saline gauze as a primary layer may help smooth out the granulation tissue bed. If the goal is to create more granulation tissue but the wound is not sufficiently exudative, the alginate may be moistened with isotonic saline. Complete gel formation of the alginate may take a few days, so leaving the bandage on for 3–5 days is recommended. Using this type of dressing is not advised for contaminated or infected wounds.

Hydrocolloids

Moderately exudative wounds may be managed with a hydrocolloid layer, such as polyurethane foam. These dressings work by absorbing exudate to form a gelatinous layer on the surface of the wound. They are great for healthy, mature granulation beds where the goal is to promote epithelialization. The dressings should be held in place with a semipermeable adherent layer, or may come with a semipermeable membrane backing. The bandages may stay on the wound bed for several days.

Hydrogels

Dry to minimally exudative wounds should be managed with a hydrogel dressing that covers and traps moisture on the wound surface. Hydrogels often come as a semipermeable sheet, an amorphous gel, or an impregnated gauze. In the authors' opinion, the preformed sheets tend to displace easily under the bandage. The sheet should be cut to the size and shape of the wound bed, and be secured in place with skin staples. Hydrogels may also be used when an eschar is present. They facilitate autolytic debridement, so the eschar sloughs off in a nonpainful manner. Hydrogels can cause maceration of the surrounding tissue, so it is important to conform the dressing to the shape of the wound bed. These dressings may be left in place for several days.

Matrix Dressings and Bio-scaffolds

The goal of this type of dressing is to provide a substrate for cellular colonization. They are often very expensive and can be rejected by host tissues. They may not be practical for management of wounds in wildlife. Oasis® Wound Matrix (Smith & Nephew, Andover, MA, USA) is one example of a naturally derived porcine small intestinal submucosa (SIS) matrix, indicated for the management of wounds.

Topical Antibacterials

Topical antibacterials include silver, triple antibiotic ointments, and aloe vera. Silver sulfadiazine 1% cream (SSD) is commonly used in veterinary medicine. Other forms of silver can be found in a variety of formulations, such as foam, alginate, mesh, and carboxymethylcellulose fiber. Incorporation of silver into hydrophilic dressings has been shown to be more effective at promoting wound healing than using silver alone. It also allows for easier application of the product. The silver reacts with exudate from the wound to release active silver ions, which exert an antimicrobial effect.

Silver-impregnated foams have become very popular in negative pressure wound therapy. Many types of foam may be obtained with silver incorporated into the material. SSD 1% cream has been shown to have negative effects on fibroblasts and on wound contraction both *in vitro* and *in vivo* (Swaim and Wilhalf 1985; Leitch et al. 1993). It is frequently the dressing of choice for burn wounds, since it can penetrate an eschar.

Healing of thermal burns treated with aloe vera gel has been proven superior to those dressed with SSD in early wound management. There is earlier pain relief and also great cost-effectiveness (Adkesson et al. 2007; Shahzad and Ahmed 2013). Aloe vera gel comes from the leaves of aloe vera plants (*Aloe vera*). It may be extracted directly from the plant leaf in a sterile environment or purchased from a medical supplier as a hydrogel-impregnated gauze (JRS Medical, Augusta, GA, USA). It possesses antimicrobial, antifungal, antiprostaglandin, and antithromboxane properties. These aid in the prevention of ischemia and infection, may stimulate fibroblastic replication, and help relieve pain.

Triple antibiotic ointments are used topically for their broad-spectrum antimicrobial activity. Topical antimicrobials are most appropriate for decreasing the bacterial burden of a chronic wound that does not appear overtly infected. When using topical products in avian species, water-soluble products are recommended to avoid damaging feather quality with oil-based products. The most common triple antibiotic ointments used contain bacitracin, neomycin, and polymyxin B (NEOSPORIN® ointment, Warner-Lambert, Morris Plains, NJ, USA). Nitrofurazone (Furacin, Vetoquinol, Lavaltrie, Quebec, Canada) should not be used since it delays epithelialization (Hedlund 2007).

Topical Enzymatic Debridement

Topical enzymatic debriding agents such as Granulex-V (Pfizer Animal Health, West Chester, PA, USA) may be useful in some cases, particularly in preventing the development of exuberant granulation tissue. Granulex contains trypsin, balsam of Peru, and castor oil and is typically in the form of an aerosol. When sprayed on wounds, it liquefies and debrides necrotic tissue, relieves pain, stimulates vascularization, and improves epithelialization. Generally, it is used in addition to lavage and surgical debridement. This product has been used in birds and rodents and can be useful in cases of myiasis but note that its ingredients (e.g., castor oil) can damage feathers, and thus the benefits should be weighed carefully (Haley et al. 2002).

Topical Yeast Extract

Topical application of yeast extract (Preparation H® with Biodyne, Whitehall-Robins Inc., Mississauga, Ontario, Canada) has shown to accelerate wound healing in diabetic mice. It is recommended to promote epithelialization when used twice daily on a healthy granulation bed. The United States formulation of Preparation H does not contain the yeast derivative and is not recommended. The Canadian formulation does, and is recommended.

Maggots

Maggot debridement therapy may be useful for areas that are difficult to debride surgically. Maggots secrete digestive enzymes that dissolve necrotic tissue. Disinfected larvae of the green blowfly (*Phaenicia (Lucilia) sericata*) are used due to their selective appetite for necrotic tissue. They will not damage healthy tissues below the epidermis. Maggots have been used experimentally in rodents and lagomorphs. (Hassan et al. 2014) (Figure 11.2). Medical Maggots™ (Monarch Labs, LLC, Irvine, CA, USA) are regulated by the FDA as a prescription-only, single-use medical device. Delivery generally takes 24–48 hours. Maggots are highly perishable and cannot be stored, reused, or returned; make sure you follow the manufacturer's recommendations.

Ancillary Therapies

Hirudotherapy (Leeches)

Leech therapy is indicated when the viability of tissue is threatened by venous congestion (Sobczak and Kantyka 2014). The saliva of a medicinal leech contains more than 100 bioactive substances. The anesthetic properties of leech saliva prevent the bitten animal from feeling the bite. In dogs and cats, the leech must stay on the skin until it satiates (30–60 minutes). Although there are no reports in the veterinary literature regarding their use in wildlife, the authors have used leeches for wildlife wounds with apparent success. Feeding time should be limited in smaller animals to prevent exsanguination. Local irritation may occur. Medicinal leeches may be purchased from a variety of sources and may be shipped overnight or take up to six business days for delivery, depending on the company. Because skin with vascular compromise can decline rapidly and become necrotic, it may be advantageous to keep leeches on hand as they are easy to house in a container with a perforated lid. Leeches can live for months on one blood meal so feeding is unnecessary if they are to be stored prior to use. Current sources include Biopharm leeches (www.biopharm-leeches.com/veterinary.html) and Leeches U.S.A. LTD (www.leechesusa.com).

Light Amplification by the Stimulated Emission of Radiation (LASER)

Therapeutic lasers (LiteCure LLC, Companion Therapy Laser, Newark, DE, USA) have become increasingly popular in companion animal medicine and in exotic species such as birds, rodents, and reptiles, but efficacy has not been well established (Demidova-Rice et al. 2007; Ritzman 2015), and one study demonstrated that laser did not improve healing in green iguanas (Cusack et al. 2018). A variety of terms have been used to describe this type of therapy including low-level light therapy, cold laser, therapeutic laser, and photobiomodulation (Anders et al. 2015). Lasers used to stimulate healing are typically class 3B and class 4. Class 3B lasers are limited to 0.5 W of power while class 4 lasers exceed those class limitations. Lasers work by emitting photons into targeted tissues and inducing a chemical change called photobiomodulation. This light energy promotes the production of adenosine triphosphate (ATP) in the cell, enhancing healing.

Indications for use include any inflammatory or traumatic conditions such as wounds, postsurgical incisions, pododermatitis, and lesions associated with myiasis. The use of therapeutic lasers on wounds reduces pain, inflammation, and edema, which promote healing. Laser treatments should be used as an adjunct therapy to medical treatment (Hamblin and Demidova 2006). Laser therapy

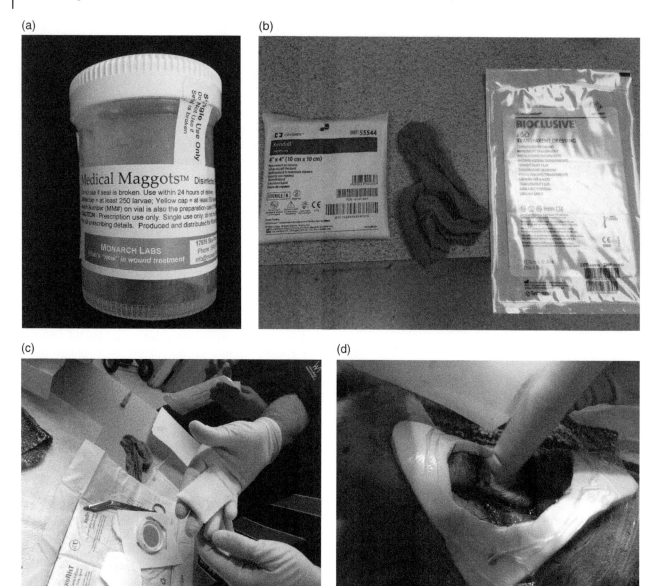

Figure 11.2 (a–d) Composite placement of maggots. Medical Maggots™ should be applied to the wound along with a sterile, moist gauze pad. After the maggots have been applied, cage them on the wound using a mesh fabric, then cover the mesh and dressing loosely with a breathable absorbent pad (i.e., two-ply cotton gauze). This permits air to reach the larvae and facilitates drainage of maggot secretions and patient exudates out from the wound. Some people find nylon stockings to be a reasonable alternative. The mesh can be affixed to a hydrocolloid pad with a central hole cut out to match the wound margins. *Source:* Information from Monarch Labs package insert.

is used in conjunction with other treatment modalities and topical therapies, making it difficult to assess how significant its role is in the healing process.

Negative Pressure Wound Therapy (NPWT)

Negative pressure wound therapy, also known as vacuum-assisted closure (VAC), has been used extensively in human medicine, and has become increasingly popular in veterinary medicine. NPWT speeds granulation tissue formation and allows wounds to heal in a shorter time than traditional bandaging

(Joseph et al. 2000). The negative pressure bandage promotes healing by creating evenly distributed subatmospheric pressures at the wound site. This reduces edema, removes exudates, and promotes granulation tissue formation while facilitating cell migration. There is increased cell proliferation and perfusion. In rodents, NPWT resulted in increased growth factor production, improved angiogenesis, collagen deposition, and earlier wound organization (Jacobs et al. 2009). In experimentally created wounds in rabbits, NPWT promoted capillary blood flow velocity, increased capillary caliber and blood volume, stimulated endothelial proliferation and angiogenesis, narrowed endothelial spaces, and restored the integrity of the capillary basement membrane. Anecdotal reports indicate this technology works well for shell defects in chelonians (Figure 11.3); however, controlled prospective studies have not been performed (Adkesson et al. 2007; Lafortune et al. 2007).

Negative pressure wound therapy has been shown to be beneficial on full-thickness skin grafts in dogs. Fibroplasia is enhanced, open meshes close more rapidly, and less graft necrosis occurs with NPWT.

Prospective studies are needed to evaluate the application of NPWT in skin grafts in exotic species. Pressures recommended for different types of wounds vary. It is best to work with the manufacturer's recommendations (Kinetic Concepts, Inc., San Antonio, TX, USA). There is also a device capable of wound irrigation under the dressing during negative pressure wound therapy (Curato®, Infiniti Medical LLC, Menlo Park, CA, USA). Curato should only be used with water-soluble topical antimicrobials, like honey, because ointments and creams will clog the foam pores.

Bandaging

The primary contact layer is held in place by a secondary layer, which also helps eliminate dead space. Secondary bandage layers are usually made of an absorbent cotton material, such as cast padding. When wrapping a limb or body part with layers, they should overlap by at least 50%. The absorbent material is compacted by using conforming gauze placed in a similar manner. The tertiary bandage layer is a self-adherent layer that provides strength to the bandage construct and protects it from the environment. Even and consistent pressure must be maintained when wrapping, and overtightening must be avoided. Wrapping around the abdomen or thorax will help maintain the bandage in place. Distraction tabs may be useful for patients who chew bandages. These can be made by placing a piece of adhesive tape over the bandage with a section pinched up, creating a tab on which the patient may alternatively chew.

Tie-over Bandage

In locations where the wound is difficult to wrap, a tie-over bandage should be considered. A tie-over bandage can be secured to the body using loose loops of nonabsorbable suture in the skin around the wound. The wound should be covered with a primary dressing appropriate for the wound type, and covered with sterile gauze as a secondary layer. A waterproof layer should be placed over the gauze. Umbilical tape is looped over the top of the bandage in a crisscross fashion, securing it in place (Figure 11.4). Bandage changes are performed by cutting the umbilical tape and removing the primary and secondary bandage layers. The suture loops are reutilized to secure the replacement bandage. Tie-over bandages are useful in all species.

Drains

If a wound is healthy enough to be closed but has a large amount of dead space, a drain should be placed to allow for the removal of exudates. This allows the tissues to adhere to each other again.

Active Drains

A closed suction drain typically consists of a fenestrated tube attached to a suction device. The system is preferable because it is more effective at removing fluid and it reduces the risk of nosocomial infection when compared to a passive drain. Collection of fluid allows for cytological

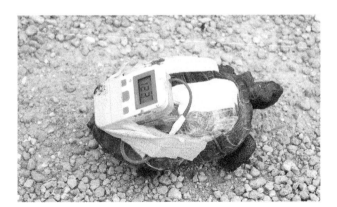

Figure 11.3 Vacuum-assisted closure of carapacial lesions is effective and smaller units allow patients to move about freely. *Source:* Courtesy of Heather Barron.

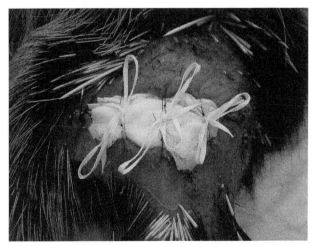

Figure 11.4 Umbilical tape was used to secure wet-to-dry bandaging over a full-thickness wound on a porcupine. *Source:* Courtesy of Sonia Hernandez.

monitoring of wound exudates and quantification of fluid production. Common active suction drains include the Jackson–Pratt drain, vacuum syringe drain, and a butterfly catheter attached to a blood collection tube (Vacutainer, Becton Dickinson, Franklin Lakes, NJ, USA). The Jackson–Pratt drain is ideal for larger wounds. It consists of a fenestrated rubber tube and a "grenade" suction bulb which creates negative pressure. As an alternative, a syringe can be used to create negative pressure when attached to a fenestrated tube implanted in the wound. The syringe plunger is pulled back, creating negative pressure, and a hypodermic needle is passed through the syringe behind the plunger to hold it in place.

A butterfly catheter may be used as an active drain by cutting off the syringe adapter and fenestrating the tube before placing it in the wound. The tube then exits through the skin adjacent to the wound. After the wound is sutured closed, the needle end of the catheter is inserted into a blood collection tube, which will provide the necessary negative pressure. When the tube is full, it may be replaced with a new tube or a needle and syringe may be used to remove the fluid and recreate a vacuum.

Studies in dogs have shown there is a greater risk of seroma formation if drains are removed while drainage is occurring at a rate >0.2 mL/kg/h (Shaver et al. 2014).

Passive Drains

The most frequently used passive drain is a Penrose drain, which consists of a flat tube of malleable latex rubber. Fluid from the wound is drawn over and through the drain by capillary action and gravitational flow. Penrose drains work well for small wounds when minimal drainage is expected. The exit point should be dependent and via a separately made stab incision through intact skin, not through the main incision. Sterile gauze and a bandage should be placed over the drain. The gauze will collect fluid, which allows for subjective quantification, as well as reducing the risk of an ascending infection. The drain should be removed when fluid production is minimal and the cytological appearance of the exudate is improving, usually after 3–5 days.

Passive drains are generally not used in avian patients, since avian heterophils lack the proteolytic enzymes present in mammalian neutrophils and thus produce more caseated pus. However, drains may facilitate flushing or keeping open an exit incision in tissue that is pocketing.

Wound Closure

Surgical closure of a wound may be considered if the wound was sustained within the previous six hours and remains clean. It may also be closed after the wound has been managed open and has developed a healthy bed of granulation tissue.

Birds

Absorbable monofilament or braided suture with a taper needle is recommended for avian muscle, subcutaneous tissues, and skin (Spearman and Hardy 1985; Coles 2007). Using absorbable suture in wild birds is particularly important for reducing stress by minimizing handling. Polydioxanone (PDS, Ethicon Inc., Somerville, NJ, USA) and polyglactin 910 (Vicryl®, Ethicon, Inc.) are both absorbed by hydrolysis and used commonly. Polyglactin 910 was shown to produce the strongest tissue reaction when compared to stainless steel, nylon, polydioxanone, or chromic gut (Bennett et al. 1997). This material was rapidly absorbed, with subsequent resolution of the inflammation. Polydioxanone produced the least inflammatory reaction.

A soft, multifilament, absorbable suture on a taper needle (Vicryl®) is used for skin closures by the authors. This material does not cause gross skin irritation and is rapidly absorbed. The soft nature of the suture allows birds to incorporate it into their preening regimen. Chromic gut should not be used because it is not absorbed well and causes severe inflammation. A taper needle is preferred for avian skin. There is a risk of tearing avian skin if a cutting needle is used. A Ford interlocking or simple continuous pattern may be used for rapid closure. A vertical mattress pattern can also be used to oppose the wound edges and relieve tension. Simple interrupted sutures are recommended for skin flaps and grafts (Stroud et al. 2003).

Reptiles and Amphibians

Reptile skin is tough and has a tendency to invert, especially in lizards and snakes. If the skin inverts, closure should be performed utilizing an everting pattern, such as an interrupted vertical or horizontal mattress pattern, or skin staples. A vertical mattress pattern can be used to evert the tissue with less disruption of the blood to the cut edge. It may take longer to place because more sutures are required to close the incision. The sutures should not be overtightened because this disrupts the blood supply to the skin edge, often resulting in necrosis of the skin at the incision. The sutures should be tightened so that the raw edges of the incision are in contact for proper healing. The raw edges should not be exposed to the environment, indicating the sutures are too tight. A liquid bandage (New-Skin, Prestige Brands Holdings, Inc., Irvington, NY, USA) may be applied over the exposed edge after closure. Either nonabsorbable (nylon; Ethilon, Ethicon, Inc., Piscataway, NJ, USA) or absorbable suture (polydioxanone, polyglactin 910) may be used (McFadden et al. 2011).

Suture removal should take place 4–6 weeks postoperatively or delayed until the first ecdysis after surgery.

Wound strength is increased after ecdysis. Small lacerations may be closed with a conservative amount of tissue adhesive (Mitchell and Diaz-Figueroa 2004).

Lagomorphs

Rabbits are fastidious groomers. Intradermal skin sutures are recommended during wound closure. The knots should be buried under the skin surface. The final knot can be hidden in the subcutaneous layer using an Aberdeen knot. The needle at the end of the suture line is directed under the skin ("Smurf") and brought out a short distance from the wound edge to bury the knot. Cyanoacrylic tissue adhesive can be used over an intradermal line. Some rabbits will chew at the glue. Skin staples are well tolerated and not easy for rabbits to remove (Bennett 2012).

Rodents

The subcutis of rodents is thick and holds sutures well. Skin staples or intradermal sutures are recommended due to the fastidious grooming nature of rodents. Cyanoacrylic tissue adhesive may be used with caution as it may be chewed out. Rodents are prone to self-mutilation of wounds. Care must be taken when handling tissues to avoid bruising and inflammation. Avoid pinching the skin with forceps, but use them for counterpressure instead.

Skin Flaps and Grafts

A skin flap is a segment of skin that maintains its blood supply and is stretched or rotated to cover an adjacent defect. Skin flaps in wildlife follow the same principles of preparation and management as in companion animals. In avian species, skin flaps have been described to cover wounds on the skull, distal extremities, and sternum (Ferrell et al. 2004; Kozar et al. 2013). These flaps usually contain feather follicles and attention should be given to the orientation of feather growth. Abnormal feather growth may stimulate excessive preening, which can lead to damage to or removal of the feathers. Single pedicle advancement and axial pattern flaps have been described for use in a variety of avian species (Hannon et al. 1993). There is no literature describing the technique of transposition flaps.

A free skin graft is a segment of skin completely detached from its location and transferred to a recipient site. A free skin graft is indicated when there is a large cutaneous defect that cannot be closed by moving adjacent skin to that site. Autogenous grafts, where the donor and recipient is the same animal, are the most successful, and are less likely to be rejected than allografts or xenografts. Full-thickness mesh skin grafts have been used in avian species to cover large skin defects. The dermis is thin and there is little subcutaneous tissue, so there is rapid revascularization of the graft. The inguinal region (flank fold) and midpropatagium are suitable donor sites. The inguinal skin covers the body wall, which is thin muscle that is meant to protect the abdominal organs. The body wall should not be disrupted when harvesting a free skin graft. The donor site is closed primarily. Abnormal healing of the propatagium can lead to wound contracture, which can inhibit flight. However, the risk of this occurring is low.

A variety of skin flaps and grafts have been performed experimentally in rabbits and guinea pigs as models for reconstructive surgery in humans. Although not commonly performed in these species, results of these experiments indicate that skin flaps and free grafts are feasible options for covering large skin defects (Figure 11.5).

(a)

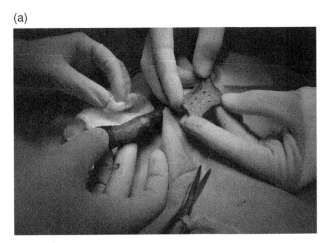

(b)

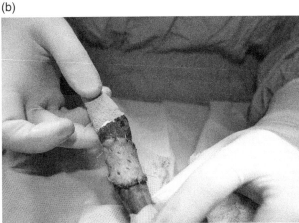

Figure 11.5 (a,b) An autogenous skin graft is prepared and sutured in place to repair a full-thickness wound on the limb of a raccoon. *Source:* Courtesy of Heather Barron.

Common Wounds Encountered in Wildlife

Burn Wounds

Thermal wounds are caused by wildfires, automobile mufflers, electrical wires, heat lamps, or other heat sources. Avian skin will not blister in response to thermal injury, as it does in mammals. Instead, the skin becomes heat-fixed to underlying tissues. Electrocution is seen mostly in large raptors. Many birds, especially raptors, select power line poles for perching. They may be electrocuted when conducting wires are placed closer together than the wingspan of the bird (Thomas 1999).

If an acute burn wound is suspected, running cold water over the area may help with pain relief, preventing further cellular damage and countering hyperthermia. Topical silver sulfadiazine is the treatment of choice for most small burn wounds due to its ability to penetrate eschars. Thermal burns treated with aloe vera gel have been proven to heal better than those dressed with SSD, with improved wound healing, pain relief, and cost-effectiveness (Shahzad and Ahmed 2013; Akhoondinasab et al. 2014). For large areas of full-thickness burns, surgical debridement may help facilitate a faster recovery. The natural separation of the burn eschar is a slow process. Hydrogels may be applied over an eschar to facilitate autolytic debridement. After a few days under the hydrogel, the eschar will typically slough in a non-painful manner.

The manifestations of electrical burns may take several days to declare themselves. Severe electrical burns to avian feet carry a poor prognosis due to the involvement of tendons and joints. Euthanasia is required by the United States Fish and Wildlife Service (USFWS) if injuries require amputation of a leg, foot, or a wing at the elbow (humeroulnar joint) or more proximal.

Bite Wounds

Most bite wounds will be deceiving. If the insult was from a dog or coyote, a majority of the damage occurs below the skin surface due to shear and compressive forces (Shamir et al. 2002). Cats and raccoons may cause lacerations below the skin surface. Primary closure is acceptable if within the first six hours after the attack. Closure should be postponed if there is any concern over the viability of the tissues, or if infected. It often takes several days for the true extent of the lesion to present itself. Delayed primary closure allows for daily assessment. If the tissues appear healthy, closure can be performed 3–5 days later. Small puncture wounds with subcutaneous pocketing can be flushed and left open to heal by second intention. However, flushing may force debris deeper into tissues, create additional subcutaneous pocketing, and induce iatrogenic edema. Only surface cleaning is recommended.

Carnivorous reptiles and amphibians may suffer from bite wounds inflicted by prey, such as rodents. Bite wounds should be lavaged and necrotic tissue debrided. Old wounds or wounds that appear infected should not be closed until the tissue appears healthy. Minor superficial wounds or abrasions may be covered with a liquid bandage (New-Skin, Prestige Brands Holdings, Inc., Irvington, NY, USA). Deeper, contaminated wounds may be treated with wet-to-dry, sugar or honey bandages. Hydrogels may be used to promote epithelialization and maintain a moist wound environment. They may need to be held in place with a semipermeable adherent layer (Tegaderm, Bioclusive). For wounds that are difficult to bandage, animals may be housed in a container lined with clean towels soaked in 0.05% chlorhexidine solution or 0.1% povidone-iodine. These towels should be changed daily.

Antimicrobials such as silver sulfadiazine cream and antibiotic ointments are good options for preventing opportunistic infections. A study comparing a polyurethane film to an antimicrobial ointment and an antimicrobial powder in experimentally induced wounds in snakes showed that ointments and powders slowed healing (Smith et al. 1988).

Myiasis (Fly Strike Wounds)

Wounds occurring during warm weather are at risk of attracting flies. Flies may also be attracted to healthy animals with urine or fecal contamination on the fur. Treatment involves removing any eggs and maggots, flushing the wound, and debriding any necrotic tissue. Fly eggs can be brushed off with a stiff brush and maggots can be flushed out with lavage solution. Animals should be treated with ivermectin or nitenpyram (see Appendix II: Formulary) to kill any missed maggots. Ivermectin should not be used on chelonians as it can cause flaccid paralysis or death. After wounds have been cleared of maggots, they should be managed as open wounds to heal by second intention or to ensure tissue is healthy prior to delayed closure. Granulex-V may be used for enzymatic debridement of necrotic tissue when the patient is a poor surgical candidate.

Pododermatitis

Sore hock is used to describe ulcerative pododermatitis in rabbits and rodents. The condition is commonly called *bumblefoot* in birds. Sore hock refers to ulcerated areas of the skin on the caudal aspect of the tarsus and metatarsus. Bumblefoot describes a degenerative, inflammatory condition of the plantar aspect of the avian foot.

Pododermatitis is secondary to avascular necrosis of the soft tissues between the bony structures of the foot and the animal's resting surface. Clinical signs include inflammation, erythema, thinning of the skin, dry crusty scabs, hyperkeratosis, and ulceration. If left untreated, severe pododermatitis can lead to erosion of the bones and ligaments of the hock, osteomyelitis, tenosynovitis, arthritis, and permanent disability.

In rabbits, the disease is classified into three types, based on tissue involved and severity of infection. Type I is a mild lesion with inflammation and thinning of fur. Type II is an extensive lesion with inflammation and infection. The skin is necrotic and ulcerated. In type III, the lesions are encapsulated in fibrous connective tissue. The tendons, joints, and bone may be involved.

Rabbits and other small mammals develop ulcerative pododermatitis as a secondary process to increased pressure on the plantar aspect of the foot. It may be caused by running on rough flooring, such as concrete, tiles, or wire cage flooring. Substrates used for bedding must be soft and kept clean and dry. A substrate that is wet and soaked with urine or feces will also predispose animals to developing lesions.

Treatment of pododermatitis in all species should be multimodal, aimed at correcting the underlying causes and treating any secondary infection. Wounds should be kept clean and dry. For small mammals, hair should be trimmed to prevent matting with discharge, but not shaved as this will decrease the natural protection of the skin. The wounds should be thoroughly lavaged. With mild lesions, liquid bandages (New-Skin) or cyanoacrylate skin protectants (Marathon Liquid Skin Protectant, Medline Industries, Inc., Mundelein, IL, USA) may be used. Please refer to Section 11.3.4 for moderate to severe cases of pododermatitis. Caution should be exercised when bandaging small mammals, as self-mutilation may occur.

In birds, the foot can be placed in a ball bandage and maintained with weekly bandage changes until the wound has closed by second intention healing (Remple 2006). A ball bandage can be made of cast padding or gauze, and placed on the plantar surface of the foot, allowing the toes to flex around the "ball." Additional cast padding and a self-adhering bandage (Petflex, Andover Healthcare, Salisbury, MA, USA; VetRap Adhesive Stretch Tape, 3 M Animal Care Products) can be wrapped around the foot, incorporating the ball of cast padding. The most recent protective foot padding available uses silicone dental impression material to create a form-fitting, flexible support shoe (Sideline Cushion Support, Kingston, NY, USA). Laser therapy has been used with anecdotal success in small mammals to encourage healing of pododermatitis lesions (Brown and Donnelly 2008; Blair 2013). Surgical debridement to remove infected tissue can be combined with other therapies to speed healing.

Closure of the wounds may be attempted after a healthy layer of granulation tissue has developed. Surgical closure is not recommended in rabbits, rodents, or birds as there is generally insufficient skin available to allow for reconstruction of tissues; however, there is one report of an advancement flap used to cover a pododermatitis lesion in a red-tailed hawk (*Buteo jamaicensis*) (Sander et al. 2013). Periods of healing are often followed by relapses if husbandry issues are not corrected. Affected areas should be bandaged for a week or more after healing to prevent relapse.

Common Wounds of Specific Animal Groups

Birds

Methods to improve the speed of wound healing in birds are of particular importance when the objective is to release them back to the wild (Riggs and Tully 2004). Avian wounds are unique in that the skin is thin and tears easily. Wound edges tend to dry out quickly, and wounds over the distal extremities, joints, axillae, inguinal regions, and propatagium heal slowly because they are less vascular (Degernes 1994; Heidenreich 1997). Avian skin is not very elastic over areas such as the skull and carpus. The skin of the pelvis is attached to the bone. The presence of feathers in the dermis further complicates wound healing. If wound closure is performed with feather pterylae in an abnormal position, the growth of the new feathers might interfere with flight.

Beak Injuries
Birds of prey and seed- or grass-eating birds have hollow beaks composed of dermal bone. The surface of the beak consists of tough keratinized epidermis. In waterfowl (ducks, geese, and swans), the beak epidermis is thinner and softer and the beak is not hollow. In these species, the beak is more vulnerable to trauma, which may occur secondary to collisions during flight. The surface of the beak heals by granulation and epithelialization, similar to the rest of the skin. The defect fills with granulation tissue and eventually becomes bone. The epithelium migrates over the granulation tissue and produces hard keratin, as in the uninjured beak. If the beak wound is clean, it can be covered with a patch, such as an acrylic material. The defect or wound will heal under the patch, which will eventually be shed as the keratin turns over. If the wound is contaminated or infected, it should be managed as an open wound. Once the tissue is healthy, the defect can be covered with a patch.

Challenges arise if the beak is regularly immersed under water and in food bowls. If the wound cannot be covered with a patch, a waterproof dressing is recommended to keep the wound clean and moist and to facilitate healing. Orabase Oral Protective Paste (ConvaTec, Greensboro, NC, USA) is a water-resistant dressing that can be placed over the injured beak. Hydrocolloid dressings can also be placed over the wound as additional protection.

If it is important to protect the beak from trauma during eating or ambulating, the beak can be secured closed (wired or taped closed) and an esophagostomy tube placed to provide nutritional support while the beak heals. If necessary, birds can be maintained on esophagostomy tube feeding for months.

Wing Wounds

Bent and Broken Feathers

Bent feathers can be straightened and stabilized with hot glue at the crease site. See Chapter 17 for information on broken feathers.

Wing Web Laceration

Wing web lacerations are a significant concern for birds that must return to flight. Closure with minimal contraction is necessary to maintain flight. A two-layer closure is required (ventral and dorsal skin layers) for full-thickness web lacerations. Once healed, physical therapy should be instituted to regain adequate extension of the laceration site. If the propatagial tendon is lacerated, it should be repaired with a three-loop pulley suture or similar tendon suture repair technique at the time of closure (Figure 11.6).

Reptiles and Amphibians

Reptile skin is dry, aglandular, firmly adhered to the subcutis, and relatively inelastic (Lock and Bennett 2003; Mader and Bennett 2006). Extensive wounds often need to heal by second intention, which may take anywhere from several weeks for small areas to over a year for larger wounds. Large defects may result in massive scarring and a change in the scale pattern, particularly in snakes. Snakes develop an obvious inflammatory response and form scabs. Lizards sustaining wounds have minimal inflammation and do not form scabs (Maderson and Roth 1972). Wounds may appear static between ecdysis in reptiles. Once the shed is complete, there is usually evidence of epithelialization. Skin around wounds may not shed easily and may require soaking and manual removal. When common garter snakes (*Thamnophis sirtalis*) were maintained at a temperature of 30 °C, epithelial cell migration occurred as early as 48 hours following an incision. Snakes held at 21 °C and 13.5 °C experienced delayed cell migration (Smith et al. 1988). A study evaluating inflammatory reactions to various suture materials and cyanoacrylate tissue adhesive in skin incisions of ball

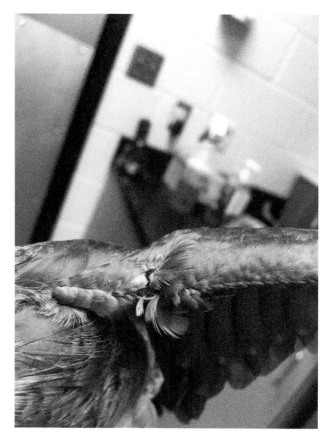

Figure 11.6 Repair of a patagial laceration with suture in a ruddy duck.

pythons (*Python regius*) found that the tissue adhesive did not cause a significant inflammatory response. All other suture materials caused significantly more inflammation when compared to the negative control group, which was left to heal by second intention (McFadden et al. 2011).

Chelonian Shell Injuries

Trauma-related injuries, particularly shell fractures, are a common reason for wild turtle and tortoise presentation. Shell fractures should be managed as an open wound initially to allow removal of dirt and debris. If they are recent and/or clean, they can be closed (patched or wired) primarily. Irrigation of wounds will help remove gross contamination. Wet-to-dry bandages with saline or 0.05% chlorhexidine can be used to help facilitate removal of minimal gross contamination or debridement of unhealthy tissues. Fractured shell fragments may be reduced and stabilized with orthopedic implants such as bone plates, interfragmentary orthopedic wire, or screws and figure-of-eight wires. Further discussion of shell repair is presented in Chapter 28. Shell fractures are unique; as the wound heals, a scab develops which should not be disturbed. The tissue under the scab turns to cartilage and finally mineralizes to bone. The epithelium migrates over the surface, creating dermal bone.

Rabbits

The thin fragile skin of lagomorphs is prone to tearing when the fur is being clipped. A #50 clipper blade is recommended when clipping rabbit fur. The teeth of the blade are closer together and less likely to traumatize skin. Rabbits are unique in that they do not have footpads like dogs and cats. The feet are covered with fur, which protects the plantar surface. Improper husbandry makes them prone to damage (Harcourt-Brown 2002).

Dermal Abscesses

Dermal abscesses are commonly seen in rabbits and rodents. They tend to be caseous in nature. Excision of the entire abscess is recommended. Lancing and draining will not resolve the infection. When the entire abscess cannot be removed, it must be opened, the pus removed, and the wound debrided and irrigated. Then it should be left open for continued debridement, daily assessment, and bandage changes.

Sore Hocks

Sore hocks refers to ulcerated areas of the skin on the plantar aspect of the tarsus and metatarsus in rabbits. The condition is generally secondary to increased pressures on the soles of the feet, brought on by rough or soiled flooring. Please refer to Section 11.4.4.

Rodents

Rodents are fastidious groomers and self-mutilate wounds so they should be closed as soon as possible. Their grooming behavior makes it very difficult to keep topical treatments on for a prolonged period of time or to place bandages. An Elizabethan collar may be tried but most wild rodents will not tolerate these devices well. Rodents and rabbits tolerate a yoke much better than an Elizabethan collar.

References

Adkesson, M.J., Travis, E.K., Weber, M.A. et al. (2007). Vacuum-assisted closure for treatment of a deep shell abscess and osteomyelitis in a tortoise. *Journal of the American Veterinary Medical Association* 231 (8): 1249–1254.

Akhoondinasab, M.R., Akhoondinasab, M., and Saberi, M. (2014). Comparison of healing effects of aloe vera extract and silver sulfadiazine in burn injuries in an experimental rat model. *World Journal of Plastic Surgery* 3 (1): 29–34.

Anders, J.J., Lanzafame, R.J., and Arany, P.R. (2015). Low-level light/laser therapy versus photobiomodulation therapy. *Photomedicine and Laser Surgery* 33 (4): 183–184.

Bennett, R.A. (2012). Soft tissue surgery. In: *Ferrets, Rabbits, and Rodents: Clinical Medicine and Surgery*, 3e (ed. K. Quesenberry and J. Carpenter), 337. St Louis, MO: Elsevier Saunders.

Bennett, R.A., Yeager, M., Trapp, A. et al. (1997). Tissue reaction to five suture material in the body wall of rock doves (*Columba livia*). *Journal of Avian Medicine and Surgery* 11: 175–182.

Blair, J. (2013). Bumblefoot: a comparison of clinical presentation and treatment of pododermatitis in rabbits, rodents, and birds. *Veterinary Clinics of North America. Exotic Animal Practice* 16: 715–735.

Brown, C. and Donnelly, T. (2008). Treatment of pododermatitis in the Guinea pig. *Laboratory Animal* 37 (4): 156–157.

Buffa, E.A., Lubbe, A.M., Verstrate, F.J.M. et al. (1997). The effects of wound lavage solutions on canine fibroblasts: an in vitro study. *Veterinary Surgery* 26: 460–466.

Coles, B.H. (2007). Surgery. In: *Essentials of Avian Medicine and Surgery*, 3e, 142–182. Oxford, UK: Wiley-Blackwell.

Cusack, L.M., Mayer, J., Cutler, D.C. et al. (2018). Gross and histologic evaluation of effects of photobiomodulation, silver sulfadiazine, and a topical antimicrobial product on experimentally induced full-thickness skin wounds in green iguanas (*Iguana iguana*). *American Journal Veterinary Research* 79 (4): 465–473.

Degernes, L.A. (1994). Trauma medicine. In: *Avian Medicine: Principles and Applications* (ed. B.W. Ritchie, G.J. Harrison and L.R. Harrison), 418–433. Lake Worth, FL: Wingers Publishing.

Demidova-Rice, T.N., Salomatina, E.V., Yaroslavsky, A.N. et al. (2007). Low-level light stimulates excisional wound healing in mice. *Lasers in Surgery and Medicine* 39 (9): 706–715.

Ferrell, S.T. (2002). Avian integumentary system. *Seminars in Avian and Exotic Pet Medicine* 11: 125–135.

Ferrell, S.T., de Cock, H.E.V., Graham, J.E. et al. (2004). Assessment of a caudal external thoracic artery axial pattern flap for treatment of sternal cutaneous wounds in birds. *American Journal of Veterinary Research* 65: 497–502.

Gall, T. and Monnet, E. (2010). Pressure dynamics of common techniques used for wound flushing. *American Journal of Veterinary Research* 71: 1384–1386.

Haley, F., Burke, B.S., Swaim, S.F., and Amalsadvala, T. (2002). Review of wound management in raptors. *Journal of Avian Medicine and Surgery* 16 (3): 180–191.

Hamblin, M.R., Demidova T.N. (2006). Mechanisms of Low-Level Light Therapy. Proceedings of SPIE, San Jose, CA (22 January 2005).

Hannon, D.E., Swaim, S.F., Milton, J.L. et al. (1993). Full-thickness mesh skin grafts in two great horned owls (*Bubo virginianus*). *Journal of Zoo and Wildlife Medicine* 24 (4): 539–552.

Harcourt-Brown, F. (2002). Skin diseases. In: *Textbook of Rabbit Medicine* (ed. F. Harcourt-Brown), 224–248. Oxford, UK: Butterworth-Heinemann.

Hassan, M.I., Hammad, K.M., Fouda, M.A. et al. (2014). The use of *Lucilia cuprina* maggots in the treatment of diabetic foot wounds. *Journal of the Egyptian Society of Parasitology* 44 (1): 125–129.

Hedlund, C.S. (2007b). Surgery of the integumentary system. In: *Small Animal Surgery*,, 2e (ed. T.W. Fossum), 136–150. St. Louis, MO: Mosby.

Heidenreich, M. (1997). *Birds of Prey: Medicine and Management*. Malden, MA: Blackwell Science.

Jacobs, S., Fomovsky, G.M., Simhaee, D.A. et al. (2009). Efficacy and mechanisms of vacuum-assisted closure (VAC) therapy in promoting wound healing: a rodent model. *Journal of Plastic, Reconstructive & Aesthetic Surgery* 62: 1331–1338.

Joseph, E., Hamori, C.A., Bergman, S. et al. (2000). A prospective randomized trial of vacuum assisted closure versus standard therapy of chronic nonhealing wounds. *Wounds: A Compendium of Clinical Research and Practice* 12: 60–67.

Katiyar, A.K., Vegad, J.L., and Awadhiya, R.P. (1992). Pathology of inflammatory-reparative response in punched wounds of the chicken skin. *Avian Pathology* 21 (3): 471–480.

Knapp-Hoch, H. and de Matos, R. (2014). Negative pressure wound therapy-general principles and use in avian species. *Journal of Exotic Pet Medicine* 23 (1): 56–66.

Kozar, M., Molnar, L., Trolova, A. et al. (2013). Application of a single vascularized skin flap in eastern imperial eagle with skin defects. *Veterinary Record* 172 (16): 425.

Lafortune, M., Wellehan, J.F.X., Heard, D.J. et al. (2007). Vacuum-assisted closure for treatment of a deep shell abscess and osteomyelitis in a tortoise. *Journal of the American Veterinary Medical Association* 231 (8): 1249–1254.

Leitch, I.O., Kucukcelebi, A., and Robson, M.C. (1993). Inhibition of wound contraction by topical antimicrobials. *Australian and New Zealand Journal of Surgery* 63 (4): 289–293.

Lock, B.L. and Bennett, R.A. (2003). Anesthesia and surgery. In: *Biology, Husbandry, and Medicine of the Green Iguana* (ed. E.R. Jacobson), 158–159. Malabar, FL: Krieger Publishing Company.

Mader, D.R. and Bennett, R.A. (2006). Soft tissue, orthopedics, and fracture repair. In: *Reptile Medicine and Surgery*, 2e (ed. D.R. Mader), 581–612. St Louis, MO: Elsevier Saunders.

Maderson, P.F.A. and Roth, S.I. (1972). A histological study of early stages of cutaneous wound healing in lizards in vivo and in vitro. *Journal of Experimental Zoology* 180: 175–186.

Mathews, K.A. and Dinnington, A.G. (2002a). Wound management using honey. *Compendium on Continuing Education for the Practicing Veterinarian* 24: 53–60.

Mathews, K.A. and Dinnington, A.G. (2002b). Wound management using sugar. *Compendium on Continuing Education for the Practicing Veterinarian* 24: 41–50.

McFadden, M.S., Bennett, R.A., Kinsel, M.J. et al. (2011). Evaluation of the histologic reactions to commonly used suture materials in the skin and musculature of ball pythons (*Python regius*). *American Journal of Veterinary Research* 72: 1397–1406.

Mitchell, M.A. and Diaz-Figueroa, O. (2004). Wound management in reptiles. *Veterinary Clinics of North America. Exotic Animal Practice* 7: 123–140.

Remple, J.D. (2006). A multifaceted approach to the treatment of bumblefoot in raptors. *Journal of Exotic Pet Medicine* 15 (1): 49–55.

Riggs, S.M. and Tully, T.N. (2004). Wound management in nonpsittacine birds. *Veterinary Clinics of North America. Exotic Animal Practice* 7: 19–36.

Ritzman, T.K. (2015). Therapeutic laser treatment for exotic animal patients. *Journal of Avian Medicine and Surgery* 29 (1): 69–73.

Sanchez, I.R., Swaim, S.F., Nusbaum, K.E. et al. (1988). Effects of chlorhexidine diacetate and povidone-iodine on wound healing in dogs. *Veterinary Surgery* 17: 291–295.

Sander, S., Whittington, J.K., Bennett, R.A. et al. (2013). Advancement flap as a novel treatment for a pododermatitis lesion in a red-tailed hawk (*Buteo jamaicensis*). *Journal of Avian Medicine and Surgery* 27 (4): 294–300.

Shahzad, M.N. and Ahmed, N. (2013). Effectiveness of *Aloe vera* gel compared with 1% silver sulphadiazine cream as burn wound dressing in second degree burns. *Journal of Pakistan Medical Association* 63 (2): 225–230.

Shamir, M.H., Leisner, S., Klement, E. et al. (2002). Dog bite wound management in dogs and cats: a retrospective study of 196 cases. *Journal of Veterinary Medicine A* 49: 107–112.

Shaver, S.L., Hunt, G.B., and Kidd, S.W. (2014). Evaluation of fluid production and seroma formation after placement of closed suction drains in clean subcutaneous surgical wounds of dogs: 77 cases

(2005–2012). *Journal of the American Veterinary Medical Association* 245 (2): 211–215.

Smith, D.A. and Barker, I.K. (1988). Healing of cutaneous wounds in the common garter snake (*Thamnophis sirtalis*). *Canadian Journal of Veterinary Research* 52: 111–119.

Smith, D.A., Barker, I.K., and Allen, B.O. (1988). The effect of certain topical medications on healing of cutaneous wounds in the common garter snake (*Thamnophis sirtalis*). *Canadian Journal of Veterinary Research* 52: 129–133.

Sobczak, N. and Kantyka, M. (2014). Hirudotherapy in veterinary medicine. *Annals of Parasitology* 60 (2): 89–92.

Spearman, R.I.C. and Hardy, J.A. (1985). Integument. In: *Form and Function in Birds*, vol. 3 (ed. A.S. King and J. McLelland), 1–52. London: Academic Press.

Stroud, P.K., Amalsadvala, T., and Swaim, S.F. (2003). The use of skin flaps and grafts for wound management in raptors. *Journal of Avian Medicine and Surgery* 17 (2): 78–85.

Swaim, S.F. and Wilhalf, D. (1985). The physics, physiology, and chemistry of bandaging open wounds. *Compendium on Continuing Education for the Practicing Veterinarian* 7 (2): 146–156.

Thomas, N.J. (1999). Electrocution. In: *Field Manual of Wildlife Disease* (ed. M. Friend and J.C. Franson). Madison, WI: US Geological Survey.

12

Principles of Initial Orphan Care

Laurie J. Gage[1] and Rebecca S. Duerr[2]

[1] *USDA APHIS Animal Care, Napa, CA, USA*
[2] *International Bird Rescue, Fairfield, CA, USA*

Ethical Considerations

Veterinary clinics are usually unsuitable places to hand raise young wild animals. Many species require frequent feeding over much of each 24-hour period, as often as every 20 minutes in some species, which may be a strain on clinic staffing. During captivity, both wild birds and mammals must develop skills and behaviors necessary for survival after release, including foraging for food, avoiding predators, breeding, and migrating. They must not be disabled such that they cannot complete these life history activities. Potential problems that may develop during captive care include poor-quality plumage or fur due to inappropriate diets or hygiene, imprinting on caregivers, habituation to humans or pets, learning undesirable behaviors that increase vulnerability to predation, inability to recognize appropriate food items, or inappropriate species-specific social skills. With certain exceptions, behavioral development affects suitability for release. Physical disabilities resulting from injuries may render an animal nonreleasable, and animals likely to be too disabled for release after treatment should be euthanized as soon as this is determined. Placement in permanent captivity is rarely available; consequently, euthanasia is an appropriate outcome for nonreleasable wild orphans.

Marine Mammals and Sea Turtles

Young marine mammals (seals, sea lions, manatees, dolphins, whales) and sea turtles require special permits for all care, even rescue from stranding locations. Consult the NOAA Fisheries website at www.nmfs.noaa.gov/pr/health/report.htm to find contact information for local permitted response organizations to report marine animals that appear to be orphaned or otherwise in distress.

Orphan or Not?

Determine if young are truly orphaned. Well-meaning individuals may incorrectly assume an animal is orphaned when it is not. If uninjured, chicks may be returned to nests and young mammals reunited with their parents. Most parents will accept returned offspring regardless of human handling. In an effort to reduce the number of unnecessary admissions into human care, many wildlife rehabilitators actively attempt to reunite wild parents with healthy offspring. Contact a local rehabilitator for assistance. If unable to be renested/reunited, neonatal wild animals entering human care have the best chance of survival if kept warm and immediately taken to a permitted wildlife rehabilitator experienced in the care of the species.

Whenever possible, raise neonates with conspecifics to avoid imprinting on humans and use methods to reduce habituation. Isolate wild infants from domestic animals to ensure appropriate wariness of potential predators, to limit stress and prevent transmission of disease; for example, never house deer fawns next to barking dogs or allow free-roaming clinic cats to stare at wild birds. The animal will either be highly stressed or become habituated to the presence of these potential predators and be inadequately wary when released.

Initial Care

Warmth, hydration, and energy are critical during initial care.

Warmth

Neonates are usually hypothermic and unable to thermoregulate when presented. Normally, most mammals and birds should feel warm to the human hand. As a

Medical Management of Wildlife Species: A Guide for Practitioners, First Edition. Edited by Sonia M. Hernandez, Heather W. Barron, Erica A. Miller, Roberto F. Aguilar and Michael J. Yabsley.

general rule, the younger the animal, the more supplemental heat must be provided and as the animal matures, less supplemental heat is needed. Infants should be warmed to normal body temperature before completing the physical examination, administering fluids, or feeding. Injured young animals may also be in shock when admitted and warming dramatically improves their condition. Provide heat using hot water bottles, heating pads, incubators, incandescent light bulbs, brooders, or other infant-appropriate sources of heat. Always insulate orphans from direct heat to prevent burns. Thermal support of nonambulatory animals must be closely monitored. Creating a heat gradient for ambulatory young allows orphans to select their own comfort zone.

Hydration

Once infants are at normal body temperature, weigh them (in grams if small, in tenths of a gram if tiny) and administer warm fluids to correct hydration deficits. Routes of administration include oral (PO), subcutaneous (SQ), interosseous (IO), intravenous (IV), and intraperitoneal (IP) (not for birds). Anatomical diversity may complicate delivery.

On admission, neonatal mammals are frequently hypoglycemic; this is also seen in hatchling precocial birds but is less common in altricial birds. Isotonic crystalloids with or without glucose are acceptable. For young mammals, SQ fluids at 50–100 mL/kg body weight, depending on species, is an appropriate initial amount. For chicks, SQ fluids may also be a good idea, especially if markedly dehydrated and an IV route is not possible (Figure 12.1). SQ fluids (50–150 mL/kg) should be administered into the folds of skin over the dorsum between the shoulder blades or the stretchable inguinal skinfold, easily accessed while keeping the bird upright, placing fluids near the stifle joint. Gravity will drive the fluids ventrally; hence, disappearance of fluids does not necessarily indicate full absorption. Check the ventral abdomen for a fluid pocket before giving more. Aiming the needle perpendicular to the body risks depositing fluids into the air sacs. SQ fluids are contraindicated if the bird has subcutaneous emphysema. If the chick is <10 g, use a 27 gauge or smaller needle; small-gauge needles also prevent leakage from needle holes. If a chick is actively gaping (begging), oral fluids may be sufficient.

Maintaining humidity of 50–70% in housing helps prevent ongoing dehydration. Dehydration may be a reason chicks cease to eat, and may contribute to lethargy in young mammals.

Feeding

Once the infant is warmed and well hydrated, species-appropriate diets may be fed. See individual species chapters for more information. Initially administer small, dilute meals until certain the infant's excretory systems are functioning. Neonates of most species have a stomach or crop capacity of ~50 mL/kg. Overfeeding may result in aspiration pneumonia or digestive upsets. Keep feathers, fur, skin, and eyes free of spilled food to avoid dermatitis and eye infections. Milk replacers and blended bird diets should be fed fresh and discarded after 24 hours in the refrigerator. Previously warmed formulas should be discarded if not consumed within two hours. Microwaving formula is not recommended; formula should be warmed to body temperature using a hot water bath.

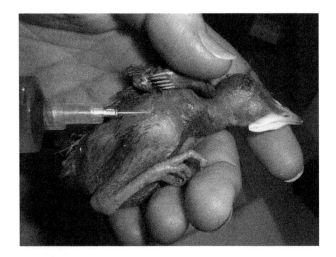

Figure 12.1 Subcutaneous fluids can be administered in the inguinal skinfold between the leg and body wall near the knee from a dorsal approach to keep the chick upright.

Birds

General information on housing, diet, and rearing of birds is provided in this section. Additional details for various species of birds can be found in Gage and Duerr (in press).

Housing

Newly arrived chicks that are too young or too debilitated to stand must be supplied with a comfortable nest substitute that allows the legs to fold normally under the body and the head to remain elevated. Growing chicks must have substrates that allow them to grip with their toes to prevent splay leg (Figure 12.2). For small birds, coiled toilet tissue inside a bowl shape works well; for larger birds, rolled towels may suffice. Do not allow chicks to lie on their sides or on flat surfaces with legs

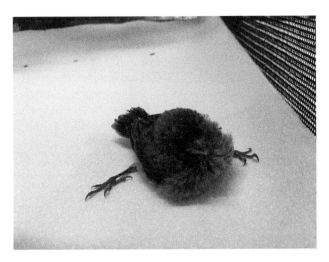

Figure 12.2 "Splay leg" is a condition that rapidly develops in chicks that are not given appropriate substrate to allow them to grip with their toes during development.

splayed. Beware of toenails becoming caught in terry cloth loops or other bedding. Natural nests vary in shape by species and are often infested with ectoparasites; consequently, these may not provide an appropriate environment for chicks in captivity.

Chicks should be weighed daily and gain weight consistently. It is normal for many species to exceed their parents' body weight before weaning begins, then decrease to normal adult weight by the end of weaning. Chicks require 8–10 hours of uninterrupted sleep in a dark, quiet area. Lack of adequate sleep can cause substantial stress. Keep lights low when working around resting chicks, as unproductive begging wastes the chicks' energetic resources.

Diet

Nutritional requirements of wild species are not well known, and are usually extrapolated from domestic species. However, with a few exceptions (e.g. house finches [*Haemorhous mexicanus*] and Columbiformes), many North American bird species primarily feed vertebrate or invertebrate prey to their chicks, even if the adult bird eats something completely different. This supports rapid growth rates and the high-protein needs of chicks.

Common Problems with Orphaned Wildlife

Parasites

Infant wildlife often present with external and/or internal parasites. In wildlife shelter nurseries, it is common to have antiparasitic protocols for infants administered on a herd health basis because individual diagnostics and treatment plans are often not feasible. Rapid social development of each animal and workload of personnel often preclude isolation of individuals until each animal tests negative for parasites. Development of herd health plans for each facility should be based on identification of which species of parasites are commonly a problem in each circumstance.

Metabolic Bone Disease

Metabolic bone disease develops quickly in wild orphans fed inadequate diets, as fast as a few days in rapidly growing species, and this is usually due to inadequate calcium in the diet. In the authors' experience, corvids, northern mockingbirds (*Mimus polyglottos*), American robins (*Turdus migratorius*), herons, gulls, killdeer (*Charadrius vociferus*) and other shorebirds, hawks, owls, opossums, and canids are especially susceptible. Deficiency may also develop when transitioned from formulas to inadequately supplemented animal protein diets prior to skeletal maturity.

Whole adult rodents and some species of fish contain an excellent balance of nutrients for growing carnivorous young, but partial carcasses (e.g., plain meat) are deficient in many nutrients. Ground mammal or poultry meat must be supplemented with 5 g of calcium carbonate/0.5 kg meat. Growing chicks require a dietary ratio of elemental calcium to phosphorus of ~2:1 by weight (Klasing 1999). Feeder insects are deficient in many nutrients, especially calcium, as are many small-bodied fish such as capelin (*Mallotus villosus*) and night smelt (*Spirinchus starksi*). Mealworms and crickets must be supplemented with approximately 550 mg elemental calcium per 100 g insects fed to meet the 2:1 Ca:P ratio (calculation based on Finke 2002). Capelin requires 455 mg Ca/100 g fish fed (McRoberts Sales Inc.) to meet that ratio.

Calcium glubionate syrup only provides 23 mg elemental calcium per milliliter while also delivering artificial sweeteners and sucrose (Dietary Supplement Label Database), which may be inappropriate for some species. Due to its low calcium concentration, using calcium glubionate to correct dietary calcium requires unrealistically large volumes to be fed. Calcium carbonate ($CaCO_3$) is a better option, as it provides 400 mg elemental calcium per gram, which would equate to supplementing mealworms and crickets with 1.4 g $CaCO_3$ per 100 g insects fed. Commercially available $CaCO_3$ pills often include vitamin D_3, which risks oversupplementation. Some rehabilitators mix calcium carbonate powder with ORA-Plus® oral suspending vehicle (Perrigo Pharmaceuticals, Dublin, Ireland) to create a no-sweetener, 100 mg Ca/mL oral supplement that can be dosed by body size, even for tiny birds. Other methods of delivery of calcium are commonly used (Bowers 2012).

Wounds and Fractures

A large proportion of chicks arrive with injuries from falls or predators such as cats. Chicks with fractures must be considered to have life-threatening injuries due to the requirement for full function in order to be releasable. Temporarily stabilize fractures to prevent worsening soft tissue damage while correcting hypothermia and dehydration. Allowing a fracture site to become open dramatically worsens the prognosis. Beak and jaw injuries must heal with well-aligned bill tips for the bird to be releasable. Skull fractures often heal well as long as the neurological function of the chick appears normal. Long bone fractures located at least the diameter of the bone away from an adjacent joint heal well; fractures or luxations that directly involve joints do not. Consider euthanasia for these chicks. Comminuted fractures may heal well if long bones are held in the correct orientation during healing. Humerus and femur fractures require pinning for best results, and pin placement is feasible for even small or young chicks with technique modification, such as using 25 or 27 gauge needles as IM pins. Threaded pins generally do not hold immature avian bone well.

In some species, different bones mature at different rates (e.g., in the author's experience [RD], tibiotarsus matures faster than tarsometatarsus or mandible in herons), and time to healing reflects this. When juvenile bone breaks, healing may not occur until the bone is ready to become skeletally mature. Use minimally restrictive splints that allow the chick to move around as normally as possible while healing. Stable callus formation occurs in approximately one week in songbird chicks, 10–28 days in larger-bodied chicks, somewhat proportional to body size. Radiographic evidence of callus formation may not reflect stability of callus, and removal of splints and pins earlier may reduce the need for physical therapy.

Many species are prone to development of joint contractures when immobilized, especially when joints are maturing. Susceptible species require careful management and access to appropriate physical therapy during and after healing to achieve normal function for release. Remove wraps frequently to perform physical therapy during treatment. Never leave wraps on more than a week without careful consideration. Placing a wrap and leaving it for several weeks is always a recipe for disaster. Bandages and splints must not impede growth of the skeleton. Wing wraps must not block, bend, or crimp emerging flight feathers.

Wounds

Chicks with bite or clawing wounds from cats are common in wild bird nurseries. Prognosis depends on location of injury and promptness of rescue. Lacerations from predators heal best if cleaned and closed primarily. Hatchling and nestling lacerations may heal well with tissue glue closure if the wound is not in an area that will be subject to excessive activity, whether due to anatomical location or age of chick. Even if skin appears devitalized, it may act as a bandage which later sloughs off with new skin beneath. Beware lavaging deep injuries because punctures may communicate with air spaces, and drowning is a risk. Extremely young chicks heal skin injuries in a small number of days, but growth may slow during healing while energetic resources are redirected to tissue repair. Older chicks also heal well, although less quickly. Emaciated or otherwise malnourished chicks do not heal well and may show poor-quality feather growth. Ample species-appropriate nutrition is an absolute requirement for optimal healing in growing birds.

Air sac ruptures are also common in traumatized chicks with or without lacerations. This may present as subcutaneous air or crepitus upon palpitation (Figure 12.3). Often, air sac ruptures heal well on their own, but require deflating the subcutaneous air by making a small skin incision to allow the skin to collapse over the air sacs. See Chapter 4 for additional details.

Chick Development

Young birds hatch at varying levels of maturity, from blind, naked, and helpless (altricial) to fully feathered and completely independent of parents (precocial), with several gradations in between. Examples of fully altricial

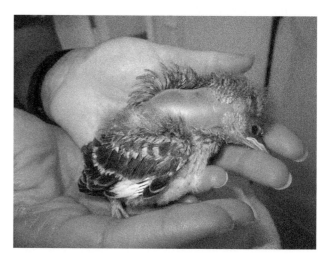

Figure 12.3 Air sac ruptures often present with distended areas consistent with subcutaneous air or crepitus upon palpation.

chicks include songbirds and parrots; fully precocial chicks include chickens, ducks, and their relatives. Altricial chicks typically have shorter but more intense growth periods with greater brain development post hatch. Precocial chicks mature at a slower pace, taking about four times longer to reach adult size.

Altricial and Semialtricial Species

Altricial and semialtricial chicks include songbirds, woodpeckers, nightjars, hummingbirds, swifts, doves, pigeons, owls, herons, ibis, pelicans, hawks, and many others. Tiny hatchlings and other small-bodied chicks require high heat 35–37.8 °C (95–100 °F) with moderate humidity (40–50%); hence a highly controlled housing environment is optimal. Animal Intensive Care Units (Lyon Technologies, Chula Vista, CA, USA) are ideal for small chicks. Empty glass aquariums can be modified into acceptable housing (Gage and Duerr in press). Chicks of larger-bodied species may do well at lower temperatures 29.4–32.2 °C (85–90 °F). Once chicks have been warmed and hydrated, begin feeding an appropriate diet (see species-specific chapters).

Comfortable, well-hydrated chicks will rest quietly in the nest between meals, eat enthusiastically when food is offered, feel warm and fleshy to the touch, and produce well-formed droppings approximately as often as fed. Hyperthermic or dehydrated chicks may have a poor feeding response, hold mouths open, appear lethargic, droop their necks over nest edges, have abnormal flesh color, and stop producing droppings (Figure 12.4).

Be aware that feeding behavior varies by species, and not all species readily gape for food. Some species have large and obvious crops but many do not. Those species with crops should empty them between meals. Digestive

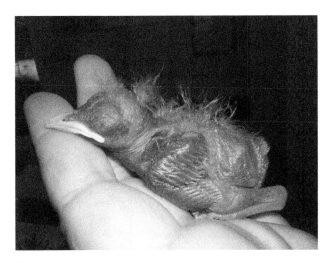

Figure 12.4 Dehydrated chicks are lethargic and do not display an active feeding response.

upsets may manifest as diarrhea, and overfeeding is a possible cause. Chicks that are too cold or hot, dehydrated, or generally weak from injury may require correction of the underlying problem prior to becoming eager eaters.

High animal protein, moderate fat, low carbohydrate diets are appropriate for most altricial species, with some exceptions. High-quality kitten diet is acceptable temporary food usually available in veterinary clinics. Soak and blend kibble or mix canned diet until it is able to go through an appropriately-sized syringe. Hills A/D® canned diet is also acceptable in the short term. Puréed or chopped whole adult vertebrate prey animals form an adequate diet for many species. Do not feed sharp bone fragments as they may cause gastrointestinal (GI) trauma or plug gavage tubes. If feeding a blended or whole frozen–thawed fish diet, supplement chicks with appropriate levels of vitamin E and thiamin, and avoid feeding old fish that has been frozen more than six months. Vitamin A, D, E, calcium, and taurine are likely deficient in 100% insect diets (Bowers 2012). Several commercial products intended for hand rearing parrots are inappropriate for wild altricial chicks, as parrot protein requirements are dramatically lower. Wild chicks fed these diets may survive care but have poor-quality plumage.

Offer fledglings ample wild-type diet in a visually engaging presentation as soon as they are old enough to stand and move about their enclosure. Food offerings and presentation will vary by species. More detailed information on each species is needed for successful weaning, and is provided in species-specific chapters. Never attempt to wean a sick or injured chick, wait until it is healthy. All species require at least 1–2 weeks in an outdoor flight cage prior to release, to exercise and build stamina, gain proficiency in foraging for natural foods, and acclimate to ambient outdoor temperatures. See Miller (2012) for minimum caging requirements for wild birds during different stages of rehabilitation. It is not appropriate to release formerly ill or injured young birds directly from a veterinary clinic, as they will be athletically deconditioned and lack life skills.

Songbirds, Swifts, and Woodpeckers

These species hatch in an extremely altricial state and grow very quickly; small species may reach adult body weight at as little as eight days of age. Larger bodied chicks take longer to reach adult size. Plumage maturation takes longer yet.

Chicks generally eat 50 mL/kg per meal and should be fed 12–14 h/day, aerial insectivores for 16 h/day (e.g., swallows). Hatchlings should be fed every 20–30 minutes, nestlings every 30–45 minutes and older birds every hour until weaned. Corvids (crows, jays, magpies) usually gape enthusiastically and stop gaping when satiated.

House finches (*H. mexicanus*) and goldfinches (*Spinus tristis*) may gape enthusiastically until dangerously over-fed. Chronic overfeeding may lead to overstretched crops with poor motility, yeast or bacterial overgrowth, diarrhea, and general unthriftiness. Swifts are difficult to feed in captivity, never self-feed in captivity, and must be hand fed until release.

In general, softly imitating a chick's begging call during feeding may assist the chick in switching from a fear response to accepting food from caregivers. This also helps redirect the inextinguishable human urge to talk to baby animals. Some species respond to tapping the feeding syringe or food on the bird's bill to stimulate the chick biting at the food. Chicks less than 20 g are best fed with a 1 cc syringe with a plastic cannula tip. Ensure the cannula tip does not get swallowed by an enthusiastic eater. Luer-Lok syringes can reduce this potential problem. Corvids do well with a slip-tip 3 cc syringe, refilled until the entire meal has been fed. Wipe the outside of the syringe each time it is filled to help keep the chick clean. To feed an entire nest of chicks, give each bird a mouthful working in a circle; moving on to the next chick allows each bird to swallow before the next mouthful arrives. Refill the syringe until the target amount has been delivered to each chick. Delivery of food far down the esophagus is safest; chicks cannot breathe and are at risk of aspiration when the oral cavity is full of food.

Many passerines (not finches) do very well on a mixed ration of mealworms, crickets, waxworms, and other miscellaneous insects but these must be adequately supplemented to correct deficiencies (Bowers 2012). A generic hand-feeding recipe is 1 cup (116 g) Purina® Pro-Plan® kitten kibble, 1.25 cup (300 mL) water, 2 tbsp (14 g) powdered egg white, 750 mg calcium from $CaCO_3$, and ½ tsp (1.4 g) Avi-Era powdered avian vitamins (Lafeber Co., Cornell, IL, USA) (Duerr in press). Do not substitute ingredients as the nutritional content of each brand differs. Soak kibble and blend until smooth and feed with an appropriately sized syringe. Adjust the water content of the diet as needed, bearing in mind that more water means fewer calories per mL. Feed hatchlings a more dilute diet, fledglings a thicker diet. Do not get birds dirty.

It is difficult to replicate the wild diet of house finch chicks, as this species is one of the only North American passerines that does not feed its chicks insects. The author's (RD) favorite current diet for house finches is a mixture of Exact® Hand-feeding Formula (Kaytee Products, Inc., Chilton, WI) and Emeraid® Carnivore® (Lafeber Co.). Feed hatchlings a higher proportion of Emeraid, fledglings a higher proportion of Exact. If shifting the fraction of each diet with age is not feasible, feed the diets mixed 50:50 by volume to all hand-fed house finches.

Passerines may have significant loads of intestinal parasites that may not appear on fecal examination until the chick is several weeks old: coccidia (*Isospora* or *Eimeria* spp.), various roundworms including *Capillaria* spp. and *Syngamus trachea*, and tapeworms. External parasites such as mites and hippoboscid flat flies are also common. Diseases of special concern in wild songbird, dove, and pigeon nurseries include avian pox, *Mycoplasma* conjunctivitis, and trichomoniasis/tetratrichomoniasis. These diseases can spread rapidly through a facility and result in large numbers of deaths, either from culling of affected birds to curtail spread in the case of *Mycoplasma* or poxvirus, or by directly causing deaths in the case of trichomoniasis/tetratrichomoniasis. Each wildlife center usually develops protocols that balance available quarantine space versus euthanasia for both symptomatic and exposed asymptomatic chicks.

Hummingbirds

Hummingbird hatchlings may weigh as little as 250 mg at hatch, and chicks that are not fully feathered require high-temperature 37.8 °C (100 °F)/moderate-humidity housing. Chicks require intensive attention and must be fed every 10–30 minutes for 12–14 h/day. An intravenous catheter (18–24 gauge) on a 1 cc syringe works well as a feeding implement. In the wild, chicks are largely fed tiny insects and spiders that provide protein to support growth; consequently, feeding hummingbird chicks commercial hummingbird nectar or sugar water rapidly leads to malnutrition. Until birds can be transferred to an experienced caregiver, feed warmed 5% dextrose every 15 minutes. Avoid spilling sugar water on the chick as this may damage plumage or require the chick to be washed later. See Elliston (in press) and Chapter 16 for more information.

Doves and Pigeons

Columbiformes (doves and pigeons) have a large crop that holds 100–120 mL/kg body weight. Hatchlings are fed crop milk manufactured by both parents, which is composed of sloughed fat-engorged crop muscle cells, and is approximately half animal protein (as free amino acids and short peptides) and half fat, with very low carbohydrate content (Vandeputte-Poma 1968). It also contains immunoglobulins and inoculates the chick with the parent's beneficial (and sometimes pathogenic) microorganisms. Crop milk is exclusively fed for the first 3–5 days of life, and then is fed in decreasing fractions mixed with parent diet until the chick is weaned at about a month of age. Fifty percent of pigeon parents stop making crop milk by day 12 of life, but some continue producing at least a small amount until the chicks are 28 days old (Vandeputte-Poma 1980).

Emeraid Carnivore is the best commercially available match for crop milk, as it is high fat, high protein, and provides the protein as free amino acids and short peptides, but it does not supply microorganisms. Older nestlings and fledglings do very well on Kaytee® Exact. As in house finches, mixing the two diets creates an excellent combination. Roudybush® Squab Diet® is another commercial option (Roudybush Inc., Woodland, CA, USA). Feed chicks 12–14h/day every 1–2 hours until the eyes open, then every three hours until walking well and eating seed. Use a syringe with a soft tube to feed into the crop, which should empty between meals. Offer dove mix seeds in a wide shallow dish as soon as chicks are able to walk. Palpate the crop before each feeding to assess crop motility and evidence of self-feeding.

Chicks may require treatment for *Trichomonas gallinae* or yeast infections. Dove chicks are very commonly caught by cats and may present with severe wounds. These chicks can be surprisingly resilient and rapidly heal soft tissue trauma, but if joints other than toes are damaged, euthanize. Missing skin heals well with hydrogel dressings; tissue glue works well for nestling and hatchling lacerations. Active fledglings heal best with sutured lacerations.

Pelicans and Cormorants

Pelican and cormorant chicks imprint on humans and habituate very easily. Always feed with puppet parents, use methods that disguise the human form, and do not talk around chicks. Never raise a single chick; transfer singletons to a rehabilitator raising conspecifics. As hatchlings, these species require thermal support until covered with down at 2–3 weeks of age. Chicks may pick food up from the floor, or may require feeding pieces of fish with hemostats or tongs. Assist the chick in learning to eat from a dish as soon as possible. When feeding frozen–thawed fish, provide vitamin E and thiamin supplementation following the manufacture's recommendations (e.g., Sea Tabs®, Pacific Research Laboratories, San Diego, CA, USA).

Pelicans and cormorants are commonly infected with several species of roundworms, tapeworms, and flukes and may have feather and pouch lice. Fledgling-age birds are at risk for fishing hook and line injuries (see Chapter 19).

Raptors

Hawks hatch with eyes open, owls do not. Hawks have a crop, owls do not. Some species imprint or habituate to humans easily; use a puppet parent to feed or disguise the human form. Feed hatchlings small pieces of warm, water-dipped meat every two hours until able to transfer to a rehabilitator to provide a more complex species-appropriate diet (see Chapter 17 for complete details on care of young raptors).

Herons and Egrets

Heron and egret chicks hatch with eyes open but are quite helpless for the first several days of life. They often arrive extremely hypothermic and dehydrated, and may have fallen from great heights. Initially, place cold chicks in a 32.2–37.8 °C (90–100 °F) brooder such as an Animal Intensive Care Unit. Provide thermal support until the chick measures cloacally >39.4 °C (103 °F), is old enough to perch, is mostly feathered, and can maintain temperature without additional warmth. Some species imprint on humans easily, so it is prudent to avoid the chick viewing humans or human hands as associated with food. However, young chicks require hand feeding until they learn to self-feed. Consequently, use puppet parents or at least disguise hands with a shapeless pillowcase when feeding, while observing unobtrusively. Use hemostats to deliver small, thawed fish (5–20g, sliced diagonally if larger) to the chick's bill hourly until it is sated. Place food right in front of the chick in a shallow dish and pick food up from the dish to feed until the chick learns to pick up food. Feeder insects and thawed, chopped mice are additional possible foods. Supplement thawed fish diets with appropriate vitamin E and thiamin. Mazuri® Auklet Vitamin #5M2G tablets (Land O'Lakes, Inc., Arden Hills, MN, USA) or Sea Tabs are available commercial supplements. Herons and egrets are highly susceptible to metabolic bone disease (see earlier discussion) and fractures from falls.

Juvenile herons and egrets often present with spaghetti-like masses of worms (*Avioserpens* spp.) within the tissues of the floor of the mouth. These worms can be difficult to kill, and cause verminous abscesses and tissue necrosis. The author (RD) has seen effective control with ivermectin and fenbendazole PO, both given once, with repeat dosing in 10 days. The author has not observed adverse effects (e.g., mortality or plumage problems) with use of fenbendazole in these species although they have been reported in other avian species (see Appendix II: Formulary). Lower doses have been ineffective. Chicks may require antibiotics for infected worm abscesses. Mouth flukes are also common. Verminous coelomitis from *Eustrongylides ignotus* infestations can be severe in fledglings and prognosis is very guarded for chicks with palpable worm masses within the coelom. Chicks may be affected by steatitis in some areas.

Precocial and Sub- or Semiprecocial Species

Precocial chicks often enter care cold, dehydrated, and starving. They may weigh less than their hatch weight at several days of age; however, if the chicks are warmed to normal body temperature, offered appropriate foods, and placed in an enclosure where they are not stressed, they will often start eating and drinking on their own.

Extremely young or small chicks such as quail and killdeer (*C. vociferus*) require high-heat brooders 35–37.8 °C (95–100 °F). For many chicks, daylight level lighting may be necessary to stimulate eating and drinking, but privacy from observation also may be necessary. Single chicks feel more secure with stuffed animals, mirrors, clean feather dusters, or other comfort objects. Monitor droppings, behavior, weight, and food dishes for evidence of eating. Closely related species may be housed together, but if ages or sizes are dramatically different, beware of food dish competition or fighting. Uncommon species and markedly debilitated chicks require close attention to housing and food presentation for a successful outcome; transfer to a rehabilitator as soon as possible if not familiar with a species.

Killdeer and Other Shorebirds

Offer food in shallow water in a wide dish or tray no higher than the chick's hock so the chick can step into and out of the dish easily. Offer tubifex worms, small bloodworms, brine shrimp, small mealworms, tiny krill, fly or mosquito larvae, or cichlid mini-pellets. Sprinkle food liberally with calcium carbonate powder. Offer fresh food trays 3–4 times daily. Extremely debilitated chicks may require feeding a few drops of nutritive liquid directly to the bill every 20 minutes. Capillary action will draw thin fluids into the mouth and stimulate swallowing. Once the chick is stronger it may start feeding on its own (see Chapter 19).

Waterfowl

Correct species identification is needed as some species of ducks (e.g., mergansers) may require different foods (e.g., live prey) and protein levels during growth. Chicks are sometimes chilled on arrival, and may have food- or droppings-contaminated plumage if kept by the finder for any length of time. Once warm and well hydrated, most duck, goose, and swan chicks will eat and drink on their own. Waterfowl starter (Mazuri Pet Nutrition) is appropriate diet for many species during the first few weeks, but other foods such as natural duckweed or watercress, small invertebrates, crushed hard-boiled egg, and small minnows should be offered. After a few weeks, they should be gradually transitioned to a grower diet. Provide a heat source such as a heat lamp for chicks to warm underneath when they exit water. Ensure tall chicks such as geese and swans cannot burn their heads on heat sources (see Chapter 18 for more details).

Gamebirds

Tiny hatchling quail and other galliform chicks are in danger of drowning in water dishes. Place pebbles or marbles in shallow water dishes to prevent chicks becoming wet and chilled or drowning. Some species do well on commercial gamebird starter, but less common species such as grouse and prairie chickens primarily consume small invertebrates. Offer small pieces of soaked puppy kibble, small-bodied invertebrates, and small clumps of grass or weeds with soil in addition to gamebird starter. Correct identification of species is crucial. See Gibson (in press) and Chapter 16.

Grebes and Rails

Grebe chicks ride on their parents' backs nestled between the wings for warmth, and are dumped into the water for eating or defecating. Pied-billed grebe (*Podilymbus podiceps*) chicks often present with wounds from cats. Close wounds to ensure rapid return to waterproof plumage (see Chapter 19). These chicks often will not eat or defecate unless swimming. Extremely young chicks require hand feeding in the water, but rarely imprint on humans. See Elliott (in press) for information on raising grebes. Rails such as black rails (*Laterallus jamaicensis*) are fed by parents for the first week or so of life but self-feed thereafter. Offer chicks chopped fish and invertebrates with forceps every 30 minutes until eating on their own. Food may need to be offered in a shallow tray of mud or in shallow water trays as for killdeer.

Gulls and Terns

These species imprint and habituate to humans easily. Like herons, gulls and terns may require hand feeding with a camouflaged human hand with forceps initially, but once chicks are warm and hydrated, they usually start eating eagerly on their own if offered thawed small fish. Moderate-temperature brooders are needed for hatchlings; older chicks do well in crèches of large numbers of chicks but competition for food can be intense. Ensure adequate dishes for the number of chicks and monitor against smaller or weaker chicks being bullied or not getting enough to eat. House these chicks with a single similarly tempered buddy to reduce aggression until strong enough to join a group.

Mammals

When found, orphaned wild mammals are usually hypothermic and dehydrated, and may be hypoglycemic. The infants must be warmed to a normal body temperature before administering anything orally. The degree of dehydration is roughly correlated to the amount of time since the infant last nursed. If the infant has not nursed in 12–24 hours, it may be as much as 7–10% dehydrated and 30 mL/kg warm electrolyte solution may be administered subcutaneously during the warming process. Hairless young should be housed in draft-free enclosures maintained at 29–32 °C (85–90 °F). Haired neonates are more likely to be capable of thermoregulation and may be housed at a cooler temperature range of 23.9–29.4 °C (75–85 °F).

Formulas have been developed to meet the needs of the more common species of orphaned wildlife. Combining the powdered formula with water and other ingredients is best accomplished using a whisk or an immersion blender; however, both can introduce air. Therefore, reconstituted powdered formulas are generally made more digestible and less apt to have excessive air if allowed to stand, refrigerated, for four hours after mixing and before feeding.

Once the neonate has been warmed to its normal body temperature and hydrated, a formula specific to the species may be given orally via nipple, syringe, or gavage (Figure 12.5). Stronger, well-hydrated babies may only need one electrolyte feeding before gradually increasing the strength of the formula from 25% to full strength over a course of 4–5 feedings. If at any time during this process the neonate develops a digestive problem (bloating, diarrhea, vomiting, or constipation), feed the dilution of formula used before the upset occurred. Severely dehydrated young may need a longer, more gradual progression to full-strength formula. Feed infants in a position of ventral recumbency; avoid feeding on their backs. Younger neonates must be stimulated to urinate and defecate by gently stroking the perineal area with a warm moist tissue, cotton ball, or gauze.

Deer Fawns

Fawns readily imprint on caregivers, and inappropriate interactions may render them nonreleasable. Raising them in groups with minimal human contact is optimal.

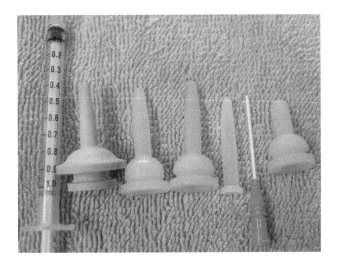

Figure 12.5 Various nipple types, shapes, and sizes are necessary when working with wildlife. *Source:* Courtesy of California Wildlife Center.

House them in a quiet enclosure away from dogs or other predators.

Initial Care

Ensure animals are warm and hydrated before giving anything orally. If mildly dehydrated, use an electrolyte solution 30 mL/kg SQ TID PRN or if moderately to severely dehydrated, place an IV catheter and give an electrolyte solution at 90 mL/kg/day IV. Newborn to two-day-old fawns require colostrum, such as Colostrx® (AgriLabs, St Joseph, MO, USA), for the first 24–48 hours. Reconstitute and administer one 454 g package via bottle or gavage over 8–10 hours (five meals/day, or one meal every two hours). Give 30–40 mL/kg/meal at one day old, gradually increasing to 50 mL/kg. Fawns will require stimulation to urinate and defecate until at least two weeks of age; continue until the fawn has been observed to urinate and defecate on its own.

Formulas

Day One Formula 30/40 Milk Replacer (Fox Valley Animal Nutrition, Inc., Lakemoor, IL, USA) for black-tailed deer (*Odocoileus hemionus*); goat's milk or Lamb Milk Replacer (Land O'Lakes, Inc.) for other fawns.

Feeding

Lamb's nipples on an 8 oz bottle work well. Dr Brown's® BPA-Free Polypropylene Newborn Feeding bottles with the internal vent system are appropriate for fawns up to three weeks old. Fawns may be fed by hand initially but as soon as they are suckling consistently, the bottles should be offered in a rack feeder (see Chapter 20). Fawns 2–7 days should be fed QID. Fawns will not overeat. From two to four weeks of age feed 240 ml (8 oz) TID or more if the fawn is still hungry. At five to eight weeks decrease frequency to BID and increase the amount to 480 ml (16 oz) per feed; add solid food such as indigenous natural browse, goat chow, calf manna, or Mazuri Wild Herbivore Plus diet (Land O'Lakes, Inc.) at about four weeks of age. By seven weeks fawns should be eating solid food and be fed one 480 mL bottle daily. By 8–10 weeks fawns should eat solid food exclusively.

For more details see Chapter 20.

Common Medical Problems

Omphalitis/omphalophlebitis should be treated locally and systemically as necessary. Fractures (from predator/dog attacks and vehicle collisions), hypoglycemia, hypothermia, and hyperthermia are frequently seen. Septicemia is commonly caused by *Escherichia coli*, *Clostridia* spp., *Salmonella* spp., *Pasteurella* spp., *Cryptosporidium* spp. or coronavirus. Treatment consists of fluids, appropriate antibiotics, and supportive care. Digestive disorders such as ruminitis or bloat may be due to inappropriate feeding practices, poor-quality feed, improper formula, or stress. Diarrhea may be acute or chronic and may originate in the small or large bowel and is most commonly caused by problems with the diet, stress, parasites (coccidiosis), and, less commonly, *Giardia*, bacteria, or viruses. Mange, ticks, fleas or lice may be seen and managed appropriately. See Chapter 20 for additional details on cervid diseases.

Rodents

Squirrels
Initial Care
Weigh the neonate. Warm it before any further handling if cool to touch. Core body temperature should be 37.8–38.9 C°(100–102 °F). Stimulate young to urinate and defecate. Urine that is dark or negligible indicates the infant is dehydrated. Ensure the neonate is warm and hydrated before feeding orally. If dehydrated, use warmed lactated Ringer's solution (LRS) at 30 mL/kg subcutaneously. If hydrated, start oral electrolytes at 4% of body weight. Start with a dilute formula and gradually increase to full strength over several feedings. Stimulate neonates with eyes still closed to urinate and defecate before and after each feeding. Eyes open at 4–5 weeks and neonates usually can eliminate on their own within one week of opening their eyes.

Formulas
Day One Formula 32/40 1 part:2 parts warm water up to four weeks. Day One Formula 20/50 1 part:2 parts warm water for squirrels over 50 g or four weeks. Two parts Esbilac®:1 part Multi-Milk™ (PetAg):4 parts water has also been used. Combine powdered formula with warm water using a whisk. Do not use a blender.

Feeding
Syringe feeding or a syringe fitted with a small nipple is the preferred method for delivering formula. Catac® nipples, Zoologic® elongated nipples, or soft catheters work well (Figures 12.5 and 12.6). Feed 5% body weight per feed initially, gradually increasing the amount as the squirrel grows. At 100 g, feed about 7% body weight per feeding. Eastern gray squirrels should be fed six times per day until two weeks of age, then five times per day until four weeks of age. Expected weight gain is 1–2 g per day. At five weeks they are fully furred and fed four times per day; at 6–7 weeks feed 2–3 times daily and offer monkey biscuits soaked in squirrel formula or feed a mix of Day One Formula 20/50 2 parts:4 parts warm water:1 part Gerber® or Beech-Nut® dry baby food. ZuPreem (Primate Dry Diet, Shawnee, KS, USA) and Mazuri (Basix Biscuit, Richmond, IN, USA) make good-quality options. When eyes are open and squirrels are ambulatory, crushed monkey biscuit, nuts, and rodent block can be offered;

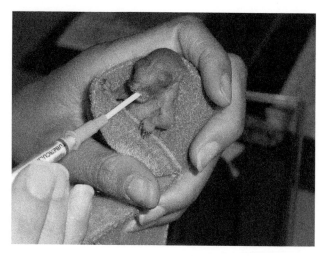

Figure 12.6 Young squirrels have a strong suckle reflex and can be successfully fed with syringes with elongated nipples or soft catheters. *Source:* Courtesy of California Wildlife Center.

chopped vegetables (squash, broccoli, greens), and a small amount of fruit (berries, apple, orange) may be offered. Monitoring the weight of neonates during weaning to solid food will help to confirm they are self-feeding. Tree squirrels wean at approximately 10–12 weeks. For information on large rodents, such as beaver, porcupine and woodchuck, refer to Chapter 14.

Rabbits and Hares

Eastern cottontail rabbits that are furred, with eyes open, ears erect and >5″ long are likely old enough to survive on their own. Weigh the neonate and warm it before any further handling if cool to touch. Normal body temperature is 37.8–39.4 °C (100–103 °F). Hares do not require stimulation to urinate or defecate while rabbits require stimulation until eyes are open. The infant is dehydrated if the urine is dark and gritty. Prepare equipment to do a quick examination and to rehydrate. Give warm electrolyte solution subcutaneously at 40 mL/kg/day. Pedialyte may be given orally using a 3 cc syringe, drop by drop up to 100 mL/kg body weight per feed. For example, a 30 g rabbit could be fed 3 mL. See Chapter 15 for additional details on feeding and care.

Opossums

Initial Care
Infants weighing <30 g have a poor prognosis and should be euthanized, particularly if they present cold to the touch or with a history of being attached to a dead jill. Opossums longer than 6″ (not including the tail) are likely old enough to survive on their own. If cool to the touch, warm the infant gradually over two hours before feeding. Weigh and check for injuries. Hydrate using a

warm electrolyte solution for haired infants at 50–70 mL/kg subcutaneously. Stimulate young less than 75 g to urinate and defecate before feeding. Provide a pouch with supplemental heat for young under 80 g. Chapter 23 has additional details on young opossum care.

Formulas and Feeding
Neonates up to 45 g, feed Day One Formula 32/40 1 part:2 parts warm water; for neonates over 45 g, Day One Formula 25/30 1 part:2 parts warm water. Other formulas include Esbilac (or Zoologic Milk Matrix 33/40) 2 parts:1 part Multi-Milk (or Zoologic Milk Matrix 30/55):4 parts water.

Feeding
Infants weighing 30–40 g, feed 50 mL/kg six times per day; those weighing 40–50 g, feed 50–60 mL/kg five times per day. Orogastric gavage (tube feeding) with a size 3.5 Fr red rubber catheter measured to the caudal rib is preferred. Start with an oral electrolyte solution and gradually increase the formula strength over the next 24 hours. A suggested formula and feeding schedule is provided in Table 23.3 in Chapter 23. Most opossums self-feed by the time they weigh 100–120 g.

Raccoons

Human Safety
Wear gloves when handling raccoons – they are hosts for rabies virus and *Baylisascaris procyonis*, a sometimes fatal roundworm which may be transmitted to humans or other animals primarily via feces. People working with raccoons should have rabies preexposure inoculations and biennial titer checks.

Initial Care
Ensure young are warm and hydrated (50–70 mL/kg of a crystalloid solution SQ) before attempting to feed. Weigh and check for injuries. Newborns weigh 60–75 g with eyes and ears sealed. Young raccoons may be bottle-fed or fed via orogastric tube if the eyes are still closed or if the neonate is too weak to lap formula from a dish. Feed 5% by volume of body weight. Use 2.5% dextrose solution subcutaneously if neonate is hypoglycemic.

Formulas
KMR® (Kitten Milk Replacer, PetAg); Zoologic Milk Matrix 42/25; Day One 40/25 (Fox Valley).

Feeding
Begin with an electrolyte solution, then gradually increase the strength of the formula at each feeding in the first 24–36 hours. Tube feed using an 8 Fr gavage tube, or feed drop by drop in the mouth using a cut, smoothed Tomcat catheter attached to a syringe until the neonate gains strength and its eyes are open. Do not overfeed. The stomach should be plump but not taut. A large Miracle nipple (Chris's Squirrels and More, Somers, CT, USA) on a 6 cc syringe may also be used. Stimulate to urinate/defecate after each feeding until they are able to eliminate without stimulation. Weigh daily. Feeding schedule options are shown in Table 21.2 in Chapter 21 but importantly, across the United States, weights of neonate raccoons vary considerably which may influence age estimates and may require adjustments to feeding schedules.

Neonates should start to defecate and urinate without stimulation at 4–6 weeks of age. Offer small pieces of solid food and a weaning formula when raccoons are about 300–400 g. A mush of formula-soaked puppy chow, mixed together with an equal part of Gerber high-protein baby cereal and using milk replacer reconstituted 1 part powder:2 parts water to combine to achieve an oatmeal consistency, is an acceptable early weaning formula. Formula should be cleaned from raccoon fur after feeding. From six to eight weeks (350–850 g), bottle feed at 5% body weight three times per day and bowl feed once a day. Supplement with soaked puppy chow, grapes, and other cut fruit. They should be weaning at 8–12 weeks of age (850 to 1850 g) and the bottle feeding should be decreased to twice daily. Offer an assortment of fruit and vegetables, high-quality dry dog food, cut meats (mice, chicks, fish), egg, and canned dog or cat food, and reduce and finally eliminate the formula feedings.

Skunks

Initial Care
Warm neonate then rehydrate with an electrolyte solution PO or LRS SQ. Start on dilute formula and gradually increase to full strength over 24 hours. Skunks need stimulation to urinate and defecate up until about 4–5 weeks of age.

See Chapter 22 for additional details on care. As with many rabies vector species, importing or possessing a wild skunk as a pet is illegal in many states. Handlers are advised to have rabies preexposure inoculations and use protective clothing and goggles.

Nine-Banded Armadillos

Age Determination
Newborns have their eyes open and physically appear to be a miniature of their parents except that the shell is soft, with a leathery texture, and pinkish-gray/brown. They are able to walk within an hour. The baby's carapace toughens, thickens, and hardens with age. They reach physical maturity in about 16 months. They weigh approximately 50–150 g at birth.

Housing

The armadillo is a burrowing animal and should be kept on a soft substrate such as soil, stringy bark mulch, wood shavings, and sand to satisfy that instinct. Hard flooring such as concrete bears a higher risk of injury because of the armadillo's constant digging attempts. There have been reports where an armadillo was given various digging opportunities and still developed pododermatitis. Substrates including artificial grass (e.g., daisy mats), horse stall mats, or modular mats will help prevent that. Outdoor facilities require wall footers extending underground for at least 1 m to keep them from escaping. If/when they are kept in pairs or groups, various hiding places should be provided to prevent aggression between individuals. Injured armadillos should be separated to prevent cannibalism. The Clinic for the Rehabilitation of Wildlife recommends the following caging suggestions based on size.

- Four inch body length (base of head to base of tail): inside. Caging such as a large aquarium, sturdy tub, or comparable sturdy enclosure that has several inches of dirt (pesticide free) at one end and abundant nonabrasive nesting material, such as shredded tissues or shredded paper towels, at the other; heating under a portion of the nest area (discontinue when the animal is self-feeding). Cover the cage securely with wire to keep the animal from escaping.
- Four to seven inch body length: inside. Large, plastic airline kennel cage that can be taken apart and the two halves placed end to end and secured, or comparable set-up equipped and covered.
- Seven inch body length to release (body length approximately 9–10 in.; approximately 0.9 kg): outside. Minimum wire cage 2 feet high by 3 feet wide by 2 feet deep with largest side down. Recess in dirt or cover the bottom of the cage with at least 4–5 in. of dirt. If a pen is used instead of a cage, it should have a bottom to keep the animal from digging out. Include a wooden nest box, natural bedding material such as leaves, grass, corn shucks (hay, straw, and sawdust can cause impaction), and a litter tray of water (approximately 2.5″ deep) for bathing and swimming. A log and rock can be provided for body scratching but should be placed in the middle of the rear of the cage since the armadillo is prone to climbing and falling, and generally climbs on the front or sides.
- Armadillos will eliminate by digging trenches in dirt, so the dirt should be turned every few days and replaced periodically. Once the animal is caged outdoors, it will generally eliminate in one area of the cage. Turn dirt once a week and replace part of it periodically. Shredded piles of newspaper also encourage the animal to eliminate.
- Cage height should not exceed more than 2 ft. If it does, you can attach a flashing to prevent the animal from climbing higher. Despite being able to climb easily, they will generally let go rather than climbing down, which can result in serious injuries.
- When caged outside, the armadillo will benefit from being taken out of its cage daily and allowed to forage on its own. A compost pile would be ideal now.

Feeding Guidelines

Young armadillos can be fed either Esbilac (20.2% solids, 8.9% fat, 7.1% protein, 3.1% carb, 1.21 kcal/cc), Fox Valley 32/40 or Zoologic Milk Matrix 33/40. Mix according to manufacturer's instructions. Young are fed every 4–5 hours during the day. The stomach should appear gently rounded, not too firm or tight after feeding. It is better to underfeed than overfeed.

Young armadillos are capable of eating soft-shelled insects such as earthworms and waxworms when they weigh approximately 370 g. Begin to wean when the animal weighs approximately 315 g or when body length reaches 6–7 in. Armadillos can generally be weaned by 340–370 g, at which time you can substitute formula mixed with Gerber High Protein Cereal or Gerber Rice Cereal, then gradually replace the cereal with soaked kitten chow.

For every 1 kg of body weight, an armadillo should be fed 50 g/day (if sufficiently active; an exercise wheel should be provided) divided into two daily feedings. Highly insectivorous xenarthrans (armadillos and anteaters) appear to require vitamin K in captive diets and potentially iron (e.g., one study showed 10 mg/animal/day of iron sulfate reversed microcytic anemia in a captive population fed a dog chow diet; Rosa et al. 2009; Aguilar and Superina 2015). Anteaters also appear to require taurine, but the requirement for armadillos is unknown. Because supplementation is inexpensive and innocuous, it is generally provided in the diet in some form. Some of the insectivore diets (e.g., Mazuri insectivore) are already supplemented with taurine. The food should contain fiber to simulate the chitin component of the insectivore diet along with vitamin C (an exogenous source is required), E, and K. Vegetables, fruit, and insects such as beetles, superworms, mealworms, crickets, hornworms, and cockroaches are additionally offered as enrichment. Enrichment items must be part of the 50 g/day or obesity may result.

Large Carnivores (Bears, Coyotes, Foxes, Bobcats, etc.) and Bats

Please see individual species-specific chapters for details on these species.

Acknowledgments

Many thanks to all the rehabilitators and wildlife veterinarians we have known who contributed content to this chapter.

Thanks to Dr Duane Tom for his assistance with the mammal section of this chapter.

References

Aguilar, R.A. and Superina, M. (2015). Xenarthrans. In: *Zoo and Wildlife Medicine*, vol. 8 (ed. R.E. Miller and M.E. Fowler), 355–369. St Louis, MO: Elsevier.

Bowers, V. (2012). *Passerine Fundamentals*. Sebastopol, CA: Native Songbird Care and Conservation.

Dietary Supplement Label Database. (n.d.) National Institutes of Health. http://dsld.nlm.nih.gov

Duerr, R.S. (in press). Passerines: hand-feeding diets. In, *Hand Rearing Birds*, 2nd Ed. (ed. R.S. Duerr and L.J. Gage). Hoboken, NJ: Wiley.

Elliott, S. (in press). Grebes. In, *Hand Rearing Birds*, 2nd Ed. (ed. R.S. Duerr and L.J. Gage). Hoboken, NJ: Wiley.

Elliston, E.P. (in press). Hummingbirds. In, *Hand Rearing Birds*, 2nd Ed. (ed. R.S. Duerr and L.J. Gage). Hoboken, NJ: Wiley.

Finke, M.D. (2002). Complete nutrient composition of commercially raised invertebrates used as food for insectivores. *Zoo Biology* 21: 269–285.

Gage, L.J. and Duerr, R.S. (eds.) (in press). *Hand Rearing Birds*, 2nd Ed. . Hoboken, NJ: Wiley.

Gibson, M. (in press). Wild turkeys, quail, grouse, and pheasants. In, *Hand Rearing Birds*, 2nd Ed. (ed. R.S. Duerr and L.J. Gage). Hoboken, NJ: Wiley.

Klasing, K.C. (1999). *Comparative Avian Nutrition*. New York: Cab International.

Miller, E.A. (2012). *Minimum Standards for Wildlife Rehabilitation*, 4e. St Cloud, MN: National Wildlife Rehabilitators Association.

Rosa, P.S., Pinke, C.A.E., Pedrini, S.C.B., and Silva, E.A. (2009). The effect of iron supplementation in the diet of *Dasypus novemcinctus* (Linnaeus, 1758) armadillos in captivity. *Brazilian Journal of Biology* 69 (1): 117–122.

Vandeputte-Poma, J. (1968). Quelques données sur la composition du "lait de pigeon". *Zeitschrift fur vergleichende Physiologie* 58: 356–363.

Vandeputte-Poma, J. (1980). Feeding, growth and metabolism of the pigeon, *Columba livia domestica*: duration and role of crop milk feeding. *Journal of Comparative Physiology* 135: 97–99.

13

The Role of Wildlife Rehabilitation in Wildlife Disease Research and Surveillance

Michael J. Yabsley

D.B. Warnell School of Forestry and Natural Resources and the Southeastern Cooperative Wildlife Disease Study, Department of Population Health, College of Veterinary Medicine, University of Georgia, Athens, GA, USA

Introduction

The abundance of animals that are admitted annually to rehabilitation centers provides a unique opportunity to conduct investigations on pathogens that may be important to the health of not only wildlife species but also domestic animals and humans. Worldwide, it is estimated that 75% of emerging human diseases originate from animals while 77% of livestock and 91% of domestic animal pathogens also infect wildlife species (Taylor et al. 2001; Cutler et al. 2010; Siembieda et al. 2011). Numerous examples of wildlife pathogens causing disease in domestic animals exist. Because of the close contact of wildlife rehabilitators with the wildlife they are caring for, transmission of zoonotic pathogens is a concern. Details of these pathogens are covered throughout this text. This chapter will review selected examples where wildlife rehabilitation centers have facilitated or conducted research on the ecology of pathogens in wildlife populations, as well as general recommendations for those interested in conducting similar studies. In addition, this chapter highlights the large number of parasites, bacteria, viruses, and other agents that animals may have upon admission, which is why proper husbandry, quarantine, and testing are critical to prevent spread and clinical disease within a center (Porter 1996).

Surveillance for Rabies

Rabies virus is an important pathogen of wildlife, domestic animals, and people. Many rehabilitation centers admit animals because they are either captured or injured due to unusual behavior. Although all neurological mammals are rabies suspects, in specific geographic regions certain hosts are more likely to have rabies virus infections. Euthanasia is generally elected for animals displaying neurological signs, but due to various factors such as finances, logistics, and human resources, these animals may not be submitted for diagnostic evaluation. For those centers that do submit animals or samples for testing, the results can represent an important contribution to understanding the ecology of rabies in wildlife, especially when data are collected over numerous seasons or years (e.g., Kelly and Sleeman 2003; Blanton et al. 2010; Patyk et al. 2012). Unfortunately, many public health agencies do not have the resources to test animals for rabies without at least a suspicion of human exposure.

Surveillance for Raccoon Roundworm, *Baylisascaris procyonis*

The raccoon roundworm is a large nematode that lives in the intestinal tract of raccoons. Eggs passed in the feces can remain infective for a long period of time; when ingested, larvae can migrate through the tissues of a wide range of avian and mammal species, many of which may develop severe disease. Prevalence of the parasite is highest in young raccoons and shedding of eggs has been noted in kits as young as eight weeks of age (Kazacos 2001). Prior to 2002, this parasite was not known to occur, or was very rare, in the southeastern United States.

During a study in Georgia, the parasite was found in raccoons from Atlanta, and this report led to the finding of the parasite in a rehabilitated raccoon (Eberhard et al. 2003). Following this, talks with rehabilitators in Florida lead to the discovery of *B. procyonis* in raccoons in several sites in Florida (Blizzard et al. 2010). This finding was facilitated by the proactive efforts of a wildlife rehabilitator

Medical Management of Wildlife Species: A Guide for Practitioners, First Edition. Edited by Sonia M. Hernandez, Heather W. Barron, Erica A. Miller, Roberto F. Aguilar and Michael J. Yabsley.

who saved large worms passed in the feces of raccoons that were treated with anthelmintics upon admission. During this study, talks at a professional wildlife rehabilitation conference led to additional collaborations that resulted in studies to better understand the knowledge and attitudes of rehabilitators for *B. procyonis*, general housing and treatment protocols for raccoons in care, and the use of personal protective equipment and hand hygiene (Sapp et al. 2018a,b). A major conclusion of the knowledge study was how important awareness and mentorship were for rehabilitators to avoid the potential risks of *B. procyonis* and other potential zoonoses, and that professional wildlife rehabilitator groups have an important role in disseminating educational materials (Sapp et al. 2018a).

Surveillance for West Nile Virus

In 1999, West Nile virus (WNV) was introduced into the United States and it spread throughout North America during the next several years. Although the virus infects a wide range of birds and mammals, corvids and raptors frequently develop more severe disease. Therefore, since its introduction, rehabilitation centers have obtained a large number of corvids and raptors infected with WNV. Data collected on birds submitted to centers have improved the understanding of this important pathogen of raptors. For example, these data have shown that the clinical presentation varies by species (Nemeth et al. 2009), that WNV is more pathogenic to raptors in the US compared to Europe (López et al. 2011), and have provided information on transmission seasonality and localities (by testing resident species) (Llopis et al. 2015; Ana et al. 2017).

Epidemiology of a Unique Parvovirus in Raccoons

Historically, parvoviruses detected in free-ranging raccoons were mostly believed to be feline panleukopenia virus (FPV) variants (Parrish et al. 1987, 1988). Among domestic dogs, canine parvovirus (CPV) emerged in 1978, spread rapidly worldwide, and mutated to CPV-2a. Since then, two additional variants, CPV-2b and CPV-2c, have emerged. This presumption changed in 2007 when a group of rehabilitated raccoons in Virginia died of parvoviral enteritis caused by a CPV-2 variant (Allison et al. 2012). This was interesting as a previous experimental study found that raccoons inoculated with CPV-2 failed to develop disease (Barker et al. 1983). After this initial finding in Virginia, numerous outbreaks in rehabilitation centers throughout the eastern United States were subsequently investigated and genetic characterization indicated most were infected with a CPV which was most similar to CPV-2a; only a single outbreak in California was associated with a FPV (Allison et al. 2012). Subsequent surveillance of free-ranging carnivores indicated that both CPV-like and FPV-like viruses were circulating, but CPV-like viruses predominated (Allison et al. 2013).

Identification of Novel Pathogens or Investigating the Epidemiology of Known Pathogens

Identification of novel pathogens in wildlife is often time-consuming and expensive. Many wildlife rehabilitators do not have the facilities to detect novel pathogens that are easily missed by the handful of commercially available tests that can be run patient-side. However, some rehabilitation facilities are associated with veterinary schools with large research programs which can investigate mortalities for novel causes of death. Independent rehabilitation centers, veterinary clinics, or individuals that have unexplained mortalities must submit animals for necropsy to private, state, regional, or federal diagnostic laboratories. Depending on the history of the animal, this is sometimes done at no cost to the submitter, while at other times there may be a charge. In addition, it is often known that certain hosts may be infected with a particular organism, but little is known about the transmission, pathogenicity, or natural history of the organism. Animals admitted for rehabilitation may be tested pre- or post-mortem for various pathogens and the resulting data increase our knowledge. Hopefully, these data can then be used to minimize morbidity and mortality caused by these pathogens in free-ranging and captive animals.

It is not possible to provide details on all the new pathogens that have been detected in wildlife admitted to rehabilitation centers. However, details from the identification of some novel pathogens or disease syndromes that have been recently published are summarized in Table 13.1. Also, a few examples of the new information on the epidemiology of pathogens using data collected from rehabilitated animals are summarized in Table 13.2.

Getting Involved in Wildlife Disease Surveillance

Pathogen surveillance is often not conducted on animals undergoing rehabilitation for numerous reasons, including time, money, lack of training, resources, and logistics.

Table 13.1 Summary of selected publications describing novel pathogens or disease syndromes detected in animals submitted for rehabilitation.

Pathogen	Host/history	References
Phocine herpesvirus 7 (PhHV-7)	Harbor seals (*Phoca virulina*). Some seals with ulcerative gingivitis and glossitis had PhHV-7 infections, although clinically normal seals were also infected	Bodewes et al. (2015)
Poxvirus	Big brown bats (*Eptesicus fuscus*). Bats had necrosuppurative osteomyelitis associated with a novel genus of poxviruses	Emerson et al. (2013)
Human enterovirus C99	Novel detection of a virus associated with acute flaccid paralysis in a chimpanzee (*Pan troglodytes troglodytes*)	Mombo et al. (2015)
Vaprio virus (VAPV)	Detection of novel rhabdovirus in Kuhl's pipistrelle bat (*Pipistrellus kuhlii*) in Italy	Lelli et al. (2018)
Nidovirus	A novel nidovirus was detected in wild shingleback lizards (*Tiliqua rugosa*) from Australia that presented with respiratory disease	O'Dea et al. (2016)
Mycoplasma gallisepticum	House finches (*Carpodacus mexicanus*) and other passerines. Conjunctivitis caused by *M. gallisepticum* has rapidly moved throughout the eastern United States	Wellehan et al. (2001b)
Mycoplasma sturni	Cliff swallows (*Petrochelidon pyrrhonota*), American crows (*Corvus brachyrhynchos*), European starlings (*Sturnus vulgaris*), blue jays (*Mimus polyglottos*), and northern mockingbirds (*Cyanocitta cristata*). Conjunctivitis, rhinitis, and sinusitis (lesions similar to lesions in passerine birds with *M. gallisepticum* infections) were noted	Ley et al. (1998), Wellehan et al. (2001a) and Ley et al. (2012)
Brucella sp.	A novel *Brucella* sp. causing osteolytic lesions was detected in a southern sea otter (*Enhydra lutris nereis*) from California, USA	Miller et al. (2017)
Brevetoxin	Double-crested cormorants (*Phalacrocorax auritus*). Data examined an association between admittance of neurological cormorants and *Karenia brevis* blooms. Birds had evidence of toxin in tissues	Kreuder et al. (2002)
Cryptosporidium baileyi	Otus owls (*Otus scopus*). Report of ocular and respiratory disease associated with this parasite	Molina-Lopez et al. (2010)
Caryospora daceloe	Laughing kookaburra (*Dacelo novaeguineae*). Routine fecal exam revealed novel coccidian parasite	Yang et al. (2014)

Table 13.2 Additional examples of known pathogens investigated in wildlife in a rehabilitation setting.

Pathogen/disease	Host/major findings	References
Ranavirus	Eastern box turtles (*Terrapene carolina*). Surveillance of turtles at several centers helped determine prevalence, clinical signs, and geographic distribution of this pathogen of frogs and reptiles	Allender et al. (2011)
Beak and feather disease virus	Eastern rosellas (*Platycercus eximius*). These birds were frequently infected and may pose a risk to other birds in center; practice strict quarantine procedures. Detected infection in various nonpsittacine Australian birds	Jackson et al. (2014) and Amery-Gale et al. (2017)
Phocine herpesvirus-1 (PhHV-1)	Harbor seals (*Phoca vitulina*). Frequent outbreaks of PhHV-1 occur in rehabilitation centers. Research determined that transmission was through direct contact and likely vertical transmission. Virus was common in free-ranging animals and disease most often occurred in neonatal and weanling pups	Goldstein et al. (2004) and Himworth et al. (2010)
Fibropapillomatosis (FP)	Various sea turtles (e.g., green turtles [*Chelonia mydas*], loggerhead turtles [*Caretta caretta*]). Seasonal and geographic location trends were noted. Animals with ocular FPs were less likely to survive. Laser-mediated tumor removal was treatment of choice	Foley et al. (2005), Page-Karjian et al. (2014) and Page-Karjian et al. (2015)
Herpesviruses	Numerous genetic types of herpesviruses, some associated with disease, were detected in various seabirds from South America	Niemeyer et al. (2017)
Clostridium difficile	Harbor seals (*Phoca vitulina*). Necrohemorrhagic enterocolitis caused by bacteria when animals were in rehabilitation was noted. To minimize risk, use antibiotics judiciously and instigate effective biosecurity and cleaning protocols	Anderson et al. (2015)

(*Continued*)

Table 13.2 (Continued)

Pathogen/disease	Host/major findings	References
Mycoplasma gallisepticum	House finches (*Carpodacus mexicanus*). Birds had conjunctivitis and it was determined that treatment of birds in care resulted in resolution of signs and lesions but birds remained asymptomatically infected	Wellehan et al. (2001b)
Chlamydophila psittaci	Blue-fronted Amazon parrot (*Amazona aestiva*). Poor husbandry and delays in diagnosis resulted in high mortality	Raso Tde et al. (2004)
Chlamydia spp.	Koalas (*Phascolarctos cinereus*). Analysis of >10 years of records for clinically ill koalas indicated that treatment protocols helped but could need improvement and that younger animals and those that received ancillary treatments were more likely to be released. More access to diagnostic tests was noted as a need to assist with koala rehabilitation	Griffith and Higgins (2012)
Leptospira interrogans	Capuchin monkeys (*Cebus* spp.). Rodent infestation in rehabilitation center lead to leptospirosis outbreak. Northern elephant seals (*Mirounga angustirostris*). Histological evaluation of leptospirosis cases in seals was provided	Colegrove et al. (2005) and Szonyi et al. (2011)
Trichomonas gallinae and *T. stableri* (novel species)	Pacific Coast band-tailed pigeon (*Patagioenas fasciata monilis*). Investigations into trichomoniasis in band-tailed pigeons and related sympatric birds revealed that two different parasite species, one of which was novel, caused clinical disease	Girard et al. (2014) and Rogers et al. (2018)
Sarcocystis calchasi	Investigation on identification of *S. calchasi* in neurological feral rock pigeons (*Columba livia*) in California	Mete et al. (2018)
Various avian parasites	Diversity and prevalence of blood parasites in (1) wading birds in Florida, USA, (2) seabirds in South Africa, (3) *Babesia* in African penguins (*Spheniscus demersus*) and cormorants (*Phalacrocorax* spp.) from South Africa, (4) schistosomes and microfilarial parasites in Magellanic penguins (*Spheniscus magellanicus*)	Coker et al. (2017), Parsons et al. (2017), Yabsley et al. (2017) and Vanstreels et al. (2018)
Spirometra erinacei	White-lipped treefrog (*Litoria infratrenata*). Previously found various *Littoria* spp. were in poor condition when they had high parasite burdens. Examination of data from frogs admitted to a care center found a lack of spatial and temporal patterns of cases which suggested that this parasite is endemic	Berger et al. (2009) and Young et al. (2012)
Avioserpens sp.	Western grebe (*Aechmophorus occidentalis*). This parasite was found well outside the normal range	Latas et al. (2016)
Tick paralysis caused by *Ixodes holocyclus*	Spectacled flying foxes (*Pteropus conspicillatus*). Investigations of tick paralysis to determine the impact of this syndrome on flying fox populations	Buettner et al. (2013)
Asian longhorn tick, *Haemaphysalis longicornis*	This tick is invasive in the United States. Because this tick uses a large number of mammalian and avian hosts in its native range, wildlife surveillance in the US has been key to identifying novel hosts that may be important in the maintenance and/or spread of this invasive tick	Southeastern Cooperative Wildlife Disease Study, ongoing research

The act of rehabilitation is extremely time-consuming and most centers utilize a team of volunteers to care for the animals. Surveillance for pathogens takes away time that people could be using to care for an animal. However, some of these pathogens may be clinically relevant to the health of these animals, so this time could be justified as it will help maintain the health of other animals in care. Some pathogen surveillance can be simple – for example, if routine fecal exams are conducted, make note of parasites found or at least those that are of importance to the health of those animals, domestic animals, or people. Surveillance of raccoons for *B. procyonis* is a great example. In some areas, little is known about the prevalence and distribution of this parasite in raccoons; therefore, these data are important.

Investigating causes of mortality can provide critical data on pathogens but often there are financial concerns with conducting investigations. However, under certain circumstances there are labs (e.g., Southeastern Cooperative Wildlife Health Study and the National Wildlife Health Center) that will investigate the cause of disease in animals that have been in care or are admitted showing signs of disease. Also, there are numerous researchers who may be interested in collaborating on certain pathogens in wildlife species. Often, supplies are provided for the collection of samples.

Conclusions

Over time, surveillance for single or multiple pathogens or investigations of mortality events can lead to data sets that allow questions to be asked regarding host-pathogen–environment interactions. This is a vital source of information on the causes of morbidity and mortality of certain wildlife species (e.g., sea turtles, raptors, penguins, white storks [*Ciconia ciconia*], common murres [*Uria*

aalge], sea otters, foxes, bats, koalas) and publication of these data allows others to have access to the data which ultimately will improve animal care (e.g., Hanni et al. 2003; Kelly and Sleeman 2003; Lierz et al. 2008; Innis et al. 2009; Mühldorfer et al. 2011; Burton and Tribe 2016; Camacho et al. 2016; Montesdeoca et al. 2016; Orós et al. 2016; Parsons et al. 2016; 2017; Gibble et al. 2018). With a little time and collaboration, great advances in our understanding of wildlife pathogens can be accomplished.

References

Allender, M.C., Abd-Eldaim, M., Schumacher, J. et al. (2011). PCR prevalence of Ranavirus in free-ranging eastern box turtles (*Terrapene carolina carolina*) at rehabilitation centers in three southeastern US states. *Journal of Wildlife Diseases* 47 (3): 759–764.

Allison, A.B., Harbison, C.E., Pagan, I. et al. (2012). Role of multiple hosts in the cross-species transmission and emergence of a pandemic parvovirus. *Journal of Virology* 86 (2): 865–872.

Allison, A.B., Kohler, D.J., Fox, K.A. et al. (2013). Frequent cross-species transmission of parvoviruses among diverse carnivore hosts. *Journal of Virology* 87 (4): 2342–2347.

Amery-Gale, J., Marenda, M.S., Owens, J. et al. (2017). A high prevalence of beak and feather disease virus in non-psittacine Australian birds. *Journal of Medical Microbiology* 66 (7): 1005–1013.

Ana, A., Perez Andrés, M., Julia, P. et al. (2017). Syndromic surveillance for West Nile virus using raptors in rehabilitation. *BMC Veterinary Research* 13 (1): 368.

Anderson, C.E., Haulena, M., Zabek, E. et al. (2015). Clinical and epidemiologic considerations of *Clostridium difficile* in harbor seals (*Phoca vitulina*) at a marine mammal rehabilitation center. *Journal of Zoo and Wildlife Medicine* 46 (2): 191–197.

Barker, I.K., Povey, R.C., and Voigt, D.R. (1983). Response of mink, skunk, red fox and raccoon to inoculation with mink virus enteritis, feline panleukopenia and canine parvovirus and prevalence of antibody to parvovirus in wild carnivores in Ontario. *Canadian Journal of Comparative Medicine* 47 (2): 188–197.

Berger, L., Skerratt, L.F., Zhu, X.Q. et al. (2009). Severe sparganosis in Australian tree frogs. *Journal of Wildlife Diseases* 45 (4): 921–929.

Blanton, J.D., Palmer, D., and Rupprecht, C.E. (2010). Rabies surveillance in the United States during 2009. *Journal of the American Veterinary Medical Association* 237 (6): 646–657.

Blizzard, E.L., Yabsley, M.J., Beck, M.F. et al. (2010). Geographic expansion of *Baylisascaris procyonis* roundworms, Florida, USA. *Emerging Infectious Diseases* 16 (11): 1803–1804.

Bodewes, R., Contreras, G.J., García, A.R. et al. (2015). Identification of DNA sequences that imply a novel gammaherpesvirus in seals. *Journal of General Virology* 96 (Pt 5): 1109–1114.

Buettner, P.G., Westcott, D.A., Maclean, J. et al. (2013). Tick paralysis in spectacled flying-foxes (*Pteropus conspicillatus*) in North Queensland, Australia: impact of ground-dwelling ectoparasite finding an arboreal host. *PLoS One* 8 (9): e73078.

Burton, E. and Tribe, A. (2016). The rescue and rehabilitation of koalas (*Phascolarctos cinereus*) in Southeast Queensland. *Animals* 6 (9): E56.

Camacho, M., Hernández, J.M., Lima-Barbero, J.F. et al. (2016). Use of wildlife rehabilitation centres in pathogen surveillance: a case study in white storks (*Ciconia ciconia*). *Preventive Veterinary Medicine* 130: 106–111.

Coker, S.M., Hernandez, S.M., Kistler, W.M. et al. (2017). Diversity and prevalence of hemoparasites of wading birds in southern Florida, USA. *International Journal for Parasitology: Parasites and Wildlife* 6 (3): 220–225.

Colegrove, K.M., Lowenstine, L.J., and Gulland, F.M. (2005). Leptospirosis in northern elephant seals (*Mirounga angustirostris*) stranded along the California coast. *Journal of Wildlife Diseases* 41 (2): 426–430.

Cutler, S.J., Fooks, A.R., and van der Poel, W.H. (2010). Public health threat of new, reemerging, and neglected zoonoses in the industrialized world. *Emerging Infectious Diseases* 16 (1): 1–7.

Eberhard, M.L., Nace, E.K., Won, K.Y. et al. (2003). *Baylisascaris procyonis* in the metropolitan Atlanta area. *Emerging Infectious Diseases* 9 (12): 1636–1637.

Emerson, G.L., Nordhausen, R., Garner, M.M. et al. (2013). Novel poxvirus in big brown bats, Northwestern United States. *Emerg Infect Dis* 19 (6): 1002–1004.

Foley, A.M., Schroeder, B.A., Redlow, A.E. et al. (2005). Fibropapillomatosis in stranded green turtles (*Chelonia mydas*) from the eastern United States (1980-98): trends and associations with environmental factors. *Journal of Wildlife Diseases* 41 (1): 29–41.

Gibble, C., Duerr, R., Bodenstein, B. et al. (2018). Investigation of a largescale common murre (*Uria aalge*) mortality event in California, USA, in 2015. *Journal of Wildlife Diseases* 54 (3): 569–574.

Girard, Y.A., Rogers, K.H., Woods, L.W. et al. (2014). Dual pathogen etiology of avian trichomoniasis in a declining band-tailed pigeon population. *Infection Genetics and Evolution* 24: 146–156.

Goldstein, T., Mazet, J.A., Gulland, F.M. et al. (2004). The transmission of phocine herpesvirus-1 in rehabilitating and free-ranging Pacific harbor seals (*Phoca vitulina*) in California. *Veterinary Microbiology* 103 (3–4): 131–141.

Griffith, J.E. and Higgins, D.P. (2012). Diagnosis, treatment and outcomes for koala chlamydiosis at a rehabilitation facility (1995-2005). *Australian Veterinary Journal* 90 (11): 457–463.

Hanni, K.D., Mazet, J.A., Gulland, F.M. et al. (2003). Clinical pathology and assessment of pathogen exposure in southern and Alaskan sea otters. *Journal of Wildlife Diseases* 39 (4): 837–850.

Himworth, C.G., Haulena, M., Lambourn, D.M. et al. (2010). Pathology and epidemiology of phocid herpesvirus-1 in wild and rehabilitating harbor seals (*Phoca vitulina richardsi*) in the northeastern Pacific. *Journal of Wildlife Diseases* 46 (3): 1046–1051.

Innis, C., Nyaoke, A.C., Williams, C.R. 3rd et al. (2009). Pathologic and parasitologic findings of cold-stunned Kemp's ridley sea turtles (*Lepidochelys kempii*) stranded on Cape Cod, Massachusetts, 2001–2006. *Journal of Wildlife Diseases* 45 (3): 594–610.

Jackson, B., Harvey, C., Galbraith, J. et al. (2014). Clinical beak and feather disease virus infection in wild juvenile eastern rosellas of New Zealand; biosecurity implications for wildlife care facilities. *New Zealand Veterinary Journal* 62 (5): 297–301.

Kazacos, K.R. (2001). *Baylisascaris procyonis* and related species. In: *Parasitic Diseases of Wild Mammals*, 2e (ed. W.M. Samuels, M.J. Pybus and A.A. Kocans), 301–341. Ames, IA: Iowa State University Press.

Kelly, T.R. and Sleeman, J.M. (2003). Morbidity and mortality of red foxes (*Vulpes vulpes*) and gray foxes (*Urocyon cinereoargenteus*) admitted to the wildlife Center of Virginia, 1993-2001. *Journal of Wildlife Diseases* 39 (2): 467–469.

Kreuder, C., Mazet, J.A., Bossart, G.D. et al. (2002). Clinicopathologic features of suspected brevetoxicosis in double-crested cormorants (*Phalacrocorax auritus*) along the Florida Gulf Coast. *Journal of Zoo and Wildlife Medicine* 33 (1): 8–15.

Latas, P.J., Stockdale Walden, H.D., Bates, L. et al. (2016). *Avioserpens* in the Western Grebe (*Aechmophorus occidentalis*): a new host and geographic record for a dracunculoid nematode and implications of migration and climate change. *Journal of Wildlife Diseases* 52 (1): 189–192.

Lelli, D., Prosperi, A., Moreno, A. et al. (2018). Isolation of a novel Rhabdovirus from an insectivorous bat (*Pipistrellus kuhlii*) in Italy. *Virology Journal* 15 (1): 37.

Ley, D.H., Geary, S.J., Berkhoff, J.E. et al. (1998). *Mycoplasma sturni* from blue jays and northern mockingbirds with conjunctivitis in Florida. *Journal of Wildlife Diseases* 34 (2): 403–406.

Ley, D.H., Moresco, A., and Frasca, S. Jr. (2012). Conjunctivitis, rhinitis, and sinusitis in cliff swallows (*Petrochelidon pyrrhonota*) found in association with *Mycoplasma sturni* infection and cryptosporidiosis. *Avian Path* 41 (4): 395–401.

Lierz, M., Hagen, N., Hernadez-Divers, S.J. et al. (2008). Occurrence of mycoplasmas in free-ranging birds of prey in Germany. *Journal of Wildlife Diseases* 44 (4): 845–850.

Llopis, I.V., Rossi, L., di Gennaro, A. et al. (2015). Further circulation of West Nile and Usutu viruses in wild birds in Italy. *Infection, Genetics, and Evolution* 32: 292–297.

López, G., Jiménez-Clavero, M.Á., Vázquez, A. et al. (2011). Incidence of West Nile virus in birds arriving in wildlife rehabilitation centers in southern Spain. *Vector Borne and Zoonotic Diseases* 11 (3): 285–290.

Mete, A., Rogers, K.H., Wolking, R. et al. (2018). *Sarcocystis calchasi* outbreak in feral rock pigeons (*Columba livia*) in California. *Veterinary Pathology*, 56: 317–321.

Miller, M.A., Burgess, T.L., Dodd, E.M. et al. (2017). Isolation and characterization of a novel marine Brucella from a southern sea otter (*Enhydra lutris nereis*), California, USA. *Journal of Wildlife Diseases* 53 (2): 215–227.

Molina-Lopez, R.A., Ramis, A., Martin-Vazquez, S. et al. (2010). *Cryptosporidium baileyi* infection associated with an outbreak of ocular and respiratory disease in otus owls (*Otus scops*) in a rehabilitation centre. *Avian Pathology* 39 (3): 171–176.

Mombo, I.M., Berthet, N., Lukashev, A.N. et al. (2015). First detection of an enterovirus C99 in a captive chimpanzee with acute flaccid paralysis, from the Tchimpounga Chimpanzee Rehabilitation Center, Republic of Congo. *PLoS One* 10 (8): e0136700.

Montesdeoca, N., Calabuig, P., Corbera, J.A. et al. (2016). Causes of admission for raptors to the Tafira Wildlife Rehabilitation center, Gran Canaria Island, Spain: 2003–13. *Journal of Wildlife Diseases* 52 (3): 647–652.

Mühldorfer, K., Speck, S., and Wibbelt, G. (2011). Diseases in free-ranging bats from Germany. *BMC Veterinary Research* 18: 61.

Nemeth, N.M., Kratz, G.E., Bates, R. et al. (2009). Clinical evaluation and outcomes of naturally acquired West Nile virus infection in raptors. *Journal of Zoo and Wildlife Medicine* 40 (1): 51–63.

Niemeyer, C., Favero, C.M., Shivaprasad, H.L. et al. (2017). Genetically diverse herpesviruses in South American Atlantic coast seabirds. *PLoS One* 12 (6): e0178811.

O'Dea, M.A., Jackson, B., Jackson, C. et al. (2016). Discovery and partial genomic characterization of a novel nidovirus associated with respiratory disease in wild shingleback lizards (*Tiliqua rugosa*). *PLoS One* 11 (11): e0165209.

Orós, J., Montesdeoca, N., Camacho, M. et al. (2016). Causes of stranding and mortality, and final disposition of loggerhead sea turtles (*Caretta caretta*) admitted to a wildlife rehabilitation center in Gran Canaria Island, Spain (1998–2014): a long-term retrospective study. *PLoS One* 11 (2): e0149398.

Page-Karjian, A., Norton, T.M., Harms, C. et al. (2015). Case descriptions of fibropapillomatosis in rehabilitating loggerhead sea turtles *Caretta caretta* in the southeastern USA. *Diseases of Aquatic Organisms* 115 (3): 185–191.

Page-Karjian, A., Norton, T.M., Krimer, P. et al. (2014). Factors influencing survivorship of rehabilitating green sea turtles (*Chelonia mydas*) with fibropapillomatosis. *Journal of Zoo and Wildlife Medicine* 45 (3): 507–519.

Parrish, C.R., Aquadro, C.F., and Carmichael, L.E. (1988). Canine host range and a specific epitope map along with variant sequences in the capsid protein gene of canine parvovirus and related feline, mink, and raccoon parvoviruses. *Virology* 166 (2): 293–307.

Parrish, C.R., Leathers, C.W., Pearson, R. et al. (1987). Comparisons of feline panleukopenia virus, canine parvovirus, raccoon parvovirus, and mink enteritis virus and their pathogenicity for mink and ferrets. *American Journal of Veterinary Research* 48 (10): 1429–1435.

Parsons, N.J., Gous, T.A., Schaefer, A.M. et al. (2016). Health evaluation of African penguins (*Spheniscus demersus*) in southern Africa. *Onderstepoort Journal of Veterinary Research* 83 (1): e1–e13.

Parsons, N.J., Voogt, N.M., Schaefer, A.M. et al. (2017). Occurrence of blood parasites in seabirds admitted for rehabilitation in the Western Cape, South Africa, 2001–2013. *Veterinary Parasitology* 233: 52–61.

Patyk, K., Turmelle, A., Blanton, J.D. et al. (2012). Trends in national surveillance data for bat rabies in the United States: 2001–2009. *Vector Borne and Zoonotic Diseases* 12 (8): 666–673.

Porter, S.L. (1996). Dealing with infectious and parasitic diseases in safari parks, roadside menageries, exotic animal auctions and rehabilitation centres. *Revue Scientifique et Technique* 15 (1): 227–236.

Raso Tde, F., Godoy, S.N., Milanelo, L. et al. (2004). An outbreak of chlamydiosis in captive blue-fronted Amazon parrots (*Amazona aestiva*) in Brazil. *Journal of Zoo and Wildlife Medicine* 35 (1): 94–96.

Rogers, K.H., Girard, Y.A., Woods, L.W. et al. (2018). Avian trichomonosis mortality events in band-tailed pigeons (*Patagioenas fasciata*) in California during winter 2014–2015. *International Journal for Parasitology: Parasites and Wildlife* 7 (3): 261–267.

Sapp, S.G.H., Murray, B.A., Hoover, E.R. et al. (2018a). Raccoon roundworm (*Baylisascaris procyonis*) as an occupational hazard: 1. Knowledge of *B. procyonis* and attitudes towards it and other zoonoses among wildlife rehabilitators. *Zoonoses Public Health* 65 (1): e130–e142.

Sapp, S.G.H., Murray, B., Hoover, E.R. et al. (2018b). Raccoon roundworm (*Baylisascaris procyonis*) as an occupational hazard: 2. Use of personal protective equipment and infection control practices among raccoon rehabilitators. *Zoonoses Public Health* 65 (5): 490–500.

Siembieda, J.L., Kock, R.A., McCracken, T.A. et al. (2011). The role of wildlife in transboundary animal diseases. *Animal Health Research Reviews* 12 (1): 95–111.

Szonyi, B., Agudelo-Flórez, P., Ramírez, M. et al. (2011). An outbreak of severe leptospirosis in capuchin (*Cebus*) monkeys. *Veterinary Journal* 188 (2): 237–239.

Taylor, L.H., Latham, S.M., and Woolhouse, M.E. (2001). Risk factors for human disease emergence. *Philosophical Transactions of the Royal Society B: Biological Sciences* 356 (1411): 983–989.

Vanstreels, R.E.T., Gardiner, C.H., Yabsley, M.J. et al. (2018). Schistosomes and microfilarial parasites in Magellanic penguins. *Journal of Parasitology* 104 (3): 322–328.

Wellehan, J.F., Calsamiglia, M., Ley, D.H. et al. (2001a). Mycoplasmosis in captive crows and robins from Minnesota. *Journal of Wildlife Diseases* 37 (3): 547–555.

Wellehan, J.F., Zens, M.S., Calsamiglia, M. et al. (2001b). Diagnosis and treatment of conjunctivitis in house finches associated with mycoplasmosis in Minnesota. *Journal of Wildlife Diseases* 37 (2): 245–251.

Yabsley, M.J., Vanstreels, R.E.T., Shock, B.C. et al. (2017). Molecular characterization of *Babesia peircei* and *Babesia ugwidiensis* provides insight into the evolution and host specificity of avian piroplasmids. *International Journal for Parasitology: Parasites and Wildlife* 6 (3): 257–264.

Yang, R., Brice, B., and Ryan, U. (2014). A new Caryospora coccidian specis (Apicomplexa: Eimeriidae) from the laughing kookaburra (Dacelo novoguinea). *Experimental Parasitology* 145: 68–73.

Young, S., Skerratt, L.F., Mendez, D. et al. (2012). Using community surveillance data to differentiate between emerging and endemic amphibian diseases. *Diseases of Aquatic Organisms* 98 (1): 1–10.

Section II

Medical Management of Specific Animals

14

Natural History and Medical Management of Squirrels and Other Rodents

Erica A. Miller

Wildlife Medicine, Department of Clinic Studies, University of Pennsylvania School of Veterinary Medicine, Philadelphia, PA, USA

Natural History

The order Rodentia comprises approximately 40% of the world's mammals, including over 2200 species, 460 genera, and 33 families (Yarto-Jaramillo 2015). While rodents live on most continents and major islands, their habitats, ranges, and distribution vary widely by species. Rodent species are diverse, including mice, rats, voles, tree, and ground squirrels, chipmunks, prairie dogs, gophers, woodchucks, marmots, muskrats, beaver, porcupines, and more. Sizes vary by species and by range, with some being extremely small, such as the harvest mouse (*Micromys minutus*) adult that weighs 6 g, while the North American beaver (*Castor canadensis*) weighs 11–30 kg as an adult (MacDonald 1985) and the capybara (*Hydrochoerus hydrochaeris*) adult weighs nearly 80 kg (Alderton 1996).

Rodent habitats are varied – and vary by species. Rodents may live in forests, plains, deserts, mountains, tundra, agricultural regions, aquatic environments, and urban areas. Many rodent species are terrestrial, while others may be specialized for underground life or mostly arboreal. Some, like beavers and muskrats, are adapted to semiaquatic life. Many rodent species, such as tree squirrels, rats, mice, and porcupines, are active year round. Some rodent species, such as chipmunks and marmots, hibernate during the winter and a few species estivate in the summer. Some are more active at night, whereas others are diurnal. Some are highly territorial and aggressively defend their territories, whereas others live in family groups or highly interactive social communities.

Some rodents that live generally solitary lives may nest together during colder weather. The types of nests used for resting, protection from weather and housing young vary widely by species. Eastern gray tree squirrels (*Sciurus carolinensis*), for example, may create a nest in either the hollow or upper branches of a hardwood tree. Fox squirrels (*Sciurus niger*) may build a nest in the branches of a deciduous tree, a conifer, or even a palm tree. Ground squirrels or woodchucks (*Marmota monax*) nest in multibranched tunnels. Beavers may nest in lodges in ponds and the young stay in the family group for two years. Some mice may only nest in wild habitats, while others may nest in buildings or agricultural fields.

Some rodent species are abundant in their range, such as house mice (*Mus musculus*) in urban areas. Other rodents are rare and protected by state and federal laws, such as the Pacific pocket mouse (*Perognathus longimembris pacificus*), Key Largo woodrat (*Neotoma floridana smalli*), Mount Graham red squirrel (*Tamiasciurus hudsonicus grahamensis*), and Vancouver Island marmot (*Marmota vancouverensis*).

Rodents are an important prey base and serve as a food source for many species. Rodents' survival requires them to be extremely alert to their environment and indicators of danger. Most rodent species are vegetarian and eat plants and seeds, although a few species may take and eat insects, eggs, fish and, in some cases, smaller mammals.

Their escape behaviors depend on the species and age of the animal. Rodents may climb, jump, run, swim, dig, hide, or all of these and more to escape. Their defensive strategies may include vocalizing, charging, scratching, biting, kicking, and other unexpected behaviors. Rodents often react to people as predators, even if the person might be trying to help. People trying to capture, handle or care for rodents need to be familiar with the escape and defensive behaviors for that particular species.

The mortality rate for young rodents is high, especially for smaller species such as mice, rats, and squirrels. Causes of rodent mortality are numerous: severe weather, parasites, injury, disease, habitat loss, collision with vehicles, trapping, hunting, poisoning, and

Medical Management of Wildlife Species: A Guide for Practitioners, First Edition. Edited by Sonia M. Hernandez,
Heather W. Barron, Erica A. Miller, Roberto F. Aguilar and Michael J. Yabsley.
© 2020 John Wiley & Sons, Inc. Published 2020 by John Wiley & Sons, Inc.

predation by both wild predators (raptors, fox, coyote, snakes, etc.) and domestic animals.

Squirrels are one of the most common wild mammals admitted for rehabilitation in North America. Adult squirrels that are found compromised and delivered to rehabilitation or veterinary clinics generally have very serious health problems since they were not able to hide or evade capture. Young squirrels that are too young to escape or recognize threats may be found and brought to rehabilitation for a variety of reasons (orphaning, falls, pet attacks, etc.). Tree squirrels brought to rehabilitation include eastern gray squirrels, fox squirrels, pine squirrels (*Tamiasciurus* spp.), Douglas squirrels (*Tamiasciurus douglasii*) and western gray squirrels (*Sciurus griseus*). Northern and southern flying squirrels (*Glaucomys* spp.), chipmunks (*Tamias* spp.,) and the many different species of ground squirrels also may be delivered for care, particularly as a result of pet attacks, poisoning, and orphaning.

Key Anatomy and Physiology

Rodents (Latin *rodere*, "to gnaw") have distinctive dentition. Their four incisors, two upper and two lower, are open rooted and grow continuously (elodont) throughout their lives (Figure 14.1). All the teeth of some rodents (including guinea pigs, chinchillas, degus, New World porcupines, and agoutis) are elodont, including molars.

Members of this group require more abrasive, voluminous diets to grind their teeth. Rodents often grind their teeth together when chewing and cutting hard materials, resulting in a beneficial wearing away of the growing teeth. Rodents do not have canine teeth but rather, a diastema, or wide space, between the incisors and cheek teeth.

Many rodents have leg bones and joints that resemble those of nonhuman primates, with the elbow joints allowing free motion of the forearms and tarsal joints allowing a swiveling motion of the hind feet (Cartmill 2010) (Figure 14.1).

Rodent joint injuries that weaken, slow, or limit movement (turning, climbing, jumping, running) quickly increase their susceptibility to predation. Rodent front feet have five fingers/toes but the thumb may be absent or vestigial. A rodent may have three to five toes on the back feet, depending on the species. Rodent front legs and claws are essential to their movement, as well as grooming, holding food, and building nests. Rodents with an amputated hindlimb are likely to be slower, weaker, and quickly vulnerable to predation, while a missing front limb could limit food gathering and feeding. Their survival does not seem reduced if they lose a couple of toes.

Rodent tail shapes, length, and function vary by species. Tails of some rodents, such as squirrels or mice, may break off when grabbed or trapped, thus allowing escape. Fortunately, despite the fact that tails are used for

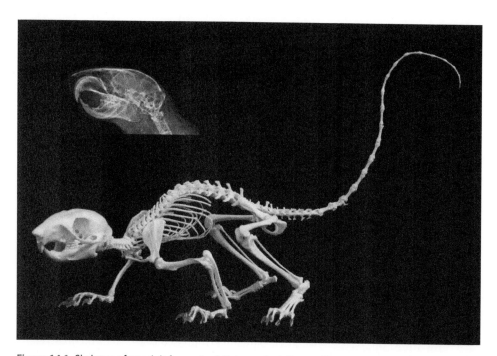

Figure 14.1 Skeleton of an adult fox squirrel (*Sciurus niger*). *Source:* Photo courtesy of Skulls Unlimited, Oklahoma City, OK. Inset: radiograph of adult fox squirrel skull illustrating size and depth of incisor roots. *Source:* Photo courtesy of Mercer County Wildlife Center, NJ.

balance, protect from precipitation, provide warmth and cooling, and are used in communication, tree squirrels can survive with very short tails.

Most rodents have acute senses of smell, hearing, and vision essential for noticing, avoiding, and escaping predators, finding mates, identifying young, and finding food.

Rodent reproduction patterns vary by species. Some larger rodent species, such as woodchucks, porcupines, and beaver, may produce a single litter in a year, while some species of mice, rats, and voles produce multiple litters per year. Pine squirrels and golden mantled ground squirrels (*Callospermophilus lateralis*) produce one litter per year, with the young born in late spring, while eastern gray squirrels and eastern fox squirrels may produce one or two litters per year, with young born in late winter (February to April) and late summer (July to September). The number of litters, length of gestation, and litter size vary by species while habitat quality, climate, weather, and other factors also may limit litter number and size. Most rodents (with the exceptions of beaver and cotton rats [*Sigmodon hispidus*]) are born hairless with their eyes closed.

Key Considerations for Rodents in Rehabilitation

Most wild rodents that are brought to veterinary clinics by either the public or a licensed rehabilitator are the common species in the local area. A few rodent species are listed as threatened or endangered by the United States Fish and Wildlife Service (USFWS) and require notification of federal authorities when admitted for care, such as the Mount Graham red squirrel, the Delmarva fox squirrel (*S. n. cinereus*), and Preble's meadow jumping mouse (*Zapus hudsonius preblei*). See Chapter 1 for legal aspects of rehabilitation.

Many rodents live near humans so people often notice them and often want to help them. In many cases, the wild rodent is fine and would *not* benefit from human intervention. It may require knowledge of the species' natural history and time to assess the situation and advise on next steps. Some young rodents do not need rescue since the mother may retrieve them if given the opportunity (Sparks and Casey 1998). You should recommend that the caller contact a rehabilitator *before* trying to capture the animal. If they already have the animal in their possession, determine whether the animal needs medical care, rehabilitation, both, or neither. It may be helpful to request that the finder/rescuer send a digital photo, to determine if the wild animal is actually injured and in need of rescue. The photo also may help with identification of the species and assist in providing options for the safe capture, restraint, and transportation of the animal. The person finding a wild rodent should be told that contact with wildlife includes risk of injury to the animal or themselves, as well as potential pathogen transmission to people or other animals (such as pets).

Handling and Restraint

Anyone capturing and handling a wild rodent needs to keep in mind that it is wild. Even young or small rodents can inflict severe bites. Wear leather gloves when handling adults or if uncertain of the animal's ability to bite or your ability to control it. Individuals with training and experience with the particular rodent species, ages, and health conditions can provide valuable information on capture and handling to reduce the risk of injury to the animal and people.

Exercise caution when opening the container or cage since the animal's condition may have improved during transport, or it may be positioned to attempt an escape. Consider how the particular species of rodent would escape in the wild and use that information to prepare for its capture and handling. For example, tree squirrels climb, jump, and hide to escape predators, and are likely to do the same in captivity. Mice, rats, chipmunks, and ground squirrels may run and hide in and under anything they access, including cabinets. If the rodent does get loose, it may be easier to direct or herd it into a cage with a towel rather than try to catch or grab it. Since rodent tails may break off, avoid trying to capture it by the tail.

The container holding the animal should be opened in a small, quiet, well-lit room with closed doors and windows and devoid of small hiding places. Any grass and leaves presented with the animal should be discarded as they may contain parasites. However, first ensure that additional young animals are not hidden among the vegetation. Materials to help hold and restrain the species (e.g., gloves, towels, nets) should be readily available. The exact capture and handling materials will depend on species, age, size, and mobility of the rodent. The container should be opened slowly and cautiously even if the animal is represented by the rescuer to be young, small, immobile, or unconscious.

Most infant rodents can be restrained safely in one gloved hand, by scruffing the nape of the animal and cradling the back of the animal in the palm of the hand (Figure 14.2). Larger/older rodents may need to be restrained by an assistant or sedated in order to safely conduct a full exam. A woodchuck, muskrat or beaver can be safely controlled by tossing a towel over the head and quickly placing a gloved hand on the nape to control the head, while using the other hand to grasp the base of

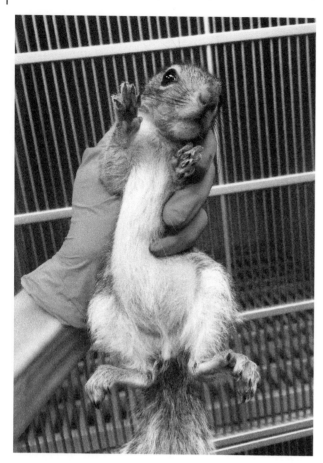

Figure 14.2 Proper restraint of a young fox squirrel (*Sciurus niger*), using a gloved hand to scruff the nape and the palm and fingers to cradle the back.

the tail. The animal can then be maneuvered into a chamber, injected with sedative or masked with an anesthetic gas.

Initial Exam

For some adult rodents, anesthesia or sedation may be required for examination. Most rodents presented for rehabilitation can be anesthetized with isoflurane in a chamber, or via mask if the animal can be manually restrained in a safe manner. Larger rodents (adult beaver, muskrats, and woodchucks) can be sedated via intramuscular injection and maintained on inhalant anesthesia delivered via mask or endotracheal tube. See Chapter 5 for details.

As with all wildlife, begin by examining the rodent at a distance. Wild rodents hide weakness and illness in order to reduce appearing vulnerable to predators and may not appear ill when in hand. Observe the body position; a hunched posture often indicates abdominal pain, a drooping head may indicate central nervous system

(CNS) trauma or general weakness, and leaning to one side may indicate a contralateral limb injury or central ataxia.

Rodent body temperatures should feel warm, and not particularly hot or cold. If a rectal temperature can be obtained safely, do so before proceeding with the exam, as handling stress may falsely elevate the values (Table 14.1). If body temperature is outside a normal range, stabilize the animal before proceeding with the exam. General triage principles apply to rodents; see Chapter 4.

Physical examinations should be conducted quickly, to minimize stress, but should be thorough and systematic. Examine the skin and fur for areas of fur loss from parasites, dermatophytes or trauma. Note any wounds, always checking both sides of the body or affected limb when animal bites are suspected, as wounds may have been inflicted by both jaws of the attacking animal. Palpate limbs for fractures, checking carefully for folding or greenstick fractures in young animals. Palpate the bladder; a distended bladder in juveniles may require stimulation to urinate. A distended bladder in an adult is not normal and may indicate spinal trauma and a poor prognosis for recovery. Pinch toes and check for pain response: withdrawal may be present, but make certain the animal senses the pain and responds appropriately by trying to bite or flee from the stimulus. Check the mouth/mucous membranes to assess hydration and note any blood or damage to the teeth or jaw. Check ears for parasites or blood, and examine eyes thoroughly with an ophthalmoscope (pupils may be dilated with a drop of 1% ophthalmic atropine solution) as head trauma may often be accompanied by retinal damage. Auscult heart and lungs; many adults with impact trauma will have hemorrhage in the lungs, and infants often have feeding-related aspiration pneumonias.

Table 14.1 Average body temperature and heart rate of several rodent species.

Species	Temperature		Heart rate
	°C	°F	beat/minute
Tree squirrels	36.7–38.9	98–102	400
Beaver	37.2–38.3	99–101	150
Chipmunk, eastern	37.2–38.3	99–101	650–700
Gopher	36.7–37.2	98–99	—
Woodchuck	37.2–37.8	99–100	—
Mouse	36.7–37.2	98–99	350–800
Porcupine	37.2–37.8	99–100	300

Source: Miller (2006).

Survey radiographs are helpful in assessing bone density in young animals, as well as early stages of folding fractures, fractured ribs, and pneumonia, which are not as easily detected on physical exam.

Because many of the rodent patients are small, blood-work is not always routine or practical. When indicated for further diagnostics, blood may be collected from the jugular, lateral tail, cephalic, femoral, saphenous veins or anterior vena cava, depending on species, usually under general anesthesia. Collection should not exceed 1% of body weight.

Captive Management

Quarantine

If newly admitted wild rodents are from the same litter, they may be housed/caged together. If there are doubts about whether they are from the same litter, keep them separate until they have been determined to be free of parasites and disease.

Caging and Bedding

After the initial quarantine period has passed and the rodent appears healthy, some rodent species (e.g., fox squirrels, eastern gray squirrels, and beaver) may be placed with others of the same species, age, size, and developmental stage in order to minimize stress and facilitate socialization. However, some rodent species (e.g., thirteen-lined ground squirrels [*Ictidomys tridecemlineatus*] and gophers [family Geomyidae]) are aggressive to others of their own species and other species, even as young animals, and should be housed alone.

A wild rodent should be kept in a secure cage of appropriate size. The cage size should allow the rodent to hide under or in bedding, to move off or on bedding, to turn around, and for older animals, a place to defecate away from the bedding. The cage should be sturdy enough to prevent escape (more secure for adult and/or larger animals). Adult or older juvenile rodents may gnaw through some plastics or squeeze through small openings, such as wire kennel doors. Cages should have ventilation, but the holes should be small enough to prevent escape or entrapment of limbs or head. For long-term housing, all rodents require hide boxes and some require vertical climbing surfaces (e.g., branches) or burrowing materials, depending on species.

For young or sick animals, soft bedding should be placed in the cage as nesting material, providing a place to hide and a way to help maintain body heat. Flannel and knit T-shirt fabric make good bedding. Avoid using fabric with holes, or terry cloth, towels or other fabric with loops since heads, claws, and limbs can become entangled. Species-specific enrichment materials are provided once the rodent has opened its eyes and is healthy enough for the types of activity the enrichment materials encourage, such as branches for climbing.

Young and sick rodents require a supplemental heat source. Cages/containers should be placed half on and half off a heat pad set on low (note most heating pads have automatic time/shutoff limits). It is best not to place a heat source inside a container or cage since a rodent may get burned or gnaw the source; however, some safe temporary heat sources that may be placed with the animal include dry rice in socks (heated in the microwave) or microwaveable heat disks (SnuggleSafe™, Pet Supply Imports, South Holland, IL, USA). When available, exotic animal incubators are the best solution as they provide the most flexibility in temperature range, humidity, and ease of cleaning and disinfection (Figure 14.3).

Covering most of the cage with a towel or sheet will help reduce stress by blocking sights of unfamiliar or threatening activity, minimizing exposure, and muffling sounds. Keep the container/cage in an area in which domestic animals and other wild animals do not have access. The sight, sound, and odor of other animals, including humans, can cause intense stress and fear for wildlife.

Rodents whose eyes are open, and who are neurologically stable, should be provided with a shallow dish of drinking water. Beaver, nutria, and muskrat seldom defecate on land; water should be provided in containers large enough for these animals to enter and defecate. If the animal has an open wound or neurological problem, water should not be left in the cage unattended, and should not be so deep that the animal could drown.

Diet and Feeding

Natural diets of rodents vary by species, age, and season (Table 14.2). Infant and juvenile rodents, like other young mammals, initially depend on their mothers for sustenance. The length of time the young suckle their mother depends on the species. As a general rule, smaller rodent species, such as voles, mice, and rats wean in less time (a few weeks) than larger rodent species such as squirrels, woodchucks, and beavers (months). Young rodents begin chewing and gnawing solid foods while they are still suckling their mothers. Weaning occurs when all teeth have erupted and are fully functional.

Milk Composition

Most wild rodents admitted to rehabilitation are orphaned young that are still dependent on their mother for nutrition. Milk composition varies by species and is

(a)

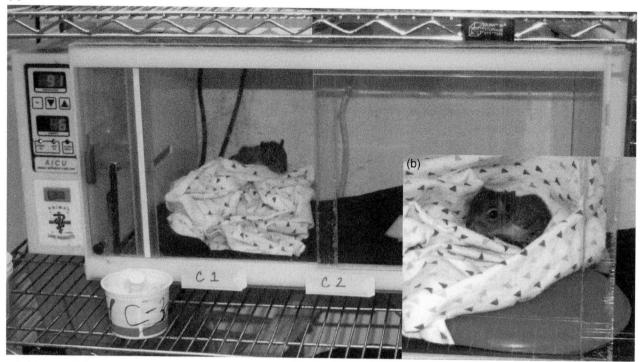

Figure 14.3 (a) Exotic animal incubator provides appropriate temperature range and humidity for young or debilitated rodents. (b) Pink microwaveable heat disk provides additional warmth. *Source:* Photo courtesy of Mercer County Wildlife Center, NJ.

Table 14.2 Natural and captive diets for several rodent species.

Species	Natural food items	Captive diets	Formula for infants	Age weaned
Beaver	Bark and twigs of various trees	Rodent chow, yams, willow, alder, birch, apples	Esbilac™: water: cream (1:2:1)	8 weeks
Porcupines	Tree bark, leaves, conifer needles, buds from conifers and deciduous trees, fruit and ground vegetation	Rodent chow, apples, yams, greens, carrots, browse, acorns, bone (Grant)	Esbilac: Multi-Milk: water (1:1:2) or Zoologic 33/40:30/55: water (1:1:2)	5 weeks
Flying squirrels	Nuts, seeds, fruit, insects, fungi	Rodent chow, seeds, apples, carrots, yams, corn, nuts, greens		6–8 weeks
Ground squirrels/ chipmunks		Rodent chow, apples, yams, broccoli, carrots, grapes, corn, nuts, greens	Esbilac: Multi-Milk: water (2:1:4) or Zoologic 33/40:30/55: water (1:1:2) or Fox Valley Day One 32/40 then 20/50	5–6 weeks
Tree squirrels	Nuts, seeds, berries, fruit, insects, tubers, fungi, occasional insects	Rodent chow, apples, yams, broccoli, carrots, grapes, corn, nuts	Esbilac: Multi-Milk: water (2:1:4) or Zoologic 33/40:30/55: water (1:1:2) or Fox Valley Day One 32/40 then 20/50	6–8 weeks
Woodchuck (groundhog)	Grasses, clover, berries, fruits, cereal crops	Rodent chow, grasses, peas, greens, apples, carrots, yams, corn	Esbilac: Multi-Milk: water (2:1:4) or Zoologic 33/40:30/55: water (1:1:2) or Fox Valley Day One 32/40 then 20/50	6–8 weeks
Muskrat	Mussels, fish, frogs, insects, aquatic vegetation	Fish, yams, corn, apples	Esbilac: water: cream (1:2:1)	4–5 weeks

Sources: Schwartz and Schwartz (1981), Grant (2004), Marcum (2002).

different from that of domestic mammals. If rodents are fed milk from another species (e.g., dog, cat, cow) or a milk replacer formula that does not match the general composition of the mother's milk, they are likely to develop potentially fatal health problems, including bloat, diarrhea, and metabolic bone disease (Casey and Casey 2012).

It is necessary to create a milk replacement formula that closely matches the milk for the species since commercial rodent species-specific milk is not available. To do this, some milk replacer products sold for domestic animals may be combined and formulated to meet the needs of juvenile wild rodents. For best results, milk replacers should be stored properly according to the product label, and not used beyond the expiry date. Additional details can be found in Chapter 12.

Infectious and Parasitic Diseases

Diseases in wild rodents vary greatly with species and geographic region. Familiarity with local wildlife diseases is important when diagnosing and treating native rodents.

Viral

Squirrel fibroma virus, commonly referred to as squirrel pox, is infectious to gray and fox squirrels and woodchucks, and is in the same genus (*Leporipoxvirus*) as the rabbit myxoma and Shope fibroma viruses. Transmission occurs via mosquitoes and arthropod ectoparasites, and via direct contact with open lesions, resulting in raised dermal nodules associated with alopecia (Kilham 1955) (Figure 14.4). Affected animals should be kept in isolation and treated for external parasites. Cleaning open nodules and applying iodine has helped to prevent secondary infections and decrease healing time (author's personal experience). Infections are usually self-limiting, provided the affected animal is given appropriate supportive care. Recovered animals maintain immunity for months to years, but may be nonclinical carriers.

West Nile virus (WNV) can cause clinical disease in rodents. Clinical signs include head tilt, uncoordinated movement, chewing at feet, paralysis, tremors, circling, fever, and lethargy (Padgett et al. 2007). While some wild rodents have recovered with supportive care and systemic nonsteroidal antiinflammatory drugs, rodents with WNV may decline quickly and prognosis is poor in advanced cases. The World Health Organization (WHO), Food and Agriculture Organization (FAO), and World Organization for Animal Health (OIE) have issued a joint statement urging "… not to use antiviral drugs in animals so that the efficacy of these drugs can be preserved for treatment of influenza infections in humans," so antiviral drugs should not be used in wildlife as their safety and efficacy have not been evaluated, and development of drug resistance is a concern.

(a)

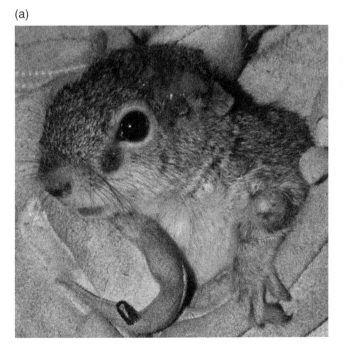

(b)

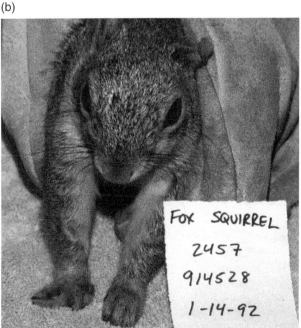

Figure 14.4 Squirrel fibroma virus. (a) Raised dermal lesions typical of pox in a fox squirrel (*Sciurus niger*). (b) Same squirrel after one month of supportive care.

Several species of rats and mice are hosts for hantaviruses and arenaviruses, but do not display clinical signs (Wobeser 2006). Although rare, beaver, muskrats, and other wild rodents may have rabies virus infections and may transmit the virus to humans (Hankins and Rosekrans 2004).

Two novel astroviruses may have been the cause of an unusually severe diarrhea event in infant squirrels at one rehabilitation center. Affected animals were acutely ill with severe mucoid diarrhea and bloating. Twenty percent of the affected animals died; the remainder were successfully treated with metoclopramide, subcutaneous fluids, trimethoprim-sulfamethoxazole or metronidazole, and simethicone gas drops (Gardner et al. 2010).

Fungal

Dermatophytoses (ringworm), generally caused by *Trichophyton* spp., may cause patchy fur loss in gray squirrels. Infections are usually self-limiting, but are highly contagious and may spread to other mammals in care and to people. With the exception of very small areas, which can be treated with topical enilconazole or a miconazole-chlorhexidine shampoo, treatment is best achieved with systemic antifungals (Yarto-Jaramillo 2015).

Bacterial

Local bacterial infections from bites, bacterial pneumonias secondary to aspiration, and bacterial gastrointestinal and urinary tract infections are common in wild rodents presented for rehabilitation. Treatment depends on the type of bacterial infection.

Important systemic bacterial infections are *Bordetella*, *Pasteurella multocida*, and *Clostridium piliforme* (Tyzzer's disease). Rodents with *Bordetella bronchiseptica* usually have fever and signs of upper respiratory infection that may progress to lower respiratory disease. Definitive diagnosis is based on culture, and treatment is usually successful using oxytetracycline and enrofloxacin (Decubellis and Shenoy 2006). Some squirrels with confirmed *Bordetella* infections also have exhibited polyuria/polydipsia (personal communication, Shirley Casey); this unusual presentation may be due to a secondary condition or disease. Treatment of laboratory rodents rarely resolves the carrier state (Harkness et al. 2010). The duration for which wild rodents still carry and potentially shed the bacteria is unknown so they should be kept isolated from other animals in care.

Pasteurella multocida is another common cause of respiratory infection and conjunctivitis in many rodent species. Presentation may resemble *Bordetella*, and strains may vary in pathogenicity, so antibiotic treatment should be based on culture and sensitivity testing. Concurrent treatment with ophthalmic nonsteroidal antiinflammatory drugs (NSAIDs) may help to reduce inflammation and improve respiration (Yarto-Jaramillo 2015).

Considered an infection of young or weanling laboratory rodents, Tyzzer's disease causes acute gastroenteritis and death in muskrats of any age and possibly other rodents. Lesions seen on necropsy include ulcerative necrotizing colitis and typhlitis, lymphadenitis, and congested lungs. Discrete white foci may or may not be present in the liver and myocardium (Wobeser 1981)

A number of bacterial infections in rodents are of zoonotic concern, including tularemia (*Francisella tularensis*), plague (*Yersinia pestis*), and *Leptospira* spp. These bacteria can also cause disease and mortality in rodents. Additional zoonoses are covered in Chapter 2.

Francisella tularensis can be found in rodents which generally do not show clinical signs and die acutely. Gross lesions include disseminated focal necrosis of the liver, spleen and lymph nodes, subcutaneous hemorrhages, and occasionally pneumonia (Davidson and Nettles 2006). Among terrestrial rodents, transmission occurs primarily through ticks and fleas, while in aquatic rodents, waterborne transmission is more common. Human infection occurs most often by contact with body fluids or via biting insects (usually ticks or deer flies). Disease in humans may vary in presentation, including ulceroglandular, glandular and pneumonic forms, and can rapidly progress to death if not treated (Jacobs et al. 1985).

Plague is enzootic among rodents in the western and southwestern USA. Many rodent species are asymptomatic reservoirs, while others (particularly ground-dwelling rodents such as prairie dogs and rock squirrels) may develop lymphadenopathy, subcutaneous hemorrhages, and rapid death, with mortality reaching 100% (Yarto-Jaramillo 2015). Transmission to humans and pets may occur through fleas, animal bites, or direct contact with contaminated tissues, further emphasizing the importance of ectoparasite control and keeping wild rodents separate from domestic animals.

Leptospira spp. may cause a wide range of clinical signs in wild rodents, including fever, lethargy, vomiting, and hematuria. Urine cultures are not always productive but may be helpful in guiding treatment protocols if the organism grows. Transmission to humans occurs via urine, and signs vary from subclinical to acute renal failure (Yarto-Jaramillo 2015).

Endoparasites

Many wild rodent species are infected with and tolerate low levels of endoparasites in their gastrointestinal tracts. However, during times of stress, injury, concurrent infection, or captivity, these parasites may cause clinical disease including bloat, soft stool or slow growth. Coccidians and *Giardia* are fairly common in wild rodents. If found, they can be treated using sulfadimethoxine (Albon™, Hoffman-LaRoche, Inc., San Francisco, CA, USA) or toltrazuril (Baycox™, Bayer Canada, Mississauga, ON, Canada, or Cocci-Cure™, Global Pigeon Supply, Savannah, GA, USA) for coccidia and metronidazole (Flagyl™, Pfizer, Inc., New York, USA) or fenbendazole (Panacur™, Hoechst-Roussel, Wiesbaden, Germany) for *Giardia* and most gastrointestinal nematodes. Note that fenbendazole toxicity has been observed in porcupines (Weber et al. 2006) so pyrantel pamoate is the preferred drug for treating nematode infections in this species.

The gastrointestinal nematode *Strongyloides robustus* is commonly found in southern flying squirrels, but rarely in northern flying squirrels. Southern flying squirrels appear tolerant of *S. robustus*, leading to one hypothesis of parasite-mediated competition between the species (Krichbaum et al. 2010). These species should be housed separately to prevent inadvertent infection across species.

Capillaria hepatica, a common cause of heptic fibrosis in rats and mice, has been reported to cause disease and fatality in porcupines and woodchucks (Hamir and Rupprecht 2000; Hilken et al. 2003). Prophylactic

deworming with fenbendazole or ivermectin and feral rodent control are important measures in preventing infection of rodent patients.

Taenia crassiceps has been reported in several rodent species, including voles, deer mice and chipmunks, but is most common in woodchucks. Carnivores are the definitive host of this tapeworm (Anderson et al. 1990). Woodchucks ingest the infective eggs from the environment, and embryos migrate to the subcutis or other tissues (brain, liver, lung) where they reproduce asexually (Anderson et al. 1990; Bröjer et al. 2002; Hilken et al. 2003). The resulting mass of larvae may become so large that they are debilitating to the woodchuck (Figure 14.5). Successful removal of these masses and treatment of the woodchucks has not been reported in the literature.

Cerebral larva migrans caused by *Baylisascaris procyonis* is commonly reported in squirrels, woodchucks, and porcupines (Roug et al. 2016). Ground foraging, communal denning with conspecifics, and using dens previously occupied by raccoons are risk factors for transmission of *Baylisascaris*. Clinical signs are consistent with central nervous system (CNS) damage, including depression, ataxia, head tilt, circling, and head pressing. Abnormalities in bloodwork or cerebral spinal fluid are not usually seen. At gross necropsy, granulomas may be observed in various organs but in many cases, no gross lesions are observed. Multifocal malacia,

(a)

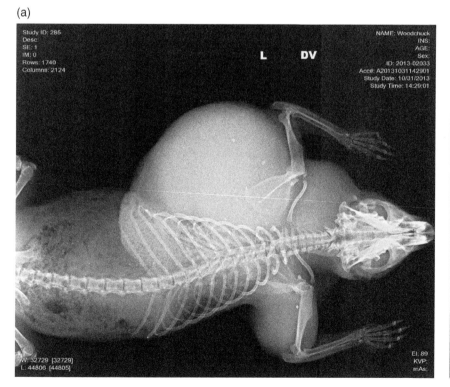

(b)

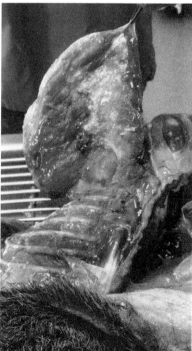

Figure 14.5 Subcutaneous cestodes. (a) DV radiograph of an adult woodchuck (*Marmota monax*) with subcutaneous cyst filled with *Taenia crassiceps* eggs. (b) Cyst removed on necropsy.

encephalitis, and sections of nematode larvae may be seen on histopathology (Medway et al. 1989).

Toxoplasma gondii has been identified in porcupines and other wild rodents, and may produce neurological signs in some infected animals (Marchiondo et al. 1976). One study found over 20% of western porcupines were seropositive for *T. gondii* (Medway et al. 1989).

Ectoparasites

A high diversity of ectoparasites may be found on rodents with fleas, ticks, lice, and mites all being common (Steele and Koprowski 2001). Rodents with compromised health that are unable to self-groom or be groomed may have large numbers, and fly eggs and maggots are often found in wounds and moist areas (axillae and body openings). Mites, fleas, and lice are easily treated with flea powders that are labeled as safe for kittens. Fipronil (Frontline™, Merial, Lyon, France) may also be used as a safe treatment for external parasites on adult rodents (Diaz 2005; Hillegass et al. 2010). Nitenpyram (Capstar™, Novartis, Broomfield, CO, USA) has been used safely in a variety of rodents for treatment of maggots as well as fleas and mites.

Mange caused by *Sarcoptes* spp. and *Notoedres* spp. is common in rodents, especially tree and ground squirrels and porcupines. Animals present with thick, yellow-white encrustations, and the problem may be severe enough to affect the ability to forage or maintain body temperature. In porcupines, *Malessezia pachydermatis* has been found on the exoskeleton of *S. scabiei*, resulting in secondary yeast infections (Salkin et al. 1980). Mange mites can be treated with systemic ivermectin and supportive care. Selamectin (Revolution™, Zoetis, Parsippany, NJ, USA) may be applied topically to adults of larger species (Snyder et al. 1991).

Cutaneous warbles (*Cuterebra* spp. larvae) are common in many small rodents and in low numbers usually present little problem for the host animal. Larvae may be carefully extracted from their cavity after enlarging the respiratory pore in the skin. The resulting cavity should be flushed with sterile saline and may be left to heal by secondary intention. In some cases, topical or systemic treatment with nitenpyram can be used to kill the larvae prior to removal.

Common Reasons for Presentation

Shock

Rodents in shock have many of the same symptoms as other mammals, including cold extremities and pale mucous membranes. A "calm, friendly" wild rodent may actually be in shock, or so young as to not recognize or react to potential predators. Shock is a common sequela to trauma, although it may also result from dehydration, hypoxia, hypothermia, excessive blood loss, or pain.

Treatment includes placing the animal in a warm, quiet chamber with subdued lighting, away from activity and excessive sensory stimuli; supplemental oxygen supplied to a chamber enclosure is also helpful. The rodent in shock should be allowed to stabilize while warm fluids and exam supplies are prepared. Handling should be kept to a minimum to avoid further exacerbating the condition. After the patient is warm, rehydration may be initiated.

Dehydration

Dehydration is common in rodents presented from the wild. Dehydration may occur in suckling young as a result of separation from the mother, diarrhea, exposure to excessive heat, or open wounds. During care, dehydration may occur or be exacerbated when the animal does not have adequate access to fluids or does not recognize a water source, spills water rather than drinks it, receives inadequate feeding amounts or frequencies, or is fed inappropriately prepared formulas. Rodents show many of the same signs of dehydration as other mammals, including sunken eyes, slow response to skin turgor test, limited urine output, and lethargy.

Treatment follows standard rehydration protocols with warm isotonic fluids, such as lactated Ringer's solution or Normosol-R™ (Pfizer, New York, USA), administered at 50–150 mL/kg/day for maintenance plus dehydration deficit (see Chapter 4), depending on the species. In cases of severe dehydration, parenteral routes such as intraosseous or intraperitoneal are advisable. Rectal administration may also be effective in smaller rodents (Girisgin et al. 2006). For mild dehydration, administration *per os* or subcutaneously is acceptable; subcutaneous fluids may be administered in divided doses between the scapulae and over the dorsal lumbar region (Mayer 2013).

Trauma

Wild rodents present with a wide variety of injuries, including general trauma, bruising, swelling, and bleeding, crushing injuries, and fractures.

Wounds
Wounds in wild rodents may result from falls, domestic animal attack, birds, traps, garden tools, gunshots, car strike, etc. Infections and abscesses often result if wounds are not treated promptly, especially bite wounds. Tiny punctures created by cat bites may be difficult to visualize,

but may still cause potentially fatal infections. If animals have known or suspected contact with cats, antibiotics should be administered prophylactically to prevent systemic infection (Casey and Goldthwait 2013).

All wounds should be cleaned and treated according to standard wound management protocols (see Chapter 11). Common antibiotics for skin wounds include trimethoprim-sulfa, enrofloxacin, or cephalosporins (see Appendix II: Formulary). However, in strictly herbivorous rodent species (e.g., beaver and porcupines), penicillins and aminoglycocides should be avoided as they often cause gastroenteritis and potentially fatal dysbiosis, but they can be used in other rodents (see Appendix II: Formulary). Wounds should also be closely checked for myiasis and treated accordingly.

Fractures and Luxations

Trauma severe enough to fracture bones may also cause spinal or head trauma, organ damage, or internal hemorrhage; animals with limb fractures should be examined carefully for other injuries. Greenstick fractures and simple, acute, closed fractures can be treated with supportive care, analgesics, restricted activity, appropriate nutrition, and time. Methods to treat fractures may include simple coaptation or surgical fixation (see Chapter 11). If the fracture is at a joint and/or chronic, open and infected or its outcome would prevent release for independent life in the wild, euthanasia is appropriate. Similarly, due to the nature of the use of their limbs, joint luxations hold a grave prognosis for rodents.

Head and Spinal Trauma

Head and spinal trauma are especially common in young tree squirrels that fall from nests, but may also result from vehicular collisions, dog attacks, gunshot, or other physical impact.

Signs of head trauma may be obvious, including bruising or swelling of head or nose, exophthalmos, bleeding from the nose or mouth, misaligned jaw or teeth, or seizures, but may also present only as subtle ataxia or head tremors that may worsen over time. Epistaxis/nasal trauma can lead to serious respiratory distress because rodents are obligate nasal breathers. To address this risk, supplemental oxygen, administration of NSAIDs, and close monitoring should be part of treatment protocols for rodents with head trauma. Treatment should also include restricting activity by housing the affected animal in a small container lacking furniture for climbing, minimizing disturbance, dimming lights (especially in the case of eye trauma), and avoiding the use of supplemental heat. Corticosteroids are generally not recommended for head trauma but may be useful in cases of acute spinal trauma (Pokras and Murray 2004).

Severe spinal trauma results in a lack of pain perception caudal to the spinal injury. Withdrawal reflexes may be present but if the animal does not react appropriately to painful stimuli (i.e., does not try to bite or escape), the prognosis is grave. A full urinary bladder with the inability to urinate is another sign of severe spinal injury and carries a poor prognosis.

In addition to trauma, differentials for neurological signs in wild rodents include infectious disease, endoparasites (e.g., larva migrans), nutritional deficiencies, and toxins. These conditions should be considered in the neurological patient with an unknown history and lack of obvious signs of trauma.

Respiratory Difficulty and Pneumonia

Respiratory problems can develop rapidly and condition can deteriorate quickly because rodents are obligate nasal breathers. Respiratory problems in wild rodents are exhibited as labored breathing, coughing, wheezing, and "clicking" sounds in the chest. In such cases, the rodent's breathing is usually shallow but may be rapid or slow. The animal is often lethargic and appetite may decrease.

One of the most common causes of respiratory problems in young rodents is aspiration of fluid during feeding; other causes include trauma to the chest, bacterial or viral infections, lengthy exposure to cold and damp conditions, or inhalation of foreign bodies (e.g., insulation) and noxious chemicals (Casey and Casey 2003). Etiology can be determined based on history, radiographs, and tracheal cultures. If the rodent aspirates fluids as a result of feeding practices, correcting the feeding method is an essential part of the treatment, in addition to appropriate antibiotic therapy. Treatment of aspiration-induced or bacterial pneumonias is most successful when based on culture; however, this may not always be feasible or cost-effective for wildlife. Trimethoprim-sulfas are sufficient for many aspiration-related pneumonias, but are generally ineffective for transmissible pneumonias such as those caused by *Bordetella* (Decubellis and Shenoy 2006).

Common supportive care for respiratory conditions includes providing oxygen supplementation in a chamber, ensuring the nares are clear (clean as needed with cotton-tipped applicators soaked in warm water), and increasing ambient humidity via a nebulizer. For suggestions on treatment of nasal congestion, see Appendix II: Formulary.

Gastrointestinal Problems

Bloat, soft stool, diarrhea, constipation, and lack of appetite are common in wild rodents in captivity. Etiologies include stress, dietary factors, intestinal parasites, astrovirus, and bacterial overgrowth. Knowing the normal shape, amount, texture, and odor of the feces for the species and age of the animal is useful in early detection of gastrointestinal problems.

Diets and feeding practices are common causes of gastrointestinal distress in wild rodents in captivity. Care should be taken to provide an appropriate diet for the species and age of the animal. Overfeeding by frequency or amount may result in bloat, soft stool, and diarrhea. An easy way to determine if overfeeding might be the problem is to reduce feeding by one per day and ensure that formula feeds are approximately 5% of body weight (Casey and Casey 2012). If the gastrointestinal problem is caused by diet or feeding practices, the condition is likely to correct when diet or practices are changed.

Penicillins, cephalosporins, lincosamides, and some macrolides may cause overgrowth of normal clostridial flora, resulting in antibiotic-induced enterotoxemia in some herbivorous rodent species, also exhibited as bloat, diarrhea, and lack of appetite. Refer to Appendix II: Formulary for antibiotics less likely to cause enteric dysbiosis in these rodents. In most wild rodent species, these antibiotics are generally safe to use. Proper antibiotic choice and possible concurrent use of a probiotic while the animal is on antibiotics, and for five days after the antibiotic treatment, may prevent this from occurring (Gardlik et al. 2012). There is anecdotal evidence on the utility of probiotics (e.g., *Saccharomyces boulardii*, a nonpathogenic yeast strain) to prevent and treat dysbiosis in rodents, some of which is supported by laboratory rodent studies (e.g., Casey and Goldthwait 2012b).

Gastrointestinal signs may be present with systemic bacterial infections (e.g., *Clostridium* spp.) or elevated burdens of intestinal parasites (see Section 14.7.4). Fecal flotations, smears, and gram stains can aid in diagnosing or dismissing these possible etiologies.

Poisoning and Exposure to Toxins

Symptoms of poisoning vary by the type of poison, and may present as hemorrhage (ecchymosis, petechiae, or bleeding from orifices), convulsions, lethargy, seizures, and/or ataxia. Small rodents, such as mice, voles, rats, and squirrels, may consume anticoagulant rodenticides directly or possibly via contaminated milk from the lactating mother or *in utero* exposure (Murphy and Talcott 2001). Affected animals exhibit petechiation in the skin, most easily seen in the pinnae of the ears or on the abdomen (Figure 14.6). If rodent exposure is suspected, vitamin K should be administered immediately and then daily for 30 days. The first dose of vitamin K should be administered as a subcutaneous injection and the remaining 29 doses may be given orally at 24-hour intervals.

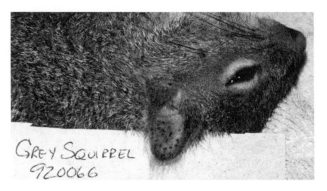

Figure 14.6 Petechiate hemorrhages in the ear of a gray squirrel (*Sciurus carolinensis*) caused by ingestion of a commercial anticoagulant rodenticide.

Carbamates are often mixed with bait to intentionally kill squirrels, woodchuck, chipmunks, and other rodents. Ingestion of these acetylcholinesterase inhibitors may produce muscarinic signs (diarrhea, miosis, salivation, emesis), nicotinic signs (ataxia, tremors, paralysis), and a variety of other CNS signs. Diagnosis can be confirmed by suppressed cholinesterase activity in heparinized whole blood or brain tissue, but treatment with atropine should be initiated immediately as the animal is likely to die before lab results are received. Supportive care, including diazepam or midazolam for seizures and supplemental oxygen, may also be required (Blodgett 2001).

Dental Problems

Rodent incisors may break as a result of head trauma from a fall or vehicle impact. Although the visible portion of the bottom incisors is longer than the top incisors, adjacent incisors need to be approximately the same length (e.g., one upper incisor should not be longer than the other upper incisor) to provide for even wear. Broken incisors that are still aligned can usually be trimmed flat, as long as the adjacent incisor is trimmed to the same length; these teeth will then wear normally as they grow. The same method used for trimming domestic rabbit and rodent teeth is used for wild rodents (Vella 2013). In some cases, it may be necessary to monitor the rodent for several weeks after the trimming to ensure the incisors align correctly and wear appropriately. Since rodent incisors are elodont, damage to an incisor or to the jaw causing malocclusion will result in overgrowth of one or more incisor. A rodent with misaligned incisors is not releasable and should be euthanized.

Urinary Tract Infections

Rodents with urinary tract infections (UTIs) may have involuntary urination (seen as a wet abdomen) or slow and/or painful urination (straining to urinate), and the urine may be cloudy or bloody. Causes of UTIs include injury, not urinating for several days (e.g., young rodents were not stimulated to urinate, were too dehydrated to urinate, or could not urinate due to neurological injury), suckling by cage mates, or blockage (due to swelling, scab, or foreign body). A urine dipstick may be useful for quickly determining the presence of bacteria, blood, ketones, etc. to help devise a treatment plan. In all cases, treatment should include ensuring the animal receives adequate fluids and initiating a sulfonamide antibiotic. If feasible, a urine culture and sensitivity should be performed and antibiotic therapy adjusted as indicated by the results.

Preputial Injuries

Young mammals, especially squirrels, may suckle the male genitalia of a sibling, or even their own genitalia, possibly because of dehydration, inadequate diet, inappropriate feeding schedule, UTI, teething, or other causes (Casey and Goldthwait 2012a). Injury can range from bruising, elongation, open sores with secondary infection, to phimosis or paraphimosis. Juvenile rodents may present for rehabilitation with this condition, or may develop these injuries while in captivity. Treatment involves addressing the behavioral component by supplying environmental enrichment (e.g., blanket, fruit, or other item on which to suckle), anxiolytics, and topical treatment for swelling and erythema. A salve composed of one part zinc oxide, one part hydrocortisone cream and one part triple antibiotic cream may provide relief and expedite healing (personal communication, Heather Barron).

Nutritional Disorders and Emaciation

Rodents with nutritional disorders may show slow or delayed growth, poor fur condition, lethargy, low energy, musculoskeletal deformities and fractures, paralysis, or seizures. Nutritional disorders often occur because of an inappropriate diet, inadequate food amounts, improper supplementation, heavy endoparasite burdens, or imbalance of intestinal flora. Loss of bone density and evidence of folding fractures on radiographs, and low serum ionized calcium and vitamin D are indicative of metabolic bone disease and carry a guarded to poor prognosis. Treatment involves feeding an appropriately nutritious diet in adequate amounts and frequency, providing supplemental calcium, exposing the animal to natural sunlight, and maintaining adequate hydration. While minor nutritional problems may be corrected, some, including advanced metabolic bone disease, may be fatal or require euthanasia.

Skin Conditions

Congenital alopecia occurs among wild rodents and is occasionally seen in tree squirrels and woodchucks presented for rehabilitation. A skin scraping can be performed to rule out mites or dermatophytoses, but an initial diagnosis can be made based on the normal, albeit hairless, appearance of the skin compared to the scaly, crusty condition seen with sarcoptic or notoedric mange and ringworm (*Trichophyton mentagrophytes*). A skin biopsy usually reveals rudimentary or complete lack of hair follicles (Davidson and Nettles 2006); these animals are not suitable for release to the wild. Idiopathic alopecia has been reported in juvenile red squirrels in Massachusetts that did eventually grow normal coats (personal communication, Mark Pokras and Christina Clark). Conversely, mange and ringworm can be easily resolved with a number of topical or systemic treatments (see Sections 14.7.2 and 14.7.5, and Appendix II: Formulary).

Euthanasia

Most regulations allow a veterinarian to euthanize a rodent with life-threatening injuries or other conditions that would prevent recovery and release to live independently in the wild. Because of the necessity for the rodent to survive in the wild, obtaining food and escaping predators, euthanasia criteria for these animals are more stringent than those applied to domestic animals.

Euthanasia is indicated for rodents whose injuries carry a poor prognosis for release; whose diseases may put other animals at serious risk; or whose injuries would require extended treatment and extensive care, placing the animal under undue stress. The following problems fit the above criteria.

1) Spinal trauma with loss of pain perception.
2) Neurological damage resulting in paralysis, inability to urinate or defecate, and/or uncontrollable seizures.
3) Severe malocclusion or jaw fracture that reduces ability to eat and/or results in overgrowth of incisor(s).
4) Damaged joints that limit mobility, agility, and strength.
5) Blindness or reduced vision in both eyes.
6) Advanced metabolic bone disease with irreversible bone and/or organ damage.
7) Severe anemia (packed cell volume <10% holds a very poor prognosis).
8) Severe maggot infestation that results in extensive tissue damage and impaired organ function.
9) Advanced disseminated cases of squirrel pox in which the animal is debilitated. If a squirrel with poxvirus cannot be adequately isolated from other rodents, euthanasia should be considered rather than risking transmission to other patients.

10) Cases of plague or tularemia that might place humans and other animals at risk of infection.
11) Identification of multiple (3+) serious conditions that each might allow recovery, but the cumulative impact of which suggests a low probability of recovery and release.

Additional injuries and circumstances frequently warrant euthanasia but may first require evaluation over several days to determine if the patient will recover or not. The injuries listed below generally hold poor prognoses, but are occasionally treatable.

1) Skull fractures and spinal injury (with pain perception still present), depending on the severity. Animals showing no improvement in any given 48-hour period (i.e., plateauing in their progress) are not likely to recover.
2) Dislocated joints that do not remain in place when reduced.
3) Fractured or dislocated jaw that does not align correctly. These injuries often require assessment over several months to make a conclusive evaluation.
4) Inability to maintain balance or coordination during daily activity.
5) Amputations that prevent full normal activity (finding food, making nests, escaping predators, etc.).
6) Fractured pelvis in a female rodent; radiographs should be evaluated closely to determine if she can undergo normal parturition. Injuries that may result in dystocia should be considered as cause for euthanasia.

Euthanasia Methods and Carcass Disposal

The American Veterinary Medical Association (AVMA) Guidelines for the Euthanasia of Animals (www.avma. org/KB/Policies/Pages/Euthanasia-Guidelines.aspx) should be consulted for appropriate euthanasia methods. Since a conscious adult rodent may be highly stressed and difficult to restrain, it is useful to place a small rodent in an enclosed chamber and administer a fatal overdose of isoflurane gas, or administer an intracardiac injection of euthanasia solution after the animal reaches a deep plane of anesthesia (McRuer 2018).

Unless the rodent is a species protected by state and/or federal law, carcass disposal methods will be determined by the euthanasia method and possible risks (e.g., disease or toxins) that might cause problems to an animal ingesting the carcass or contribute to environmental contamination. Cremation and burial are two common disposal methods, but state and local laws may affect which method is used where (see Chapter 1 for additional information).

Release

Animals should be evaluated using multiple criteria including health, age, development, behavior, strength, independence, and acclimation to weather. The appropriate release location, including habitat, proximity to others of its own species, territoriality, and regulatory requirements (many states have strict release regulations), must also be considered. Finally, the season, time of day the rodent is most active, extent to which nesting materials are available, possibility of hibernation, and weather must also be considered (see Chapter 9).

Acknowledgement

Thank you to Shirley Casey for background research regarding rodent natural history, her contribution to content and references used in this chapter, and her many years of advancing the care of squirrels and other native wildlife.

References

Alderton, D. (1996). *Rodents of the World*. London, UK: Banford.

Anderson, W.I., Scott, D.W., Hornbuckle, W.E. et al. (1990). *Taenia crassiceps* infection in the woodchuck: a retrospective study of 13 cases. *Veterinary Dermatology* 1: 85–92.

Blodgett, D.J. (2001). Organophosphate and carbamate insecticides. In: *Small Animal Toxicology* (ed. M.E. Peterson and P.A. Talcott), 640–652. Philadelphia, PA: W.B. Saunders.

Bowen, L.E. (2007). Hairless red squirrel (*Tamiasciurus hudsonicus*) case study. *Wildlife Rehabilitation Bulletin* 25(2): 16–19.

Bröjer, C.M., Peregrine, A.S., Barker, I.K. et al. (2002). Cerebral cysticercosis in a woodchuck (*Marmota monax*). *Journal of Wildlife Diseases* 38 (3): 21–624.

Cartmill, M.A.T.T. (2010). Pads and claws in arboreal locomotion. In: *Primate Locomotion* (ed. F.A. Jenkins), 45–83. New York: Elsevier.

Casey, S. and Casey, A. (2003). *Squirrel Rehabilitation Handbook*, 3e. Evergreen, CO: WildAgain Wildlife Rehabilitation, Inc.

Casey, A. and Casey, S. (2012). Utilizing squirrel natural history in making rehabilitation decisions. In: *Wildlife Rehabilitation Resources: Squirrels* (ed. L. Davis), 1–11. St Cloud, MN: National Wildlife Rehabilitators Association.

Casey, S. and Goldthwait, M. (2012a). Etiologies and treatments of genital injuries of juvenile squirrels in rehabilitation. In: *Wildlife Rehabilitation Resources: Squirrels* (ed. L. Davis), 101–109. St Cloud, MN: National Wildlife Rehabilitators Association.

Casey, S. and Goldthwait, M. (2012b). Twelve common causes of stool problems in squirrels. In: *Wildlife Rehabilitation Resources: Squirrels* (ed. L. Davis), 111–119. St Cloud, MN: National Wildlife Rehabilitators Association.

Casey, S. and Goldthwait, M. (2013). When pets attack wildlife – part 2: what to do. *Wildlife Rehabilitation Bulletin* 31 (2): 18–25.

Davidson, W.R. and Nettles, V.F. (2006). *Field Manual of Wildlife Diseases in the Southeastern United States*, 3e. Athens, GA: Southeastern Wildlife Disease Cooperative Study.

Decubellis, J. and Shenoy, K. (2006). Bordetella in young rabbits and squirrels. *Wildlife Rehabilitation Bulletin* 24 (2): 33–34.

Diaz, S.L. (2005). Efficacy of fipronil in the treatment of pediculosis in laboratory rats. *Laboratory Animals* 39 (3): 331–335.

Gardlik, R., Palffy, R., and Celec, P. (2012). Recombinant probiotic therapy in experimental colitis in mice. *Folia Biologica (Praha)* 58 (6): 238–245.

Gardner, A.L., Schneider, R.M., & Wellehan, J.F.X. (2010). Astrovirus-associated disease in orphaned grey squirrels (Sciurus carolinensis). Proceedings of the AAZV AAWV Joint Conference, South Padre Island, TX (23–29 October 2010), pp. 32–33.

Girisgin, A.S., Acar, F., Cander, B. et al. (2006). Fluid replacement via the rectum for treatment of hypovolaemic shock in an animal model. *Emergency Medicine Journal* 23 (11): 862–864.

Grant, K. (2004) Nutrition of the North American Porcupine, *Erethizon dorsatum*. Association of Zoos and Aquariums Rodent Taxon Advisory Group, Silver Spring, MD.

Hamir, A.N. and Rupprecht, C.E. (2000). Hepatic capillariasis (*Capillaria hepatica*) in porcupines (*Erethizon dorsatum*) in Pennsylvania. *Journal of Veterinary Diagnostic Investigation.* 12: 463–465.

Hankins, D.G. and Rosekrans, J.A. (2004). Overview, prevention, and treatment of rabies. *Mayo Clinic Proceedings.* 79: 671–675.

Harkness, J.E., Turner, P.V., van de Woude, S., and Wheler, C.L. (2010). Specific diseases and conditions. In: *Harkness and Wagner's Biology and Medicine of Rabbits and Rodents*, 5e, 264. Ames, IA: Wiley-Blackwell.

Hilken, G., Büttner, D., and Militzer, K. (2003). Three important endoparasites of laboratory woodchucks (*Marmota monax*) caught in the wild: *Capillaria hepatica, Ackertia marmotae*, and *Taenia crassiceps*. *Scandinavian Journal of Laboratory Animal Science* 3 (30): 151–156.

Hillegass, M.A., Waterman, J.M., and Roth, J.D. (2010). Parasite removal increases reproductive success in a social African ground squirrel. *Behavioral Ecology* 21: 696–700.

Jacobs, R.F., Condrey, Y.M., and Yamauchi, T. (1985). Tularemia in adults and children: a changing presentation. *Pediatrics* 76 (5): 818–822.

Kilham, L. (1955). Metastasizing viral fibroma of gray squirrels: pathogenesis and mosquito transmission. *American Journal of Hygiene* 61: 55–63.

Krichbaum, K., Mahan, C.G., Steele, M.A. et al. (2010). The potential role of *Strongyloides robustus* on parasite-mediated competition between two species of flying squirrels (*Glaucomys*). *Journal of Wildlife Diseases* 46 (1): 229–235.

MacDonald, D. (1985). *The Encyclopedia of Mammals*. New York: Facts on File Publications.

Marchiondo, A.A., Duszynski, D.W., and Maupin, G.O. (1976). Prevalence of antibodies to *Toxoplasma gondii* in wild and domestic animals of New Mexico, Arizona and Colorado. *Journal of Wildlife Diseases* 12 (2): 226–232.

Marcum, D. (2002). Mammal nutrition: substitute milk formulas. In: *Principles of Wildlife Rehabilitation: The Essential Guide for Novice and Experienced Rehabilitators*, 2e (ed. A.T. Moore and S. Joosten), 295–353. St Cloud, MN: National Wildlife Rehabilitators Association.

Mayer, J. (2013). Fluid therapy in rabbits and rodents. In: *Clinical Veterinary Advisor: Birds and Exotic Pets* (ed. J. Mayer and T.M. Donnelly), 355–360. St Louis, MO: Elsevier Saunders.

McRuer, D. (2018). Euthanasia in wildlife rehabilitation. *Wildlife Rehabilitation Bulletin* 36 (1): 6–17.

Medway, W., Skand, D.L., and Sarver, C.F. (1989). Neurologic signs in American porcupines (*Erethizon dorsatum*) infected with *Baylisascaris* and *Toxoplasma*. *Journal of Zoo and Wild Animal Medicine.* 20 (2): 207–211.

Miller, E. (ed.) (2006). *Quick Reference*, 3e, 108. St Cloud, MN: National Wildlife Rehabilitators Association.

Murphy, J.J. and Talcott, P.A. (2001). Anticoagulant rodenticides. In: *Small Animal Toxicology* (ed. M.E. Peterson and P.A. Talcott), 406–419. Philadelphia, PA: W.B. Saunders.

Padgett, K.A., Reisen, W.K., Kahl-Purcell, N. et al. (2007). West Nile virus infection in tree squirrels (Rodentia: Sciuridae) in California, 2004–2005. *American Journal of Tropical Medicine and Hygeine.* 76 (5): 810–813.

Pokras, M. and Murray, M. (2004). Throw away your dex!! A polemic on why rehabilitators should NOT use dexamethasone. *Wildlife Rehabilitation Bulletin* 22 (1): 4–6.

Roug, A., Clancy, C.S., Detterich, C., and van Wettere, A.J. (2016). Cerebral larva migrans caused by *Baylisascaris* spp. in a freeranging north American porcupine (*Erethizon dorsatum*). *Journal of Wildlife Diseases* 52 (3): 763–765.

Salkin, I.F., Stone, W.B., and Gordon, M.A. (1980). Association of *Malassezia* (*Pityrosporum pachydermatis*) with sarcoptic mange in New York state. *Journal of Wildlife Diseases* 16 (4): 509–514.

Schwartz, C.W. and Schwartz, E.R. (1981). *The Wild Mammals of Missouri*. Columbia, MO: University of Missiouri Press and Missouri Department of Conservation.

Snyder, D.E., Hamir, A.N., Hanlon, C.A., and Rupprecht, C.E. (1991). Notoedric acariasis in the porcupine (*Erethizon dorsatum*). *Journal of Wildlife Diseases*. 27 (4): 723–726.

Sparks, B. and Casey, S. (1998). Reuniting young wild mammals with their mothers. *Journal of Wildlife Rehabilitation* 21 (3–4): 3–8.

Steele, M.A. and Koprowski, J. (2001). *North American Tree Squirrels*. Washington, DC: Smithsonian.

Vella, D. (2013). Rabbits, dental disease. In: *Clinical Veterinary Advisor: Birds and Exotic Pets*, (ed. J. Mayer and T.M. Donnelly), 355–360. St Louis, MO: Elsevier Saunders.

Weber, M.A., Miller, M.A., Neiffer, D.L., and Terrell, S.P. (2006). Presumptive fenbendazole toxicosis in north American porcupines. *Journal of the American Veterinary Medical Association* 228 (8): 1240–1242.

Wobeser, G.A. (1981). Tyzzer's disease. In: *Infectious Diseases of Wild Mammals* (ed. J.W. Davis, L.H. Karstad and D.O. Trainer), 347–351. Ames, IA: Iowa State University Press.

Wobeser, G.A. (ed.) (2006). Disease shared with humans and domestic animals. In: *Essentials of Disease in Wild Animals*. Ames, IA: Blackwell Publishing.

Yarto-Jaramillo, E. (2015). Rodentia. In: *Fowler's Zoo and Wild Animal Medicine*, vol. 8 (ed. R.E. Miller and M.E. Fowler), 384–422. St Louis, MO: Elsevier Saunders.

15

Natural History and Medical Management of Lagomorphs

Florina S. Tseng

Wildlife Clinic, Cummings School of Veterinary Medicine, Tufts University, North Grafton, MA, USA

Introduction

The lagomorphs include the hares/rabbits (family Leporidae) and the pikas (Ochotonidae) which occupy numerous habitats throughout North America. Only two of 30 pika (*Ochotona* spp.) species are found in North America. The Leporidae family (58 species in 11 genera) can be broadly divided into two groups: the cottontails and the jackrabbits/hares (Chapman and Litvaitis 2003). This chapter focuses on cottontails (*Sylvilagus* spp.) since they are more widely distributed than jackrabbits/hares and pikas and are more likely to be encountered and brought in for rehabilitation. Finally, there is much more information available about captive care and medical/surgical concerns in cottontails than for other North American lagomorphs.

Natural History

Species Identification, Habitat, and Conservation Status

The 17 species of cottontails are widely distributed throughout the New World. In general, they utilize disturbed, early successional, or shrub-dominated habitats with abundant forage and dense understory cover (Chapman and Litvaitis 2003). The Eastern cottontail (*Sylvilagus floridanus*) is the most widely distributed, with a broad range extending from southern Canada throughout the United States into Mexico (Chapman and Litvaitis 2003). Of the nine other closely related species, the New England cottontail (*Sylvilagus transitionalis*), restricted to small populations from Maine to Massachusetts and southern New York, is considered to be vulnerable in its conservation status. It is nearly impossible to morphologically distinguish this species from eastern cottontails. The eastern cottontail is generally lighter in color and may have a white spot on the forehead as opposed to the New England cottontail, which rarely has a white spot on the forehead and often has a black spot between the ears (Chapman and Litvaitis 2003).

Of the other North American species, the Appalachian cottontail (*Sylvilagus obscurus*) is listed as near threatened by the International Union for the Conservation of Nature (IUCN). The robust cottontail (*Sylvilagus robustus*) is listed as endangered by the IUCN (IUCN Red List of Threatened Species 2014). The pygmy rabbit (*Brachylagus idahoensis*) is listed by the Federal government as endangered. Five other *Sylvilagus* species living in Mexico or Central America are also considered threatened or endangered by the IUCN. Other North American *Sylvilagus* species reside in the desert southwest and high deserts extending into northern Montana (*Sylvilagus audubonii*), the intermountain regions of the western US (*Sylvilagus nuttallii*), the Pacific coast south of the Columbia River (*Sylvilagus bachmani*), and the southeastern US (*Sylvilagus aquaticus* and *palustris*).

Diet

Cottontails are herbivorous and consume a wide variety of plants. During the spring and summer, they will consume herbaceous plants such as grasses and wild carrot, then transition during the fall to woody plants such as apple, sumac and berry bushes. In the wintertime, cottontails mostly consume small trees, including birch, maple, and cherry or shrubs and vines (Chapman and Litvaitis 2003). Knowing the natural diet during a certain time of the year will help to determine an appropriate diet when the animal is in captivity.

Medical Management of Wildlife Species: A Guide for Practitioners, First Edition. Edited by Sonia M. Hernandez, Heather W. Barron, Erica A. Miller, Roberto F. Aguilar and Michael J. Yabsley.

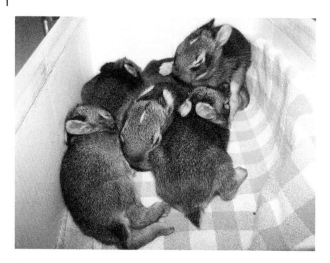

Figure 15.1 Young rabbits of approximately one week of age are furred and weigh between 25 and 35 g.

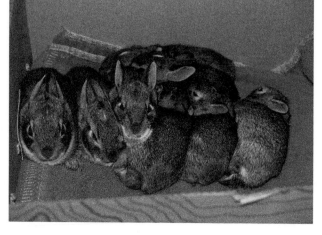

Figure 15.2 Young rabbits wean at around 15 days old and are able to leave the nest and self-feed.

Reproduction and Development

The breeding season for cottontails is generally early spring through early fall in most of the US. Like all lagomorphs, cottontails are induced ovulators and the mean gestation period is about 28 days. Mean litter size varies from three to five young and as many as 7–8 litters per year can be produced (Chapman and Litvaitis 2003). Nests are built on the ground and the females give birth to altricial young (kits). Neonates range from 15–25 g, have no fur and tightly closed eyes and ears. By days 4–7, fur is starting to develop, the young are about 3–4 in. in length, and weights are 25–35 g (Figure 15.1). By 7–10 days, the eyes and ears usually start to open, weights range from 35 to 40+ g, and the young are fully furred.

While the female is nursing young, she will feed a high-fat milk formula once or twice a day, at dawn and dusk. During the daytime, she stays away from the nest so that predators will not be attracted to the young. Young rabbits may start to eat vegetation as early as day 10 and are usually weaned by about day 15, at which time they are able to leave the nest and self-feed (Figure 15.2). Weights are generally 55–70 g by two weeks of age and will double by 3–4 weeks of age. Generally, the young disperse from the nest by 6–7 weeks after birth (Chapman and Litvaitis 2003).

Behavior

One of the most important considerations in working with cottontail rabbits is that they are prey species so their natural behavior has evolved in order to avoid predation. For instance, they prefer to forage in areas with cover, where they are less likely to be seen by predators, and have highly developed senses of sight, smell, and sound in order to detect nearby threats. When in danger, they are liable to either freeze in place or, if possible, flee from predators or other threats. These adaptations and behavior should always be considered when working with cottontails in the captive setting.

Clinically Relevant Anatomy and Physiology

Rabbit eyes are directed more laterally than most mammals and the rabbit cornea occupies approximately 30% of the globe, giving them a wide field of vision for predator detection. Rabbit pinnae are prominent and, in addition to enhancing their sense of hearing, serve as an area of heat exchange with large arteriovenous shunts (Donnelly 2004).

Rabbits have a relatively delicate skeletal structure, with the skeleton representing only 7–8% of body weight. In contrast, the skeletal muscle comprises >50% of body weight (Cruise and Brewer 1994). Rabbits have very powerful hind legs that can kick off strongly if the animal is trying to flee a dangerous situation. These attributes can easily lead to fractures as a result of trauma, including vertebral fractures if handling and restraint are done improperly.

Rabbit skin is extremely thin and easily torn with any trauma (Bensley 2009). This can result in severe degloving injuries that will require immediate treatment or euthanasia. If possible, it is best to avoid clipping wild rabbit fur as the skin is easily torn.

Because rabbits are obligate nasal breathers, mouth breathing is a poor prognostic sign, and any inflammation of the upper respiratory tract will increase the risk of anesthetic mortality in animals that are not intubated (Donnelly 2004). The thoracic cavity is relatively small, in marked contrast to the large abdominal cavity. Because rabbits are diaphragmatic breathers, thoracic wall excursions may not be that noticeable as an indication of respiratory rate.

Rabbit teeth grow continuously with hypsodont dentition, meaning that they have open-rooted teeth. The dental formula is 2(I 2/1, C 0/0, P 3/2, M 3/3). Malocclusion can occasionally be seen in wild rabbits, usually as a result of trauma to the opposing teeth. The oral cavity is small, narrow, and deep, thus making endotracheal intubation a challenge.

The gastrointestinal tract is relatively long and can make up 10–20% of total body weight, with the stomach and cecum holding most of the ingesta. Muscular contractions in the colon lead to separation of fiber from nonfiber components of colonic contents. Fibrous material is excreted in the hard feces while nonfibrous material is moved in a retrograde direction into the cecum, where fermentation of these contents takes place. Following fermentation, the cecum contracts and the fermented material is expelled through the colon to the anus, where the rabbit directly consumes it in a process called coprophagy. The consumed cecal contents are called cecotropes and appear as a cluster of soft pellets surrounded by a mucous membrane that acts as protection against the acid stomach pH (Donnelly 2004).

Serum calcium in rabbits is not maintained in a narrow range, as in most mammals, but reflects the level of dietary calcium. Excess calcium is excreted in the urine (up to 45–60% of urine content). This high calcium content can lead to thick, creamy white urine. This is more often seen in pet rabbits with high levels of dietary calcium than in their wild counterparts. Urine color can also vary from yellow to red, depending on pigments associated with various diets, and can be falsely diagnosed as hematuria (Donnelly 2004).

Captive Husbandry Guidelines

Captive wild rabbits experience tremendous stress. Captivity-related stress could result in immune suppression, thus exacerbating any infectious disease problems, decreasing gastrointestinal motility, reducing renal blood flow and increasing gastric acidity (Harcourt-Brown 2002). The most important consideration in caring for captive lagomorphs is to decrease this stress by proper diet and caging while minimizing handling and any clinical procedures. Young rabbits will benefit from being raised with conspecifics as their presence will help considerably to decrease stress.

Housing Guidelines

It is vitally important that rabbits of any age be protected from visual and auditory stress. Thus, rabbit caging should always be set up in a quiet area, as far away from people and domestic animals as possible. Cage fronts should be covered with a visual barrier and a hide box should be provided, facing away from the cage front (Figure 15.3). This hide box will enable the rabbit to feel that it is in a more protected environment while in care.

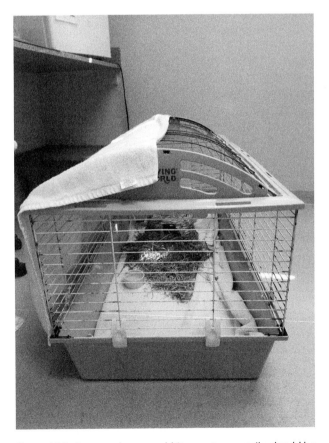

Figure 15.3 A cage to house a rabbit, even temporarily, should be partially covered with a visual barrier, contain a hide box and have plenty of forage.

Cages should always be constructed such that they are escape-proof.

Neonatal rabbits less than two weeks of age will always require supplemental heat. An incubator set at 26–29 °C (80–85 °F) is ideal; however, a heating pad set on low, covered by a towel, and placed under half of the cage can also be used. Minimum standards for infant rabbit housing are the size of a 10 gal aquarium or a 12″ × 12″ × 12″ tote (Miller 2012). Line the bottom of the cage with soft towels or fleece, making sure that there are no loose strings or holes which could wrap around or trap the young rabbits. Using light-colored bedding will make it easier to detect any abnormalities in urine and fecal appearance. Neonatal rabbits under two weeks of age should also be placed in a "nest" within the larger cage. If the original nest is available, this can be used as a means to keep the babies in a familiar environment, thus decreasing stress. An alternate nest can be made from a smaller box lined with soft material, such as fleece, that enables these very young rabbits to snuggle together.

Juvenile rabbits greater than two weeks of age no longer need a nest structure but should still have a hide box. At this stage, supplemental heat can be lowered to 21–24 °C (70–75 °F), though this will depend on the status of individual rabbits. Depending on their level of activity, these rabbits will often need a larger indoor enclosure than that recommended for the infant stage. If they are old enough to be moved outside, the minimum standard for outdoor caging of juvenile rabbits is a 6′ × 6′ × 4′ pen (Miller 2012). Any lagomorph caging should not be made of wood, as rabbits can easily chew through this material. In addition, do not use chain link, wire mesh or hardware cloth as rabbits cannot easily visualize these barriers. Shade cloth or mesh screening can be used on the exterior of the cage to form a visual barrier that should be at least 12–24″ high. Cover the bottom of the enclosure with hay to prevent pododermatitis and make sure that there are no protruding objects along the interior cage wall. A free-standing shelter, such as a crate, placed facing away from the entrance, will serve as a hide area. Natural shrubs, hollow logs, and branches with edible bark should also be provided (Miller 2012). Avoid using bark from trees, such as wild black cherry or black locust, that contain toxic compounds.

Adult rabbits can easily injure themselves when panicking if they are housed incorrectly. In addition to the general recommendations for housing them indoors in a quiet area and decreasing their visual stress by keeping the cage front covered, it is helpful to house them in a cage that allows cleaning without having to handle the rabbit, if at all possible. For example, a cage with wire

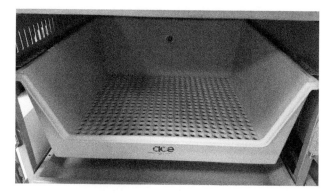

Figure 15.4 Cages to house rabbits should allow for feces and urine to drop through to a pull-out tray for ease of cleaning.

mesh floors that allow feces and urine to drop through to a pull-out tray can be used for easy cleaning (Figure 15.4). High-quality hay can be used for nutritional purposes as well as to help cushion the feet to avoid pododermatitis. This hay should be replaced on a daily basis to avoid accumulation of feces and urine. A hide box that can be easily closed is also a good idea as most rabbits feel safer inside this box. Once closed, the box enables the handler to move the rabbit from the cage to another location without hands-on contact. Minimum standards for housing adult rabbits indoors are 12″ × 18″ × 12″. Minimum standards for outdoor adult housing is a 6′ × 6′ × 6′ pen, following the same guidelines for cage construction as for juvenile rabbits (Miller 2012).

Dietary Guidelines

Nutritional needs and feeding protocols for neonatal and juvenile cottontail rabbits will be discussed in the orphaned young section of this chapter.

Adult rabbits are generally not that difficult to feed during captivity in the spring and summer months. They should be offered a variety of grasses and other greens, such as clover, wild carrot or dandelion greens, freshly picked from a pesticide-free area. In addition, they can be given legumes, succulent annuals, and small amounts of garden vegetables. During the fall and winter months, rabbits transition to a diet of small twigs, bark, and buds of shrubs and trees. In captivity, these items can also be obtained from foraging in the wild but fresh vegetables, such as dark, leafy greens, carrots, and winter peas, may also be given. Avoid feeding large quantities of starchy root vegetables, such as carrots, or items with large amounts of sugar, such as fruit. Commercial timothy-based pellets may be offered but are not always consumed by wild cottontails. Critical care diets (Critical Care for Herbivores, Oxbow Pet Products, Murdock, NE, USA) may occasionally be consumed in captivity and the palatability of any of these diets can be enhanced by mixing in small amounts of plain apple sauce. Fresh timothy hay and access to fresh water are recommended at all times (Brooks 2004).

Handling, Restraint, and Clinical Techniques

Handling and restraint of young rabbits is generally not as difficult as working with their adult counterparts. Young rabbits should be gently held in a cupped hand for examination or other procedures, taking care not to let the rabbit jump out and injure itself. Keeping the eyes covered and minimizing contact time are essential (Figure 15.5). Adult cottontails can be challenging because of their extreme stress and drive to escape the handler. In order to handle adult cottontails, a towel can be used to quickly wrap around the entire body and head, using one hand to encircle the rabbit to the handler's body and the other to firmly support the rear quarters and prevent hindquarter hyperextension. When carrying the rabbit, lift the thorax first and then the hindquarters. The rabbit can then be placed on a surface covered with a nonslip material for examination or other procedure, taking care to lower the rabbit's hindquarters first. The patient can also be quickly transported, if necessary, by staying wrapped in the towel and tucking the head under the handler's arm while the other arm supports the back and feet.

If any procedure needs to be accomplished that will take more than a few minutes, it is recommended that the rabbit be sedated or anesthetized (see Chapter 5).

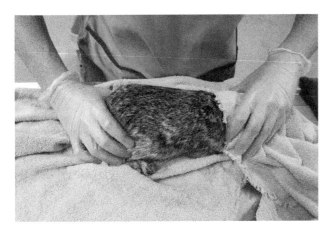

Figure 15.5 Keeping the eyes covered is essential when working with rabbits.

Venipuncture sites include the lateral saphenous, cephalic, and jugular veins. Wild rabbits should be sedated or anesthetized for blood collection. Subcutaneous injections are relatively easy given the large space over the dorsum in rabbits. Intramuscular injections can be given in the quadriceps or epaxial muscles, while intravenous injections can be given in the cephalic or lateral saphenous veins. Ear veins in wild cottontails are not as well developed as in domestic rabbits and should not be used for venipuncture or intravenous injections.

Oral medications or commercial tube feeding formulations can be administered through the diastema, the space on the side of the mouth between the incisors and the premolars. Alternatively, oral medications can be mixed into a small amount of apple sauce, which is palatable enough for most rabbits to eat on their own.

Daily fluid requirements are 100–150 mL/kg and should be divided into 2–3 different treatments (Donnelly 2004). Fluid amounts may need to be increased for dehydrated rabbits or those with ongoing fluid losses, such as with diarrhea. Fluids are most easily administered via subcutaneous injection since most wild rabbits do not readily tolerate intravenous (IV) or intraosseous (IO) catheters. However, in critical cases, IV catheters can be placed in the cephalic or saphenous veins and IO catheters can be placed in the greater trochanter of the femur or the tibial crest (Mader 2004).

Nasoesophageal or pharyngostomy tubes can be placed to assist with enteral feeding in the anorexic rabbit. The technique is similar to that done with cats (Chan 2009). However, these are better tolerated in domestic rabbits than in their wild counterparts.

Unfortunately, euthanasia is a relatively common procedure when presented with wild cottontails. Young rabbits may suffer from severe traumatic injuries or show critical signs associated with dehydration and gastrointestinal disease. Adult rabbits can be admitted with traumatic injuries leading to a poor prognosis, thus warranting euthanasia. Euthanasia of wild rabbits should only be done with the animal sedated or anesthetized. Sodium pentobarbital is administered through intravenous or intracardiac injection, the latter being an easier technique for most practitioners. Euthanasia options are discussed in the AVMA Guidelines for the Euthanasia of Animals (www.avma.org/KB/Policies/Documents/euthanasia.pdf).

Infectious and Parasitic Diseases of Concern

Rabies has not been documented in wild rabbits, but any mammal showing neurological signs with evidence of bite wounds should be considered a rabies suspect and appropriate personal protective equipment (PPE) should be used. A survey of rodents and lagomorphs submitted for rabies testing in the US between 1995 and 2010 found confirmed rabies only in pet rabbits (*Oryctolagus* spp.) (Fitzpatrick et al. 2014).

Myxomatosis is caused by the myxoma virus (family Leporipoxvirus). It was first described in laboratory rabbits in Uruguay in 1896 and has spread to North, Central and South America. In the US, it is found in the brush rabbit (*S. bachmani*), in California and Oregon. In this species, the virus causes a cutaneous fibroma, usually on lips or feet or at the base of the ears, but does not develop into a systemic disease as happens in the European rabbit (*Oryctolagus cuniculus*). The eastern cottontail has been experimentally infected but levels of virus in the ensuing lesions are too low for mosquito transmission (Robinson and Kerr 2001). Blood-feeding arthropods are the most common means of virus transmission although the virus can also be spread via close contact with shed discharges or contaminated fomites.

In affected *O. cuniculus*, there is swelling of the eyelids, ears and head and mucopurulent nasal discharge. Nodules can be found on the head and may sometimes be seen over the remainder of the body. The anogenital region is often severely swollen.

Treatment is supportive and often unsuccessful. Control in wild European rabbits is undertaken in some areas of the world with large-scale vaccination programs. However, myxomatosis is regarded as an important means of rabbit control in Australia.

Cottontail rabbit papillomavirus (or Shope papillomavirus) is an oncogenic, DNA virus of the Papovaviridae family. It is transmitted via biting arthropods and primarily affects wild cottontail rabbits, hares, and jackrabbits. Viral infection causes dark red, wart-like, highly keratinized lesions around the head, neck, and shoulders.

In domestic rabbits, it can cause lesions around the hairless areas of the ears and eyelids. Lesions may disappear after several months in immunocompetent individuals or may progress to squamous cell carcinoma, most often in domestic rabbits. Treatment involves surgical removal of larger lesions though most will regress on their own over time. Control of arthropod vectors is important in facilities housing domestic rabbits (Hess 2004).

The rabbit (Shope) fibroma virus is a member of the Leporipoxvirus family. The natural host is the eastern cottontail; natural infections have not been reported in other *Sylvilagus* species. *Oryctolagus* spp. may occasionally be infected. This virus is generally transmitted by biting arthropods and affects young rabbits more severely than adults. Shope fibroma virus causes large wart-like tumors of the face, feet, and legs. High viral concentrations can be found in these tumors for many months after inoculation (Robinson and Kerr 2001). The overlying epidermis may slough and secondary bacterial infections may occur. The lesions may regress over several months. In young rabbits, a systemic disease may develop and lead to death.

Rabbit hemorrhagic disease virus (RHDV) is a calicivirus endemic in Australia, New Zealand, Cuba, parts of Asia and Africa, and most of Europe. The virus usually causes an acute disease characterized by inappetance, depression, and fever followed by death within 24 hours. The first reported occurrence in the United States was in a backyard rabbitry in Iowa in 2000. Other outbreaks in domestic rabbits in the US have occurred since this time, most recently in Minnesota in 2010 (USDA-APHIS 2013). Both wild and domesticated European rabbits are susceptible to RHDV but other wild North American rabbits and hares, including cottontail species, have not been affected to date and are thought not to be susceptible. However, any suspected RHDV cases should be immediately reported to USDA.

Tularemia ("rabbit fever") is primarily a disease of lagomorphs and rodents caused by the bacterium *Francisella tularensis*. The distribution of this disease is throughout the northern hemisphere. The bacteria can be inoculated by blood-feeding arthropod vectors, passed by contact with blood and tissues of infected animals, by inhalation of infected aerosol particles and by ingestion of contaminated water or meat.

Francisella tularensis (Type A) is the primary pathogen of cottontail rabbits in North America. Infection in high-density rabbit populations can quickly lead to steep declines in numbers. An experimental infection with *F. tularensis* in wild cottontail rabbits showed that each of the Type A strains used in the study was highly virulent, causing microabscesses in the liver and spleens of most affected rabbits (Brown et al. 2015). Type A tularemia is responsible for about 70% of the US human cases, with a mortality rate of about 5–7% in untreated people (Morner and Addison 2001). Most people are exposed during the summer months from tick bites or during the fall and winter rabbit-hunting season. A geographic focus of the pneumonic form of tularemia is present on Martha's Vineyard, Massachusetts.

Clinical signs in affected animals are rarely observed due to the acute nature of disease progression. Signs include severe weakness followed by fatal septicemia. Postmortem diagnosis is based on demonstrating the causative agent in tissues such as liver, spleen, kidney or lung.

Treatment of wild rabbits with tularemia is not attempted because it is acutely fatal. Anyone working with cottontail rabbits in endemic areas should always wear proper PPE, such as gloves and masks, in order to reduce possibility of transmission.

Leptospirosis is caused by the bacterium *Leptospira* spp. and is more often found in wild rodents than other small mammals. However, it should still be considered as a possible zoonotic disease when handling wild lagomorphs and cleaning cages. Antemortem diagnosis may be made with antibody testing and culture of blood or urine, though false negatives are not uncommon. Appropriate antibiotic therapy may not completely eliminate infection and treated animals may continue to shed bacteria in the urine. Additional details are given in Chapter 2.

Staphylococcus spp. are common bacteria of lagomorphs, usually causing local abscesses but occasionally leading to severe and fatal disease (Wobeser 2001). Most disease is attributed to *Staph. aureus*, a gram-positive coccus that inhabits the skin and mucous membranes of warm-blooded vertebrates. The organisms are opportunistic pathogens that become established in underlying tissues with a break in the skin or mucous membranes.

Infected areas of skin show pustules, exudate, and inflammation. Superficial lymph nodes may be swollen and abscessed. Less commonly, visceral organ infection can be seen with abscess formation in spleen, liver, kidneys, and other organs. Treatment of skin infections involves thorough cleaning of infected areas, appropriate wound care and antibiotic therapy based on culture and sensitivity.

Colibacillosis, a severe intestinal disease, can develop in neonatal rabbits if they have *Escherichia coli* overgrowth secondary to malnutrition, stress, or concurrent endoparasitism. Morbidity and mortality are high (Vennen and Mitchell 2009). Clinical signs include profuse watery diarrhea, weight loss, and bloat. Treatment centers around fluid therapy, antibiotics based on culture and sensitivity, proper nutrition, and other supportive care measures.

Coccidial infections can be a problem in young or immunocompromised cottontail rabbits. *Eimeria* spp. can infect both the intestinal tract and the liver. Transmission of this parasite is via the fecal–oral route and is enhanced by poor sanitary conditions in captivity. Clinical signs include inappetence and subsequent weight loss, dehydration, and diarrhea. Hepatic infection can lead to ascites, hepatomegaly, icterus, and encephalopathy (Vennen and Mitchell 2009). Diagnosis is via fecal flotation, direct smear, polymerase chain reaction (PCR) or with histopathology of affected organs. Treatment with sulfa drugs (sulfadimethoxine 50 mg/kg PO once, then 25 mg/kg q24h × 10–20 days) (Carpenter 2013) may need to be given over an extended period of time in order to clear infection. Fluid therapy and nutritional support are also indicated.

Baylisascaris procyonis, the raccoon roundworm, has been associated with fatal neurological disease in rabbits (Jacobson et al. 1976). Clinical signs include torticollis, ataxia, and circling without obvious external signs of trauma. Transmission is by ingestion of larvated eggs passed in the feces of infected raccoon. Most clinical signs are a result of neural larval migrans (Kazacos et al. 1983). Antemortem diagnosis is difficult, and most infections are diagnosed postmortem by histological examination of tissues. While treatment with anthelmintics, such as albendazole, may help to ameliorate some of the clinical signs, prognosis is poor for release back to the wild. Additional details are provided in Chapters 2 and 21.

Cuterebra infestation is often seen in cottontail rabbits, especially during the summer and fall months. It is easily diagnosed by observation of a subcutaneous swelling with an associated breathing hole (Figure 15.6). Many affected rabbits show multiple nodules and parasitism is especially heavy in younger rabbits (Jacobson et al. 1978). Adult flies lay their eggs near rabbit burrows and the larvae enter the host via the mouth, nares or small skin wounds. Larval development is most commonly found around the genital region or around the head and neck. Oftentimes, the fur is matted around the swelling because the rabbit has been overgrooming in response to the presence of this parasite. Treatment requires gentle removal of the larvae. The entire larval cyst should be removed to prevent anaphylactic reaction or secondary infection.

Fly strike, or myiasis, is sometimes observed in wild lagomorphs, especially if the animal is debilitated or has wounds that provide an environment for egg and larval development. This condition is usually seen during the warmer summer and fall months. Initial signs of fly strike are the appearance of off-white to yellow eggs surrounding the wound. The eggs will then develop into larvae,

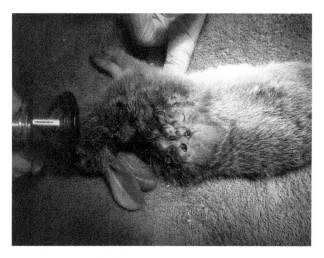

Figure 15.6 *Cuterebra* infestations are common in rabbits. It can be easily diagnosed by observing if subcutaneous swellings move and looking for a small opening (the breathing hole for the larvae).

called maggots, which can burrow into the wound and adjacent tissue. Treatment involves aggressive wound debridement under anesthesia, manual removal of maggots and flushing with nitenpyram (Capstar®, Novartis, Greensboro, NC) solubilized in saline (11 mg tablet in 250 mL saline). Multiple sessions of wound debridement and flushing are often necessary to resolve the myiasis. Antibiotic and analgesic therapy are also recommended.

Sarcoptic mange, caused by *Sarcoptes scabiei*, is infrequently seen in cottontail rabbits. The mite may be passed directly from an infected individual or via contamination of rabbit burrows. Once the mite burrows into the skin and lays its eggs, the rabbit experiences an intensely pruritic dermatitis, resulting in crusty, inflamed skin particularly in areas around the head and external genitalia (Vennen and Mitchell 2009). Diagnosis is by deep skin scrape of the lesion and treatment involves the use of topical ivermectin (0.2–0.4 mg/k SQ q10–14 days), appropriate wound care, possible antibiotics for secondary bacterial infection and analgesics, such as meloxicam (0.3 mg/kg PO SID or 0.2 mg/kg IM or SQ SID) (Carpenter 2013).

Common Reasons for Presentation

Orphaned Young

Young cottontail rabbits are often abducted from their ground nests by well-meaning members of the public who falsely assume that the mother has abandoned them. If they are plump, hydrated, and not injured, they should be immediately returned to the nest. The mothers will readily return to them if humans are not nearby. When returning young cottontails to the nest, arrange the bedding in a recognizable pattern that, if disturbed, will indicate that the mother has tended to her young. In addition, cats should be confined indoors and dogs should be leash walked until the young rabbits are old enough to disperse from the nest. Once juvenile rabbits are old enough to try to evade capture, they do not need to be brought in for care.

If neonatal or juvenile rabbits are orphaned (i.e., mother has been found dead) or if there is obvious illness or injury, then they should be brought to an experienced wildlife rehabilitator or veterinarian. The veterinary staff should work closely with licensed and experienced wildlife rehabilitators to provide optimal care.

Physical examination of the neonatal or juvenile rabbit should be done in order to assess hydration status, body temperature and whether any injuries are present. Always wear examination gloves, as the possibility of bite wounds from a rabid animal should not be forgotten. Try to minimize the time required for this examination because these animals are so easily stressed. Puncture wounds and other injuries may be difficult to visualize underneath the dense hair coat. Criteria for euthanasia include animals with severe injuries such as head trauma, open extremity fractures, amputations, penetrating bite wounds, and degloving wounds that extend over a large area of the body surface. In addition, neonates with severe gastrointestinal bloat from malnutrition or those that are moribund on presentation have a poor prognosis for survival.

Most young cottontails presented for care are initially hypothermic, hypoglycemic, and dehydrated. These issues must be addressed prior to any feeding. Warmed subcutaneous fluids, such as lactated Ringer's solution or normal saline, should be given at a rate of 80–100 mL/kg/day, divided into 2–3 treatments. If the animal is very thin and likely hypoglycemic, 2.5% dextrose in lactated Ringer's solution can be given subcutaneously. Normal body temperature is 37.8–39.4 °C (100–103 °F). Hypothermia should be addressed by placing these animals into an incubator or on a heating pad as previously discussed.

Neonatal rabbits have very few microorganisms in the stomach and small intestine. In healthy neonates, a unique fatty acid in the stomach reacts with the doe's milk to inhibit bacterial infection up until three weeks of age. Young rabbits acquire gastrointestinal microorganisms by consumption of the doe's cecotrophs beginning at two weeks of age (Johnson-Delaney 2006). Because very young rabbits lack the adult's ability to digest and absorb carbohydrates, inappropriate feeding may lead to overgrowth of pathogenic *E. coli* and *Clostridia* spp.

Once the young animal is warmed and hydrated, it can be started on oral feeding. It is best to start oral feeding with a balanced electrolyte solution and gradually transition to feeding full-strength formula over a 24–48-hour period. Since wild rabbits only suckle their young 1–2 times in a 24-hour period, their milk has a high nutritional value with low lactose content. The composition of the milk changes toward the end of lactation as fat and protein levels increase (Bewig and Mitchell 2009).

There is much debate within the rehabilitation community about the best formula to feed orphaned baby cottontail rabbits. Fox Valley (Fox Valley Animal Nutrition Inc., Lake Zurich, IL, USA) Day One 32/40 (powder), Zoologic Milk Matrix (PetAg, Hampshire, IL, USA) 33/40 (powder), and Zoologic Milk Matrix 42/25 or KMR (PetAg) have all been used successfully with rabbits. To increase fat content, Multi-Milk (PetAg) may be added to formulas once the rabbits have become stable. A sample recipe is 1 part Esbilac powder to 1 part MultiMilk powder to 1.5 parts water (2.01 kcal/mL). Zoologic Milk Matrix 33/40 mixed 1 part powder with 1 part water yields a formula that is 1.6 kcal/mL. Fox Valley

Day One 32/40 is considered a medium-protein and high-fat content milk that is mixed 1 part powder with 2 parts water (1.25 kcal/mL). Studies have demonstrated that these formulas with high fat content will mix more readily and not show separation if they are mixed with hot water (175 °F, 80 °C) and then allowed to sit for at least four hours prior to feeding (Casey and Casey 2012). Any reconstituted formula should not be kept for longer than 24 hours and only the amount used at each feeding should be warmed up.

The amount and frequency of feeding are determined by the size of the young rabbit. Calculate the caloric needs of the animal by using the following formula: $2 \times (70 \times BW[kg]^{0.75})$, then divide this number by the caloric content of the formula being fed. This should yield the total volume that needs to be fed in a 24-hour period. As a rough estimate, the neonatal rabbit stomach can hold up to 100–125 mL/kg of body weight at each feeding. Calculate the amount of formula that can be fed at one feeding then divide this number into the total 24 hours volume that needs to be fed. This will determine the number of times/day the baby should be fed. For example, for a cottontail rabbit that weighs 50 g:

$$2 \times \left(70 \times 0.05^{.75}\right) = 14.8 \, kcal / 24 \, hours$$

If feeding Zoologic Milk Matrix 33/40 (1.6 kcal/mL), then: 14.8 kcal/24 hours divided by 1.6 kcal/mL = 9.25 mL/24 hours.

If we assume that the rabbit's stomach can hold 100 mL/kg of body weight, then the 50 g baby's stomach can hold 5 mL in one feeding. In this case, we can feed the rabbit 5 mL of full-strength formula every 12 hours. Keep in mind, however, that you may not be able to feed the maximum stomach capacity at each feeding. If the rabbit is even younger, the formula might be raised to: $3 \times (70 \times 0.05^{.75}) = 22.2 \, kcal$ needed in a 24-hour period.

Syringe feeding with a 1 cc non-Luer-Lok syringe placed in the corner of the rabbit's mouth is one method that can be effective if the baby has a good suckling response. However, many young rabbits, especially when first fed, have a poor suckling response and so tube feeding is recommended. A red rubber catheter (3.5–5 Fr) is attached to the syringe. Starting with the tip of the catheter at the last rib, measure the distance from the last rib to the tip of the nose and mark this distance on the catheter. This is how far the tube should be passed in order to reach the stomach of the rabbit. Prime the feeding tube and lubricate the tip with a sterile lubricant, then gently pass it into the back of the oral cavity and advance it as the rabbit swallows. Administer the formula slowly and stop if the rabbit starts to regurgitate milk into the oropharyngeal area. Neonatal and juvenile rabbits should be weighed daily and caloric needs recalculated every 2–3 days.

Infant cottontails require stimulation of the anogenital region in order to urinate and defecate. Gently stroke a moist cotton tip applicator or small gauze sponge in this area prior to feeding the babies. Depending on the degree of dehydration, feces may not be produced for as long as 24–48 hours after the initial feeding. However, urine should be produced before the second feeding (Taylor 2002).

Young rabbits will generally start weaning by about two weeks of age. Even before this time, once the eyes are open, juvenile rabbits should have formula provided to them in a shallow dish, which they will start lapping on their own. Once they are starting to self-feed, provide them with greens and other food items, as previously discussed. Fresh water should also be provided in a shallow dish once the eyes are open. By two weeks of age, formula may only need to be fed once/day or even stopped if the rabbit is readily self-feeding. If healthy, older rabbits are available, cecotrophs should be collected and offered to weanling young 2–3 times per week. Most juvenile cottontail rabbits are ready to be released by about 4–5 weeks of age, once they reach ~120 g.

Bacterial Dysbiosis

Wild rabbits, similar to their domestic counterparts, have a balanced gastrointestinal ecosystem of aerobic and anaerobic bacteria. This delicate microbiome is extremely sensitive to the misuse of orally administered antibiotics, including clindamycin, lincomycin, ampicillin, amoxicillin, amoxicillin-clavulanic acid, cephalosporins, penicillin derivatives, and erythromycin (Jenkins 2004). The use of these antibiotics can lead to alterations in the normal intestinal microflora, resulting in pH changes, an increase in volatile fatty acids, and proliferation of *Clostridium spiriforme* (Vennen and Mitchell 2009). Endotoxins produced by *C. spiriforme* lead to peracute death of the animal. Probiotics are sometimes used to decrease the risk of dysbiosis, though their value has not been proven. Cecotrophs from healthy adult rabbits free of known parasites/pathogens can be mixed into solution and force fed to the rabbit with dysbiosis in order to encourage colonization of normal gut flora. Treatment for dysbiosis is supportive and includes fluid therapy, proper nutrition and, of course, discontinuing the use of the inappropriate antibiotic. Antibiotics which are safe to use in lagomorphs include trimethoprim-sulfa, fluoroquinolones, and parenterally administered penicillin G. Another factor contributing to gastrointestinal abnormalities is captive stress. Stress in wild rabbits held in captivity can lead to an epinephrine-induced inhibition of gut motility, leading to enteritis (Jenkins 2004).

Predator Injuries

Lagomorphs are prey species for many different kinds of predators. Carnivores, such as fox, bobcat, coyote, and many raptors, ingest rabbits as a regular part of their diet. Domestic dogs and cats, despite being well fed, will also predate on rabbits if they are allowed to roam freely. If the wild rabbit is not killed, it may sustain serious injuries from these attacks. Superficial and deep puncture wounds, lacerations, and degloving injuries as a result of predator attacks are commonly encountered in rehabilitation of these species. Spinal injuries and fractures are also a frequent occurrence. In general, the prognosis with extensive soft tissue wounds, spinal injuries, and extremity fractures in rabbits is poor. Because rabbit skin is so thin, it can tear easily with any kind of trauma and, oftentimes, what looks like a small wound will reveal itself to be more extensive when explored thoroughly. In this author's experience, degloving injuries that involve more than 10% of the rabbit's skin surface do not usually result in a favorable outcome.

If the degloving injury is not very extensive, it should be treated as quickly as possible once the animal is stabilized enough for anesthesia. The wound should be thoroughly flushed with a dilute disinfectant solution, such as 0.2% chlorhexidine, followed by a saline flush until all visible contamination is eliminated. If the underlying tissue is healthy, any viable skin edges can be brought together with tissue adhesives. Attempting to close the very thin skin edges with sutures often results in the suture material tearing through the skin. If skin edges cannot be directly apposed, keep the wound bed clean, cover with an appropriate wound dressing and allow it to heal by secondary intention. Silver sulfadiazine cream is useful for its antibacterial action though this product may interfere with wound healing. Antibiotics and analgesics should also be administered.

Other Traumatic Injuries

Rabbits may also be admitted with traumatic injuries from other causes, such as being hit by vehicles or encounters with lawnmowers or weed whackers. Treatment of soft tissue trauma is similar to that described above, including the use of appropriate antibiotics and analgesics. Wound care should be performed under sedation and/or anesthesia and may require multiple procedures before a healthy wound bed is established. Limiting activity by housing in quiet, confined areas and minimizing handling will aid in more rapid wound healing. Drains are rarely used in infected wounds due to the viscous nature of pus formation in rabbits and because these animals will often chew them out. Chronic abscess formation is common in rabbits and these are often refractory to treatment

(Harcourt-Brown 2002). Wound dressings should be kept as small as possible in order to reduce discomfort.

Refrigerated hydrogels have been shown to have analgesic effects in humans and may be effective in rabbit wounds to prevent dessication and hydrate necrotic tissue, which facilitates debridement (Brown and Pizzi 2012). Hydrogels should be covered by a semipermeable dressing in order maintain a moist wound environment. Medical-grade honey has been used in the initial stages of wound healing in order to promote a moist wound bed and decrease bacterial growth and for its antiinflammatory effect. Honey has been effective in the treatment of chronic abscesses in rabbits (Harcourt-Brown 2002). A product called Collasate® (PRN Pharmaceuticals, Pensacola, FL, USA) is useful in areas in which it is difficult to place a dressing. This is a collagen gel that serves as a biomatrix for cell regrowth, decreases wound infection, and forms a tissue adhesive covering over the wound.

Spinal and extremity fractures in wild rabbits can be a result of a traumatic episode or improper handling and restraint in captivity. Diagnosis of spinal trauma can be made by clinical presentation of hindquarter paresis or paralysis and confirmation with radiographic evidence of vertebral luxation or fracture. Treatment in wild rabbits should not be attempted and euthanasia is recommended. Surgical repair of long bone fractures in wild rabbits is possible though postoperative care is difficult. Wild lagomorphs, particularly adults, are prone to further traumatizing themselves in captivity when panicking during handling procedures. Nondisplaced scapular and hip fractures can heal well given enough time to cage rest.

Neurological Abnormalities

Wild rabbits can sometimes be seen with clinical signs such as head tilt, ataxia, and circling. While many of these cases may be as a result of head trauma, other reasons include *Baylisascaris* larval migration, middle or inner ear infection with pathogens such as *Pasteurella*, and neoplasia. *Encephalitozoon cuniculi* is a consideration for these neurological signs in pet rabbits (*Oryctolagus* spp.) but only one report of this parasite in cottontail rabbits has been published and it was in eastern cottontail rabbits that had been introduced to northwestern Italy for hunting purposes (Zanet et al. 2013). In general, the prognosis for a wild rabbit with neurological signs is poor though it may be possible to treat otitis infections with appropriate antibiotic therapy.

Release Considerations

Pre-release conditioning of rabbits that have resolved any medical and/or surgical problems is best done in conjunction with rehabilitators experienced in working with these species (see Chapter 9). Prior to release, all animals should be acclimatized to ambient outdoor temperatures and have a full covering of fur in order to withstand weather conditions at the time of release. Wild rabbits must show behavioral fitness prior to release back into the wild. In particular, juvenile rabbits should be appropriately wary of predators, be able to recognize and forage effectively for natural food items, and interact normally with conspecifics.

Release site selection is also critical to postrelease success. Adult animals should be released at a safe site as close as possible to where they were found. Juvenile animals may be "soft" released, that is, releasing them from the location where they were raised directly into adjacent suitable habitat. Food, shelter, and water are still provided in the captive caging set-up post release so that the animal can return as necessary. As the young animal learns survival skills in the wild, it will gradually decrease its visits to the captive cage.

Rabbits are best released earlier in the day or at dusk in favorable weather conditions and into edge habitat with available natural forage, such as open grassland, and dense understory cover. Postrelease monitoring is rarely done with wild rabbits as most techniques significantly increase stress and decrease survival rates in this group of animals.

References

Bensley, B.A. (2009). *Practical Anatomy of the Rabbit: An Elementary Laboratory Textbook in Mammalian Anatomy*. Charleston, SC: BiblioBazaar.

Bewig, M. and Mitchell, M.A. (2009). Wildlife. In: *Manual of Exotic Pet Practice* (ed. M.A. Mitchell and T.M. Tully), 493–529. St Louis, MO: Elsevier Saunders.

Brooks, D.L. (2004). Nutrition and gastrointestinal physiology. In: *Ferrets, Rabbits and Rodents*, 2e (ed. K.E. Quesenberry and J.W. Carpenter), 155–160. St Louis, MO: Elsevier Saunders.

Brown, V.R., Adney, D.R., Bielefeldt-Ohmann, H. et al. (2015). Pathogenesis and immune responses of *Francisella tularensis* strains in wild-caught cottontail rabbits (*Sylvilagus spp.*). *Journal of Wildlife Diseases* 51 (3): 564–575.

Brown, D. and Pizzi, R. (2012). Surgical nursing. In: *BSAVA Manual of Exotic Pet and Wildlife Nursing* (ed. M. Varga, R. Lumbis and L. Gott), 222–242. Gloucester, UK: British Small Animal Veterinary Association.

Carpenter, J.W. (2013). *Exotic Animal Formulary*, 4e. St Louis, MO: Elsevier Saunders.

Casey, A.M. and Casey, S.J. (2012). Solubility issues with milk replacer powders – an easy fix. *Wildlife Rehabilitation Bulletin* 30 (1): 36–40.

Chan, D. (2009). The inappetent hospitalized cat: clinical approach to maximizing nutritional support. *Journal of Feline Medicine and Surgery* 11: 925–933.

Chapman, J.A. and Litvaitis, J.A. (2003). Eastern cottontail. In: *Wild Mammals of North America*, 2e (ed. G.A. Feldhammer, B.C. Thompson and J.A. Chapman), 101–125. Baltimore, MD: Johns Hopkins University Press.

Cruise, L.J. and Brewer, N.R. (1994). Anatomy. In: *The Biology of the Laboratory Rabbit*, 2e (ed. P.J. Manniung, D.H. Ringler and C.E. Newcomers), 47–61. San Diego, CA: Academic Press.

Donnelly, T.M. (2004). Basic anatomy, physiology and husbandry. In: *Ferrets, Rabbits and Rodents*, 2e (ed. K.E.

Quesenberry and J.W. Carpenter), 136–146. St Louis, MO: Elsevier Saunders.

Fitzpatrick, J.L., Dyer, J.L., Blanton, J.D. et al. (2014). Rabies in rodents and lagomorphs in the United States 1995–2010. *Journal of the American Veterinary Medical Association* 245 (3): 333–337.

Harcourt-Brown, F. (2002). *Textbook of Rabbit Medicine*. Oxford, UK: Butterworth Heinemann.

Hess, L. (2004). Dermatologic diseases. In: *Ferrets, Rabbits and Rodents*, 2e (ed. K.E. Quesenberry and J.W. Carpenter), 194–202. St Louis, MO: Elsevier Saunders.

IUCN Red List of Threatened Species (2014) www.iucnredlist.org

Jacobson, H.A., McGinnes, B.S., and Catts, E.P. (1978). Bot fly myiasis of the cottontail rabbit, *Sylvilagus floridanus mallurus* in Virginia with some biology of the parasite, *Cuterebra buccata*. *Journal of Wildlife Diseases* 14 (1): 56–66.

Jacobson, H.A., Scanlon, P.F., Nettles, V.F. et al. (1976). Epizootiology of an outbreak of cerebrospinal nematodiasis in cottontail rabbits and woodchucks. *Journal of Wildlife Diseases* 12 (3): 357–360.

Jenkins, J.R. (2004). Gastrointestinal disease. In: *Ferrets, Rabbits and Rodents*, 2e (ed. K.E. Quesenberry and J.W. Carpenter), 147–154. St Louis, MO: Elsevier Saunders.

Johnson-Delaney, C. (2006). Anatomy and Physiology of the Rabbit and Rodent Gastrointestinal System. Proceedings of the Association of Avian Veterinarians, Teaneck, NJ, pp. 9–17.

Kazacos, K.R., Reed, W.M., Kazacos, E.A. et al. (1983). Fatal cerebrospinal disease caused by *Baylisascaris procyonis* in domestic rabbits. *Journal of the American Veterinary Medical Association* 183: 967–971.

Mader, D.R. (2004). Basic approach to veterinary care. In: *Ferrets, Rabbits and Rodents*, 2e (ed. K.E. Quesenberry and J.W. Carpenter), 147–154. St Louis, MO: Elsevier Saunders.

Miller, E. (ed.) (2012). *Minimum Standards for Wildlife Rehabilitation*, 4e. St Cloud, MN.: National Wildlife Rehabilitators Association and International Wildlife Rehabilitation Council.

Morner, T. and Addison, E. (2001). Tularemia. In: *Infectious Disease of Wild Mammals*, 3e (ed. E.S. Williams and I. Barker), 303–309. Ames, IA: Iowa State Press.

Robinson, A.J. and Kerr, P.J. (2001). Poxvirus infections. In: *Infectious Disease of Wild Mammals*, 3e (ed. E.S. Williams and I. Barker), 179–201. Ames, IA: Iowa State Press.

Taylor, K.H. (2002). Orphan rabbits. In: *Hand-Rearing Wild and Domestic Mammals* (ed. L.J. Gage), 5–12. Ames, IA: Iowa State Press.

USDA-APHIS, Veterinary Services (2013). *Rabbit Hemorrhagic Disease Standard Operating Procedures: Overview of Etiology and Ecology*. Riverdale, MD: Veterinary Services, Animal and Plant Health Inspection Service, U.S. Department of Agriculture.

Vennen, K.M. and Mitchell, M.A. (2009). Rabbits. In: *Manual of Exotic Pet Practice* (ed. M.A. Mitchell and T.M. Tully), 375–405. St Louis, MO: Elsevier Saunders.

Wobeser, G. (2001). *Staphylococcus* infection. In: *Infectious Disease of Wild Mammals*, 3e, 509–510. Ames, IA: Iowa State Press.

Zanet, S., Palese, V., Trisciuoglio, A. et al. (2013). *Encephalitozoon cuniculi, Toxoplasma gondii* and *Neospora caninum* infection in invasive eastern cottontail rabbits *Sylvilagus floridanus* in northwestern Italy. *Veterinary Parasitology* 197 (3–4): 682–684.

16

Natural History and Medical Management of Passerines, Galliformes, and Allies

Sallie C. Welte[1,2] *and Erica A. Miller*[2]

[1] *Tri-State Bird Rescue and Research, Inc., Newark, DE, USA*
[2] *Wildlife Medicine, Department of Clinic Studies, University of Pennsylvania School of Veterinary Medicine, Philadelphia, PA, USA*

Natural History of Passerines and Allies

Passerines are a phenomenally large and diverse order, encompassing almost 60% of all living bird species. They are the dominant land birds globally, with over 5100 species in 59 families. The 29 families found in North America include many backyard songbirds (Macwhirter 1994). Passerines range in size from kinglets (6.5 g) to ravens (1230 g). They are defined by their perching feet – that have three forward toes and one hind toe (anisodactyl). Although this is a feature shared with other orders, it is useful in distinguishing them from similarly sized birds in allied orders. They are considered to be the evolutionarily most advanced order, intelligent and adapted to a wide variety of niches (Prum et al. 2015; Terres 1982). Many are specialized feeders and/or long-distance migrants, traits that may present challenges in their rehabilitation. Their foraging behaviors can predispose them to certain types of injuries: wrens are frequently caught in glue traps, while doves collide with windows, rupturing their distended crops. Shoulder injuries can render an aerial insectivore or hummingbird incapable of foraging or migration. Unlike domestic animals, most cannot modify their behavior to survive with a deficit.

Passerine nesting strategy is variable; these birds may nest in open cups, weave hanging baskets, utilize cavities or chimneys, and a few species – including oven birds (*Seiurus aurocapilla*) and nightjars (Caprimulgidae) – may nest on the ground. Mourning doves (*Zenaida macroura*) are notorious for building flimsy nests of pine needles, grass stems, and twigs on branches, in gutters, or even on the ground. With the exception of the semialtricial young of nightjars, young are altricial, hatching naked, blind, and helpless; all require intensive parental care in the nest until they fledge at a few weeks of age.

Cavity nesting species such as chickadees and tree swallows (*Tachycineta bicolor*) are developmentally more mature at fledging than are young of open cup nesters such as robins and sparrows; almost all species continue to receive parental care after fledging as they master their flight and foraging skills.

Feeding Adaptations and Diets

While passerines typically feed their young arthropod invertebrates during their rapid growth phase, their diets may vary seasonally and at different life stages. Birds are classified on the basis of the adult's primary diet, which is reflected in structural and behavioral feeding adaptations such as beak shape and foraging strategy (Proctor and Lynch 1993). Identification of the beak shape and species is thus an important step in determining the food type(s) to offer the passerine patient.

Generalist feeders, including omnivores such as crows, thrushes, and blackbirds, have less specialized beaks than niche feeders. Nectivorous hummingbirds use long, slender beaks to access nectar deep inside flowers. Carnivorous northern shrikes (*Lanius excubitor*) have hooked beaks that tear prey into small pieces, and piscivorous belted kingfishers (*Megaceryle alcyon*) use long, sturdy beaks to seize fish and crayfish.

Seed eaters' beaks reflect both the size of seeds eaten and feeding technique. The thick, conical beak of cardinals and grosbeaks can crack large seeds, and the crossbite of crossbills is used to pry open pinecones. Titmice and chickadees hammer at seeds with short, sturdy beaks, while the smaller, light beaks of white-throated sparrows (*Zonotrichia albicollis*) are adapted for small seeds and plant material. Doves have short, "soft" beaks, and rely on well-developed gizzards and grit to crush ingested seeds.

Medical Management of Wildlife Species: A Guide for Practitioners, First Edition. Edited by Sonia M. Hernandez,
Heather W. Barron, Erica A. Miller, Roberto F. Aguilar and Michael J. Yabsley.
© 2020 John Wiley & Sons, Inc. Published 2020 by John Wiley & Sons, Inc.

Aerial insectivores snatch insects from the air using broad flat beaks (martins and flycatchers), or scoop-like mouths with tiny beaks and fragile jaws (swifts, night hawks, and nightjars). Arboreal insectivores, including warblers and kinglets, use slender beaks to glean insects from foliage and branches. Woodpeckers are specialized insectivores that use chisel-like beaks to drill into wood, extending a long, sticky tongue to retrieve ants and insect larvae. Many nonmigratory insectivorous birds also eat seeds and/or fruit, particularly in the winter.

In addition to beak shape, foot and leg structure, stiffness and length of tail, and shape and length of wings aid in identification. Several excellent field guides and online guides are available; two easy-to-use online resources are Inside Birding and Merlin Bird ID, available through Cornell's Lab of Ornithology website (www.allaboutbirds. org). An excellent natural diet reference is *Songbird Diet Index* (Scott 2013), which also has recommendations for diets in captivity.

Migratory Patterns

Knowing the migratory status is important when establishing a patient's prognosis for rehabilitation. Migration patterns vary by species and sometimes within a species. Birds that are able to find adequate food supplies throughout the winter may remain as permanent residents in part or all of their range, while some subpopulations may change elevation, move regionally, or undergo long migrations. Species with large ranges may remain in North America, following a north–south pattern of movement. Nectivores and many obligate insectivores are long-distance neo-tropical migrants breeding in North America and wintering in the Caribbean, Central, and South America (Terres 1982).

Natural History of Galliformes

Gallinaceous birds compose an order of seven families with 256 species; of these, four families are native to North America. These large-bodied, fowl-like birds live and forage on the ground and roost in trees. Common species include pheasants, quail, grouse, partridges, ptarmigans, prairie chickens, turkeys, peafowl, and jungle fowl. While some species may include short-distance migrants, most are resident (nonmigratory) game species that fall under state rather than federal regulations (Gibson in press).

Gallinaceous birds have strong legs and feet and will generally run and flap when threatened. Capable of short bursts of flight, they will use their nails, spurs, and powerful wings to defend themselves. Many species are secretive in the wild and most have cryptic coloration.

The adults are sexually dimorphic, and some species have unusual skin appendages on their head and neck. These are most dramatic in wild turkeys where dewlaps can change color and size, and snoods decrease and increase in length. Gallinaceous birds have well-developed crops, which in some species can be inflated for display. Hybridization between related species has been documented (Schales and Schales 1994).

Adults nest on the ground and have large clutches of highly precocial, downy young. Chicks can self-feed soon after hatch but rely upon adults to locate food, although wild turkeys have been observed feeding their young (Terres 1982). Until the chicks can thermoregulate, they are brooded by adults; young birds require supplemental heat in captivity, as do compromised adults, particularly smaller species such as quail. Rapidly growing gallinaceous chicks require large amounts of animal protein, and chicks are attracted to moving insects.

Gallinaceous birds are generalist feeders whose diets reflect seasonal food availability; large amounts of browse provide needed crude fiber. Their anisodactyl feet have sturdy nails for scratching as they forage, and thick down-turned beaks, grinding gizzards and well-developed ceca enable them to process everything from worms and small vertebrates to clover, acorns, and twigs.

Captive Management

General Housing Principles

These birds should be housed away from routine noises; use of a natural sounds recording or white noise machine is helpful to mask background sounds. Prey species should not be in close proximity to predators, including other avian species such as grackles, crows, and raptors. Visual blocks, in the form of hide boxes and/or towels draped over the front of cages or containers, help reduce stress.

Follow a routine when providing care so that patients are undisturbed most of the day; minimizing handling will encourage self-feeding, which in itself is stress reducing and often stimulates other natural behaviors (preening, bathing, etc.). Encourage species-typical behavior whenever possible by incorporating natural objects and familiar foods that provide foraging opportunities (Bowers 2014).

Housing for Adult Birds

House adult birds individually; social behavior in many species is seasonal or nonexistent, and pecking orders exist even in captivity. A ventilated cardboard box, solid-sided or mesh carrier, incubator, or aquarium with a screened lid are suitable housing depending upon the species, age, size, and condition of the bird (e.g., dark boxes may be suitable for juvenile cavity nesters) (Figure 16.1). Soft lids should be used for mourning doves and other species predisposed to explosive flight.

Do not use wire cages that can damage feathers or metal hospital cages that are not only reflective and noisy, but also serve as heat sinks. Housing should be large enough that the bird can maintain normal postures without damaging feathers or injuring itself.

Place paper towels, newspapers or other tightly woven, absorbent material on the cage bottom; add a perch if appropriate for the species and condition of the bird (Miller 2012). If sternal, seizuring or profoundly neurological, drape the insides of the container with towels or linens, and do not add cage furniture (perches, greenery) or food/water. Perching birds should be provided with a single well-secured perch of appropriate diameter; a general guideline is to use a pencil-sized perch for a finch-sized bird. Natural twigs and branches provide slight variations in diameter/texture and can reduce stress through their familiarity. Position the perch low enough to provide head room and far enough from the walls of the container to prevent tail damage; this is especially important with long-tailed species such as thrashers and cuckoos.

Birds that do not normally perch vertically, such as nightjars, are more comfortable resting on a wide, stable, textured surface, such as a half-round log or section of bark, placed on the bottom of the container. Species that cling to vertical surfaces, such chimney swifts (*Chaetura pelagica*), should have a securely draped section of tightly woven fabric covering one wall of the container; a sturdy log wedged at a gradual angle from floor to ceiling serves a similar purpose for woodpeckers, brown creepers (*Certhia americana*), and nuthatches. Avoid using terry cloth – the loops can trap nails, toes, tongues, and feathers.

Small boxes turned on their sides and lined with paper towels provide "hides" for secretive species and/or cavity nesters such as wrens; adding a chunk of bark, hollow log, and/or a branch of dense foliage will decrease any inclination to escape. Ground-dwelling gallinaceous species should be provided with larger hide boxes and/or sufficient leafy vegetation to provide visual security.

Mirrors can be used to encourage self-feeding in young birds and social species such as mourning doves. These should be placed behind the food containers and secured to prevent possible injury. Monitor the bird's reactions: social behavior varies seasonally and male cardinals almost universally attack their reflection during the breeding season.

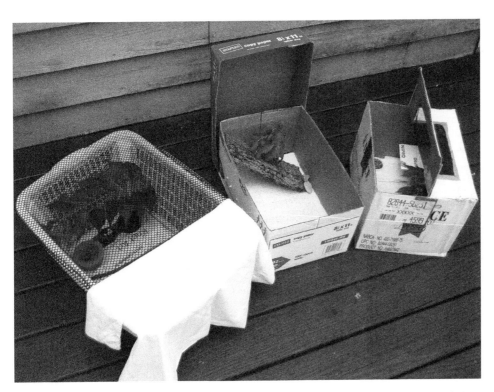

Figure 16.1 Examples of temporary caging for songbirds. Laundry basket lined with netting (*left*); box with solid lid and vent holes cut in sides; good for keeping bird calm and quiet during transport (*center*); box with screening in top for ventilation (*right*). All three are lined with paper, natural foliage, a branch or bark to provide a perch, and a hide area.

Partially cover the top and one end of the container with a light-colored cloth to provide privacy while enabling enough light for the bird to feed. Supplemental heat is needed for all nestlings, hummingbirds in torpor, and chilled, wet or debilitated birds. A heat lamp placed above, or a warm heating pad placed under half of the container, allow mobile birds to select the desired thermal zone; a 29.4°C (85°F) incubator can decrease energy demands on a compromised bird (Quesenberry and Hillyer 1994). Monitor for open-mouth breathing or panting, both signs of overheating. Note the position of the bird relative to the heat source and adjust accordingly.

For hummingbirds, a well-ventilated shoebox or an aquarium with a net or screen top can serve as temporary housing; use a paper towel substrate and secure a slender branch in place as a low perch. The entire container can be placed inside an incubator or on a heating pad to provide supplemental warmth. Once the hummingbird begins to drink on its own, secure a syringe to the container wall at a comfortable feeding height and angle; this should be checked hourly to make sure the bird is feeding (Figure 16.2a,b).

Housing for Nestling Birds

Because neither nestling songbirds nor the downy young of galliformes can thermoregulate, supplemental heat is always required. Ambient temperatures of 21.1°C (70°F) are typically satisfactory for healthy, feathered fledglings and adults. Some species differences exist, and the health of the bird must be considered, but regardless of their age or species, all young birds should feel warm to the touch and their hydration status should be closely monitored (Duerr in press). Once warmed and rehydrated, food should be provided (see Chapter 12).

With a few exceptions, young birds may be safely housed with conspecifics and/or other birds of similar type, size, and age. Precocial young can be housed in boxes or plastic containers similar to those for adults. Altricial nestlings need replacement nests to properly support the developing skeleton and keep feathers and skin clean (see Chapter 12 for information on nest construction). Nests of cavity nesting species should be placed underneath a "hide" box placed on its side, leaving just enough head clearance for easy access. Fledglings can be housed similarly to adults with appropriate perches/perching substrate; low perches and supplemental heat should be provided, and hand-feeding continued, for recently fledged birds.

Diets of Nestling Birds

The nutritional demands of growing passerines are extraordinary. With a few exceptions, a calorie-dense, high-protein, arthropod-based diet is required for normal feather, muscle, and bone development. The protein requirement is so high that amino acid deficiencies can result in permanent stunting, and irreversible metabolic abnormalities can develop if fed an inappropriate diet even for a 24-hour period (Hoggard 2007; Klasing 1999). Further information on hand feeding young birds is found in Chapter 12.

Diets for Compromised Adult Birds

With emaciated patients, gastrointestinal function may be compromised and a gradual transition to whole foods

(a)

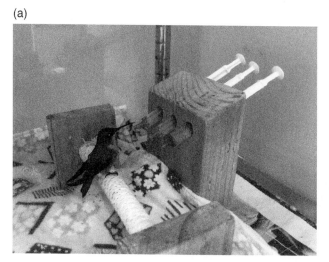

(b)

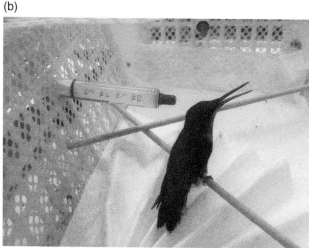

Figure 16.2 Syringe feeding set-up for hummingbirds. (a) Syringe is placed through netting in side of basket. (b) Syringes are placed through slanted holes drilled in a block of wood. Note: syringe types are painted red with fingernail polish to attract the bird to feed.

is needed; these birds require gavage feeding following the techniques used with oral rehydration. Regardless of their "normal" adult diets, emaciated birds have been utilizing body stores to provide needed energy; ideal critical care diets for emaciated birds are both elemental and low in carbohydrates (Donoghue 2006; Remillard et al. 2000). Because many birds lack sucrase, human products containing sucrose should be avoided. Enteral veterinary products such as CliniCare® Canine/Feline liquid diets (Abbott Veterinary Diets, Abbott Nutrition, Columbus, OH, USA) are lower in carbohydrates and higher in protein and fats. Emeraid® products (Lafeber Co., Cornell, IL, USA) are designed for wildlife species and the four formulations can be reconstituted and combined in various ratios to meet the nutritional profile of specific patients.

Adult passerines have high metabolic needs, with basal metabolic rates (BMR) up to 65% higher than larger non-passerine species, and correspondingly increased caloric and fluid requirements (Macwhirter 1994). Very small birds (<25 g) are fasting intolerant and can rapidly deplete their energy reserves, often dying within a few days (Klasing 1999). Active adult hummingbirds feed almost constantly, depending upon the caloric concentration of the food, environmental temperature, and their activity level (whether hovering or perching). If not self-feeding, they can be *temporarily* offered a 1:4 sugar water solution (boiled then cooled) or warmed 5% dextrose in water by syringe at 30–60-minute intervals to maintain their caloric and fluid balances (Elliston in press).

When elemental diets are not required but the bird is in very poor body condition and/or not eating adequate amounts on its own, semisolid veterinary products can be temporarily gavage fed to most adult passerines (e.g., Hill® Prescription Diet® Canine/Feline a/d®; Hill Pet Nutrition, Inc., Topeka, KS, USA). The nutritional content of passerine hand-feeding diets is also appropriate for gavage feeding adult insectivores and omnivores, and ZuPreem® (Premium Nutritional Products, Inc., Shawnee, KS, USA) and/or Exact® (Kaytee Products, Inc., Pottsville, PA, USA) hand-feeding formulas are appropriate for doves, finches, and gallinaceous birds. Many passerines do not have true crops; depending upon their species, overall condition, and feeding status, adults that are not self-feeding may be gavage fed 3–5% of their gross body weight (GBW) 2–4 times daily. Obligate insectivores (swifts, swallows) are fed smaller amounts at shorter intervals, while adult doves are given a larger amount (5–10% GBW) twice daily (Kudlacik and Eilertsen in press).

Feeding Techniques for Gavage and Hand Feeding

Both force feeding and gavage feeding are stressful, and the risk of injury to the bird is high. Minimize handling time by having supplies ready before restraining the bird. Small birds can be held by an assistant or placed in the nondominant hand. Gentle pinching pressure on the skin at the commissure of the beak often results in an open mouth; take extreme care with the fragile, easily broken jaws of nightjars and swifts. Gently sliding a thumb into a nightjar's mouth will distribute the pressure over a wider area while holding the mouth open. For many seed eaters, a thumbnail inserted between the rhinotheca and rhamphotheca will open the mouth. Continuing light pressure or inserting a swab near the commissure will keep the beak open while the gavage tube is carefully threaded well into the mouth or the food bolus placed behind the glottis. In small birds, it is not possible to visualize the glottis; palpation of the throat or very slight movement of overlying neck coverts may be used to confirm correct placement of the feeding tube. With the exception of birds having true crops (doves, gallinaceous species), feeding tubes should be inserted far enough to reach the proventriculus. The diet is then slowly expelled while monitoring the bird for gagging or regurgitation.

Because swifts and nightjars are not anatomically designed to pick up food, they must be hand fed while in captivity. When possible, enlist the bird's natural behavior and use natural foods to facilitate hand feeding. Many insectivores will open their mouths or snap when their vibrissae are stimulated or beaks tapped with a feeding stick, or a small food item is zoomed in a circular motion near their faces; blowing on them may also trigger a feeding response. Nightjars will sometimes "gape" when cornered; if force feeding is necessary, feeding on a flat surface with one hand cupped over the bird may help. Swifts and swallows will snap at fingers, enabling a 1 cc syringe, gavage tube or insect/food bolus to be inserted quickly. Clustering hand feedings near times of normal activity for these species (dawn and dusk) may facilitate acceptance. Because many of these birds drink in flight, hydrating their food will decrease frequency of handling (Hufford in press; Scott 2013).

Diets for Adult Birds: Encouraging Self-Feeding

Even in a brief hospital stay, it is important to encourage self-feeding in birds physically able to do so. Birds with diverse diets and feeding strategies can more easily adapt, and even specialized feeders often eat when knowledge of their natural history is used. Aerial insectivores are typically the most difficult to get to self-feed.

Recognizable foods must be presented in a way adapted to their foraging strategy to trigger a feeding response. However, unless a ready supply of natural plant foods and invertebrates is available, substitute foods of appropriate nutritional quality must be used. Combinations of soaked kitten kibble, crumbled hard-boiled egg yolks, diced sprouts, soaked raisins, finely chopped grapes and/or appropriately sized seeds can be offered with a sprinkling of natural food items, such as mealworms, freeze-dried crickets, and/or seasonal berries (grapes, raspberries, and cherries are low in sucrose). A small chunk of suet or a crumbled peanut butter mix (1 part peanut butter to 2 parts wheatgerm) are readily accepted by many seed- and insect-eating birds. Canned dog or cat food can provide a temporary diet for larger omnivores and faunivores. Freeze-dried mealworms and seed mixtures are available at many grocery stores, while live feeder insects are often available at pet stores.

Food for most ground-feeding birds can be placed in shallow containers such as small jar lids. Use two containers, one for dry food (seed) and one for moist foods (fruit). To avoid contamination, do not place feeding containers under perches. Sprays of millet can be provided for seed eaters, while arboreal insectivores and swallows may self-feed from easily accessible containers of feeder insects secured at perch level. Woodpeckers require deeper dishes, or peanut butter crumbles can be rubbed deep into bark crevices for foraging. Shallow jar lids of water containing stones are suitable for most small passerines, and larger birds require correspondingly larger water bowls, also weighted with stones to prevent tipping and inadvertent bathing. Doves need deeper bowls (small rodent crocks are ideal) because their ability to siphon water requires beak submergence. Food and water should not be placed in cages with swifts or nightjars.

Gallinaceous birds are encouraged to eat by providing a diverse menu on a wide, flat dish, small tray, or sprinkled on the ground. Options include unmedicated game and turkey starter, crushed or moistened kitten or puppy kibble, crumbled hard-boiled egg yolk, finely chopped greens, sprouts, small berries, seeds, clumps of wild grasses or weeds (with roots and soil), and tiny mealworms, bloodworms, and/or ants. A light-colored flooring substrate provides contrast and sprinkling food on their backs also may encourage feeding (Gibson in press).

Clinically Relevant Anatomy and Physiology

Galliformes and some passeriformes have distinct crops, usually on the right side of the neck, cranial to the thoracic inlet. Columbiformes have extensive, bilobed crops that extend across the neck and produce "crop milk" from desquamated crop epithelial cells to feed to their hatchlings. They also have a vascular plexus cranial to the crop that is used in thermoregulation and production of crop milk. The plexus and crop may complicate jugular access.

Feather quality is essential for flight, insulation, waterproofing, and protection, as well as mate attraction and territorial defense. Emerging feathers are particularly fragile and easily damaged by soiling or inappropriate housing. Flight feathers are not replaced until the follicle is empty, typically at the next molt cycle, so care must be taken to avoid damaging feathers when handling birds of any age. Most columbiformes and many passerines readily drop feathers as a defense mechanism to escape predators. Because of this, one or two primaries can be carefully pulled if damaged or broken. Broken tail feathers can also be pulled in smaller species without risking follicle damage. Galliformes remain flighted while molting. Adult grouse, which molt in summer, may lose all of their tail feathers at once, and some species molt the horny sheath to replace worn nails (Schales and Schales 1994).

Providing appropriate warmth, nutrition, and fluid support is critical for the initial survival and long-term care of all passerines. Their small body size and high BMR result in narrower thermoneutral zones and higher body temperatures (e.g., $42.5 \pm 0.4\,°C$ [$108.5 \pm 0.7\,°F$] in black-capped chickadees, *Poecile atricapillus*) than larger species (Wojciechowski and Pinshow 2009). The high BMR in turn necessitates higher drug doses than in larger species. Some species have evolved mechanisms for conserving energy, including controlled hypothermia (body temperature drops to $25–35\,°C$ [$77–95\,°F$]) and noctivation or torpor (body temperature $<25\,°C$ [$<77\,°F$]) (Klasing 1999). The latter is most commonly observed in hummingbirds but is also documented in highly migratory species: swifts, swallows, and nightjars. Noctivating birds may appear dead but will gradually recover with increased ambient temperatures. Birds should have ready access to a food source upon recovery.

A lower metabolic rate and large body size enable galliformes to tolerate fasting better than passerines. Pheasants have been known to survive a week without eating when snow is deep (Environment Canada 1973).

Handling, Restraint, and Clinical Techniques

Passerines can stress easily, so handling should be minimized. Young and small passerines chill quickly, so warm hands prior to restraint. Most passerines can be restrained in one hand using a bander's hold: index and middle finger on either side of the neck, with thumb and ring finger wrapped lightly around the wings and body (Figure 16.3). Covering the bird with a light tea towel or pillowcase further reduces stress and protects feathers. Avoid using terry towels that are likely to snag toenails. Some species (e.g., jays and doves) readily lose tail

An assistant is needed when examining larger birds such as crows, ravens, and upland game birds to minimize injury to bird, feathers, and people. Such birds can be restrained against the handler's body for transport, then placed sternally on an exam table, using the towel to cover the head and torso and to snug wings to the body (Figure 16.4). Game birds can inflict painful scratches, while the claws and beaks of crows and ravens are vise-like.

Examination

Passerines and galliforms are examined in a similar manner, beginning with observation from a distance (i.e., before taking the bird in hand). Observations at a short distance allow you to evaluate the respiration, attitude, and posture of the bird that may not occur or be noted when the bird is being held.

Attitude

Observe the bird's activity and response to noise and motion.

Respiration

Note respiratory rate and pattern. Abnormal conditions include open-mouth breathing, rapid and shallow breathing, breathing with extreme effort, irregular/gasping patterns, moist or harsh respiratory noises. Any bird with moist respiration, especially songbirds, should be *minimally handled*. In a bird with a respiratory problem, stress from excessive handling can result in rapid death; if available, place dyspneic birds in an oxygen

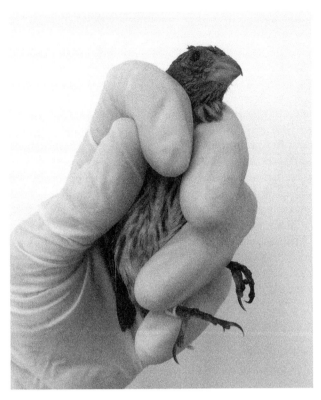

Figure 16.3 Bander's hold for restraining songbirds. The index and middle finger prevent movement of the neck but allow access to the head; the legs are held between the fourth and fifth digit, allowing access to the pectoral muscle.

feathers when stressed. Seed eaters (e.g., cardinals, buntings, and grosbeaks) have heavy bills and can inflict painful bites. Allowing these birds to clamp onto a cotton swab will allow for a safer examination.

(a)

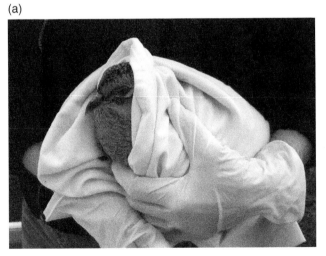

(b)

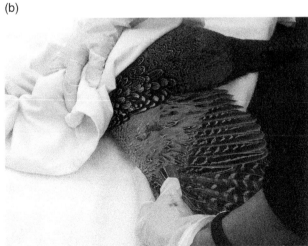

Figure 16.4 Galliform restraint. (a) Pheasant restraint against handler's body, using a pillowcase to control the wings while the hands support the body and control legs and feet. (b) Restraint technique for a sternal bird. Gentle pressure on the back controls the covered head and torso while a wing is examined.

chamber and conduct the exam in intervals, allowing the bird to rest between handling.

Posture/Nervous System

Seizures, head tremors, and abnormal body postures may be indicative of a nervous system problem, and are often best evaluated at a distance. Note any abnormal postures/positions of the bird or its body parts (e.g., wing droop, torticollis, head droop, wing extended for balance, lateral or sternal recumbency), and evaluate leg use and response when touched.

Droppings

Check for feces and urates. Fecal smears and flotations should be performed on all underweight birds.

Hands-On Exam

All efforts should be made to examine the bird as quickly as possible in order to minimize handling. Have all necessary equipment and supplies ready before picking up the bird. A second person should be used to hold during the exam of any bird larger than a pigeon in order to prevent injuries to the examiner and to minimize stress on the bird.

After weighing the bird, assess the body condition by palpating the keel. If you can pinch the ridge of the keel, the bird is lean to underweight. If the keel is very prominent, the bird is emaciated. Hydration is most easily assessed in naked nestlings, but any bird with squinty or sunken eyes, thickened saliva, dry mucous membranes, tented skin or blood loss can be considered dehydrated to some degree. Check if the feathers around the nares are damp or crusted with dried discharge. Any feathers matted over the nares should be cleaned with a moist cotton swab to allow the bird to breathe and the nares to drain.

Check for any recent or healed beak damage. For most species, the oral mucosa should look moist and pink. Note any paleness, odor, dryness, thickened saliva, fresh blood, or parasites. If plaques or lesions are seen (most frequently in doves or galliforms), perform a swab and wet mount to look for protozoans or yeast cells. Palpate the crop for contents and consistency and note the odor.

Check the skin over the crop for lacerations or punctures. Clean any wounds carefully to assess the extent of the damage. To determine if the crop has been perforated, insert a small amount of clear, sterile fluids with a soft gavage tube after the bird has been stabilized. If fluid leaks out of the neck wounds, see the section on crop lacerations. Gently palpate the caudal coelom for any abnormalities including firm distention from an enlarged liver, impactions, or egg binding. The area caudal to the sternum should be visually inspected for any blood under the skin or bruising. A concave abdomen may indicate emaciation. Check the vent for impaction due to matted feathers and clean with warm water as needed.

A complete fundic exam should be done to check for hemorrhage within the globes and to assess response to visual stimuli. Vision can be difficult to evaluate as birds will often react stoically rather than demonstrate menace responses and have voluntary control over pupil size. Each ear is located at the point of a triangle between the lateral canthus and the commissure of the mouth. Note any bruising or the presence of blood or parasites.

Check for broken, missing, or in-sheath feathers. Damaged feathers may need to molt before the bird can be released. Check for lice, mites, hippoboscid flies, ticks, or maggots and consider treating accordingly. Carefully examine the skin by gently brushing or blowing the feathers back until the skin is visible. Look for puncture wounds or hidden lacerations on any bird with a history of possible contact with a cat; avoid wetting the bird with alcohol as rapid hypothermia may result.

Examine all digits and the plantar surface of the feet for wounds. Compare the feet to check for swelling. If the bird is standing, place it on the floor of a secure area to observe how it walks. If the bird has decreased function of both legs and the vent area is soiled or impacted, a complete neurological exam is indicated. Evaluate the spinal column for bruising, abnormal movement, or displacement. If neurological deficits are suspected, check for cloacal tone (should be closed, not open or flaccid). Pinching the edge of the cloaca should elicit a puckering response. Assess for withdrawal reflex versus pain response by gently pinching the toes. When palpating, evaluate the range of motion of the joints.

To evaluate bones for fractures, hold one end of the bone securely and apply gentle pressure down the length of the bone. Check for symmetry with the opposite leg/wing. End by palpating the spinal column, keel, synsacrum, and pelvic and pectoral girdles. Consider the prognosis of any injuries found, keeping in mind the species, natural history, and overall condition of the bird.

Anesthesia

Potentially painful or long procedures (e.g., invasive orthopedics, some wound management) are best performed under general anesthesia. See Chapter 5 for specific recommendations.

Due to their small size and rapid metabolic rates, general anesthesia in passerines and their allies is most commonly achieved with isoflurane or sevoflurane administered via a modified facemask (Hawkins and Pascoe 2007). Most passerines can be manually restrained and anesthetized in this manner using a nonrebreathing circuit with an oxygen flow rate of 0.5–1% L/min and 5% isoflurane. A surgical plane of anesthesia is usually obtained in 30–90 seconds and maintained at 2–3% isoflurane. Anesthesia depth can be monitored using a Doppler probe on the brachial, medial metatarsal or carotid artery (Hawkins and Pascoe 2007), an ECG using 25–27 gauge needles for lead attachments, or a respiratory/apnea monitor (Medical Engineering and Development, Horton, MI, USA). Larger passerines and galliformes may benefit from presedation with a benzodiazepine.

Local anesthetics may be used in conjunction with inhalant anesthetic to provide additional analgesia and muscle relaxation for orthopedic procedures. For example, a brachial plexus nerve blockade can be achieved rapidly using 2% lidocaine and is useful when reducing overriding wing fractures. For lengthy procedures or surgeries requiring access to the beak or face, small birds can be intubated using an 18–14 gauge indwelling Teflon catheter with the stylet removed as a modified endotracheal tube (see Chapter 5 for further details on avian anesthesia).

Manual restraint and topical anesthetics such as benzocaine spray (Cetacaine™, Cetylite Industries, Inc., Pennsauken, NJ, USA) may be used for short procedures in galliformes and larger passerines less prone to handling-induced stress (Clubb 1998). Topical ophthalmic anesthetics such as tetracaine drops may be used in wounds to provide some analgesia in smaller passerines without a high risk of overdosing (authors' personal experience).

Rehydration

Before offering or force feeding any nutritional items that require digestion, the patient must be properly hydrated (Hoggard 2007). Existing deficits are normally replaced over 48–72 hours; these are added to the daily maintenance requirement plus any ongoing loss. The total amount required per day is then divided up and administered several times daily. While the general rule for adult birds is 100 mL/kg/day, it can be up to 250–300 mL/kg/day for passerines (Myers 2007). Additional details are provided in Chapter 4. Fluid needs must be balanced against the stress of frequent handling; the sooner birds self-feed, the better.

With the exception of hummingbirds, rehydration with an isotonic electrolyte solution such as lactated Ringer's solution or Normosol®-R (Abbott Laboratories, Lake Bluff, IL, USA) is recommended. Also, B-vitamins should be added for debilitated birds (Remillard et al. 2000) at 1 mL injectable B-complex per liter of fluids or 1–2 mg/kg SID dosed according to the amount of thiamine (Tseng 2005). This is customarily given

subcutaneously or orally, or both, depending on the age, size, injuries, and hydration status of the bird.

Oral fluids are preferred, especially for young songbirds that readily gape, as oral fluids also flush the gastrointestinal tract (GIT) of inappropriate food items and avoid complications when subcutaneous (SQ) emphysema is present. If alert and gaping, these birds may be given small amounts of fluids every 15–20 minutes. In very young/small birds, a 1 cc syringe with a teat cannula or similarly blunt tip can be passed over the tongue to place 1–2 drops into the esophagus (Hoggard 2007). In larger/older birds, a 1 cc syringe can be similarly placed and 0.1–0.2 mL of fluid expressed. Hand-feeding formula can generally be introduced after three rounds of hydrating fluids if the bird is bright, swallowing well, and/or produces droppings (see Chapter 12).

Because of differences in esophageal structure, recommended oral fluid volumes for most adult passerines are based on a conservative estimate of stomach capacity, or roughly 3–5% GBW; this should be halved in debilitated patients with compromised GIT function (Hoggard 2007).

Subcutaneous fluids are indicated if birds are moderately dehydrated, and may be given concurrently with oral fluids to minimize handling. Subcutaneous fluids can be safely administered in boluses of 3–5% GBW. Unless the bird is hyperthermic, all fluids should be warmed to 29.4 °C (85 °F) prior to administration. For hyperthermic birds, room temperature fluids are recommended.

In passerines and allies, SQ fluids are given between the shoulders (dorsal intrascapular apteria) or in the inguinal area, using a fine (25–30) gauge needle. Because the lungs and cervicocephalic air sacs lie close to the skin in small birds, oral administration of fluids is often preferable, using tubing cut from a butterfly catheter or IV extension set; the cut end should be flamed to round sharp edges. Avoid subcutaneous fluids if SQ emphysema is present.

In doves, fluids are given orally using 3–4 in. of a soft rubber gavage tube, or SQ in the inguinal fold. The intrascapular apteria are not utilized due to the large vascular plexus (Miller 1996). Because of the undue levels of restraint and skill required, the authors do not recommend parenteral fluids in hummingbirds, or IV and IO fluid administration in small wild birds.

In gallinaceous birds, oral fluids are administered via an 18 Fr feeding tube, and SQ fluids in the inguinal folds or intrascapular apteria. Intravenous fluid boluses (2% GBW) can be given to larger species via the medial metatarsal vein.

Replacement fluid support may be continued for up to three days, based upon response of the bird. Fluids are generally administered 2–3 times per day, but more is sometimes needed. Appropriate nutritional support must be initiated for passerines within 24 hours. If hydrated and provided the correct diet, most passerines will begin to self-feed quickly (Hoggard 2007).

Infectious and Parasitic Diseases

The information presented here is a quick reference regarding the more commonly encountered diseases and parasites. Diagnosis in small passerines is realistically often based on clinical signs alone, but diagnostic tests are listed for definitive purposes. Most diseases can be controlled through careful management of vectors; by disinfecting cages, dishes, and furnishings with 10% bleach solution; and washing hands well after handling birds with suspected infections.

Bacterial Diseases

Mycoplasmal conjunctivitis has been a concern in many North American passerines since the early 1990s. The causative agent, *Mycoplasma gallisepticum*, most commonly affects immature house finches (*Haemorhous mexicanus*), but also occurs in American gold finches (*Spinus tristis*), blue jays (*Cyanocitta cristata*), and

occasionally other passerine species (Ley et al. 2016). Transmission occurs both vertically and horizontally at some types of bird feeders (Hartup et al. 1998). Affected birds present with conjunctivitis, periocular inflammation, dyspnea, sinusitis, and ocular discharge from secondary bacterial conjunctivitis (Figure 16.5). Diagnosis can be confirmed by culture or polymerase chain reaction (PCR). Treatment consists of rinsing the eyes with saline, followed by topical application of antibiotic ophthalmic drops for secondary bacterial infections and systemic treatment of tylosin tartrate for 21 days (Mashima et al. 1997). Concern for the possible creation of subclinical carriers that may remain PCR positive after treatment has caused several states to prohibit the rehabilitation and release of affected birds (Dhondt et al. 2013; Luttrell and Fischer 2007).

Salmonellosis (most often caused by *Salmonella typhimurium*) is commonly spread at winter bird feeders, with large outbreaks reported in pine siskins (*Spinus pinus*) and finches. Signs include sudden death, ataxia, and poor flight, ingluvitis, crop abscesses, enteritis, weakness, and emaciation. Individuals may also present with multiple joint infections (arthrosynovitis). Transmission is fecal–oral, so contaminated tray-style feeders often serve as a fomite. Diagnosis is most commonly made on necropsy (abscesses of the upper GIT, hepatomegaly,

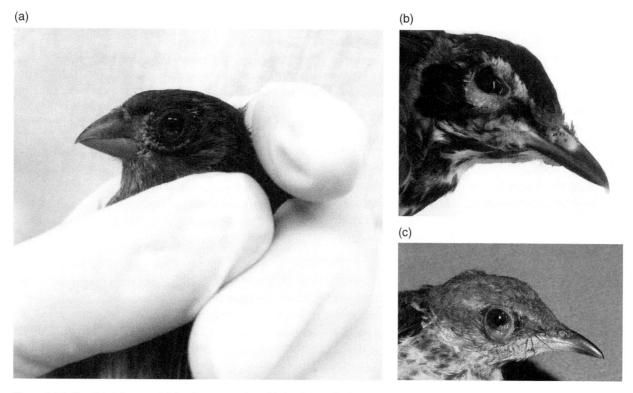

(a)

(b)

(c)

Figure 16.5 Songbird diseases. (a) Swollen, crusted eyelids in a house finch (*Haemorhous mexicanus*) with conjunctivitis caused by *Mycoplasma gallisepticum*. (b) Papular skin lesions in an American Robin (*Turdus migratorius*) with avian poxvirus. (c) Sinusitis in a northern mockingbird (*Mimus polyglottos*) caused by *Tetratrichomonas* spp.

splenomegaly, and necrotic foci in the GI tract) and by culture. Treatment consists of long-term antibiotic therapy, but is rarely successful and may create subclinical carriers (Daoust and Prescott 2007).

Bacterial sinusitis is most commonly seen in hand-reared passerines, usually from food entering the upper respiratory tract. Facial sinuses distend with caseous material and/or mucoid fluid; swelling may distort the face and upper palate. Gram stains and/or bacterial culture and sensitivities should be performed as these infections often contain a mixture of bacteria. Treatment consists of appropriate systemic antibiotics in conjunction with nasal flush and broad-spectrum ophthalmic drops applied into nares until clinical signs resolve. Note that the right and left nasal sinuses do not communicate, so drops must be applied to both nares if infection is bilateral.

Viral Diseases

Pox virus (Avipoxvirus) is commonly seen in doves, crows, thrushes (including robins and mockingbirds), and finches, but may occur in any species. Birds generally present with one of three forms: cutaneous, neoplastic, or diphtheritic. The cutaneous form (dry pox) is most common, with nodules appearing first on the featherless areas of the skin: cere, eyelids, commissures of the beak, carpi, legs, and feet (Figure 16.5b). Very large tumor-like lesions develop in the neoplastic form, and these growths readily recur if removed. Membranes develop in upper gastrointestinal and respiratory tracts in the diphtheritic form (wet pox), often resulting in anorexia and cyanosis. Viral transmission occurs via mosquitoes, mites and direct contact, with lesions appearing 7–9 days after infection. Diagnosis may be confirmed by finding intracytoplasmic inclusions (Bollinger bodies) on smears or histopathology of lesion biopsies.

The dry form is often self-limiting and treatment is largely supportive. Topical iodine on open skin lesions has helped to dry lesions and prevent secondary infections. Broad-spectrum systemic antibiotics may be indicated if secondary infections occur. Treatments of the neoplastic and wet forms are rarely successful. Scabs and open lesions are highly infectious; the virus may remain latent for years. However, recovered birds are usually immune to reinfection with that virus strain (van Riper and Forrester 2007). Because it is highly contagious, infected birds should be isolated and cages clearly marked so that all materials are disinfected. If birds cannot be adequately separated, euthanasia should be considered to prevent rapid spread within the facility.

Passerines are susceptible to and serve as subclinical reservoirs for numerous arboviruses, including the three equine encephalitis viruses (eastern, western, and Venezuelan), and the flaviviruses St Louis encephalitis and West Nile virus (WNV) (Smith 2015). Most arboviruses have little direct effect on passerines, their allies and galliformes, but several groups (e.g., corvids, shrikes, and raptors) may develop severe clinical disease from WNV infections (Gerhold et al. 2007; Travis 2008). Clinical signs include ataxia, paralysis, tremors and seizures, diarrhea, and sudden death. Several passerine species are likely reservoirs, responding with high viremias but low morbidity (Komar et al. 2003). Transmission occurs via mosquitoes (biological vector), hippoboscid flies (mechanical vectors), and direct contact of all body fluids (Doyle et al. 2011; Gancz et al. 2004; Hubálek 2004; Komar et al. 2003). Diagnosis is confirmed via positive antibody titer or PCR.

The authors treat suspected cases with supportive care and systemic antiinflammatories; some avian species have been treated successfully with supportive care alone but should be monitored for neurological sequelae (Nemeth et al. 2009). Affected birds should be isolated from other patients and treated for external parasites to reduce transmission.

Avian influenza virus (Orthomyxoviridae) rarely causes morbidity or mortality in passerines and wild galliforms, but has been isolated from a number of species in these groups. However, there is no evidence supporting their role as natural reservoirs for the virus (Slusher et al. 2014). House finches may develop splenomegaly, pancreatic lesions, perivascular edema, and neuronal necrosis, while European starlings (*Sternus vulgaris*) appear refractory to the virus. Galliform species may develop these same lesions, in addition to respiratory lesions (Stallknecht et al. 2007).

Fungal Diseases

Candidiasis or thrush is caused by *Candida albicans*, a yeast that is part of the normal GI flora of most birds. Overgrowth may occur in young birds, especially hand-fed passerines (most commonly swifts), as a result of improper diet temperature, antibiotic use, and/or stress. *Candida* has also been seen by the authors in conjunction with beak deformities in hummingbirds (possibly from fungal overgrowth at feeders). Clinical signs include vomiting, anorexia, weight loss, diarrhea, and crop stasis. A white coating is often seen on the oral mucosa and/or crop, and is often malodorous. Diagnosis may be confirmed with a fungal culture or stain of an oral swab, or increased yeast on a fecal gram stain. Early infections respond well to nystatin or fluconazole.

Aspergillosis, most commonly caused by *Aspergillus fumigatus*, is usually secondary to an underlying immunosuppressive condition and is rarely diagnosed antemortem in passerines. Clinical signs are nonspecific and include weight loss, anorexia, vomiting, diarrhea, large buffy coat, and sometimes dyspnea. Serology and endoscopy are useful diagnostic tools in larger passerine allies (such as crows) and galliformes. Treatment options include a combination of terbinafine and voriconazole (Smith 2015). Lesions seen on necropsy include granulomatous nodules, filamentous forms, and/or fibrinous plaques within the respiratory tract and/or on serosal surfaces of internal organs.

Parasites and Parasitic Diseases

Ectoparasites

Wild songbirds and galliformes may be affected by ectoparasites, including chewing lice (order Phthiraptera), ticks (most commonly *Argas* spp.), flat flies (order Hippoboscidae), scaly leg mites (*Knemidokoptes jamaicensis*), skin mites (*Ornithonyssus* sp.), feather mites (*Dermanyssus* sp., and others), and follicular mites (*Harpyrhynchus* sp.). Most will cause feather damage or loss, anemia, or cyst-like dermal lesions. Scaly leg mites cause hyperkeratosis of the skin on the legs and feet, and occasionally the face. Diagnosis is based on observation of the parasites, sometimes requiring a skin scraping if the mites are buried.

Because most can act as mechanical and, in some cases, biological vectors of blood-borne diseases (*Haemoproteus* spp., *Leucocytozoon* spp., *Plasmodium* spp., WNV, and Avipoxvirus), identification and treatment are important. With the exceptions of follicular mites and scaly leg mites, they can be treated with a pyrethrin-based avian mite and lice spray. The spray is applied to a cloth and the bird is wrapped in it; this avoids accidental application to eyes and oral mucosae. Pyrethrin-based spray may be repeated twice daily if live parasites continue to be observed. Affected birds should be isolated until all external parasites are gone. Hand washing after handling prevents transmission to other patients.

Scaly leg mites and follicular mites burrow into the skin. Topical application of ivermectin or Scalex™ (Gimborn Pet Specialties, LLC, Atlanta, GA, USA) is usually effective. A single dose of ivermectin may also be administered orally or subcutaneously for systemic treatment.

Passerines do not present with myiasis as commonly as galliformes, but any species may have fly eggs or larvae in moist tissues of wounds, blood feathers, eyes, nares, mouth, cloaca, or ventral patagia, especially during warm weather. Maggots and eggs may be physically removed with forceps or flushed away with water or saline. A final rinse with dilute ivermectin or nitenpyram kills any remaining larvae within hours. Ivermectin and nitenpyram can also be given orally (either in addition to or in lieu of topical route), but both act more rapidly via direct application.

Endoparasites – Intestinal

Wild passerines, galliforms, and their allies are often infected with intestinal parasites, including cestodes, trematodes, acanthocephalans, and various nematodes and protozoans. Weight loss and/or diarrhea are the most common clinical signs, and all are easily diagnosed via direct fecal smear or flotation. At least two species of trematodes infect passerines outside the GI tract: *Collyriculum* spp. may encyst in the skin and *Diplosomum* spp. may migrate to the ocular conjunctiva, appearing as conjunctivitis. Cestode infections respond well to praziquantel, as do most intestinal trematode infections. Acanthocephalans are resistant to most anthelmintics, but infections may respond to loperamide (Mehlhorn 1990). Cestodes, trematodes, and acanthocephalans all require intermediate hosts, so contamination of the environment and transmission between patients is not generally of high concern.

Nematodes of greatest concern include *Baylisascaris procyonis*, whose larvae migrate through the brain and spinal cord causing neurological signs; gapeworms (*Syngamus* spp. and *Cyathostoma* spp.), whose adults pair and attach to the tracheal mucosa causing gaping and dyspnea; and threadworms (*Capillaria* spp.), that often cause diarrhea, weight loss, and anemia. Most nematodes can be treated with ivermectin, fenbendazole or pyrantel pamoate, although some species of columbiformes are sensitive to fenbendazole (Howard et al. 2002).

Coccidia of the genera *Isospora* and *Eimeria* are commonly associated with diarrhea (with or without blood), anemia, emaciation, and dehydration. Most infections respond to treatment with sulfadimethoxine, toltrazuril, or ponazuril. The rotating use of the coccidiostats amprolium and sulfamethazine in water sources in outdoor cages may reduce infection from local wild birds.

Trichomoniasis (*Trichomonas gallinae*) results in lesions in the upper GIT of doves and, less commonly, other passerines and galliformes (Anderson et al. 2009). The parasite may spread rapidly among young birds in rehabilitation, especially if hand-feeding implements are not cleaned well. Outbreaks have been reported in finches and sparrows (NWHC 2002). White, caseous exudates appear on oral and esophageal mucosae; birds are dysphagic and often present in an emaciated condition with distended, malodorous crops. Flagellated protozoans are seen on wet mount of crop swabs or washes, and sometimes in direct fecal smears. Minor infections respond well to carnidazole or other nitroimidazoles (Forrester and Foster 2008), while more advanced cases may require surgical debulking in addition to systemic drugs.

Tetratrichomonas gallinarum is associated with sinus infections in passerines, particularly the Turdidae and

Mimidae families (Anderson et al. 2009; Welte 2000). Infection results in distension of the sinuses, nasal discharge, periorbital inflammation, blepharosis, and/or chemosis (Patton and Patton 1996) (Figure 16.5c). Flagellated organisms may be seen in scrapings of the choana or in sinus aspirates, and/or in a direct fecal smear (St Leger and Shivaprasad 1998). Treatment requires both surgical debridement of the sinuses and a combination of a systemic nitroimidazole and topical antibiotics and supportive care (Welte 2000).

A *Cryptosporidium*-like disease has been reported in cliff swallows (*Petrochelidon pyrrhonota*) that presents similarly to *T. gallinarum* and *M. gallisepticum* infections (Jackman and Meier 2013). Treatment with paromomycin, effective in some cases of mammalian cryptosporidiosis, provided only temporary remission in the swallows.

Noninfectious Reasons for Presentation

Predator Attacks

Wounds inflicted by wild predators and domestic dogs and cats are one of the most common causes for wild birds being brought for rehabilitation (Frink et al. 1994). Injuries may present as punctures, lacerations, degloving wounds, feather loss or damage, fractures, dislocations, organ damage, subcutaneous emphysema, hemorrhage, and shock (Casey and Goldthwait 2013). After the bird is stabilized, traumatic injuries should be treated accordingly, including the use of a broad-spectrum antibiotic, as cats and dogs carry a large number of oral bacteria (August 1988).

Head Trauma

As with other avian species, head trauma resulting from collisions with windows, wires, vehicles, or other objects is common in galliforms, passerines, and their allies. Birds may present with seizures, obtundation, head tilt, torticollis, nystagmus, paresis or paralysis, ataxia, beak fractures, scalping of the crown, and/or eye trauma. Immediate care should be focused on patient stabilization: providing supplemental oxygen, elevating the head, keeping the patient in a dark and quiet environment (to reduce stress), and administering systemic nonsteroidal antiinflammatories. Additional injuries and secondary problems are not uncommon; birds should be carefully evaluated every 24 hours for delayed effects that may preempt release.

Entrapment in Adhesives

Insectivorous passerines may get stuck to glue traps or fly strips in their pursuit of prey. Fractures commonly occur as the bird struggles to free itself; care must be taken in removing the bird from the adhesive. Cover the bird's head to reduce stress, then apply flour or talcum powder to exposed adhesive to prevent additional body parts from adhering. Using a syringe, apply small drops of canola oil to points of contact between the feathers and adhesive, allow to sit for 30–60 seconds, then gently peel the adhesive away from the bird. The now oiled bird should be given fluids and allowed to stabilize before bathing in 3–5% (0.5–0.8 cups/gal) Dawn™ dish detergent in 104–106 °F water (40–41 °C), followed by spray rinse with water at the same temperature to remove all detergent; dry under a heat lamp, then encourage preening by misting (Frink and Miller 1998).

Toxins

Passerines may be incidentally exposed to pesticides applied to yards or crops (usually cholinesterase inhibitors) or intentionally via avicides (usually 4-aminopyridine or 3-chloro-4-methylaniline hydrochloride). Birds present with ataxia, tremors, torticollis, seizures, and/or acute death. Cholinesterase inhibition responds well to atropine. For avicides or unknown toxins, midazolam may control seizures and activated charcoal may prevent further absorption.

Cedar waxwings (*Bombycilla cedrorum*) and other species may collide with objects (windows, fences) as a result of ethanol toxcity from gorging on overripe berries of certain plants (*Schinus terebinthifolius* and *Ampeloposis brevipedunculata*; Woldemeskel and Styer 2010) or consuming berries of invasive species such as *Nandina domestica* which contain cyanide (Kinde et al. 2012).

Albendazole and fenbendazole are toxic to pigeons and doves and possibly other species and should not be used in columbiformes, and used with caution in other species (Howard et al. 2002).

Fractures

When presented with a passerine with a fractured limb, assess the bird's overall condition and stabilize it with fluids, analgesics, heat, etc., as indicated before any further treatment. For severe or open fractures that appear treatable, apply a quick body wrap to keep the affected limb from incurring further damage during stabilization. The limb should be positioned as normally as possible – do not overflex the joints. The wrap and/or splints should immobilize the fracture but not the circulation. Additional details can be found in Chapter 4.

Flush wounds of open fractures thoroughly with dilute antiseptic solution, being careful to avoid soaking the bird. Topical ointments should be avoided, as they may damage waterproofing and impede healing. If the bone end is protruding and cannot be easily manipulated into alignment, apply a sterile gel (e.g., Surgilube®, HR Pharmaceuticals, York, PA, USA) over the wound and cover it to prevent desiccation. Open fractures require surgical reduction as soon as the bird is stable. The bird should be started on antibiotics immediately (e.g., amoxicillin-clavulanic acid or clindamycin) and an antiinflammatory/analgesic.

Surgical reduction of long bone fractures in songbirds can be accomplished under general anesthesia using hypodermic needles for intramedullary pins (Figure 16.6). All pins are placed proximal to distal (normograde). In robin-sized songbirds, 22 g needles work well: generally 3.8 cm (1.5 in.) for tibiotarsal and ulnar fractures and 2.5 cm (1 in.) for humeral and femoral fractures. Smaller gauges (25 g) work well for most finch-sized songbirds. After placing the needle, the hub is bent 90° and the excess is trimmed and taped against the bird's limb.

Curled Digits

Nestlings and fledglings may present with flexed digits, attempting to stand on the lateral aspects of the foot or holding the digits closed and standing on the "knuckles." A stiff splint cut from the lid of a plastic food container (e.g., a pint-sized deli container) taped to the plantar surface of the foot with the digits extended will usually remedy this problem in 4–7 days (see Duerr 2010 for illustrations and instructions of splint preparation).

Wounds

Punctures, lacerations, and degloving wounds are all common, especially in birds that have been injured by cats (Casey and Goldthwait 2013). General wound care should be administered. Primary closure may be accomplished with tissue glue or 5-0 to 7-0 suture on a taper needle.

Beak Injuries

Many beak fractures in passerines can be repaired using tissue glue to affix external splints directly to the maxillary or mandibular rhamphotheca. The thin but rigid aluminum of many suture packages can be easily cut and molded to the appropriate size and shape for this purpose. The glue generally holds long enough for fractures to heal, and falls off or is manually removed after 14 days.

Crop Rupture

Traumatic crop injuries occur most often in doves and pigeons, as these birds have large, bilobed crops

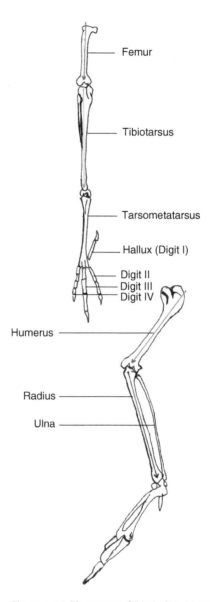

Figure 16.6 Placement of IM pin (22–25 g needles) for fracture stabilization in songbirds. All pins are placed normograde.

that are easily distended with seed. Acute impact may cause rupture from the inside outward, while lacerations from predator claws or talons cause rupture from the outside inward. The crop, as part of the esophagus, should be sutured as such, separately from the skin.

Domestic Species

Many "rescued" galliforms have been captive raised, resulting in feather damage, decreased wariness, and inability to survive in the wild. These birds as well as exotic species should never be released to the wild (Gibson in press).

Phlebotomy

Blood collection is easily obtained from the right jugular vein, located in the dorsal apteric region. Pigeons and doves lack this apteric tract, and their extensive crop and vascular plexus make jugular access difficult. Small quantities of blood may be collected from the medial metatarsal vein. The brachial vein is best accessed under anesthesia to avoid hematoma formation. Passerine size may limit blood collection, and the necessity to use a needle of 27 g or smaller may result in cell lysis (see Appendix I for clinical pathology references).

Euthanasia

Euthanasia is indicated for wild passerines and gamebirds whose injuries carry a poor prognosis for release (injuries cannot be treated or will not resolve to the extent that the bird would be able to survive in the wild); whose diseases may put other birds at serious risk; or whose injuries will require extended treatment and extensive care, such that care of other patients may be compromised.

Wild passerines and gamebirds are commonly euthanized by intravenous injection with a sodium pentobarbital solution. Birds may be sedated or anesthetized via mask or chamber induction with isoflurane, or intranasal or IM injection with midazolam.

Euthanasia solution may also be administered intraosseously, or into the liver/hepatic sinus or coelomic cavity in very small birds provided they are unconscious or anesthetized (AAZV 2006; AVMA 2013). Cervical dislocation is sometimes used in the field for birds under ~70 g. For other methods, consult the AVMA Guidelines for Euthanasia of Animals 2013 edition.

Release

The last critical step in the rehabilitation process is preparing an animal – physically and psychologically – for survival *after* its release. The natural behavior and adaptations of each species must be considered.

All juvenile and adult birds must be in good feather condition, waterproof, flighted, and capable of foraging and (if appropriate) migrating, when evaluated for release. Selection of the release location is influenced by available food supply, site fidelity, and migratory status.

Healthy passerine and galliform chicks can often be reunited with their families or, in the case of some species, adopted by foster families with young of similar age. Wildlife rehabilitators often have a network of volunteers trained to renest young birds and monitor their success.

Corvid (jays, crows, etc.) and galliform chicks easily become imprinted on humans and, unable to interact appropriately with others of their species, cannot then be released. Minimizing contact and early renesting/fostering are priorities.

Birds of social species benefit from release into a flock; this is particularly true for young chimney swifts and cedar waxwings where individuals are readily assimilated and their survival enhanced by access to food sources and roosting sites. Coordinating the release time with the bird's natural diurnal cycle and migratory schedule enhances postrelease survival (Bowers 2014).

Acknowledgement

The authors would like to thank the many staff and volunteers of Tri-State Bird Rescue and Research, Inc., past and present, whose combined knowledge formed the foundation of this chapter and provided care for thousands of wild birds in need.

References

American Association of Zoo Veterinarians (AAZV) (2006). *Guidelines for Euthanasia of Nondomestic Animals*, 100–102. Yulee, FL: American Association of Zoo Veterinarians.

American Veterinary Medical Association (AVMA) (2013). *Guidelines for the Euthanasia of Animals*, 65–67. Schaumberg, IL: American Veterinary Medical Association.

Anderson, N.L., Grahn, R.A., van Hoosear, K., and BonDurant, R.H. (2009). Studies of trichomonad protozoa in free ranging songbirds: prevalence of *Trichomonas gallinae* in house finches (*Carpodacus mexicanus*) and corvids and a novel trichomonad in mockingbirds (*Mimus polyglottos*). *Veterinary Parasitology* 161: 178–186.

August, J.R. (1988). Dog and cat bites. *Journal of the American Veterinary Medical Association* 193: 1394–1398.

Bowers, V. (2014). *Passerine Fundamentals*. Sebastopol, CA: Native Songbird Care & Conservation.

Casey, S. and Goldthwait, M. (2013). When pets attack – part 1: what can happen. *Wildlife Rehabilitation Bulletin* 31 (2): 8–16.

Clubb, S.L. (1998). Round table discussion: pain management in clinical practice. *Journal of Avian Medicine and Surgery* 12 (4): 276–278.

Daoust, P.Y. and Prescott, J.F. (2007). Salmonellosis. In: *Infectious Diseases of Wild Birds* (ed. N.J. Thomas, D.B. Hunter and C.T. Atkinson), 270–288. Ames, IA: Wiley.

Dhondt, A.A., Dhondt, K.V., Hochachka, W.M., and Schat, K.A. (2013). Can American goldfinches function as reservoirs for mycoplasma gallisepticum? *Journal of Wildlife Diseases* 49: 49–54.

Donoghue, S. (2006). Nutrition. In: *Reptile Medicine and Surgery*, 2e (ed. D. Mader), 251–298. St Louis, MO: Saunders Elsevier.

Doyle, M.S., Swope, B.N., Hogsette, J.A. et al. (2011). Vector competence of the stable fly (Diptera: Muscidae) for West Nile virus. *Journal of Medical Entomology* 48: 656–668.

Duerr, R. (in press). General care. In: *Hand Rearing Birds*, 2nd Ed. (ed. R.S. Duerr and L.J. Gage). Hoboken, NJ: Wiley.

Duerr, R. (2010). *Splinting Avian Fractures*, 2e, 23–24. Cordelia, CA: International Bird Rescue Research Center, Inc.

Elliston, E. (in press). Humming birds. In: *Hand Rearing Birds*, 2nd Ed. (ed. R.S. Duerr and L.J. Gage). Hoboken, NJ: Wiley.

Environment Canada Wildlife Service (1973). *Hinterland Who's Who: Ring-Necked Pheasant*. Ottawa: Information Canada.

Forrester, D.J. and Foster, G.W. (2008). Trichomonosis. In: *Parasitic Diseases of Wild Birds* (ed. C.T. Atkinson, N.J. Thomas and B.N. Hunter). Ames, IA: Wiley.

Frink, L. and Miller, E.A. (1998). Cleaning (s)oiled songbirds. *NWRA Quarterly* 16 (1): 8–9.

Frink, L., Smith, L., and Frink, J.A. (1994). Cat attacks in wild birds: prevalence, characteristics, and treatment of injuries. In: *Wildlife Rehabilitation*, vol. 12 (ed. D. Ludwig), 55–66. St Cloud, MN: National Wildlife Rehabilitators Association.

Gancz, A.Y., Barker, I.K., Lindsay, R. et al. (2004). West Nile virus outbreak in North American owls, Ontario, 2002. *Emerging Infectious Diseases* 10: 2135–2142.

Gerhold, R.W., Tate, C.M., Gibbs, S.E. et al. (2007). Necropsy findings and arbovirus surveillance in mourning doves from the southeastern United States. *Journal of Wildlife Diseases*, 43 (1): 129–135.

Gibson, M. (in press). Wild turkeys, quail, grouse, and pheasants. In: *Hand Rearing Birds*, 2nd Ed. (ed. R.S. Duerr and L.J. Gage). Hoboken, NJ: Wiley.

Hartup, B.K., Mohammed, H.O., Kollias, G.V., and Dhondt, A.A. (1998). Risk factors associated with mycoplasmal conjunctivitis in house finches. *Journal of Wildlife Diseases* 34: 281–288.

Hawkins, M.G. and Pascoe, P.J. (2007). Cagebirds. In: *Zoo Animal & Wildlife Immobilization and Anesthesia* (ed. G. West, D. Heard and N. Caulkett), 269–297. Ames, IA: Wiley.

Hoggard, C. (2007). Nutritional considerations for critical wildlife patients. In: *Topics in Wildlife Medicine: Emergency and Critical Care,* (ed. F.S. Tseng and M.A. Mitchell), 112–126. St Cloud, MN: National Wildlife Rehabilitators Association.

Howard, L.L., Papendick, R., Stalis, I.H. et al. (2002). Fenbendazole and albendazole toxicity in pigeons and doves. *Journal of Avian Medicine and Surgery* 16 (3): 203–210.

Hubálek, Z. (2004). An annotated checklist of pathogenic microorganisms associated with migratory birds. *Journal of Wildlife Diseases* 40 (4): 639–659.

Hufford, L. (in press). Goat suckers. In: *Hand Rearing Birds*, 2nd Ed. (ed. R.S. Duerr and L.J. Gage). Hoboken, NJ: Wiley.

Jackman, T. and Meier, J.E. (2013). A case study of cryptosporidium-like disease in American cliff swallows. *Wildlife Rehabilitation Bulletin* 31 (1): 31–35.

Kinde, H., Foate, E., Beeler, E. et al. (2012). Strong circumstantial evidence for ethanol toxicosis in cedar waxwings (*Bombycilla cedrorum*). *Journal of Ornithology* 153 (3): 995–998.

Klasing, K.C. (1999). *Comparative Avian Nutrition*. New York: CAB International.

Komar, N., Langevin, S., Hinten, S. et al. (2003). Experimental infection of North American birds with the New York 1999 strain of West Nile virus. *Emerging Infectious Diseases* 9 (3): 311–322.

Kudlacik, M. and Eilertsen, M. (in press). Pigeons and doves. In: *Hand Rearing Birds*, 2nd Ed. (ed. R.S. Duerr and L.J. Gage). Hoboken, NJ: Wiley.

Ley, D.H., Hawley, D.M., Geary, S.J. et al. (2016). House finch (*Haemorhous mexicanus*) conjunctivitis, and *Mycoplasma* spp. isolated from North American wild birds, 1994–2015. *Journal of Wildlife Diseases* 52 (3): 669–673.

Luttrell, P. and Fischer, J.R. (2007). Mycoplasmosis. In: *Infectious Diseases of Wild Birds* (ed. N.J. Thomas, D.B. Hunter and C.T. Atkinson), 317–331. Ames, IA: Wiley.

Macwhirter, P. (1994). Passeriformes. In: *Avian Medicine: Principles and Application* (ed. B.W. Ritchie, G.J. Harrison and L.R. Harrison), 1172–1189. Lake Worth, FL: Wingers Publishing Inc.

Mashima, T.Y., Ley, D.H., Stoskopf, M.K. et al. (1997). Evaluation of treatment of conjunctivitis associated with *Mycoplasma gallisepticum* in house finches (*Carpodacus mexicanus*). *Journal of Avian Medicine and Surgery* 11 (1): 20–24.

Mehlhorn, H.E.A. (1990). Loperamid, an efficacious drug against the acanthocephalan *Macracanthorhynchus hirudinaceus* in pigs. *Parasitology Research* 76: 624–626.

Miller, E.A. (1996). Captive care of mourning doves. *NWRA Quarterly* 14 (2): 1–6.

Miller, E.A. (2012). *Minimum Standards for Wildlife Rehabilitation*, 4e. St Cloud, MN: National Wildlife Rehabilitators Association.

Myers, D. (2007). Fluid therapy considerations for wildlife. In: *Topics in Wildlife Medicine: Emergency and Critical Care* (ed. F.S. Tseng and M.A. Mitchell), 26–39. St Cloud, MN: National Wildlife Rehabilitators Association.

Nemeth, N.M., Kratz, G.E., Bates, R. et al. (2009). Clinical evaluation and outcomes of naturally acquired West Nile virus infection in raptors. *Journal of Zoo and Wildlife Medicine* 40 (1): 51–63.

NWHC (2002). *Epizootic Files*. Madison, WI: United States Geological Survey, National Wildlife Health Center,.

Patton, C.S. and Patton, S. (1996). *Tetratrichomonas gallinarioum* encephalitis in a mockingbird (*Mimus polyglottos*). *Journal of Veterinary Diagnostic Investigations* 8: 133–137.

Proctor, N.S. and Lynch, P.J. (1993). *Manual of Ornithology*, 66–69. New Haven, CT: Yale University Press.

Prum, R.O., Berv, J., Dornburg, A. et al. (2015). A comprehensive phylogeny of birds (Aves) using targeted next-generation DNA sequencing. *Nature.* 526 (7574): 569–573.

Quesenberry, K. and Hillyer, E. (1994). Supportive care and emergency therapy. In: *Avian Medicine: Principles and Application* (ed. B.W. Ritchie, G.J. Harrison and L.R. Harrison), 383–416. Lake Worth, FL: Wingers Publishing Inc.

Remillard, R., Armstrong, P., and Davenport, D. (2000). Assisted feeding in hospitalized patients: enteral and parenteral nutrition. In: *Small Animal Clinical Nutrition* (ed. M. Hand, C. Thaytcher, R. Remillard and P. Roudenbush), 351–399. Topeka, KS: Mark Morris Institute.

van Riper, C. and Forrester, D.J. (2007). Avian pox. In: *Infectious Diseases of Wild Birds* (ed. N.J. Thomas, D.B. Hunter and C.T. Atkinson), 131–176. Ames, IA: Wiley.

Schales, C. and Schales, K. (1994). Galliformes. In: *Avian Medicine: Principles and Application* (ed. B.W. Ritchie, G.J. Harrison and L.R. Harrison), 1219–1236. Lake Worth, FL: Wingers Publishing Inc.

Scott, M.R. (2013). *Songbird Diet Index*. St Cloud, MN: National Wildlife Rehabilitators Association.

Slusher, M.J., Wilcox, B.R., Lutrell, M.P. et al. (2014). Are passerine birds reservoirs for influenza a viruses? *Journal of Wildlife Diseases* 50 (4): 792–809.

Smith, J.A. (2015). Passeriformes (songbirds, perching birds). In: *Fowler's Zoo and Wild Animal Medicine*, vol. 8 (ed. R.E. Miller and M.E. Fowler), 236–246. St Louis, MO: Elsevier Saunders.

St. Leger J. & Shivaprasad, H.L. (1998). Passerine Protozoal Sinusitis: An Infection You Should Know About. Proceedings of the Association of Avian Veterinarians Annual Conference.

Stallknecht, D.E., Naby, E., Hunter, D.B., and Slemons, R.D. (2007). Avian influenza. In: *Infectious Diseases of Wild Birds* (ed. N.J. Thomas, D.B. Hunter and C.T. Atkinson), 108–130. Ames, IA: Wiley.

Terres, J.K. (1982). *The Audubon Encyclopedia of North American Birds*. New York: Alfred A. Knopf, Inc.

Travis, D. (2008). West Nile virus in birds and mammals. In: *Zoo and Wild Animals Medicine: Current Therapy*, 6e (ed. M.E. Fowler and R.E. Miller), 2–9. St Louis, MO: Elsevier Saunders.

Tseng, F. (2005). Refeeding syndrome: how to avoid killing your patients with kindness. Poster presented at Wildlife Rehabilitators Association of Massachusetts (WRAM) Conference, Tufts University.

Welte, S.C. (2000). Protozoal sinusitis in passerines. In: *Wildlife Rehabilitation*, vol. 18 (ed. D. Ludwig), 109–116. St Cloud, MN: National Wildlife Rehabilitators Association.

Wojciechowski, M.S. and Pinshow, B. (2009). Heterothermy in small migrating passerine birds during stopover: use of hypothermia at rest accelerates fuel accumulation. *Journal of Experimental Biology* 212 (19): 3068–3075.

Woldemeskel, M. and Styer, E.L. (2010). Feeding behavior-related toxicity due to Nandina domestica in cedar waxwings (Bombycilla cedrorum). *Veterinary Medicine International* 2010: 1–4.

Web Resources

- All About Birds – this easy-to-use online resource for North American species is available from the Cornell Lab of Ornithology. Birding Basics leads the user through a series of questions based on external features; users can also search by common name or taxonomic grouping to confirm identification and basic information needed for captive care. www.allaboutbirds.org/guide/browse_tax/12

- Birds of North America online – this membership-supported resource is available from the Cornell Lab of Ornithology and provides comprehensive life histories for each of the 716+ species of birds breeding in the USA (including Hawaii) and Canada. http://bna.birds.cornell.edu
- Lafeber's Emeraid Critical Care System Formulations for North American Wild Animals. www.lefebervet.com

17

Natural History and Medical Management of Raptors

David Scott

Carolina Raptor Center, Huntersville, NC, USA

Natural History

Birds of prey are a very diverse group. Natural habitat requirements vary from open fields and dry desert to dense woods and waterways. Correspondingly, their diet and normal prey also vary, so it is imperative that the rehabilitator or clinician fully understand these aspects of natural history. Sibley (2000, 2001) provides an excellent overview of many avian species, including birds of prey.

Birds of prey generally fall into four major categories or groups: hawks and their allies, falcons, owls, and vultures. In general, birds of prey are characterized by hooked beaks and sharp talons, both of which are used for grasping and tearing flesh. Identification and aging of birds of prey are both difficult and crucial to proper care while in captivity. Scott (2010) provides a quick aging guide for some common raptor species.

Accipitridae

The family Accipitridae includes the majority of the diurnal raptors worldwide with greater than 230 species, ranging from the *Buteo* hawks, the *accipiters*, to the kites and eagles. Habitat ranges across the globe with the exception of the extreme Arctic and Antarctic.

Members of this family are usually monogamous and often pair for life. Stick nests are typically built or used, oftentimes lined with leaves, grass or other material to help protect the eggs. Nest placement varies depending on the species and nests can be found on the ground, in low bushes, on cliffs or in trees. Usually one clutch of eggs is laid each year and both sexes will incubate them, although this is typically the responsibility of the female. The incubation period ranges from 28 to 35 days depending on the species and clutch size varies widely, with 2–3 eggs being most typical. The young are altricial but their eyes open quickly after hatching and the young of smaller species can fledge as early as 3–4 weeks of age. During the nestling period, the male does most of the hunting and the female stays near the nest to protect and feed the chicks.

Most species in this family display reverse sexual dimorphism in that the female is typically larger than the male. In general, plumage coloration is designed to blend into the environment with a predominance of beiges and browns in streaks and bars. The plumage of juveniles is somewhat uniform across many species but the adult plumage is quite varied and is generally apparent by the end of the first molt in the second year. Sexual dimorphism is rare.

Diet is highly variable and includes birds, fish, amphibians, reptiles, and invertebrates as well as the opportunistic use of carrion. Some species are generalists and others, such as osprey (*Pandion haliaetus*) and snail kites (*Rostrhamus sociabilis*), have very specialized diets. The preferred prey often determines the hunting range. Accipiters hunt in forests, making short flights between concealed perches. Buteos such as red-tailed hawks (*Buteo jamaicensis*) often soar from a high elevation scanning for prey and can also be seen on a tall perch waiting for prey. Some species such as the Mississippi kite (*Ictinia mississippiensis*) will hunt on the wing and most species hunt alone. However, hunting in packs is well documented in the Harris hawk (*Parabuteo unicinctus*).

Many raptor species migrate in the fall. The migrations occur by day and can often involve synchronized groups of thousands of birds. The migration can span thousands of miles, with many North American species wintering as far south as Argentina. The migration routes usually follow topographic features that support thermals on which they soar. Migration over open water is avoided.

Medical Management of Wildlife Species: A Guide for Practitioners, First Edition. Edited by Sonia M. Hernandez, Heather W. Barron, Erica A. Miller, Roberto F. Aguilar and Michael J. Yabsley.

Falconidae

The family Falconidae includes the true falcons such as the peregrine falcon as well as the caracaras. The true falcons range in size from the American kestrel (*Falco sparverius*) at 100–130 g all the way up to the peregrine falcon (*Falco peregrinus*) and the gyrfalcon (*Falco rusticolus*) which can weigh over 1000 g. These birds typically have long pointed wings and are known for very high speeds in level flight and during a stoop. Because of this, they are well liked in the falconry community.

Many falcon species have a dark vertical bar in their plumage beneath each eye. They also have a small "tomial" tooth on the edge of the upper beak and many have a small protuberance in the center of each nare that is thought to assist in airflow when flying at high speed.

Habitat ranges widely from northern frozen tundra to arid desert. Many falcons, such as the peregrine, catch prey in flight and birds can make up a large portion of the diet of many falcon species. Prey can be grabbed in flight or stunned with a high-speed, midair impact and are grabbed in a second pass as they fall to the ground.

Many falcons nest on cliffs or rock ledges but some will use cavities in trees (American kestrel) or old nests (merlin, *Falco columbarius*) built by other species.

Owls

The owls include the typical owls in family Strigidae as well as the barn owls in family Tyonidae. Owls are mainly nocturnal, although there are several exceptions, including the short-eared owl (*Asio flammeus*), that are diurnal. They range in size from the insectivorous elf owl (*Mirathene whitneyi*, 40 g) to the Eurasian eagle owl (*Bubo bubo*) and the snowy owl (*Nyctea scandiaca*) that can weigh in excess of 2000 g. Most owls share many characteristics including forward-facing eyes, facial discs surrounding the eyes, zygodactyl feet, and feather adaptions that decrease or even eliminate sound during flight. Many owls have horn-like feather tufts that function for camouflage and display purposes. The barn owl (*Tyto alba*) is the most widespread owl species worldwide and is also morphologically and behaviorally distinct from most other owls. They have long, thin legs, heart-shaped facial discs and can breed year-round.

Owls live in a diverse set of habitats ranging from the Arctic tundra and rainforests to farmland and urban areas. Diet and desired prey vary widely from small insects, rodents, crayfish, and even fish to large mammals. Whereas hawks and their allies are mostly visual hunters, owls rely on sound as well as sight. Owls are more apt to swallow their prey whole rather than tearing it up into smaller pieces before swallowing. Owls do not have a crop (ingluvies) and their pellets, unlike those of diurnal birds of prey, contain undigested bones.

Small owls generally use a cavity for nesting. Larger species will reuse a stick nest built by another species and the burrowing owl (*Athene cunicularia*) will nest in tunnels dug by other animals. With the exception of the barn owl, one clutch of eggs is produced each year and incubation is typically performed by the female.

Many owls maintain permanent territories. Some do migrate, although not to the extent or distance of diurnal raptors. Irruptions are winter movements in which northern species such as the snowy owl move south in search of more abundant prey. The most common form of movement is the dispersal when young owls are forced away from their nest territory in the fall.

Vultures

The New World vultures of family Cathartidae are similar to Old World vultures but are actually more closely related to storks. They are large, soaring scavengers, with a wingspan of up to 9 ft (2.7 m) in the California condor (*Gymnogyps californianus*). The diet consists mostly of carrion, but black vultures (*Coragyps atratus*) and turkey vultures (*Cathartes aura*) have been known to take live prey such as nestlings or newborn calves. Carrion is normally found by sight while soaring on thermals but the turkey vulture has an strong sense of smell as well. Large groups will often form around a carcass to feed, with black vultures being the more dominant species. The head and neck are bare as adults in order to help keep clean while feeding on a carcass. The feet are adapted for walking and, unlike those of other raptors, are relatively weak with short talons.

Nests are often built on cliffs, in caves or on horizontal man-made structures. Since vulture feet are not adapted for carrying food, vultures must carry food in their crop and regurgitate at the nest site to feed their chicks. Fledging takes much longer than in most other raptors (three months in vultures and six months in condors). In additions, these birds are particularly easy to malimprint when young and therefore present a significant challenge when in a rehabilitation setting.

Husbandry

Proper husbandry practices are critical to successfully work with birds of prey. This includes providing appropriate caging, perching, and diet, as well as making all attempts to minimize stress. Arent (2007) is the definitive guide covering all aspects of captive management for birds of prey.

Indoor Housing

In general, birds of prey do well, at least initially, in dog or cat carriers or standard veterinary hospital caging, as long as they are modified to include a perch. The appropriate-sized cage should be provided so there is space above the bird's head when it is on the perch. Table 17.1 lists kennel sizes for typical species. Once the patient has begun to recover, it will likely need to be moved to a larger enclosure. It is very important to keep birds of prey in a location free from loud noises, barking dogs, and even human speech. Raptors are also very visual animals, thus providing a visual barrier in front of their cage/kennel will aid in lowering stress.

Outdoor Housing

There are several factors to consider when designing and building an outdoor enclosure for birds of prey. In addition, the size of the enclosure is very much determined by the species. This is especially important when needing to exercise and evaluate flight.

- All cages for flighted birds must have a double-door system to prevent escapes and accidental release.
- Appropriate predator proofing must be incorporated into the construction and includes using materials of sufficient strength to keep predators out. It also must include a barrier to prevent predators from burrowing under the cage perimeter. Chainlink fence secured on or under the ground around the perimeter is very effective.
- The walls should be made of vertical slats of wood or another similar material. The important detail is that the openings are vertical and will not snag or catch the tail feathers if and when the bird grabs onto the walls. If chainlink or any other mesh is used, the tail feathers will get caught and can be severely damaged.
- It is critical that all cages have adequate ventilation, with direct access to sunlight as well as shaded areas.

- Ideally, in areas where mosquitoes or other biting insects are a problem, appropriately sized netting or mesh should be used. This netting should be attached to the outside of the slats so that the feathers will not be damaged.
- The substrate on the ground should be a nonorganic material to decrease the risk of fungal diseases such as aspergillosis. Smooth pea gravel 1/4 to 1/2 in. in diameter is ideal and is easy on the feet. Gravel with jagged edges should never be used. The one exception to the "no organic" rule is in cages used for live prey testing. In these cages, it is important to use natural ground cover such as leaf litter in order to provide hiding places for the mice and to ensure that the live prey test is as realistic as possible.
- Feeding hatches are important for orphans so food can be provided without requiring entry into the cage. This is most crucial in young birds at risk for habituation or improper imprinting.

Perches

Perches of various sizes and textures should be provided. It is very important that birds be given several different choices to minimize the risk of bumblefoot. Perches should be installed at various heights and provide enough space so that all the birds in an enclosure can find a comfortable place to perch without having to gather too closely together. Floor standing perches should be provided for birds that are unable to fly. Birds should never be forced to stand on the ground. Perches can be made from many different materials including natural branches or 2 × 2 stock covered in AstroTurf or "daisy mat" material. Perch diameter is also very important. In general, the perch should be of sufficient diameter that the talons are not curled under too much or spread out too flat. The key is to provide variety. If a perch is too small, bumblefoot tends to develop on the sole/center pads. If a perch is too large, bumblefoot tends to develop on the toes.

Tail Wraps and Wrist Protection

Feather damage is not uncommon in captivity but it can be avoided or minimized. This is especially true of the tail feathers which are often damaged or broken. Placing a tail wrap is an inexpensive and easy way to protect the tail feathers. This is particularly important in species that are known to be more stressed in captivity, or that have long tails, or that are unable to stand. The Cooper's hawk is an example of a species that should have a tail wrap placed immediately upon admission. Tail wraps are also useful to prevent feather damage when a bird is being shipped or transported in a kennel.

Table 17.1 Kennel sizes for various species.

Species	Kennel size (L × W × H in inches)
American kestrel, screech owl	18 × 12 × 15
Cooper's hawk	24 × 17 × 18
Red-shouldered hawk, barred owl	32 × 21 × 24
Red-tailed hawk, great-horned owl	32 × 21 × 24
Vulture	36 × 24 × 30
Eagle	36 × 24 × 30

The wrap can be made by folding and cutting a piece of radiograph film or a manila office folder. The wrap is attached to the bird with masking tape secured to the downy covert feathers on the dorsal and ventral side of the tail. It is important that the feathers around the vent are not taped into place in such a way as to block the vent.

Carpal wounds are another common problem that can occur in captivity. Trauma to the carpus can easily result in an open wound over the carpal joint or metacarpal bones. These wounds can take a long time to heal and may result in irreparable joint damage, so prevention is imperative. A simple, padded "bumper" can be made by securing a few layers of gauze or nonadherent pad (Telfa, Kendall/Tyco Healthcare, Mansfield, MA, USA) to the cranial edge of the carpal joint with Tegaderm (3M Health Care, St Paul, MN, USA). This bandage provides good protection but does not limit range of motion or flight.

Diet

Birds of prey are obligate carnivores. Although many species do scavenge carrion for a significant part of their diet, the majority hunt live prey. Despite this, most species do quite well on a diet of thawed frozen prey. While the majority of birds of prey eat rodents, osprey are strictly piscivorous and accipiters primarily eat other birds. Bald eagles will eat rodents or fish but also scavenge from carcasses. Table 17.2 outlines the daily food requirements for many species. Supplementation with vitamins (Vitahawk, D.B. Scientific, Oakley, CA, USA) is recommended 2–3 times per week and is especially important when feeding exclusively fish diets since many species of fish contain thiaminase.

Birds that are on twice-daily medicationss should have their diet split in two portions. This is important as medications should be given in the food if the bird is reliably eating in order to minimize the stress of handling. Birds that are only fed once daily should be fed in the morning or afternoon if diurnal or early evening if nocturnal.

Handling and Restraint

Proper restraint is important for the patient's well-being and for handler safety. Always remember that the talons, in most cases, are the most dangerous part of the bird and should be restrained at all times.

- Appropriately sized leather gloves should always be worn. They must be thick enough to protect the wearer but not too thick as they can make handling cumbersome. Goggles should be worn to protect the handler's eyes, especially when grabbing a bird of prey from a small enclosure like a kennel.
- The legs should be held with the index finger between them. This is more comfortable for the bird (the legs will not rub) and the grip is much more secure (Figure 17.1).

Table 17.2 Daily food requirements for various species.

Species	Daily food requirements
American kestrel, screech owl	20–30 g mouse
Red-shouldered hawk, barred owl	60–75 g mouse, rat, chick
Cooper's hawk	80–90 g mouse, chick, quail
Red-tailed hawk, great-horned owl	110–120 g mouse, chick, rat
Black vulture, turkey vulture	175–200 rat
Osprey	200–225 g fish
Bald eagle	250–300 rat, fish

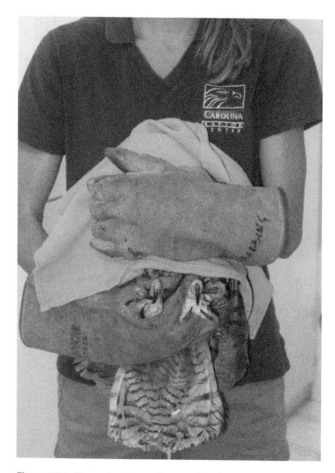

Figure 17.1 Proper handling of raptors involves restraining the legs by keeping one finger between them.

- The legs should always be grabbed as close to the body as possible (i.e., above the stifle joints) to avoid iatrogenic fractures. This is especially important in birds with long, thin legs such as Cooper's hawks. Once the bird is adequately restrained, the grip should be moved closer to the feet for better control of the talons.
- When transporting a bird, secure the legs with an underhand grip, cover the bird's head with a light towel or hood and place the bird's back to your chest. Gently place your other hand across the chest (be careful not to interfere with respiration) to hold the beak up. This method effectively protects the bird's face from its talons and also restrains both wings.
- The eyes and head should be covered with a light towel or hood whenever possible as this can have a dramatic calming effect.
- To decrease stress, consider using general anesthesia or anxiolytics (e.g., midazolam) when doing examinations or treatments.
- Vultures use their beak for defense so their head must be gently restrained at all times. This can be done by covering the head with a towel and loosely encircling the neck with your fingers just under the mandible.
- Young birds should be handled with extreme caution. In most cases, these birds should be handled as little as possible, should not be manipulated onto their back unless absolutely necessary and should be transported in a box, rather than hand-carried. Young birds and hatchlings should never be grabbed by the legs. Always use a body grab from behind with the wings carefully folded up against the body.

Clinically Relevant Anatomy and Physiology

Physical Examination

The majority of the physical exam can be achieved with the bird restrained on its back and a complete exam can be done in under 5 minutes. Most procedures involving birds of prey, including examinations, require two people. This allows the process to be most efficient and safe and, most importantly, minimizes stress to the patient. A methodical approach covering the entire body should be followed each time. Pay particular attention to the following points.

- The eyes are of critical importance to raptors. In a recent study, 40% of admitted wild raptors had significant damage in at least one posterior chamber (Scott 2015) (Figure 17.2). Typical findings include retinal detachment as well as large amounts of fresh blood and floating fibrinous debris. Detached areas often appear as a bright white, smooth area with a sharp margin. It is also very common to see evidence of

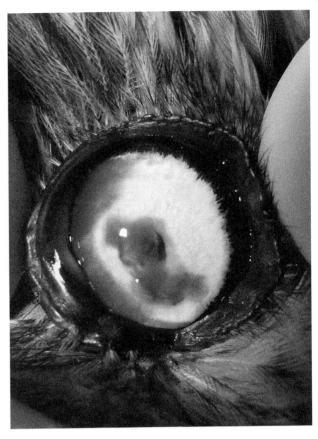

Figure 17.2 Ocular lesions in both the posterior segment and/or the anterior chamber, like the hyphema in this individual, may be seen in raptors presenting for traumatic injuries.

chronic retinal damage including rough or blotchy dark areas without overlying floating debris. Note that damage to the anterior chamber and cornea is less common so it is very important that a careful fundic exam be performed on admission.
- Examine the mouth and look for caseous, necrotic lesions or thick ropy mucus as these can indicate an infection with *Trichomonas* spp.
- The body condition score (BCS), in combination with the weight, is critical when evaluating an avian patient's overall health. The BCS typically ranges from 1 to 5 where 1 is severe emaciation, 3–4 is a healthy individual and 5 indicates a potentially overconditioned animal. Therefore, the keel bone along the midline will be clearly visible in a healthy bird unless it is covered by a layer of subcutaneous fat.
- Coracoid bone fractures are very common but are also very difficult to palpate during an exam. A radiograph (ventrodorsal view) is required in order to diagnose this fracture.
- The feathers are often damaged secondary to trauma, barbed-wire fences, and, unfortunately, inappropriate care and handling while in captivity. It is very important

that all attempts be made to protect the feathers, especially in younger birds whose feathers are still developing. Feather condition can be graded from best to worst as: normal, frayed, tipped, bent, broken but repairable, broken and not repairable, or missing entirely. Whenever possible, the condition of all primary wing feathers and tail feathers should be recorded accurately. Feather condition in owls is particularly important as they rely on stealth and silence in flight and even minor damage can affect their sound level enough to make an owl nonreleasable. The feathers can be protected in many ways.

- Proper handling: be very careful with the tail and primary wing feathers when handling and during exams.
- Proper caging: avoid any sort of mesh that allows the feathers to slip through and become damaged.
- Place a tail wrap, especially in high-stress species such as Cooper's hawks.

Radiographs should be taken if possible, but proper positioning is critical in order for them to have any diagnostic value. For the ventral/dorsal (VD) view, the keel and spine must be perfectly overlaid, the wings should be stretched out symmetrically and the legs should be pulled down to ensure that the elbow and stifle joints are not overlapped. The VD view can sometimes be taken without anesthesia but best results are obtained with anesthesia. The lateral view, however, cannot be taken without anesthesia. In order to align this view properly, the wings are both pulled back dorsally and the legs are pulled back caudally. The shoulders and coxofemoral joints should be overlaid as much as possible.

Bloodwork can be very useful in cases where the cause of injury or illness is not obvious. This is especially true for aspergillosis where the patient can appear relatively normal initially. Blood can be collected from the jugular vein, from the basilic vein on the ventral side of the elbow joint or from the medial metatarsal vein. A minimum database should include a packed cell volume (PCV) and total solids (TS) as well as an estimated complete blood count (CBC) (Table 17.3).

Treatments and Triage

There are many conditions and injuries that can be managed with a reasonable chance of successful release. However, the opposite is also true. In general, the following injuries would necessitate immediate, humane euthanasia.

- Severe or total loss of vision in one or both eyes. Owls are an exception and can sometimes be released if blind in one eye (Scott 2013).
- Severe degloving wounds such as from barbed-wire injuries.
- Loss of the first or second digit on either foot (except for vultures which do not rely on grasping of prey items).
- Any amputation of any part of the wing.
- A fracture with dry, devitalized exposed bone, extensive necrotic tissue or involving a joint. In addition, chronic fractures with a significant amount of fibrous scar tissue and poor range of motion generally cannot be repaired.

Antibiotics are appropriate for severe soft tissue wounds or open fractures. A combination of enrofloxacin and clindamycin works well to prevent osteomyelitis.

Common Reasons for Presentation

Infectious and Parasitic Diseases

Aspergillosis
Aspergillosis is a very common disease in raptors and should be a top differential for any animal that is systemically ill and presents with emaciation and/or lethargy. It is particularly common in juvenile red-tailed hawks. It is caused by a fungus (*Aspergillus* spp.) which is a ubiquitous, saprophytic, opportunistic organism. It is not contagious or zoonotic.

This disease can cause a primary illness or can be secondary to any condition (such as trauma or a fracture) that leads to debilitation. The disease can also occur while an animal is in captivity as a result of immunosuppression

Table 17.3 Changes seen on the complete blood count (CBC) and total solids.

Indices	Increase	Decrease
Packed cell volume	Dehydration	Chronic disease, emaciation
Heterophil	Inflammation or infection	Acute or overwhelming infection
Lymphocyte	Chronic antigenic stimulation, leukemia	Stress, corticosteroid use
Monocyte	Chronic, granulomatous infection (aspergillosis, *Mycobacterium*), tissue damage	
Eosinophil	Unknown – function unclear. Possibly related to parasitism	

secondary to stress. Diagnosis can be difficult but endoscopic examination of the air sacs is the best way to get a definitive diagnosis. Radiographs may be helpful and a CBC may show a marked leukocytosis with a heterophilia and/or monocytosis. An elevated total solids (TS) is also very common. It is important to note that respiratory signs are not typically seen until very late in the disease.

Early diagnosis is key to successful outcome. Treatment consists of supportive care as well as use of an antifungal such as amphotericin B, itraconazole, terbinafine, or voriconazole. Surgical removal of granulomas may be indicated for focal infections. Prevention is very important and steps should be taken to minimize stress while in captivity. Use of antibiotics should be avoided unless needed and prophylactic treatment with itraconazole and oral terbinafine has been useful in the author's experience (Bechert et al. 2010).

West Nile Virus

This virus primarily causes encephalitis. The vectors are mosquitoes but consumption of infected animals can also lead to infection (Ip et al. 2014). Birds are reservoirs but often develop clinical disease due to infection. It was first seen in the western hemisphere in 1999 but has now been reported in most states and it affects many species of birds. Corvids are highly susceptible but many species of raptors (especially great-horned owls and Cooper's hawks) have also been seriously affected. This disease is zoonotic but is not transmitted directly from birds to humans.

Clinical signs develop 10–12 days post infection and can include any type of neurological signs, including ataxia and seizures, vision loss from retinal pathology, feather growth abnormalities including a "pinched-off" calamus, or sudden death. Although many raptor infections result in mortality, some birds with milder clinical signs may recover but should be monitored for neurological sequelae (Nemeth et al. 2009).

Definitive diagnosis is typically made using a polymerase chain reaction (PCR) test on a combined choanal/cloacal swab or blood sample. However, false negatives are not uncommon as the period of viremia can be very short (2–7 days) (Redig 2010a). Since this virus is usually transmitted by mosquitoes, this disease would only be expected in the warmer months of the year. Note that bird-to-bird transmission is possible so appropriate measures should be taken (Banet-Noach et al. 2003).

Trichomoniasis

This disease is caused by flagellated protozoa (*Trichomonas* spp.) which infect the oral cavity and upper gastrointestinal tract. Pigeons and other columbiformes as well as some passerines are common hosts and may develop a disease known as "canker." Raptors are usually infected after eating fresh pigeons and the disease is known as "frounce."

Large, caseous lesions are commonly found in the mouth, under the tongue and around the choana (Figure 17.3). The masses can get so large that eating and breathing can be difficult and it is not uncommon for birds to become emaciated as a result. In addition, lesions in the roof of the mouth can erode through the hard palate and into the sinuses. Dysphagia and "food flicking" are also common. Diagnosis is based on physical findings and the motile organisms may be seen on a saline wet-mount from an oral swab. Treatment includes use of either metronidazole or carnidazole as well as surgical debridement. Supportive care is also necessary in emaciated cases.

Emaciation

Emaciation is not a disease in itself but the result of some other underlying problem such as systemic disease (aspergillosis, West Nile virus, etc.), poor hunting ability in a young bird, or traumatic injury such as a fracture. Severely emaciated birds are in a hypometabolic state and they need to be slowly and gradually returned to a normal physiological state. These birds are suspected at risk for "refeeding syndrome" so it is vitally important that they are not fed calorically dense diets immediately (for a more in-depth review see Murray (2014)). While not previously defined in raptors, it is the author's experience that refeeding syndrome usually occurs within 3–7 days of starting to feed. Patients can develop fluid and electrolyte disorders, especially hypophosphatemia, along with systemic complications.

A typical treatment protocol consists of the following.

- Rehydration with large volumes of fluids. As a rule of thumb, starting with twice maintenance split three times daily for 2–3 days works well. Monitoring of the

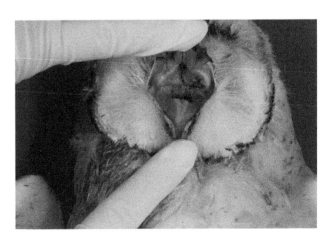

Figure 17.3 Trichomoniasis lesions in the mouth of a barn owl (*Tyto alba*).

PCV and TS can be helpful. Values below 15% and 1.0 g/dL, respectively, have a very poor prognosis and such animals may need to be euthanized. Care must be taken when giving fluids via the IV or IO route as substantial hemodilution of an already hypoproteinemic/anemic bird can result.

- Use of an oral gel such as Nutri-Cal (Vetoquinol, Fort Worth, TX, USA) may provide temporary benefit in hypoglycemic animals.
- Vitamin B-complex can be added to the fluids.
- Iron dextran given intramuscularly on admission and repeated again in 10 days in birds that have or are at risk for anemia.
- Provide heat support as needed.
- An antifungal, such as itraconazole or terbinafine, is often given preventively, especially in juvenile red-tailed hawks or other high-risk species or facilities.
- After 24 hours of rehydration, start feeding small amounts of clean (furless, with large bone fragments removed) meat. An initial amount is typically 10 g/kg q8h. This can be ramped up slowly over the following 3–4 days. Alternatively, a carnivore formula diet can be provided via stomach tube.

Recovery can be dramatic but it is not uncommon for these birds to appear to improve for a few days only to die on day 3 or 4. Even in the best of circumstances, only about 50% of these birds will survive (Scott 2015).

Lead Toxicosis

Lead toxicosis is most commonly caused by the ingestion of prey containing lead shot (Redig 2009), fragments from bullets or fishing sinkers. It is usually seen in bald eagles which often scavenge deer carcasses but could also be seen in osprey and vultures due to their eating habits. The disease causes physical damage to nervous tissue which is thought to be secondary to a vasculitis and resulting hemorrhage/necrosis (Redig 2010b). It is important to realize that lead embedded in muscle tissue subsequent to a gunshot injury typically does not result in lead toxicity.

These patients may present with either the acute or chronic form. The acute form is less common and these birds will likely be in good body condition but may exhibit severe neurological signs like tremors, seizures, paralysis, and blindness. The chronic form is characterized by generalized weakness and emaciation. In either case, the diagnosis is made by measuring the blood lead level. A level of 20 μg/dL (0.2 ppm) is generally considered a toxic level but this does vary with species and with the individual. Note that ingested lead may have already been broken down and absorbed and thus would not be visible on a radiograph. Orthogonal views will improve the ability to accurately localize any suspected metallic foreign bodies.

Treatment includes supportive measures (fluids, nutritional support, etc.) and chelation in order to remove the heavy metal from the blood as well as from depot tissues such as bone. Calcium EDTA is an injectable chelation agent that should be used initially. Once the patient is self-feeding, dimercaptosuccinic acid (DMSA) can be administered in the food. Any macroscopic metallic foreign bodies seen that are suspected to be in the lumen of the gastrointestinal tract need to be removed. This can be accomplished in many ways, including stomach lavage, the use of cathartics or laxatives, or through endoscopic/surgical removal. Luckily, birds of prey produce and expel a pellet or cast and in some cases, lead fragments in the ventriculus can be expelled with the pellet.

Chelation therapy is a multistep process in which the patient is chelated for 2–4 weeks, with intermittent "off" periods. During these periods it is not uncommon for the blood lead level to rebound as more lead leaches out of bone stores. For this reason, it can take several rounds of chelation and testing before the lead has reduced to a sufficiently low level.

Maggot Infestation

Maggot infestations are commonly seen in the summer months. The infestation may be located on an existing wound or be centered around actively growing blood feathers in younger birds. These infestations should be treated as an emergency since they can produce a staggering amount of damage in a very short period of time. Contrary to popular belief, many maggots do indeed consume healthy tissue. In addition to the actual maggots, there may be clumps of fly eggs attached to the feathers. All wounds and blood feathers should be carefully inspected for maggots or fly eggs. Areas such as the vent, the base of the tail, and the elbows seem to be preferred locations for maggots.

Maggots and fly eggs must be physically removed. Removal can sometimes take a great deal of time and general anesthesia is helpful. The infestation can be very severe and require that feathers be plucked. Clumps of eggs can simply be crushed if they are too numerous or difficult to remove. All wounds should be thoroughly flushed and debrided. Application of topical nitenpyram (Capstar, Novartis Animal Health, Greensboro, NC, USA) is very effective in killing the maggots quickly and will help greatly in their removal. The tablets can be crushed, mixed with water and sprayed directly on maggots in the wounds. In addition, Capstar may be given orally to affected birds.

Trauma

Trauma secondary to vehicular collision is the most common identifiable cause of injury. Collisions with windows and gunshot are also very common causes of injury (Scott 2015).

Fractures

Fractures of the long bones and coracoid are frequently diagnosed, as well as fractures of the spine with trauma to the spinal cord.

All fractures should be stabilized with a wrap or splint until surgery, if indicated, can be performed. Fractures distal to the elbow joint (i.e., ulna, radius, or metacarpal) should be stabilized with a figure-of-eight wrap. Fractures proximal to the elbow (humerus, coracoid, scapula, and clavicle) should be stabilized with a figure-of-eight wrap that is extended with a body wrap. Fractures of the leg distal to the hock joint are stabilized with a modified Robert Jones splint. The splint can be stiffened with the use of metal (i.e., coat hanger) rods on the cranial and lateral aspects. The splint can be extended below the foot by incorporating a ball wrap or foam shoe. Foam shoes can be made by slicing off sections of "water noodles" used in swimming pools. Fractures of the distal to mid-tibiotarsus can be stabilized in a similar fashion with a Robert Jones splint but fractures of the proximal tibiotarsus or femur cannot be effectively splinted and generally require surgery as soon as possible.

The decision to repair a fracture surgically depends on several factors.

- The location of the fracture and the characteristics of the fracture. Well-aligned/transverse fractures can often be treated with a simple wrap or splint. Poorly aligned or oblique fractures usually require surgery. Fractures of the humerus and femur almost always require surgery.
- The chronicity of the fracture. Fractures older than 5–7 days tend have significant contracture and scar tissue which can make them difficult or impossible to repair.
- The proximity of the fracture to a joint. Fractures very close to a joint can be much more difficult to repair and also will lead to a lower chance of successful release.
- The age of the patient. Younger birds often heal faster and may require a simpler repair than adults.
- The skill of the surgeon. More comminuted fractures or fractures that are closer to a joint are significantly more difficult to repair.

In most cases, a combination intramedullary pin with an external skeletal fixation (IM-ESF) tie-in is the best choice as it affords very good stability, provides for an excellent range of motion and does not require the use of a bandage which can lead to contracture and stiffness at the joints (Figure 17.4). Samour (2008) and Scott (2010) provide a good description of the procedures for the most common fractures. There are a few exceptions where an IM-ESF fixation is not indicated.

- The radius is repaired with an IM pin only.
- The tarsometatarsus is repaired with an ESF only as an IM pin is not possible.
- The coracoid is better treated with conservative therapy. This includes a body wrap and once- or twice-weekly physical therapy (PT) for two weeks followed by two more weeks of cage rest. Scheelings (2014) has also found that simply using cage rest (without a wing wrap) for several weeks works just as well. Either way, once the cage rest period is over, the bird can be slowly introduced to exercise and moved to a progressively larger flight cage until full flight and conditioning are regained. The entire process can take less than eight weeks unless complications are encountered.

Regardless of whether surgery is performed or not, PT will be required. PT is generally done under general anesthesia. For the wing, the elbow and wrist should be repeatedly extended and flexed. The elbow and carpal

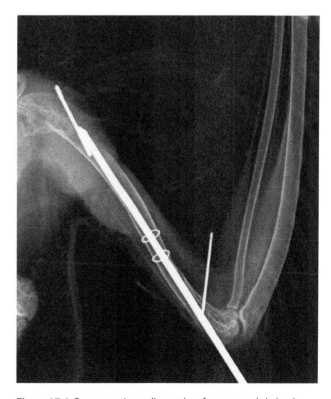

Figure 17.4 Postoperative radiographs of an external skeletal fixation with IM tie-in to repair a humeral fracture.

joints should generally extend to approximately 140° and 180°, respectively. In some species, such as osprey, the elbow can extend much further. If in doubt, always compare to the other wing. Use of a goniometer can assist in making accurate measurements. A typical protocol may involve doing PT three times weekly for 2–3 weeks or until full range of motion can be easily and repeatedly achieved (see Chapter 9). Implants are typically removed when the fracture feels stable on palpation and a callus is visible on radiographs. In some cases, staged removal of implants is warranted. In most cases, this process typically takes from four to five weeks, depending on the fracture. Once the implants are removed, cage rest is continued for two weeks before active flight conditioning is begun. Flight conditioning can be achieved with either a creance line or flight cages (Table 17.4).

Barbed-Wire Injuries

Barbed-wire injuries are usually very serious and can result in extensive degloving injuries that extend over large areas of the wing. Severe flight feather damage as well as fractures of the ulna and radius are also common. Owls, especially great-horned owls, are most commonly affected due to their preference for hunting in farm fields which are often bordered with barbed-wire fences.

The barbs are often deeply embedded in the skin of the propatagium and adjacent feathers. After anesthetizing the patient, the wire is most easily removed by cutting off the long ends and then derotating the remaining length to relieve the tension that has twisted the feathers and soft tissue around the barbs. Begin supportive care with antibiotics and analgesics as well as wound care and a figure-of-eight bandage. These injuries never display the full extent of the damage on admission so it is best to wait 7–10 days before any serious debridement or surgical repair is attempted.

Repeated debridements and PT will be required during the healing process. Scar tissue formation is very likely so every attempt must be made to prevent contracture and to maintain full range of motion. Damage to feathers and feather follicles can be significant. This is especially important in owls as their sound level in flight

Table 17.4 Minimum flight cage sizes for various species.

Species	Cage size (L × W × H in feet)
American kestrel, screech owl	30 × 8 × 8
Red-shouldered hawk, barred owl	50 × 12 × 12
Cooper's hawk	60 × 12 × 12
Great-horned owl	60 × 20 × 20
Red-tailed hawk, vulture, eagle	100 × 20 × 20

is critically important to survival. While the initial wound may heal, the resultant feather damage may still result in a nonreleasable bird.

Head Trauma

Trauma to the head, including the brain and eyes, is very likely, especially after impact with a vehicle or window.

Chorioretinitis, damage to the choroid and retina, is very common. The retina is avascular, so any damage is generally considered to be irreversible. The extent of the damage is what is important, and this can be very difficult to assess.

Treatment with meloxicam and supportive care can be beneficial and significant improvement can sometimes be seen in 2–3 weeks. Treatment with a single dose of corticosteroids (e.g., dexamethasone) is still recommended (Korbel, personal communication) if it can be administered within the first 24 hours after the injury. It is particularly important to note that large amounts of floating debris in the posterior chamber can make it impossible to adequately assess the retina. Because of this, enough time (i.e. 2–3 weeks) should be allowed for the inflammation to resolve so that the retina can be clearly visualized. It is not uncommon for cases to resolve significantly so that successful release can occur (Scott 2015). This can be true with diurnal raptors (specifically red-tailed hawks) but rarely for owls as the damage to the nocturnal retina tends to be much more severe.

Release of birds of prey that are blind in one eye is a controversial subject. Since diurnal raptors rely on binocular vision much more than a nocturnal bird, release would not be a good option. Nocturnal raptors, on the other hand, rely on hearing in addition to vision so they can potentially be released with damage to one eye. A recent study (Scott 2013) showed that one-eyed owls have a relatively good chance of survival and release can be considered in these cases. One must ensure that the remaining eye is perfect and it is suggested that these birds be released in a very rural environment so that the likelihood of encountering a vehicle is minimized.

Brain damage resulting in extreme lethargy, head tilt, and tremors is common and can be accompanied by ocular abnormalities as described above. Treatment is supportive and includes use of supplemental oxygen, meloxicam and mannitol, or hypertonic saline. Midazolam can be used as needed for tremors and seizures. Prognosis is guarded and depends on the extent of the initial damage. Birds that have recovered should have their neurological state tested thoroughly in a flight cage or by other means before release.

Orphans

Many hatchling and nestling birds of prey are presented at rehabilitation centers in the spring. While these birds are often referred to as "orphans," this terminology is usually incorrect as it is rare for the actual parents to be missing. These animals usually present after falling out of the nest or, more likely, after simply being found on the ground. It is important to realize that all birds of prey will spend some time on the ground as they develop and learn to fly. If left alone, the parents will provide for them and protect them. Because of this, most of these birds are best served by simply returning them to the location in which they were found.

However, the situation is complicated by the presence of dogs, cats, and wildlife as well as automobile traffic and other human activity which can clearly cause harm. In addition, actual injuries are not uncommon so a careful examination is required before planning a course of action. Remember to carefully check for fly eggs as well as fractures of the long bones in the legs and wings. Particular care must be taken during handling as the bones and blood feathers are extremely delicate and the liver normally extends beyond the borders of the sternum.

If the bird is healthy, it should be returned to the nest site. A downy hatchling or nestling must be returned to the nest and this may require the assistance of a skilled tree-climber or arborist. Birds that are branching (just learning to perch outside the nest) should also be returned to the nest site and should be placed on a branch off the ground in the original or nearby tree even though they are very likely to jump right back to the ground. Artificial nests can be made and secured to a nearby tree if the actual nest cannot be found or reached.

If a young bird is injured and/or cannot be returned to the nest site, then it will have to be raised in captivity. While this can be done successfully, there are several challenges that must be addressed.

Proper Development and Imprinting

The first four weeks of life are crucial as this is when a young bird gains important knowledge about its identity. Through a process of "imprinting," the young bird receives visual and auditory cues from its parents, siblings, and surrounding. This is an irreversible process that allows them to, among other things, socialize and find a suitable mate later in life. If raised improperly, these birds may imprint incorrectly on humans. When this happens, these birds will be unable to survive in the wild and must be considered nonreleasable. To prevent improper imprinting, the following steps should be taken.

- Renest any and all birds, if possible.
- House them with a surrogate parent and/or other young birds of the same species and similar age.

- Limit all contact while treating and feeding. Use camouflage and species-appropriate feeding puppets (Figure 17.5). Keep in a quiet place away from all sounds of human origin.

Feeding

Hatchlings and nestlings must be fed with long forceps/tweezers. When very young, they may require a meal every 2–3 hours. The feedings can be spread out as the bird develops but camouflage and a feeding puppet must be used at all times (Figure 17.5). Initially, it is very important to obtain a weight every day at the same time of day (generally in the morning before the first feeding). The bird's weight should increase daily until an adult weight is reached. Any reductions in weight should be treated seriously and the treatment plan should be adjusted immediately. In these cases, force feeding and fluid replacement may be necessary. In the peak growth phase, it is not uncommon for a young bird to consume

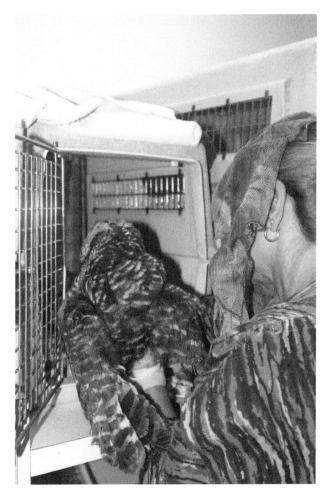

Figure 17.5 Feeding puppets should be used when feeding young birds of prey, such as owls, to avoid imprinting.

20–25% of its total body weight each day. In general, a young bird may eat 2–3 times the amount of an adult. Note that peak body weight is typically reached just prior to fledging and it is not uncommon for the weight to drop by as much as 10% after fledging.

Once a bird is self-feeding, make every attempt to minimize contact, place in groups and move into an enclosure with a surrogate adult. Food must be provided in skinned, bite-size pieces, with the bones pulverized until the bird is able to cast. This generally occurs at approximately the same time the bird develops pin feathers. Specific details on feeding and schedules are provided in Chapter 12.

Further Development

By 6–7 weeks of age, most of the smaller species have reached adult size and have fully developed flight feathers. They can fly at this point but may still have some downy feathers. They should also have transitioned to a "whole" prey diet (no longer cut up in small chunks) at this point. Note that larger species such as vultures and eagles will take considerably longer to develop and mature. Active exercise/flight training should begin and it is highly recommended that every young, inexperienced bird be tested with live prey.

Pre-release Conditioning and Evaluation

In preparation for release, there are several potential problems and issues that must be checked. Failure to meet the requirements of any one should disqualify a bird from release until all issues can be resolved.

Feather Condition

The feathers must be in very good condition with minimal damage. They should be clean and waterproof and any broken flight feathers should be repaired if possible. If too many feathers are damaged, the bird may have to overwinter and wait for a molt cycle to replace the damaged feathers. Alternatively, selected flight feathers can be repaired through a process call "imping." Imping involves the process of splicing in a corresponding feather from a cadaver using a bamboo rod and five-minute epoxy. A step-by-step guide can be found in Scott (2010) (Figure 17.6).

Feather condition is especially important for owls as this dramatically affects the amount of sound generated in flight. Owls rely on stealth when hunting and should be almost completely silent in flight.

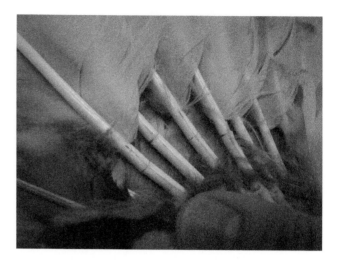

Figure 17.6 Feather imping is achieved by inserting and gluing a wooden dowel into the recipient feather shaft, which will allow joining of the donor feather.

Flight Evaluation

The ability to fly well is a critical requirement for release and survival in the wild. Once a bird's injuries have been resolved, the reconditioning process must begin in order to rebuild endurance and strength. This can be done in free flight on a creance line or in flight cages of the appropriate size (Table 17.4).

Evaluation of flight is not a simple matter and many factors must be considered. It is often helpful to have more than one bird together in a flight cage as differences in ability can be more obvious.

- A bird should appear effortless in flight. Any signs of exercise intolerance, labored breathing or breathing with an open mouth should be investigated.
- Inability to maintain level flight is commonly seen in birds that need more conditioning.
- Any asymmetry in flight, such as a full body tilt or the tail skewed to one side, is an indication that the bird is compensating for either weakness or a lack of range of motion.
- A wing droop that persists or develops during exercise can indicate pain and can make a bird nonreleasable if it is severe or does not resolve sufficiently.
- Most birds will fly readily when approached. Unwillingness to fly can be simply behavioral, as in great-horned owls and vultures, or it can be due to lack of conditioning or pain. Some birds may have to be physically prodded to leave the perch.

The flight style varies dramatically with species and the evaluator must be familiar with each species. It is very important that adequate flight space is provided in order to condition and evaluate birds of prey properly. Vultures and large hawks glide a great deal and it is common to see them glide for 30 or 40 ft to a perch. Accipiters are quick, with a fast wing beat and maneuver sharply. Owls typically pounce on prey from above and should be silent in flight.

Vision

A bird's vision should be thoroughly evaluated, especially if there was evidence of trauma on admission. While clinical signs of traumatic chorioretinitis can decrease or resolve over time, vision in the eye can still be affected. Evaluation of the menace response, pupillary light response and testing birds in a flight cage with obstacles to maneuver around can be useful in determining if any visual deficits exist. Note that any obstacles placed in the flight path should be constructed such that the bird will not be harmed after a collision. Use of long, flexible plastic strips hanging from the ceiling works well for this.

Behavior

Abnormal behavior can have many causes, including neurological disease (Scott 2014), visual problems or improper imprinting in young birds raised in captivity. In addition, stress and fear can cause certain species and individuals to act abnormally so recognizing abnormal behavior requires that normal behavior be understood.

Improper imprinting behavior in juveniles is particularly important because these birds are not releasable under any circumstances. Food begging is a classic sign of malimprinting. In addition, a normal bird should display a healthy fear of humans and should flee when approached. A bird that displays a lack of fear or an overly aggressive stance should be evaluated carefully as this is not normal behavior.

Body Condition and Overall Health

A quick physical exam should be performed before release to check for any major problems and feather damage. A weight and BCS should be evaluated and all birds should be released with a BCS of 3.5–4 on a five-point scale. In some cases, a recheck of the PCV and TS may be warranted.

Release

The actual release should be carefully planned. Factors to consider include the habitat, time of day, current weather, and season. The release site should be of the appropriate habitat for the species and this requires an in-depth understanding of natural history and ecology. It is usually preferable to release animals where they were found but there are some exceptions. These include sites where the animal was injured by gunshot or in areas where there are obvious sources of danger, including vehicle traffic or barbed-wire fences.

Diurnal birds should be released in the daytime and owls should be released at dusk. It is also important to consider season in migratory species. In cases where the species has left the area for the winter, for example, the bird will need to be held over until the spring before it can be released.

References

Arent, L. (2007). *Raptors in Captivity: Guidelines for Care and Management.* Surrey, Canada: Hancock House Publishing.

Banet-Noach, C., Simanov, L., and Malkinson, M. (2003). Direct (non-vector) transmission of West Nile virus in geese. *Avian Pathology* 32 (5): 489–494.

Bechert, U., Christensen, J.M., Poppenga, R., Fahmy, S.A., and Redig, P. (2010). Pharmacokinetics of terbinafine after single oral dose administration in red-tailed hawks (*Buteo jamaicensis*). *Journal of Avian Medicine and Surgery* 24 (2): 122–130.

Ip, H.S., van Wettere, A.J., McFarlane, L. et al. (2014). West Nile virus transmission in winter: the 2013 great salt lake bald eagle and eared grebes mortality event. *PLoS Currents* 6: ii.

Murray, M. (2014). Raptor gastroenterology. *Veterinary Clinics of North America: Exotic Animal Practice* 17 (2): 211–234.

Nemeth, N.M., Kratz, G.E., Bates, R. et al. (2009). Clinical evaluation and outcomes of naturally acquired West Nile virus infection in raptors. *Journal of Zoo and Wildlife Medicine* 40 (1): 51–63.

Redig, P. (2009). Lead from Spent Ammunition: A Source of Poisoning in Bald Eagles. Proceedings of the 30th Conference of the Association of Avian Veterinarians, Milwaukee, WI (10–13 August 2009), pp. 427–428.

Redig, P. (2010a). Use of MRI and Histological Methods for Detection of Lead-Induced Lesions in the CNS of Bald Eagles. Proceedings of the 31st Conference of the Association of Avian Veterinarians, San Diego, CA (2–5 August 2010), pp. 33–34.

Redig, P. (2010b). Raptors: Practical Information Every Avian Practitioner Can Use. Proceedings of the 31st Conference of the Association of Avian Veterinarians, San Diego, CA (2–5 August 2010), pp. 33–34.

Samour, J. (2008). *Avian Medicine*, 2e. St Louis, MO: Mosby-Elsevier.

Scheelings, T. (2014). Coracoid fractures in wild birds: a comparison of surgical versus conservative treatment. *Journal of Avian Medicine and Surgery* 28 (4): 304–308.

Scott, D. (2010). *Handbook of Raptor Rehabilitation.* Morrisville, NC:: Lulu Press.

Scott, D. (2013). A Retrospective Look at the Survival of Birds of Prey Released from a Rehabilitation Center in North Carolina. Proceedings of the First International Conference of Avian, Herpetic, and Exotic Mammal Medicine, London, England (28 April–2 May 2013), p. 365.

Scott, D. (2014). A Retrospective Look at Outcomes of Raptors with Spinal Trauma. Proceedings of the 35th Conference of the Association of Avian Veterinarians, New Orleans, LA (2–6 August 2014), p. 43.

Scott, D. (2015). RaptorMed™. https://raptormed.com/

Sibley, D.A. (2000). *The Sibley Guide to Birds.* New York: Alfred A. Knopf, Inc.

Sibley, D.A. (2001). *The Sibley Guide to Bird Life & Behavior.* New York: Alfred A. Knopf, Inc.

18

Natural History and Medical Management of Waterfowl

Michele Goodman

Elmwood Park Zoo, Norristown, PA, USA

Waterfowl Taxonomy and Natural History

The family Anatidae is a complex and frequently revised group including duck, goose, and swan species along with several aberrant or monotypic species. The subfamily classification "tribes" breaks this extensive family into related species groups. This discussion of waterfowl taxonomy follows Livezey (1997). For detailed accounts on the natural history of North American waterfowl, see Baldassarre (2014). For worldwide species accounts see Kear (2005).

Tribe Dendrocygnini

This tribe includes the whistling ducks, commonly referred to as tree ducks, although only a few members perch or nest in trees. Two species occur in southern North America: the black-bellied whistling duck (*Dendrocygna autumnalis*) and the fulvous whistling duck (*Dendrocygna bicolor*). All whistling duck species are sexually monomorphic and both parents participate in incubation and rearing of offspring. They are especially gregarious, prone to forming large flocks and are thought to mate for life. Whistling ducks are primarily herbivorous and prefer to feed in shallow water, collecting submerged seeds and aquatic vegetation with occasional aquatic insects. Whistling ducks are adept divers and will submerge to collect food. They also consume agricultural waste grains, especially pregerminated rice. In captivity, they are prone to frostbite when kept outside their native range.

Tribe Anserini

Seven members of this true goose tribe occur in North America in two genera: *Anser* and *Branta*. Anser include the arctic nesting snow goose (*Chen caerulescens*) and the white-fronted goose (*Anser albifrons*) and are characterized by a thick bill with a "grinning patch" used for plucking and grubbing vegetation and roots. *Anser* species are capable of biting through a typical red rubber catheter used for gavaging, which may necessitate endoscopic retrieval (Miller, personal communication). *Branta* members include the Canada goose (*Branta canadensis*), brant (*Branta bernicla*), and Hawaiian goose or nene (*Branta sandvicensis*). Most *Branta* spp. prefer to graze on pasture grass and agricultural fields; however, *B. bernicla* have a more specialized diet and rely on eelgrass and other marine vegetation as their primary food.

True geese are sexually monomorphic and do not breed until at least two years. Both parents participate in rearing offspring and family bonds extend through their first winter and often into the next breeding season.

Tribe Cygnini

This tribe contains the swan species, including the native tundra (*Cygnus columbianus*) and trumpeter (*Cygnus buccinator*) swans as well as the nonnative, invasive mute swan (*Cygnus olor*), which has restrictions placed on possession and rehabilitation in many states. The sexes are monomorphic and both sexes participate in rearing of offspring. Family bonds are long, with offspring remaining with their parents through their first winter until their return to breeding grounds in the spring. During the breeding season, the yearling cygnets are often forced by their parents to disperse from their natal territory and are potentially more susceptible to injury during this time. In general, swans do not breed until at least three years. They prefer to feed on plant material, including roots and tubers of aquatic plants, and generally feed by submersing their head and neck, or by

Medical Management of Wildlife Species: A Guide for Practitioners, First Edition. Edited by Sonia M. Hernandez, Heather W. Barron, Erica A. Miller, Roberto F. Aguilar and Michael J. Yabsley.

"tipping up" in deeper waters. They have been reported to use their feet to loosen rhizomes by paddling or treading (Baldassarre 2014). Some species, particularly tundra swans, are seasonally observed feeding in agricultural fields.

Tribe Anatini

This large tribe includes dabbling ducks, occasionally referred to as puddle ducks. Twelve species occur in North America, including mallards (*Anas platyrhynchos*) and northern pintails (*Anas acuta*). North American members are generally sexually dimorphic with males having brightly colored alternate plumages (e.g., northern shoveler [*Anas clypeata*] and mallard). Dabbling ducks tend to occupy shallow marsh and wetland habitats. They typically feed on the water's surface, just below it, or tip up to feed on deeper vegetation and small aquatic invertebrates. Most species are sexually mature at one year and form seasonally monogamous pair bonds that end during incubation (Baldassarre 2014). They are capable of springing to flight directly out of the water without a running start.

Tribe Aythyini

These are the diving ducks or pochards; five species are found in North America, including canvasback (*Aythya valisineria*) and ring-necked ducks (*Aythya collaris*). Pochards are sexually dimorphic with a generally rounded shape. Their heavy bodies and short wings with a high wing load necessitate that they run along the surface of the water prior to take-off (Baldassarre 2014). These ducks feed on a combination of vegetation and aquatic invertebrates by diving up to 60 ft, using their large feet with lobed hallux to propel them underwater (Baldassarre and Bolen 2006). They generally breed at one year, and form seasonally monogamous pair bonds.

Tribe Mergini

This tribe consists of the "sea duck" species, including eiders, scoters, mergansers, goldeneyes, and a few other monotypic species. These sexually dimorphic ducks mainly winter on coastal waters but many move inland during the breeding season. Mergini spend most of their time on water and are not well adapted to land, with their feet being positioned more caudally on their bodies than Anatini. While most species within this tribe utilize their large feet to propel them under water, some species also use their wings to paddle under water.

Sea ducks are generally not sexually mature until 2–3 years. Most species are seasonally monogamous but there is evidence birds will pair up with the same mate each winter after a brief hiatus during offspring rearing, which is done by the females exclusively (Baldassarre 2014).

Members are often thought of as fish eaters, but only the mergansers are truly adapted to consume fish, with serrated bills to facilitate fish capture. The remaining members feed primarily on aquatic invertebrates and mollusks, and are extremely skilled at diving to obtain food.

Tribe Oxyurini

These are stiff-tailed ducks, which in North America include only the ruddy duck (*Oxyura jamaicensis*) and the masked duck (*Nomonyx dominicus*). They are extremely awkward on land and often dive to escape danger rather than fly. Oxyurini feed on submerged aquatic vegetation and invertebrates and rely on their feet and long, rigid tail feathers to facilitate diving and maneuvering under water. They are sexually dimorphic, with most males developing bright blue bills during breeding season.

Captive Management

Waterfowl care starts with proper identification of orphans and adults. When faced with an unknown injured adult, it can be helpful to try to determine the tribe or family of the bird by looking at bill shape, foot color, foot shape, leg position on the body, and stance. Madge and Burn (1988), Nelson (1993), and Baldassarre (2014) are useful references to assist with proper identification of waterfowl.

Once properly identified, appropriate nutrition is critically important and can vary widely by species. Most commercial diets are designed for generic "fowl" or for meat birds, and have elevated protein levels and inadequate vitamin and mineral content compared to the requirements of wild waterfowl. These deficiencies can lead to several developmental problems in young waterfowl, discussed later. Whenever possible, natural food items should be offered, including greens (grass, duckweed, lettuces), aquatic invertebrates (krill, bloodworms, brine shrimp), and live insects (gut-loaded mealworms and crickets).

Neonatal Waterfowl

Neonatal waterfowl are typically presented within the first 48 hours of hatching, after becoming separated from their parent(s). Neonates should be properly identified on arrival (Figure 18.1a–h) and can be maintained temporarily in a converted 30 gal plastic tub with lid, placed on a heating pad set on low. Ambient temperature for

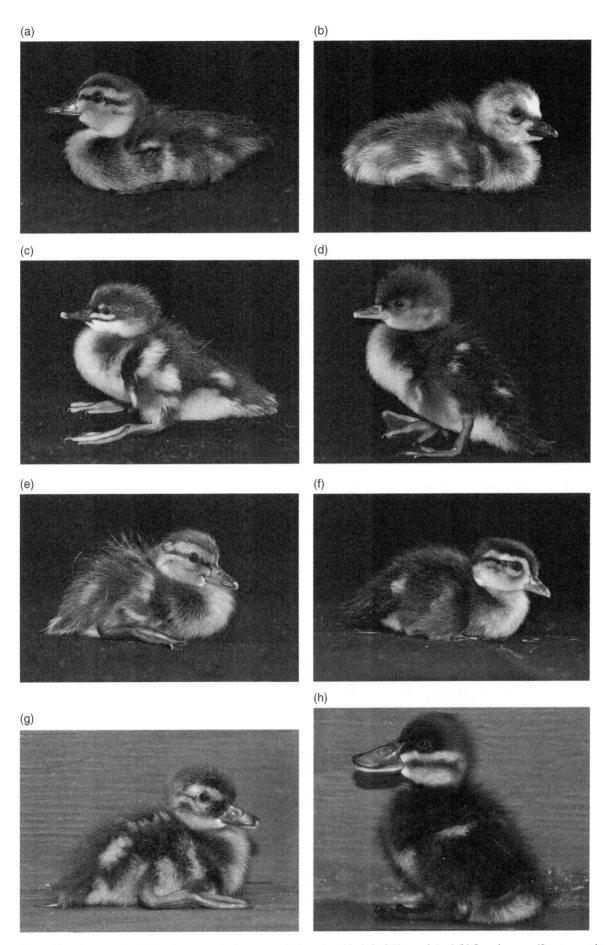

Figure 18.1 Common North American waterfowl neonates. (a) American black duck (*Anas rubripes*). (b) Canada goose (*Branta canadensis canadansis*). (c) Common merganser (*Mergus merganser*). (d) Hooded merganser (*Lophodytes cucullatus*). (e) Mallard (*Anas platyrhynchos*). (f) American wood duck (*Aix sponsa*). (g) Northern pintail (*Anas acuta*). (h) Ruddy duck (*Oxyura jamaicensis*). *Source:* Photos courtesy of Ian Gereg.

hatchling waterfowl should be around 85 °F (29.4 °C). Temperature should be gradually decreased to 70 °F (21.1 °C) by the time the birds are three weeks old; monitor for signs of hyperthermia (heat avoidance, open mouth breathing, lethargy) and adjust the temperature as needed. A secure covering over the tub limits human contact, offers privacy to high-stress species, and prevents escape. Several species of waterfowl are strong jumpers and many easily imprint or habituate to humans. Plastic tubs should be cleaned at least twice daily and disinfected between uses.

In general, waterfowl have nutrient requirements that are dissimilar from other poultry species, specifically an increased need for the B vitamins niacin, choline, and biotin (NRC 1994). These differences make commercially available turkey, game bird, chicken or "all flock" diets inappropriate for waterfowl in general, especially wild species, and have been linked to developmental abnormalities like angel wing and perosis (Olsen 1994). Pelleted or extruded diets are preferable to crumbled or mash forms because of improved feed efficiency and decreased risk of impacted feed under the tongue or in the upper bill (NRC 1994; Olsen 1994). For wild waterfowl, nutritional requirements are extrapolated from information available on commercial species (NRC 1994). Whenever possible, natural food items should be incorporated into captive diets to stimulate natural foraging behavior. It is generally accepted that protein content of commercially available feed should not exceed 22% for ducklings, goslings, or cygnets (NRC 1994). The only commercially available diet specifically designed for wild waterfowl is the line of waterfowl feeds from Mazuri® (St Louis, MO, USA). While there are numerous species differences, the author's experience is that Mazuri waterfowl starter can safely be fed to all waterfowl for the first month of life.

Despite being precocial, neonatal waterfowl can be reluctant to eat; this reluctance is likely due to being cold, stressed, or unable to recognize food items offered in captivity (Goodman 2017). Weight loss should be avoided, as this can rapidly lead to death. Neonates can be gavage fed 1–2% of their body weight of commercially available formula (e.g., Mazuri Nestling Handfeeding Formula mixed according to manufacturer instructions) 4–6 times daily, adjusting formula volume based on frequency and body weight. For ducklings, a 1 mL syringe can be used with an 8 or 10 Fr feeding tube attached, cut to approximately 2 in. in length so it passes beyond the glottis to the level of the thoracic inlet. The syringe and tube size can be scaled up for goslings and cygnets, and Lafeber's® (Cornell, IL, USA) Omnivore Care should be used as their formula.

Another technique to establish self-feeding is "drip feeding," where a mixture of aquatic invertebrates are thawed in water, drawn up into a 1 mL syringe and then dripped onto the bills of the ducklings; this provides the birds with both fluid and nutrition. Drip feeding works particularly well for all species of mergansers but may be counterproductive in other higher-stress species such as wood ducks.

Perhaps the most practical technique for getting young waterfowl to self-feed in captivity is to offer food items in a way they recognize. All food items should be offered on light-colored substrates (white paper towels, shallow white trays or lids). Food offered should closely mimic items they would encounter in the wild, such as duckweed and aquatic invertebrates (frozen or freeze-dried bloodworms, brine shrimp, and tubifex work well for ducklings). Mazuri Waterfowl Starter, can be offered dry or as a thin layer floating in water in conjunction with natural items. Orphaned waterfowl should not be offered anything with a mash or paste consistency as these can disturb feather quality and can form concretions on the upper palate.

Neonates are often not waterproof on presentation and can easily become chilled when placed in swimming water. They should nevertheless have limited access to swimming water so that they can become waterproof. Initially, swimming in cool water should be limited to a utility sink or shallow bathtub for 5–10 minutes at a time, several times a day. If ducklings become wet, they should be removed, towel dried and returned to their dry tub set-up. As their waterproofing improves, they can be left in swimming water for extending periods of time but should always have access to a dry area or float where they can easily leave the water. Food items described above should be offered floating in water during swimming time as many reluctant eaters will begin to peck at floating food items.

Housing

Neonatal waterfowl can be housed in a plastic tub (Figure 18.2a–d). A large hole is cut in the lid of a 30 gal tub, leaving a 2 in. rim. The hole is covered with fiberglass screening attached by cable ties. A heating pad is set on low over half of the tub bottom. The entire tub floor is covered with a soft towel. A "hide pocket" is arranged of rolled towels with an additional towel covering the heated section of the container. The hide pocket gives orphans a secure resting place that simulates brooding. On the unheated half of the container, three layers of white paper towels are placed over the cloth towel. White paper towels can be changed easily and allow for high contrast of food items to be visible to the birds. Mazuri Waterfowl Starter is sprinkled on top of the paper towels. A small poultry fount no deeper than 0.5 in. (1.3 cm) is provided with small pebbles added inside the lid of the fount so that waterfowl cannot

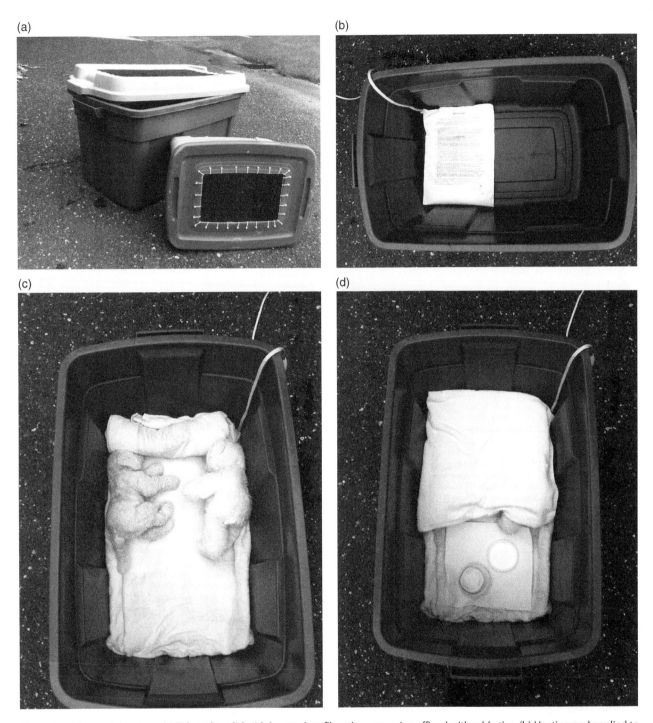

Figure 18.2 Plastic tub set-up. (a) Tub and cut lid with heavy-duty fiberglass screening affixed with cable ties. (b) Heating pad applied to half of the tub. (c) Towel covering entire bottom of the tub and rolled towels or stuffed animals inserted at the heated end. (d) Towel draped over rolled towels or stuffed animals to create a "hide pocket" and white paper towels placed on nonheated side of the tub. Shallow white dish for food and quail fountain for water.

submerge themselves. A shallow white lid less than 0.5 in. deep can be used to provide species-appropriate natural food items (aquatic invertebrates, mealworms, duckweed) suspended in a small amount of water. This tub set-up can house up to six mallard ducklings for up to one week. For larger clutches of ducklings or for goslings and cygnets, a 50 gal tub can be configured the same way. Neonatal waterfowl species with more aquatic lifestyles should be housed in a wet brooder as soon as waterproof for constant access to swimming water.

Adult Waterfowl

Depending on species, adult waterfowl can be temporarily housed in stainless steel or Vari Kennels (Pet Mate®, Conroe, TX, USA) readily found in most veterinary hospitals. They should be housed on cloth towels or rubber matting to provide a textured surface to reduce the incidence of pododermatitis. Diving ducks and ducks with pelvic limb or spinal injuries should be housed on a net bottom to reduce the incidence of keel lesions (Holcomb 1988). Newspaper should be avoided as it provides no padding and is easily soiled with food, water, and fecal material. Hay and straw should also be avoided as the fungal spores in these substrates may increase the incidence of aspergillosis.

For initial critical care and stabilization, waterfowl can be offered food and water in shallow ceramic bowls not prone to tipping. Most waterfowl will attempt to swim in even the smallest amount of water; to prevent this, place small, rounded stones in water bowls. Unless medical management prohibits access to swimming water, provide clean swimming water at least twice daily to maintain feather condition. As a staple diet, Mazuri Waterfowl Maintenance can be provided in dry dishes or floated as a thin layer on water. Reluctant eaters can be fed nonoily foods (e.g., gut-loaded mealworms, krill, or other aquatic invertebrates) during swim time to facilitate self-feeding. For species that naturally consume plant material, chopped lettuce can be provided. Grains should consist of white millet and whole corn, and should comprise no more than 5% of the diet in captivity.

Restraint, Anesthesia, and Clinical Techniques

Restraint

Proper restraint of anseriformes is essential for the safety of both the handler and the bird being restrained. All species of waterfowl are capable of scratching and biting; bites can be painful, especially from snow geese and mergansers. Geese and swans will use their wings to strike if not adequately restrained (Kearns 2003).

Smaller waterfowl species can be restrained by wrapping hands around both wings and body of the bird with the legs and feet tucked up against the body (Figure 18.3a). Birds presenting for care should not be held by the wings alone, as they can sustain nerve or orthopedic injuries (Backues 2015). Larger species of waterfowl can be restrained under the arm of the handler so that the arm and body of the handler act to keep the wings tight to the bird's body; the bird should also be positioned with its head pointing backward, making it more difficult for it to bite (Backues 2015) (Figure 18.3b).

Anesthesia

Fasting for 4–6 hours prior to general anesthesia is recommended for adult waterfowl (Backues 2015). Intubation is recommended for even short procedures as the dive response can interfere with normal respiration via stimulation of trigeminal nerve receptors when the bill is closed; manual positive pressure ventilation may be necessary for the duration of any anesthetic procedure (Machin 2004; Echols 2013). Intubation is generally straightforward as in other avian species although some species possess a crista ventralis, or septum, within the glottis that can make intubation difficult and necessitate the use of a smaller diameter tube (Echols 2013). An uncuffed endotracheal tube or Cole tube should be used in all cases except for gastric lavage procedures. Airway patency should be assessed frequently during every anesthetic procedure as waterfowl are prone to thick tracheal mucous secretions that occlude the lumen of the endotracheal tube during anesthesia (Mulcahy 2007; Backues 2015). Neck extension is important in all avian species, but is essential in waterfowl to ensure that the

(a)

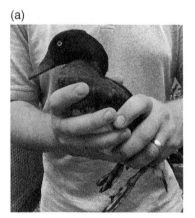

(b)

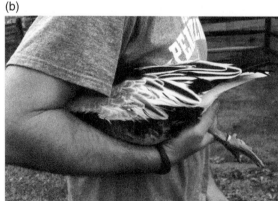

Figure 18.3 Waterfowl restraint. (a) Smaller waterfowl: one hand supports under the bird's sternum while the other hand is placed securely over the bird's back and wings. (b) Larger waterfowl: the bird is placed under the arm, supporting the sternum, with the head directed backwards. The elbow and side of the restrainer's body are used to prevent wing flapping.

trachea is not kinked (Olsen 1994). In contrast to most avian species, waterfowl, especially sea ducks and arctic waterfowl, are prone to hyperthermia during anesthesia so cloacal temperature should be monitored throughout the procedure. If hyperthermia occurs, the animal may be cooled by wetting legs and feet with isopropyl alcohol (Mulcahy 2007). Isoflurane is commonly used for waterfowl induction but is associated with cardiorespiratory depression (Machin 2004).

Waterfowl should be recovered from anesthesia in lateral to slightly ventral recumbency and the handler should be prepared for periods of flapping and struggling during reorientation (Mulcahy 2007). Information on injectable anesthetic agents and their use in waterfowl is published in detail elsewhere (Machin 2004; Mulcahy 2007).

Clinical Techniques

Venous Access
Compared to other avian species, venous access is easy in waterfowl. For small blood samples, the medial metatarsal vein is readily accessible and offers few complications. For larger samples, the right jugular vein can be accessed but the dense covering of down over the entire neck often makes this a blind stick.

Intravenous catheters can be placed in the medial metatarsal, right jugular vein, and, if necessary, cutaneous ulnar vein. The shortest available catheter should be used in the most distal access point on the metatarsal vein to prevent feeding the catheter over the hock joint. For cutaneous ulnar vein catheterization, the feathers can be wet with alcohol for vessel identification, and a waterproof transparent dressing applied. The intravenous catheter is then placed through the dressing into the vessel, with half-inch paper or porous tape used to secure the catheter. The transparent dressing helps anchor the tape and secure the catheter. The wing can be wrapped in a figure-of-eight to further secure the catheter. Techniques for jugular and intraosseous catheter placement are similar in waterfowl to other species (Tully et al. 2009).

Gastric Lavage
Gastric lavage is a technique used to remove foreign objects (such as lead) from the gastrointestinal (GI) tract, is less invasive than a ventriculotomy, and requires less equipment and training than endoscopic retrieval.

A gastric lavage is done on a fully anesthetized bird, intubated with a cuffed endotracheal tube gently inflated to avoid damage to the tracheal rings (Miller 2007). The bird is secured on a tilted surgical table in ventral recumbency with head and neck extended downward at 45–60°. Flexible hosing long enough to reach the proventriculus and approximately twice the diameter of a normal gavage tube is lubricated with a water-based gel and passed into the proventriculus. Warm water is delivered into the proventriculus with sufficient force to dislodge the foreign material while not so forceful as to damage the proventriculus, which can be prone to rupture in cases of impaction (Degernes 1995). The water can be administered via a series of 60 mL catheter tip syringes (Samour and Naldo 2005), a manual pump, or a garden hose attached directly to a threaded sink faucet. The movement of the water dislodges the gastric contents, which flow by gravity out of the mouth and into a collection bucket. The contents can be sifted or radiographed to ensure all foreign objects have been successfully recovered, or the bird can be radiographed to check for the persistence of radiopaque materials.

Clinically Relevant Anatomy and Physiology

Waterfowl have several unifying features differentiating them from other groups of birds. They all have downy young that leave the nest shortly after hatching and are capable of eating, swimming, and diving almost immediately. In rehabilitation, downy young often present wet and hypothermic and can be reluctant eaters, requiring innovative food presentation and feeding techniques. Due to family social structures, young are at high risk for inappropriate imprinting on humans and care must be taken to limit visual and auditory contact.

Waterfowl undergo a complete or eclipse molt after breeding where all flight feathers are replaced at once, rendering them flightless for 1–5 weeks depending on species (Kear 2005). Swans, geese, and whistling ducks undergo one molt per year; other ducks, in addition to a complete molt, will molt in the fall or early winter, replacing contour and inner wing feathers (Kear 2005). Biannual molts allow ducks to display breeding plumage for the breeding season alone. During these molts, waterfowl often lose body mass, thought to be an adaptation in reducing the flightless period (Kear 2005).

Waterfowl have bills that are specifically adapted to each species' feeding habits. Bills are generally broad or conical, covered by a soft membrane with a nail at the tip, and serrated lamellae which interdigitate with the lateral bristles of their tongues (Kearns 2003). A bill tip organ containing mechanoreceptors assists with food gathering (Gottschaldt and Lausmann 1974). Lamellae are of greatest density in the northern shoveler that feeds on invertebrates by filtration. There is no ongoing bill growth; traumatic injuries to the bill can adversely affect a bird's ability to obtain food or to preen feathers appropriately to maintain waterproofing.

Waterfowl have a nasal or supraorbital salt gland just dorsal to the eye, which includes a duct opening into the nasal cavity. The gland helps with osmoregulation and is most developed in species living in saline environments, such as sea ducks. Waterfowl from marine environments may benefit from exposure to salt water prior to release to restimulate the gland function (see Chapter 19).

The respiratory systems of some species have adaptations for vocalization. The swan sternum contains an excavated cavity for elongated tracheal coils, which increases dead space during anesthesia procedures. Male ducks possess a cartilaginous enlargement of the syrinx forming a syringeal bulla, which is often asymmetrical and is readily visualized on radiographs (Kearns 2003).

Male ducks, geese, and swans have a phallus that utilizes a lymphatic erectile mechanism to facilitate eversion during copulation. The phallus is covered by keratinized papillae; the size and shape vary extensively by species. The presence of a phallus is useful in determining gender; trained aviculturists and bird banders routinely use "vent sexing" in waterfowl. Penile prolapse may result from trauma affecting innervation to the phallus or from herpes infection (duck viral enteritis [DVE]).

Infectious Diseases

A number of infectious diseases may result in large outbreaks in waterfowl species and because some may have important implications for domestic fowl, appropriate authorities should be contacted.

Bacterial Diseases

A wide variety of bacterial infections have been described in waterfowl. Many affect primarily domestic species, such as *Reimerella anatipestifer*, also known as "new duck disease," which causes a septicemic disease of ducklings and goslings as well as annual die-offs of wild mallards and American black ducks in the Chesapeake Bay. Others, including the causative agent of avian cholera, *Pasteurella multocida*, are associated with large-scale die-offs involving thousands of wild birds (Wobeser 1997). Bacterial infections of waterfowl are extensively covered elsewhere (Wobeser 1997; Friend and Franson 1999a; Pello and Olsen 2013).

Waterfowl may present for care with any number of bacterial infections associated with trauma or other causes of debilitation. When possible, cultures should be obtained and submitted for aerobic culture and sensitivity to direct appropriate treatment with antimicrobials.

Viral Diseases

Numerous viruses are associated with large mortality events in waterfowl. Many of these viral diseases are covered in detail elsewhere (Wobeser 1997; Friend and Franson 1999a; Hess and Paré 2004; Pello and Olsen 2013) and only those clinically relevant viruses are discussed here.

Avian pox occurs in waterfowl worldwide and is caused by an avipoxvirus. The disease is transmitted by mosquitoes and other biting arthropods and results in either a "cutaneous" or "wet/diphtheroid" form of disease (Hess and Paré 2004). The cutaneous form presents with multiple papillomatous fleshy nodules on featherless areas, primarily the bill, face, legs, and feet. These nodular plaques often ulcerate and can be colonized by secondary bacteria (Wobeser 1997). Intracytoplasmic acidophilic inclusion bodies, known as Bollinger's bodies, along with hypertrophied epithelial cells, are pathognomonic for avian pox infection (Hess and Paré 2004). The wet form affects primarily the respiratory and GI tracts and can cause obstruction by formation of diphtheritic plaques in the airway and esophagus resulting in dyspnea (Hess and Paré 2004; Pello and Olsen 2013). As there is no treatment for avian pox but infections are usually self-limiting, supportive care is essential (Pello and Olsen 2013).

Duck viral enteritis, a highly transmissible herpesvirus, is distributed throughout the Americas, is regularly associated with waterfowl mortality events, and is reportable in most states (Hess and Paré 2004). DVE is an epitheliotropic virus and causes vasculitis, with grossly visible lesions on necropsy consisting of multifocal areas of hemorrhage within the intestines and often throughout the peritoneal cavity (Hess and Paré 2004). Development of clinical signs varies with species. Some duck species are highly susceptible to developing disease (e.g., mallards) while others may develop disease but also can be asymptomatic (e.g., Muscovy ducks). Live birds may present with photosensitivity and bloody discharges, and males may exhibit penile prolapse (Friend 1999a). When DVE is suspected, authorities should be notified and affected birds euthanized, as a prolonged carrier state exceeding four years has been reported (Burgess et al. 1979).

Avian influenza viruses (family Orthomyxovirus) are widespread, with waterfowl often considered as reservoir hosts which rarely develop clinical disease (Pello and Olsen 2013). However, highly pathogenic avian influenza (HPAI H5N2 and H5N8) was identified in wild waterfowl in British Columbia, Canada, in December 2014 and has since been identified in multiple states and several Canadian provinces. The viruses are believed to have entered North America through the Pacific flyway, where migratory birds from the United States seasonally mix with migratory birds from Asia (Rao 2014). While most commonly impacting commercial poultry, HPAI has been shown to cause clinical disease in raptors as well as wild waterfowl. Clinical signs in affected waterfowl include respiratory signs of sneezing and coughing and neurological signs of depression, tremors, torticollis, and opisthotonus (Converse 2007). Historically, HPAI fails to persist long-term in wild bird populations, but the epidemiology of avian influenza in waterfowl is constantly evolving. Both the USDA and FAO websites provide updated information on this pathogen.

Fungal Diseases

Waterfowl are susceptible to cutaneous, mucosal, and systemic fungal disease. *Aspergillus fumigatus* commonly infects the respiratory tract of waterfowl, especially sea ducks out of their natural aquatic environment. While not considered contagious, aspergillosis can manifest as an acutely fatal disease or may be associated with chronic disease (Friend 1999). This saprophytic fungus is ubiquitous in the environment; birds may be more susceptible to clinical disease when immunosuppressed, stressed in captivity or housed in poorly ventilated areas (Orosz 2000; Pello and Olsen 2013). Clinical signs of acute infection include dyspnea, gasping, open mouth breathing, and cyanosis (Converse 2007). Chronically infected birds may not show respiratory signs until later in the disease process but will often show signs of emaciation and general debilitation (Converse 2007).

Prevention is easier than treatment; the prophylactic use of itraconazole is slowly being replaced by the fungicidal triazole voriconazole (Kline et al. 2011). Sea ducks kept out of water for even short periods of time should be treated prophylactically, especially if concurrently treated with another antimicrobial agent. Voriconazole in mallard ducks at a recommended dosing interval of 8–12 hours resulted in no signs of toxicity and higher bioavailability than reported in other avian species (Kline et al. 2011). Voriconazole has been associated with auto-induction of cytochrome P450, which may necessitate periodic dose increases if given for extended periods of time (Kline et al. 2011). Terbinafine has been reported as an effective treatment of aspergillosis in birds but evidence is lacking in waterfowl. Treatment of aspergillosis is difficult and consists of endoscopic debridement of fungal lesions along with both topical and systemic antifungal therapy (Hess and Paré 2004; Pello and Olsen 2013).

Candida albicans has been implicated as the cause of ocular lesions in sea ducks deprived of access to salt water (Crispin and Barnett 1978). *C. albicans* and other opportunistic fungal organisms can also cause esophageal, follicular, and venereal lesions in waterfowl and are often found in association with mixed bacterial infections (Wobeser 1997; Kline et al. 2011).

Parasitic Diseases

External Parasites

Leeches from the genus *Theromyzon* may be found attached to the nasal passages, pharynges, and nictitating membranes of dabbling ducks and swans, causing head shaking, sneezing, and constant scratching at the head (Tuggle 1999; Ballweber 2004). Leeches can cause tissue damage to the nasopharynx, cornea, and trachea and may cause mortality of affected birds. When possible, leeches should be manually removed with forceps; if not, ivermectin should be administered (Carpenter 2013). Debilitated waterfowl are commonly infested with chewing lice of the genus *Mallophaga*. Lice can be removed with forceps or with pyrethrin spray or dust (Ballweber 2004). Fly larvae are capable of causing fatal myiasis in newly hatched wild waterfowl by initiating infection at the umbilicus, or in adult waterfowl in association with open wounds (Wobeser 1997). Initially, the infestation is locally invasive with affected waterfowl often exhibiting lethargy and anorexia.

Internal Parasites

Waterfowl may be infected with a number of protozoal parasites including coccidia, *Giardia*, *Hexamita*, and *Sarcocystis* (Ballweber 2004). Intestinal coccidiosis in neonates can manifest as blood-tinged, mucoid diarrhea, emaciation, and anemia (Friend and Franson 1999b). Waterfowl are commonly infected with *Eimeria* spp., less commonly with other coccidians. Intestinal coccidia can be transmitted rapidly between birds and good husbandry and sanitation practices are essential to prevent spread. Effective therapeutics include ronidazole, clazuril, and ponazuril. Renal coccidiosis is frequently reported in waterfowl, most often associated with *Eimeria* spp., although its presence is not often associated with clinical disease in infected birds (Cole 1999b). *Sarcocystis* is an intramuscular protozoal parasite of waterfowl and is generally only seen at necropsy. *Giardia* and *Hexamita* are commonly seen in dabbling ducks and geese and on occasion may be associated with watery diarrhea and weight loss, especially when combined with concurrent disease or when the infection is overwhelming. Both can be treated with either metronidazole or fenbendazole.

Hemoparasites, including *Plasmodium*, *Hemoproteus*, and *Leucocytozoon* spp., are routinely identified in blood. Of these, *Leucocytozoon* and *Plasmodium* are most likely to be pathogenic, especially in young waterfowl. *Leucocytozoon* has been implicated in several large waterfowl die-offs (Atkinson 1999; Ballweber 2004). *Hemoproteus* and *Plasmodium* can be treated with chloroquine, primaquine, or mefloquine; *Leucocytozoon* is less likely to respond to these treatments; even with treatment, some birds may remain subclinically infected (Carpenter 2013).

Waterfowl are susceptible to numerous helminth parasites including nematodes, cestodes, trematodes, and acanthocephalans. Diagnosis in many cases is made by direct smear or for increased sensitivity, centrifugation flotation or sedimentation (for trematodes). However, intermittent shedding or prolonged prepatent periods may make detection challenging.

Common nematodes infecting waterfowl include tracheal worms (*Syngamus trachea*), gizzard worms (*Amidostomum* spp. and *Epomidiostomum* spp.), hookworms and ascarids (Cole and Friend 1999). Infection is diagnosed by finding eggs in the feces or sputum and may be treated with ivermectin, fenbendazole or pyrantel pamoate (Carpenter 2013).

Trematodes can be found in the oral cavity, trachea, bile duct, eyes, and intestinal tract in a wide variety of waterfowl (Wobeser 1997). Certain species have been associated with significant mortality events; the small *Sphaeridiotrema globulus* can be lethal, causing severe blood loss and hypovolemic shock (Cole and Friend 1999). Schistosomes, or blood flukes, are associated with obliterative endophlebitis, granulocytic enteritis, and neurological signs relating to aberrant larval migration or the release of eggs by adult worms (Huffman and Fried 2008). Schistosomes are also associated with the zoonotic disease cercarial dermatitis or "swimmer's itch" in humans. While most trematodes respond to praziquantel (Carpenter 2013), schistosomes often require much higher doses in some, but not all waterfowl (Blankespoor et al. 2001).

Cestodes are frequently present in waterfowl and are rarely associated with pathology in adults. When present in heavy burdens in juveniles, particularly Canada geese, they may cause decreased body condition, incoordination, and inability to stand. Following rehydration with intravenous fluids and oral administration of praziquantel, affected geese shed dozens of worms and regain normal function within 24 hours. Waterfowl are commonly infected with cestodes of the order Cyclophyllidea. When mature, cyclophyllideans release gravid terminal segments unlike other orders of cestodes that release senile terminal segments. This is clinically relevant as cestode eggs are rarely found in waterfowl feces, resulting in a negative fecal examination unless terminal segments are identified grossly (Huffman and Fried 2008).

Acanthocephalans (thorny-headed worms) are routinely found in sea ducks, with more than 50 species reported in waterfowl (Cole 1999a). The link between parasite burden and clinical disease (primarily emaciation and diarrhea) has not been made definitively as histopathologically the proboscis causes only a localized inflammatory response when embedded in the intestine (Bender et al. 2015). Acanthocephalans rely on an indirect life cycle for transmission and the prepatent period can be several months; a negative fecal examination does not rule out parasite infection (Hollmen 1999). Loperamide, a synthetic opiate, has been effective at reducing acanthocephalan burdens in both pigs and fish; initial studies in waterfowl have been promising but additional research is needed (Mehlhorn et al. 1990; Tarachewski et al. 1990; Bender et al. 2015).

Common Reasons for Presentation

Soft Tissue Injuries

Bill Injuries
Waterfowl are prone to traumatic bill injuries, affecting the maxilla, mandible or the associated soft tissue structures. For fractures of the maxilla or mandible, surgical repair techniques are described elsewhere and are associated with a poor prognosis if compound (Olsen 1994; Wheler 2002). Soft tissue injuries can be corrected surgically with simple interrupted monofilament suture if the bird is presented within 12–24 hours post injury and the underlying blood supply is viable. Waterfowl may present with traumatic amputation of a portion of the bill. Numerous prosthetic techniques have been described but none are permanent, requiring that the animal remain in captivity; even then, they may not regain sufficient function of the bill to maintain feather condition and waterproofing and to remove ectoparasites (Olsen 1994; Wheler 2002). Euthanasia should be considered for any bird with loss of the nail of the maxilla or with soft tissue loss over the mandible leading to destabilization.

Fishing Hook or Line Ingestion
Waterfowl encounter fishing hooks and discarded monofilament line frequently in their aquatic environments. If they present with line hanging out of the bill, it is important not to tug on the line before obtaining a radiograph to rule out the presence of a fishing hook in the GI tract. Surgical removal of fishing hooks is similar in waterfowl as it is in other species and is addressed in Chapter 11.

Perosis/Achilles Tendon Luxation
Perosis results from medial or lateral luxation of the gastrocnemius, or Achilles tendon, from the condylar groove of the hock joint, preventing extension of the affected limb (Kirkwood 2008). Malnutrition, more specifically manganese deficiency, over-crowding, and lack of exercise, have been associated with the condition (Olsen 1994; Goodman et al. 2016). Perosis commonly affects young, rapidly growing birds but can present following trauma in adults. Surgical correction has been described (Olsen 1994; Bowles 2003; Kirkwood 2008) but in the author's experience, outcomes have been poor, especially in birds younger than five weeks.

An alternative approach using a lightweight splint has been successful in several cases, facilitating swimming and walking during treatment (Goodman et al. 2016). A splint can be fashioned from padded aluminum material or porous thermoplastic material measured to the length of the tibiotarsus and tarsometatarsus with a smoothly curved notch cut out on either side for the hock joint (Figure 18.4a). Cover the exposed edge with tape to prevent abrasions. Porous thermoplastic material may be better tolerated for more aquatic species as the splint will be less buoyant while swimming. The splint is bent to hold the leg in a naturally flexed position (approximately 60°). The splint is applied to the cranial surface of the leg with notches lined up with the hock joint. The luxated tendon is manually replaced in the condylar groove; several minutes of physical therapy and gentle massage may be required to accomplish this. The proximal and distal portions of the splint aligned with the tibiotarsus and tarsometatarsus, respectively, are bent caudally around the leg and secured with paper tape (Figure 18.4b). When properly placed, the position of the Achilles tendon can be visualized (Figure 18.4c). For birds weighing less than 150 g, 2 mm foam can be used to fashion the splint as above, with the addition of a score line connecting the two notches to facilitate bending the hock joint.

The splint should be checked daily to make sure the tendon is correctly positioned. In young waterfowl, the splint will have to be resized frequently to allow for growth. Due to limited vascular supply to the tendon, the affected leg should remain splinted for at least 10 days in growing birds, 30 days in adults. Birds should receive meloxicam for the first 72 hours and may require a broad-spectrum antimicrobial such as clindamycin if the hock joint is hot or swollen. The addition of a vasodilator may speed healing.

Angel Wing

Angel wing, also known as droop wing or airplane wing, is a carpal joint deformity that occurs in rapidly growing birds. The condition is thought to relate to a nutritional imbalance and may result from deficiencies in manganese and vitamin D3 as well as feeding a diet with excessive protein (Olsen 1994). Inadequate exercise may also be involved in the development of this condition. The weight of developing flight feathers places excessive stress on weak muscles of the carpal joint, leading to an outward or downward deviation of this joint. If not corrected before the primary feathers reach their terminal length, the condition will be permanent and the bird will be flightless.

To correct this condition, the wing is splinted with a lightweight flexible material such as padded aluminum, foam or perforated thermoplastic that can bend slightly to follow the natural contours of the wing (Figure 18.5a). The splint is secured with paper tape or cohesive bandage in a figure-of-eight wrap, being careful not to impinge upon the patagium, to keep the wing in a normal anatomical position, and not cause the growing primary feathers to bend (Figure 18.5b). The splint should remain in place for five days, then removed for two days, during which time physical therapy should be performed (Goodman 2017). The splint can be replaced for another five days if needed, and if not corrected after this time, the condition is likely permanent.

Scalping and Mating Injuries

Waterfowl often present with degloving injuries over the cranium, which may occur more frequently during the breeding season as a result of forced mating (Baldassarre and Bolen 2006) (Figure 18.6a). A dorsal cervical single

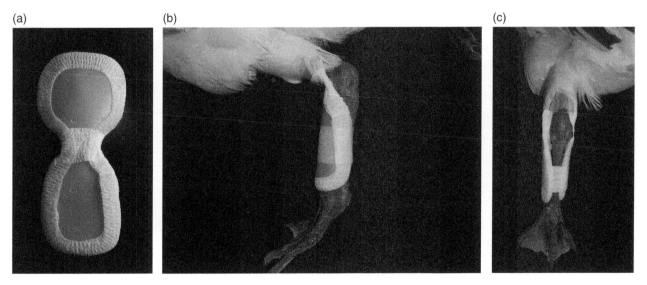

(a)   (b)   (c)

Figure 18.4 Padded aluminum splint for the treatment of perosis. (a) Splint with smooth notches and edges covered with tape to prevent abrasions; (b) applied splint, lateral view; (c) applied splint, caudal view.

(a)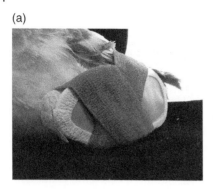

(b)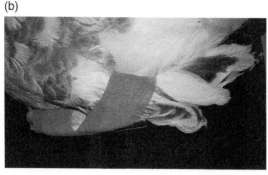

Figure 18.5 Figure-of-eight wrap with padded aluminum splint for correction of angel wing. (a) Cranio-lateral view; (b) dorsal view of same splint.

pedicle advancement flap can be used to close the skin defect over the cranium, which prevents eyelid deformation that would result from second intention healing or surgical apposition of the lateral wound margins (Gentz and Linn 2000; Duerr, personal communication) (Figure 18.6b).

Orthopedic Injuries

Fracture management in waterfowl is similar to that of other avian species. Due to their aquatic lifestyle, splinting and bandaging materials for closed fractures should be waterproof whenever possible to enable swimming during recovery (Goodman et al. 2016). The buoyancy of materials should be considered when treatment permits swimming; buoyant materials can place unnatural stresses on the pelvic limb.

While the etiology is still poorly understood, sea ducks are prone to ischemic necrosis of the hock and plantar toe surfaces (Duerr, personal communication). Lesions may not be apparent on presentation, but depending on lesion depth, tendons and bone may be involved which necessitate surgical intervention. Complete digit amputation may render a bird nonreleasable if it interferes with diving and food acquisition. Salvage procedures involving removal of just the bone of the affected digit, with preservation of associated webbing, have been performed successfully and described in both domestic and wild waterfowl (Duerr, personal communication; Olsen 2015).

Neurological Injuries

Traumatic injuries to the hock or tarsus may become secondarily inflamed or infected, often as a result of inappropriate weight bearing, resulting in neurological damage. With hock injuries, waterfowl may walk on the plantar aspect of the hock joint, unable to extend the leg. In tarsal joint injuries, they may walk on the dorsal aspect of the foot, unable to flex the foot.

(a)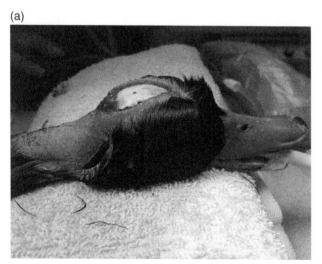

(b)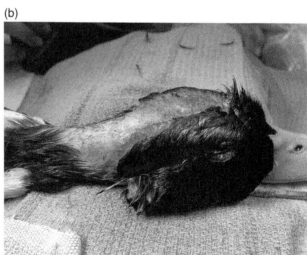

Figure 18.6 Pedicle advancement flap surgery to repair scalping injury common in waterfowl. (a) Debrided scalp wound on a mallard drake (*Anas platyrhynchos*). (b) Flap suture in place to cover the exposed skull. *Source:* Photos courtesy of Rebecca Duerr, DVM, PhD.

Neurological injuries to the hock may be corrected by modifying the splinting technique previously described for perosis. The splint should be applied to the caudal aspect of the leg and the hock joint lightly padded with foam. For injuries to the tarsus, a boot can be constructed of padded aluminum or foam and secured to the plantar aspect of the foot and the caudal aspect of the tarsometatarsus using cohesive bandage or waterproof tape. The splint should be secured with the toes spread. Nylon suture can be used to sew a tension line from the bandage covering the tarsometatarsus to the bandage covering the foot (Figure 18.7a,b). These splints should remain for 5–7 days (in young waterfowl, splints may have to be replaced more frequently to allow for growth).

Vascular Injuries

Several conditions commonly seen in waterfowl affect the vascular supply to the legs, feet, or digits. Discarded monofilament line is frequently encountered and can easily become entangled around any part of the body. As the bird struggles, the line tightens and constricts circulation, and can cause ischemic necrosis of portions distal to the ligature. Waterfowl can be affected by frostbite of the feet, which can occur when they do not have access to open water in freezing temperatures. As with monofilament line entanglement, frostbite compromises the circulation to the feet, leading to areas of necrosis. The full extent of tissue damage resulting from either monofilament line entanglement or frostbite can take several days to become evident; affected birds should be held and monitored prior to release.

Treatment for birds with vascular compromise consists of multimodal pain management (meloxicam and an opioid such as buprenorphine or tramadol), a vasodilator (isoxsuprine or pentoxifylline) and, if indicated, a broad-spectrum antibiotic with distribution to the bone (e.g., clindamycin).

Captivity-Induced Lesions

Keel Lesions

Waterfowl are prone to the development of ischemic keel lesions secondary to abnormal weight placement on the keel (Duerr 2016) or, less commonly, from trauma (Samour 2008). Any species of waterfowl can develop a keel lesion when forced to spend time sternally recumbent due to inappropriate housing or pelvic limb or spinal injury (Duerr 2016). Highly aquatic species, such as sea ducks, are prone to developing keel lesions when housed in a dry environment for even short periods of time. To prevent such lesions, sea ducks, and waterfowl with injuries of the pelvic limb or spine, should be housed on net bottom pens when not in water (Holcomb 1988).

Once a keel lesion has formed, surgical intervention is required as conservative management is associated with poor cure rates (Hochleithner and Hochleithner 1996). Surgical debridement and closure should be performed under general anesthesia (see Chapter 19), and is often curative in most species of ducks. In the author's experience, lesions in heavy-breasted birds like geese and swans carry a poorer prognosis.

Pododermatitis

Pododermatitis, or bumblefoot, is a condition commonly affecting waterfowl in captivity. Poor housing is often

(a)

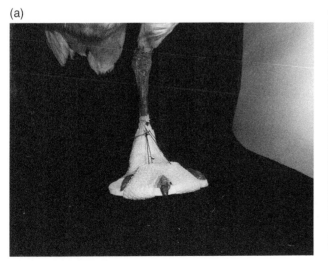

(b)

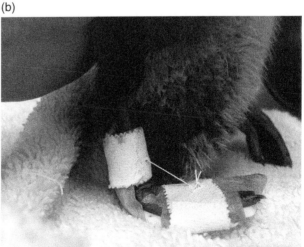

Figure 18.7 Foam tension line boots to keep foot in normal position following neurological injury. (a) Boot with cohesive bandage and braided nylon tension line on a gull. (b) Boot modified for use in duckling by using 2 mm foam and porous tape.

implicated, especially when birds are housed on hard, smooth surfaces such as linoleum, concrete, wood, plastic, or newspaper without padding (Backues 2015). To prevent this condition from developing, waterfowl should be housed on a variety of substrates that provide both cushion and traction. When housed indoors, waterfowl should be on textured rubber matting such as Dri-dek™ (Kendall Products, Naples, FL, USA) or unbacked Nomad™ (3 M™, St Paul, MN). Sea ducks should be housed on net-bottom pens (Holcomb 1988). Treatment for the condition is difficult and often unsuccessful and may include surgical debridement, padded bandages and lengthy courses of systemic antibiotics, depending on the severity (Backues 2015) (see Chapter 11 for more information).

Carpal Wounds

Carpal wounds occur in waterfowl as in other species and are treated similarly (see Chapter 19).

Common Waterfowl Toxicities

Waterfowl may be impacted by a wide variety of natural and synthetic toxins. Toxicities affecting waterfowl are discussed at length elsewhere (Wobeser 1997; Degernes 1995; Friend and Franson 1999a; Miller 2007). Approaches to treatment for common toxicities relevant to clinical practitioners are discussed here.

Natural Toxins

Treatment for natural toxicities, including those caused by blue-green algae, red tides and mycotoxins, focuses on gastric decontamination and supportive care (Miller 2007). Activated charcoal should be administered orally along with isotonic fluids to birds sufficiently stable to protect their airways. Parenteral fluids may be required in unstable patients. Supplemental oxygen and barbiturates may be necessary for dyspneic or seizuring birds. Patients with dermal exposure should be washed with water to reduce the risk of oral intoxication from preening.

Avian Botulism

Waterfowl affected by botulism are classified into three groups based on the severity of clinical signs (Rocke and Friend 1999).

- Stage 1: Mild clinical disease, unable to fly and may walk using their wings for propulsion; capable of self-feeding and will recover with minimal supportive care.

- Stage 2: More severely affected and unable to fly, walk, or feed; are reluctant to hold their heads upright and may have a slow nictitans response; fair to guarded recovery with supportive care.
- Stage 3: Critically ill and almost completely paralyzed; are at risk of suffocation and are unable to hold their heads upright; guarded to poor recovery despite intensive treatment.

Treatment varies by clinical stage, but all birds should have the following done on intake: clean feces and urates from vents, flush eyes with sterile saline and apply lubricating ointment, and gavage isotonic fluids and activated charcoal (Miller and Brunner 2013). The key to treatment is gastric decontamination via copious volumes of oral isotonic fluids. While stage 2 and 3 birds may not be fully capable of holding up their heads, they still require oral fluids to flush the toxin from their GI tracts. When providing oral fluids to these birds, their head and neck should be placed in a normal position with the help of rolled towels, with their beaks angled downward to facilitate drainage of nasal secretions. They should be gavage fed in place so that they do not risk aspirating while being transferred from a treatment table to holding cage. These birds are extremely susceptible to aspiration as they often have difficulty swallowing. Nares should be checked frequently in all birds for patency. Subsequent treatments are adjusted based on response to initial therapy and consist largely of fluids and caloric support via gavage.

Heavy Metal Poisoning

Lead poisoning is not uncommon in wild waterfowl; any bird with clinical signs consistent with heavy metal poisoning (ataxia, drooped wings, GI stasis) should be radiographed and have blood submitted for lead analysis. Other heavy metals, including zinc and mercury, can also be associated with clinical disease in waterfowl; these metals have been discussed in detail elsewhere (Miller 2007). When evaluating radiographs with metallic densities, soft lead shot will often have irregular edges compared to harder nontoxic shot which is usually perfectly round. The presence of metallic densities on radiographs, along with clinical signs, supports a diagnosis of heavy metal poisoning. In waterfowl, a definitive diagnosis is based on elevated blood lead concentrations exceeding 0.35 ppm (Miller 2007).

Treatment for lead poisoning has three components: supportive care, chelation therapy and removal of toxic materials (Degernes 2008). Chelation therapy should begin promptly following diagnosis. Retrieval of toxic materials is often best achieved with gastric lavage under general anesthesia (see Section 18.3.3). When gastric lavage is not successful, endoscopy, or ventriculotomy may be required to remove foreign materials. Sea ducks and swans (species susceptible to aspergillosis) should receive prophylactic treatment with itraconazole or voriconazole for the first 10 days of therapy (Degernes 2008). The two most common drugs used for chelation therapy are calcium disodium ethylenediamine tetraacetic acid (CaEDTA) and succimer (meso-2,3-dimercaptosuccinic acid [DMSA]) (Miller 2007; Degernes 2008). CaEDTA should be administered orally only after radiographic confirmation that all lead materials have been successfully removed from the GI tract as oral administration may actually enhance lead absorption (Miller 2007). Succimer (DMSA) is an effective oral chelator that does not enhance absorption if lead is still present in the GI tract. DMSA is administered for five days, followed by 2–4 rest days, and repeated until lead levels have returned to normal and clinical signs have resolved (Miller 2007).

Pre-release Conditioning and Postrelease Monitoring

When evaluating waterfowl for release, they must be completely waterproof and able to recognize and obtain appropriate food items. Pre-release conditioning enclosures should be adequate for the given species to acquire food in a way that mimics the feeding challenges encountered in the wild. Captive-reared, orphaned waterfowl should exhibit behaviors appropriate for the species and show normal fear of humans. Ages for release vary by species and circumstance, but the author recommends releasing them approximately a week prior to their becoming fully flighted, to ensure that they remain in the appropriate release habitat for several days.

When transporting waterfowl to an appropriate release location, soft-sided kennels should be utilized to prevent feather and carpal trauma. Sea ducks, pochards, and stifftails will benefit from a net-bottom transport pen to reduce feather contamination with fecal material.

References

Atkinson, C. (1999). Hemosporidiosis (avian malarias). In: *Field Manual of Wildlife Diseases: General Field Procedures and Diseases of Birds* (ed. M. Friend and J.C. Franson), 193–200. Madison, WI: USGS.

Backues, K.A. (2015). Anseriformes. In: *Fowler's Zoo and Wild Animal Medicine*, vol. 8 (ed. M.E. Fowler and R.E. Miller), 116–126. St Louis, MO: Elsevier:.

Baldassarre, G. (2014). *Ducks, Geese, and Swans of North America*. Baltimore, MD: Johns Hopkins University Press.

Baldassarre, G.A. and Bolen, E.G. (2006). *Waterfowl Ecology and Management*. Malabar, FL: Krieger Publishing.

Ballweber, L.R. (2004). Waterfowl parasites. *Seminars in Avian and Exotic Pet Medicine* 13 (4): 197–205.

Bender, S., Goodman, M.D., and Nolan, T.J. (2015). *Histopathology of Acanthocephalans in Sea Ducks and Brant*. Philadelphia, PA: University of Pennsylvania School of Veterinary Medicine.

Blankespoor, C.L., Reimink, R.L., and Blankespoor, H.D. (2001). Efficacy of praziquantel in treating natural schistosome infections in common mergansers. *Journal of Parasitology* 87 (2): 424–426.

Bowles, H.L. (2003). Repair of displaced flexor tendon in two ducks. *Exotic DVM* 5 (3): 91–94.

Burgess, E.C., Ossa, J., and Yuill, T.M. (1979). Duck plague: a carrier state in waterfowl. *Avian Diseases* 23 (4): 940–949.

Carpenter, J.W. (2013). *Exotic Animal Formulary*, 4e. St Louis, MO: Saunders.

Cole, R.A. (1999a). Acanthocephaliasis. In: *Field Manual of Wildlife Diseases: General Field Procedures and Diseases of Birds* (ed. M. Friend and J.C. Franson), 241–243. Madison, WI: USGS.

Cole, R.A. (1999b). Renal coccidiosis. In: *Field Manual of Wildlife Diseases: General Field Procedures and Diseases of Birds* (ed. M. Friend and J.C. Franson), 215–218. Madison, WI: USGS.

Cole, R.A. and Friend, M. (1999). Miscellaneous parasitic diseases. In: *Field Manual of Wildlife Diseases: General Field Procedures and Diseases of Birds* (ed. M. Friend and J.C. Franson), 249–258. Madison, WI: USGS.

Converse, K.A. (2007). Aspergillosis. In: *Infectious Diseases of Wild Birds* (ed. N.J. Thomas, D.B. Hunter and C.T. Atkinson), 360–374. Ames, IA: Wiley.

Crispin, S.M. and Barnett, K.C. (1978). Ocular candidiasis in ornamental ducks. *Avian Pathology* 7 (1): 49–59.

Degernes, L.A. (1995). Toxicities in waterfowl. *Seminars in Avian and Exotic Pet Medicine* 4 (1): 15–22.

Degernes, L.A. (2008). Waterfowl toxicology: a review. *Veterinary Clinics of North America: Exotic Animal Practice* 11 (2): 283–300.

Duerr, R.S. (2016). Surgical Repair of Keel Lesions and Lacerations in Aquatic Birds. Association of Avian Veterinarians Annual Conference at ExoticsCon, Portland, OR.

Echols, M.S. (2013). *Backyard Poultry and Waterfowl Anesthesia and Surgery*. Gainesville, FL: North American Veterinary Conference.

Friend, M. (1999a). Aspergillosis. In: *Field Manual of Wildlife Diseases: General Field Procedures and Diseases of Birds* (ed. M. Friend and J.C. Franson), 129–134. Madison, WI: USGS.

Friend, M. and Franson, J.C. (1999a). *Field Manual of Wildlife Diseases: General Field Procedures and Diseases of Birds*. Madison, WI: USGS.

Friend, M. and Franson, J.C. (1999b). Intestinal coccidiosis. In: *Field Manual of Wildlife Diseases: General Field Procedures and Diseases of Birds* (ed. M. Friend and J.C. Franson), 207–214. Madison, WI: USGS.

Gentz, E.J. and Linn, K.A. (2000). Use of a dorsal cervical single pedicle advancement flap in 3 birds with cranial skin defects. *Journal of Avian Medicine and Surgery* 14 (1): 31–36.

Goodman, M.D. (2017). *Ducks, Geese, and Swans: An Introduction to Waterfowl Medicine*. Washington, DC: Association of Avian Veterinarians Annual Conference.

Goodman, M., Schott, R., and Duerr, R. (2016). Waterfowl (ducks, geese, and swan). In: *Topics in Wildlife Medicine, vol. 4: Orthopedics* (ed. R.S. Duerr and G.J. Purdin), 99–119. St Cloud, MN: National Wildlife Rehabilitators Association.

Gottschaldt, K.M. and Lausmann, S. (1974). The peripheral morphological basis of tactile sensibility in the beak of geese. *Cell and Tissue Research* 153: 477–496.

Hess, J.C. and Paré, J.A. (2004). Viruses of waterfowl. *Seminars in Avian and Exotic Pet Medicine* 13 (4): 176–183.

Hochleithner, M. and Hochleithner, C. (1996). Surgical treatment of ulcerative lesions caused by automutilation of the sternum in psittacine birds. *Journal of Avian Medicine and Surgery* 10: 84–88.

Holcomb, J. (1988). Net-bottom caging for waterfowl. *Wildlife Journal* 11 (1): 3–4.

Hollmen, T. (1999). An experimental study on the effects of polymorphiasis in common eider ducklings. *Journal of Wildlife Diseases* 35 (3): 466–473.

Huffman, J.E. and Fried, B. (2008). Schistosomes. In: *Parasitic Diseases of Wild Birds* (ed. C.T. Atkinson, N.J. Thomas and D.B. Hunter), 246–260. Ames, IA: Wiley.

Kear, J. (2005). *Ducks, Geese and Swans*. Oxford, UK: Oxford University Press.

Kearns, K.S. (2003). Anseriformes (waterfowl, screamers). In: *Zoo and Wild Animal Medicine*, 5e (ed. M.E. Fowler and R.E. Miller), 141–149. St Louis, MO: Elsevier Science.

Kirkwood, J. (2008). Slipped tendon, angel wing and rolled toes. In: *Avian Medicine*, 2e (ed. J. Samour), 260–261. Edinburgh, UK: Elsevier.

Kline, Y., Clemons, K.V., Woods, L. et al. (2011). Pharmacokinetics of voriconazole in adult mallard ducks (*Anas platyrhynchos*). *Medical Mycology* 49 (5): 500–512.

Livezey, B.C. (1997). A phylogenetic analysis of basal Anseriformes, the fossil Presbyornis, and the interordinal relationships of waterfowl. *Zoological Journal of the Linnean Society* 121 (4): 361–428.

Machin, K. (2004). Waterfowl anesthesia. *Seminars in Avian and Exotic Pet Medicine* 13 (4): 206–212.

Madge, S. and Burn, H. (1988). *Wildfowl: An Identification Guide to the Ducks, Geese and Swans of the World*. London: Christopher Helm.

Mehlhorn, H., Tarachewski, H., Zhao, B. et al. (1990). Loperamid, an efficacious drug against the acanthocephalan *Macracanthorhynchus hirudinaceus* in pigs. *Parasitology Research* 76: 624–626.

Miller, E.A. (2007). Common toxicoses of wildlife. In: *Topics in Wildlife Medicine: Emergency and Critical Care*, vol. 2 (ed. F.S. Tseng and M.A. Mitchell), 71–97. St Cloud, MN: National Wildlife Rehabilitators Association.

Miller, E.A. and Brunner, E. (2013). Botulism or is it? *Wildlife Rehabilitation Bulletin* 31 (1): 1–12.

Mulcahy, D.M. (2007). Free-living waterfowl and shorebirds. In: *Zoo Animal and Wildlife Immobilization and Anesthesia* (ed. G. West, D. Heard and N. Caulkett), 299–324. Ames, IA: Wiley.

National Research Council (1994). Nutrient requirements of ducks. In: *Nutrient Requirements of Poultry*, 9th revised edn., 42–43. Washington, DC: National Academies Press.

Nelson, C.H. (1993). *The Downy Waterfowl of North America*. Deerfield, IL: Delta Station Press.

Olsen, J. (1994). Anseriformes. In: *Avian Medicine: Principles and Application* (ed. B.W. Ritchie and G.J. Harrison), 1237–1275; 1343–1344. Lake Worth, FL: Wingers Publishing.

Olsen, G. (2015). Web Sparing Amputation of the Third Digit of a Duck. Proceedings of the Association of Avian Veterinarians, Oakley, CA, p. 169.

Orosz, S.E. (2000). Overview of aspergillosis: pathogenesis and treatment options. *Seminars in Avian and Exotic Pet Medicine* 9 (2): 59–65.

Pello, S.J. and Olsen, G.H. (2013). Emerging and reemerging diseases of avian wildlife. *Veterinary Clinics of North America: Exotic Pet Practice* 16 (2): 357–381.

Rao, D.M. (2014). Enhancing epidemiological analysis of intercontinental dispersion of H5N1 viral strains by migratory waterfowl using phylogeography. *BMC Proceedings* 8 (Suppl 6): S1.

Rocke, T.E. and Friend, N. (1999). Avian botulism. In: *Field Manual of Wildlife Diseases: General Field Procedures and Diseases of Birds* (ed. M. Friend and J.C. Franson), 271–281. Madison, WI: USGS.

Samour, J. (2008). Keel injuries. In: *Avian Medicine*, 1e (ed. J. Samour), 207–208. Edinburgh, UK: Elsevier.

Samour, J. and Naldo, J.L. (2005). Lead toxicosis in falcons: a method for lead retrieval. *Seminars in Avian and Exotic Pet Medicine* 14 (2): 143–148.

Tarachewski, H., Mehlhorn, H., and Raether, W. (1990). Loperamid, an efficacious drug against fish-pathogenic acanthocephalans. *Parasitology Research* 76: 619–623.

Tuggle, B.N. (1999). Nasal leeches. In: *Field Manual of Wildlife Diseases: General Field Procedures and Diseases of Birds* (ed. M. Friend and J.C. Franson), 245–248. Madison, WI: USGS.

Tully, T.N., Dorrestein, G.M., and Jones, A.K. (2009). *Handbook of Avian Medicine*. Philadelphia, PA: Elsevier.

Wheler, C.L. (2002). Orthopedic conditions of the avian head. *Veterinary Clinics of North America: Exotic Animal Practice* 5 (1): 83–95.

Wobeser, G.A. (1997). *Diseases of Wild Waterfowl*, 2e. New York: Springer Science + Business Media.

19

Medical and Surgical Management of Seabirds and Allies

Rebecca S. Duerr

International Bird Rescue, Fairfield, CA, USA

Natural History

The lifestyle of living in aquatic habitats is shared by genetically and behaviorally diverse groups of birds, including grebes, loons, herons, egrets, pelicans, cormorants, boobies, alcids (murres, puffins, murrelets, auklets), gulls, terns, shorebirds, procellariiformes (tubenoses: albatrosses, fulmars, shearwaters, petrels), rails, and a few others (e.g., American dipper). The anseriformes (ducks, geese, swans) are covered in Chapter 18 although many of the issues discussed in this chapter also apply to diving ducks such as scoters and buffleheads. Taxonomic relationships of these species are beyond the scope of this chapter. Care of aquatic birds contaminated by oil is covered in Chapter 6 and care of chicks is discussed in Chapter 12.

Aquatic habitats span both freshwater and marine environments. Herons and other wading birds breed and forage in freshwater areas, but may also forage in salt water. Pelican and cormorant species vary in preferring fresh versus saltwater habitats; some individuals move between the two extremes routinely. Many loons and grebes migrate between fresh and marine habitats seasonally, breeding in inland lakes but wintering in coastal marine areas. Most alcids, tubenoses, and some species of gulls, terns, and shorebirds live entirely in marine habitats year round. As discussed in Padilla (2015), loons, grebes, and tubenoses are rarely kept in captivity and are difficult to manage for even short-term care. For information on the natural history of North American wild bird species, see Birds of North America Online at http://bna.birds.cornell.edu/bna. This resource is invaluable when species-specific information, such as timing of molt or wild diet, is needed. These species consume a varied diet, including vertebrate and invertebrate prey.

For all aquatic bird species, plumage condition and maintenance of a waterproof state are of critical importance because the plumage provides buoyancy, thermal homeostasis, and aero- and hydrodynamics, among other functional attributes. Poor-quality plumage, damaged feathers, plasma-weeping dermal conditions, and plumage contamination are serious enough problems that they may result in the death of the bird; hence, plumage condition must be a primary concern during all aspects of medical care for these species. Management or restoration of waterproofing in highly aquatic birds can be logistically challenging at typical veterinary clinics.

Reasons for Entering Care

Many of the reasons why aquatic birds enter care are anthropogenic: fishing hook or line injuries, gunshot injuries, heavy metal toxicity, habitat loss and resultant conflicts with humans over nest locations, attack by human pet predators, exposure to plumage contaminants, injuries from other wild animals due to conflicts over human fish waste disposal, ingestion of inappropriately discarded refuse, or collisions with vehicles. Other causes include disease outbreaks, harmful algal blooms, adverse weather events, or starvation related to food supply. Chicks also enter care due to parental separation, parental feeding of inappropriate foods, or injuries due to falling from nests.

Husbandry

Housing

Miller (2012) reviews housing requirements while in temporary captivity. To minimize stress, keep birds in a quiet area away from disturbances or view of potential predators. Species that normally stand (e.g., gulls,

Medical Management of Wildlife Species: A Guide for Practitioners, First Edition. Edited by Sonia M. Hernandez, Heather W. Barron, Erica A. Miller, Roberto F. Aguilar and Michael J. Yabsley.

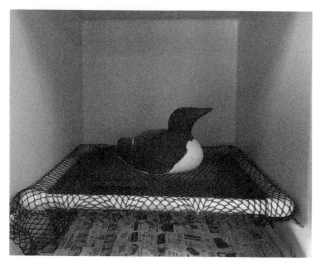

Figure 19.1 Net-bottom wall cage insert made from netting stretched across a PVC pipe frame, attached by hooking net onto screws placed on bottom of frame. Netting allows droppings to fall away from the bird and provides cushioning to keel and legs.

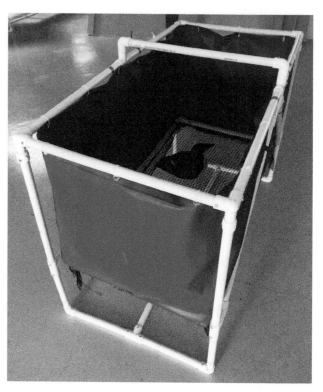

Figure 19.2 Net-bottom, soft-sided caging made from PVC pipe frame, with tarpaulin walls, and floor of netting stretched across PVC frame as in wall cage insert. Use fabric sheeting or shade cloth as cage ceiling. Netting allows droppings to fall away from the bird and provides cushioning to keel and legs while soft-sided walls reduce carpal lesions.

pelicans, herons) and are able to stand may be temporarily housed in standard veterinary wall cages with towel or coated wire substrates, but are at risk for injuring wings on caging. Application of preventive carpal and metacarpal wraps (aka "bumper pads") is advisable for agitated birds. Application of protective foot wraps when out of water helps reduce the development of foot lesions in grebes, loons, alcids, and diving ducks. Use 2″ cotton tubular stockinette stitched or taped shut at one end to form soft booties; attach with Vetrap™ (3M, St Paul, MN, USA) mid-tarsometatarsus. Do not apply proximal to the hock as this causes foot edema. Nonstanding pelicans, gulls, and herons may benefit from padded hock wraps to prevent pressure lesions. Keel cushions may be used to reduce the development of keel lesions in grebes, loons, and diving ducks, but poor application technique or inappropriate design for a given species may cause harm.

When too young, too disabled, or too hypothermic for standard housing, loons, grebes, and others require specialized housing to avoid rapid development of lesions on bony prominences (e.g., keel, hocks, toes, carpometacarpus). Standard veterinary wall cages are not considered appropriate by the author for more than short-term use; house in net-bottom, soft-sided caging to prevent injuries. Net bottoms decrease formation of pressure lesions on keels or legs, reduce plumage contamination with droppings or food, and help prevent injuries to the carpus and wingtip joints (Figures 19.1 and 19.2) (Holcomb 1988). Net-bottom pens also work well for pelicans unable to stand due to injuries.

Lesions may develop even when birds unable to stand are kept on seemingly adequately padded hard surfaces, and may rapidly progress to life-threatening severity.

Housing on towels often leads to loss of waterproofing due to plumage contamination and damage by droppings; fleece is better but still problematic. Agitated birds may injure themselves against hard cage walls or break feathers off in caging holes. Caregivers should think of plumage as an organ that must be in top-functioning condition for the bird to remain alive, rather than thinking of the feather coat as clothing that can be replaced. With certain exceptions (e.g., pelicans, gulls), it can very difficult to maintain these species in captivity long enough for new feather growth to occur.

Long-billed shorebirds (e.g., acovets, ibises) are at risk for breaking bill tips in hard-walled caging. If soft-sided caging is not available, an open-topped cardboard box may suffice short term. Cover with screen to allow daylight-level lighting necessary for self-feeding. House small-bodied shorebirds or rails in appropriately sized caging. Clear plastic solid-walled pet containers are adequate for short-term care of shorebirds but cover clear walls to give privacy while allowing light in at the top. These birds may be frantically stressed while being observed.

If birds are brought to a veterinary clinic for surgical procedures, minimize residence time at the clinic to prevent development of additional problems. At 24-hour facilities, house the bird in an area where it can rest undisturbed overnight. Some species are nocturnally active and may eat when humans are absent. Debilitated birds must be allowed adequate hours to rest. Diurnal day/night cycles are optimal.

Warmth, Fluids, and Nutrition

Providing thermoregulatory support, reducing stress, correcting dehydration, and providing nutritional support are the backbones of supportive care. Despite the large size of many of these species, debilitated individuals are often hypothermic and thermally unstable for the first few days of care. Cloacal temperature monitoring is useful in birds >100 g, but hand-held human digital thermometers may not fully assess hypo- or hyperthermia. Care must be taken when inserting thermometers as there is risk of cloacal perforation. Normal temperature in these species is 39.4–42.2 °C (103–108 °F) (International Bird Rescue [IBR], in-house data). Although certain species have body temperatures cooler than others, most aquatic birds are cold if cloacal temperature is <39.4 °C (103 °F). If a bird is bright, alert, responsive, and temperature is >38.6 °C (101.5 °F), it may be sufficiently warm. Provide supplemental heat if quiet or lethargic and <39.4 °C (103 °F). Handling stress may elevate body temperatures of birds, especially if the bird is well-fleshed, struggling, and covered with a restraint cloth (Greenacre and Lusby 2004). Handle hyperthermic birds as little as possible. Sick birds often exhibit hypothermia; febrile states are uncommon.

Deliver heat by placing the bird in a warm room (29.4 °C/85 °F), heated via radiant heat from hot pads on walls or under containers, or use space heaters or pet dryers directed into cages. Space heaters and pet dryers may exacerbate dehydration but may be the best option for delivering heat in circumstances such as warming cold pelicans housed in wall cages or plastic kennels. Pet dryers work well for birds in net-bottom housing, as the warm air can be directed up from below, which also helps dry wet ventral feathers. Animal Intensive Care Units (Lyon Technologies Inc., Chula Vista, CA) or other incubator-type housing are useful for short-term warming of adult birds but can lead to severe hyperthermia. Overnight housing of this type without frequent monitoring is inadvisable, except for young chicks.

Birds unable to eat for any reason become emaciated very quickly (Shapiro and Weathers 1981; Jeffrey et al. 1985; Herzberg et al. 1988). Carnivorous birds primarily fulfill requirements for water by catabolism of food (Goldstein and Skadhauge 2000) so once nutritional stores are depleted, debilitated birds become significantly dehydrated. Consequently, wild birds are usually presented for care cold, emaciated, and dehydrated, especially those that are wet or become debilitated in cold environments (Duerr and Klasing 2015). Carnivorous birds maintain blood glucose through obligate gluconeogenesis (Migliorini et al. 1973; Meyers and Klasing 1999), so are rarely hypoglycemic and are at risk of hyperglycemia when fed glucose (Pham 2004).

Consider all newly admitted birds as being at least mildly dehydrated and rehydrate through oral, subcutaneous (SQ) and/or intravenous (IV) routes after the bird has been warmed to normal body temperature. Intraosseous (IO) administration is another option, but anatomical variation may complicate placement of catheters (e.g., pneumatized ulna and tibiotarsus in pelicans). Most wild aquatic birds present with isotonic to hypotonic dehydration due to moderate to severe anorexia or cachexia, and often have wounds; consequently, replace electrolytes during rehydration. Warm (40.5 °C/105 °F) tap water given orally is only appropriate for birds in generally good condition or during extenuating circumstances such as mass stranding events.

New birds usually do well when orally hydrated once and then started on a feeding schedule until self-feeding. For SQ fluids, sterile isotonic fluids, such as lactated Ringer's solution, can be given into the inguinal skinfold with a 23–27 gauge needle (see Appendix II: Formulary). Avoid excessive perforation of skin as this may impact waterproofing in swimming species. Never use the pre- or postpatagium for fluid administration. The dorsal scapular back may provide sufficiently stretchy skin in some species. Once- or twice-daily SQ fluid administration is extremely helpful for management of inappetent birds, especially species or individuals that tend to regurgitate (e.g., herons).

In addition to subcutaneous air cells ("bubble wrap skin"), pelicans have large extracoelomic air spaces at pectoral (between the pectoralis and supracoracoideus muscles) and inguinal (cranioventral and medial to the muscles of the tibiotarsus) locations that communicate with the clavicular air sac. Avoid administering fluid into these air spaces.

Warmed parenteral fluids may improve the thermoregulatory status of markedly debilitated birds. Catheters are difficult to manage, so IV fluids are often administered as intermittent boluses of 10–20 mL/kg via a 25–27 gauge butterfly catheter infusion set; colloids given at up to 20 mL/kg/day are also helpful for extremely debilitated birds, especially if hypoproteinemic. The medial metatarsal vein is the primary venous access in aquatic birds. Pelicans also have easily accessible veins at the medial side of digit 3, dorsal side of digit 2 at the foot joint crease, and the ventral mandible. Midmandible, this vessel easily accepts a 24–26 gauge over-the-needle indwelling catheter for use with either an intermittent access port or a drip set; use tape or suture to secure. Basilic and jugular veins should be avoided in most species, as hemorrhage at these locations may adversely affect waterproofing due to dermal weeping of subcutaneous hematomas. Unlike most aquatic species, herons, egrets, and gulls have a large apteria over the jugular vein, which is easily accessible for administration of emergency drugs or blood collection.

Gavage feeding is administered into the proventriculus with size 8–16 Fr red rubber catheters on appropriately sized syringes. These species do not have crops. No tube is necessary for pelicans; hold the bill upward and deposit fluid or diet into the pouch base past the glottis, massaging down the esophagus. Gavage volumes are typically 50–70 mL/kg every 1.5–2 hours, 6–7 times/day when the sole source of nutrition. Begin with smaller volumes until you are certain the bird can handle higher volumes. Measure daily body weights until the bird is eating reliably and housed outside.

Most aquatic birds do well on critical care gavage diets intended for obligate carnivores (e.g., cats). However, extremely emaciated birds may have impaired digestion and are benefitted by feeding diets that contain hydrolyzed proteins and low to moderate levels of fat rather than higher calorie (higher fat) diets (Duerr and Klasing 2017). Once birds are housed in pools, feed low-fat diets to avoid excreted excess fat contaminating the plumage. Acceptable gavage diets include blended small whole fish slurry (with appropriate vitamin E and thiamin supplementation; see Appendix II: Formulary), Emeraid Piscivore (Lafeber Co., Cornell, IL, USA) fed at 11% fat (Duerr and Klasing 2017), Carnivore Care (Oxbow Animal Health, Murdock, NE, USA), or blended Hill's canned feline A/D diet (Hill's Pet Nutrition Inc., Topeka, KS, USA). Only the Lafeber product provides hydrolyzed proteins; the others are whole-protein diets and rather high fat. Feeding hydrolyzed protein diets may be beneficial in emaciated birds to allow immediate absorption of nutrients rather than additional energetic expenditures on digestive processes. Consider treatment of warmed whole-protein diets with pancreatic enzymes (Viokase-V, Fort Dodge Animal Health, Overland Park, KS, USA) 30 minutes prior to feeding if extremely debilitated patients are having digestive problems.

Marine species such as tubenoses and alcids housed full-time on fresh water require salt supplementation. Without supplementation, plasma sodium may drop as low as 117 mEq/L in northern fulmars (Frankfurter et al. 2012). Hyponatremic behavior includes inappetence, lethargy, and obtundation that worsens the longer the bird remains in fresh water. Salt supplementation at IBR's clinics is 500 mg/kg NaCl PO every 48–72 hours for alcids and 1000 mg/kg once daily for tubenoses. Salt is given as portions of salt tablets, or mixed as a 3%

solution and gavaged. Dry housing and housing in salt water negate the need for supplementation. Over-supplementation may lead to hypernatremia, dehydration, and seizures.

Pelicans and gulls eat well from simple presentations of thawed smelt or capelin in a dish of water, but others such as ibis or shorebirds may be more difficult. Long-billed mud- or sand-foraging species may eat well when presented with plentiful food items in a large shallow platter; offering food in mud is helpful for ibis. Prey items should include a diversity of commercial insects plus brine shrimp, bloodworms, krill, and other small invertebrates. Birds offered mud trays should also have access to clean water for bathing unless treatment for a problem (e.g., wing wrap) precludes access to bathing water. Wing wraps should be changed if they become wet, as feathers may mildew. Small grebes and some diving ducks eat well when offered krill. Small-bodied minced fish or tiny whole fish may also be eaten by long-billed shorebirds. Invertebrate eaters consume vast quantities of food and need new food platters several times a day. Gulls respond well to fish plus soaked dog kibble, scrambled egg, or other natural food items. Unenthusiastic herons may respond to a bowl of live and frozen/thawed fish in water. The presence of live prey can stimulate birds to start taking frozen/thawed fish.

Handling and Restraint

Eye and face protection is necessary during handling, and other personal protective equipment may be prudent depending on circumstances. The bill presents the greatest danger to handlers, although scratches from toenails may break the skin. Pelicans and large herons have a long bill-striking distance and will target the eyes. Nondebilitated loons and cormorants may aggressively launch attacks, including speeding towards doors to stab or bite caretakers.

In general, aquatic birds may be restrained with a size-appropriate towel or sheet with the head restrained, wings folded against the body, and the feet prevented from kicking. Restrain the bird quickly to prevent injuries during capture. Many birds will calm when eyes are covered and feet are supported. Ensure the bird can move the keel to breathe. Restrainers should hold birds at waist level when walking to keep them out of striking distance of the face. Herons and egrets may catch and avulse toenails or luxate toe joints on terry cloth; ensure toenails are free when changing patient position. Loons may luxate or fracture toes during restraint if allowed to kick against hard surfaces. Always restrain the beak of obligate mouth breathers (e.g., pelicans) with the beak slightly open.

Anesthesia and Surgery

Veterinarians should have postoperative care arranged with an experienced aquatic bird rehabilitator prior to performing surgical procedures. When possible, delay procedures until birds are in improved nutritional condition, while minimizing development of captivity-associated lesions. A two-hour presurgical fast is sufficient for grebes, shorebirds, and most diving ducks as they rarely regurgitate. Pelicans, gulls, herons, egrets, and tubenoses are highly prone to regurgitation during induction and recovery from anesthesia and longer fasts are prudent, at least 4–6 hours, or even overnight for known binge feeders.

Dog or cat masks are effective for induction of gas anesthesia for many species, although unusually shaped bills benefit from custom creation of better-fitting masks made of items such as plastic syringe cases. See Chapter 5 for information on pain management and anesthesia. Intubate during procedures expected to last more than 10 minutes. Because birds may passively regurgitate due to gravity, keep the head elevated above the body during surgical procedures. Use endotracheal tubes designed for birds whenever possible; do not inflate cuffed mammal tubes. Tubenoses may regurgitate defensive oil early and late in anesthesia and may aspirate. Intubate quickly and tape endotracheal tubes securely. The trachea of northern fulmars bifurcates approximately 2 cm from the glottis, hence unilateral intubation is a risk. Unfamiliar species may have anatomy that complicates anesthesia. Pelicans and some shorebirds may have a rigid septum just inside the glottis (the crista ventralis) which limits the size of tube used; this septum may bleed if bent or broken.

Use intermittent positive pressure ventilation (IPPV) to ensure adequate ventilation during anesthesia, at least every 30 seconds, or 6–10 ×/minute if the bird is not breathing on its own, which many diving birds will not. When providing IPPV to pelicans, minimize leakage by gently clamping a hand over the glottis from outside the pouch during inspiration. The trachea is soft and collapsible in many species of diving birds such as loons, but rigid and noncollapsible in others such as grebes.

Diving birds often exhibit marked bradycardia during anesthesia but usually respond well to atropine or glycopyrrolate. Many gull species display atropine-responsive arrhythmias during anesthesia. Most aquatic birds will show a heart rate of 150–200 bpm under anesthesia and, as is typical of vertebrates, heart rate is inversely proportional to body size. In general, bradycardias under 100 bpm or nonsinus arrhythmias should trigger concern by the clinician. Continuous monitoring is recommended as this allows deleterious changes to be noticed and treated immediately.

Prevent intraoperative hypothermia, especially in young, wet, or debilitated surgical patients. Hypothermia may dramatically increase anesthetic recovery times. Extubation should not occur until birds have a swallow reflex and are breathing well. Respiratory stimulants are rarely needed in these species. Do not consider the bird out of danger of anesthetic complications until it is holding its head up and fully awake; a responsible person should stay with the animal until fully conscious. Do not allow groggy birds to thrash around in caging as severe injuries may occur.

Anesthetic monitoring equipment is always desirable, but many rehabilitation centers lack technological monitoring devices and small animal practitioners may lack avian equipment. However, esophageal stethoscope attachments are within the budget of nearly everyone (<$25) and are extremely useful, especially when the surgical field requires complete draping of the bird. These are available from many veterinary medical supply companies.

Pluck feathers minimally to prepare surgical sites; a 3 mm margin is adequate. Never cut feathers; plucked feathers begin regrowing immediately. Hold feathers away from the surgical site by applying paper tape (e.g., 3M Micropore™) or other tapes that will not leave a residue on feathers. Swimming species must have enough contour feathers remaining to waterproof without growth of replacement feathers.

Minimize application of surgical skin disinfectants to avoid postoperative waterproofing problems in swimming birds. Betadine solution (not scrub) and 70% ethanol are typical presurgical disinfectants.

Loons, grebes, and alcids may present with large lacerations and necrotic skin may extend under plumage that appears normal, resulting in an irregularly shaped lesion with necrotic subcutaneous fat or muscle. Pluck feathers from around the margin of healthy skin, dissect all damaged tissue, trim wound contours, and close with a horizontal mattress pattern that creates a narrow everted lip that will exfoliate in time, as described in the Keel Repair section. Even when large, these repairs heal very well as long as subcutaneous fat is kept out of the closure. Strive to have swimming birds as waterproof as possible prior to surgery. If the animal is returned to its pool immediately after waking from surgery, surgical incisions will stay cleaner, fewer secondary problems will erupt, and healing will progress faster.

After foot surgery in standing species, bandage the foot to keep surgical incisions free of droppings and food. Waterproof outer wraps and food dish modification may be needed. Pelicans do well keeping foot incisions dry for three days then going back into an aviary if the bird will spend ample time swimming and bathing. Gulls and herons heal best when the foot is kept dry and clean until the incision heals in 10–14 days. Herons do not usually dunk foot wraps in fish dishes but gulls do. Change wraps daily. Housing cleanliness and species behavior drive the need for bandaging. Consider the effect of loss of webbing on swimming ability when deciding on toe amputation versus euthanasia. IBR in-house guidelines are to remove no more than 25% of total foot surface area for grebes, loons, or diving ducks. Swimming species should return to a pool promptly after foot surgery.

Selected Surgical Procedures

Pelican Pouch Lacerations

Use surgical staples to secure the mouth temporarily so that the bird can eat (Figure 19.3). Repair can wait until the surgeon's convenience, but generally within 10 days of injury. Substantial reductions in pouch size often stretch in time, and even enormous lacerations heal well. If the laceration is very large, plan on more than one procedure to keep anesthesia time <3 hours per procedure. Allow the animal a day or more to eat and recover between procedures, especially if still debilitated.

Pouch tissue consists of inner and outer stratified squamous epithelium with central skeletal muscle (William et al. 1988). Repair involves splitting the inner and outer layers and closing separately such that no epithelium is sutured inside the closure. Trim tissues to create a fresh edge, removing jagged, edematous, devitalized areas, and rounded granulating edges. Prior to cutting, ligate any large vessels that will be affected by the cut. Stretch the skin edge between fingers to create tension on the edge. Use a #11 scalpel blade to slice the inner and

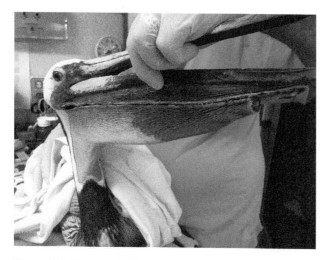

Figure 19.3 Temporarily close large pouch lacerations with skin staples to allow the bird to eat and become medically stable prior to surgery. Even extremely large lacerations have an excellent prognosis. Note the thickened granulating edge which will be trimmed off at surgical repair.

outer layers apart to a depth of 5 mm around the entire laceration. Avoid accidental cuts through epithelium. Simple digital pressure usually controls hemorrhage. To prevent mismatches and puckering when suturing this extremely elastic tissue, identify landmarks such as the ventral midline and tack in place with simple interrupted sutures at several locations.

Begin the closure at the caudal aspect of the laceration. Invert the inside layer with a segmentally continuous horizontal mattress (Connell) pattern, with knots every 5–10 cm. Once a section of the inside layer has been sutured, close the matching outer layer with a continuous everting horizontal mattress pattern (Figure 19.4). The author uses 4-0 Monocryl suture on a taper needle, with ophthalmic instruments such as Bishop Harmon forceps. The split edge tissue tends to roll, so excellent visualization of the edge is needed to ensure correct placement of sutures to avoid the epithelial side of the skin being inside the closure. Place sutures 1–2 mm from the edge and 3 mm apart. Wider spacing allows gaps that may lead to dehiscence. Moisten laceration edges periodically with warm sterile fluids, and flush small blood clots from the suture. Avoid overtightening sutures, and also avoid too little tension so that there are gapped areas between stitches. Adjust sizes of opposing bites as needed to gradually tailor mismatched lengths. Y-shaped junctions are often unavoidable when tailoring large pouch repairs but minimize when possible.

Limit access to water and offer frequent small meals for five days post repair to prevent pouch stretching. After this time, house in a large aviary with pool. Expect the suture line to heal in 10–14 days. Never release until the repair has healed as starvation may ensue if dehiscence occurs once out of human care.

If the laceration involves avulsion of pouch from the mandible or an area of exposed bone adjacent to the pouch, thoroughly debride all exposed bone. Scrape with the flat back of a scalpel blade to remove debris and devitalized tissue from the mandible. Trim damaged keratin to create a perpendicular interface between the flat bone face and vital keratin. Freshen the edge of the pouch skin. Use small blunt-tipped tissue scissors to dissect pouch layers apart as deeply as needed to provide a graft with minimal tension. Beware of creating tears in the pouch skin. Start in the defect's center and suture from skin up under the wall of keratin (Figure 19.5), using a simple continuous pattern. The author uses 4-0 Monocryl on a taper needle. Pouch skin knits well to bill keratin and with time modifies into heavily keratinized bill.

Keel Repair

Loons, grebes, and diving ducks are prone to the development of keel lesions. Emaciated birds are at especially high risk.

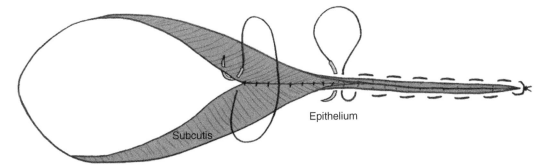

Epithelium

Subcutis

Figure 19.4 Suture patterns used for pelican pouch repair. Split into inner and outer epithelium with #11 scalpel blade. Use a segmentally continuous horizontal mattress (Connell) pattern to close the inner layer and a continuous everting horizontal mattress pattern to close the outer layer. Place stitches 1–2 mm from skin edge and 3 mm apart, place knots every 5–10 cm. Do not allow any epithelium to be on the subcuticular side of the closure.

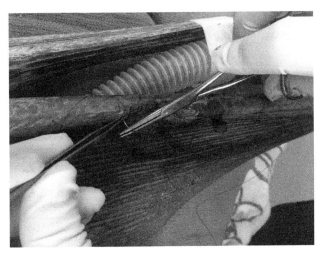

Figure 19.5 Advancement graft of pouch skin to cover exposed mandible. Debride bone and devitalized keratin aggressively, split pouch tissue to create flap, and freshen skin edge. Pass taper needle through skin, then up under lip of keratin, gently apposing skin to keratin edge.

Lesion severity is graded as follows.

- Grade 1 mild: simple linear necrotic skin, not adhered to underlying bone.
- Grade 2 moderate: thickened, linear scabrous lesion, not adhered to underlying bone, but may weep plasma.
- Grade 3 severe: linear necrotic skin adhered to underlying bone, may be dry or weep plasma.
- Grade 4 open: may involve ripped pectoral muscle.

Grade 1 and 2 lesions may slough off as linear scabs and not cause clinical problems. Some grade 2 and all grade 3 lesions are likely to split open during vigorous flapping and require surgery. Grade 4 lesions require immediate repair.

Prior to surgery, birds should be well hydrated and well nourished, and as waterproof as possible. Birds with grade 2 and 3 lesions should be waterproof for several days prior to surgery so that regaining a waterproof state occurs quickly after surgery. Birds with grade 3 or 4 lesions may require washing after surgery to remove dried plasma and blood if the bird has difficulty waterproofing the surgical site.

Closed Keel Repair

Grade 1 and 2 lesions can be repaired preemptively without opening the skin by application of closely spaced, horizontal mattress sutures that evert the necrotic skin into a protuberant lip of tissue that will slough off as a scab. Space sutures 2–3 mm apart and 2–3 mm between halves of the mattress stitch, 1–2 mm into healthy skin from the necrotic skin border.

Open Keel Repair, Simple

Pluck a 3 mm margin into healthy skin along the lesion edges and hold feathers away with tape. Remove necrotic skin by sharp dissection. If the live/dead interface is irregularly shaped or not distinct, trim skin as needed to obtain a healthy skin margin in an elliptical shape. Avoid trimming the skin too close to the plucked border or feathers may be problematic when suturing. Bluntly dissect skin and pectoral muscle to a depth of 3 cm along the pectoral fascial plane, to allow closure with minimal tension on the incision. Subcutaneous fat should remain with the visceral side of the skin. Do not separate layers of muscle or separate fat from skin. In chronic lesions, fibrin, and granulation tissue may obscure the separation of tissue planes; freshening the lesion edge usually reveals the layers.

Excise unhealthy-looking subcutis. If possible, suture fascia between the keel and skin. To close skin, place interrupted horizontal mattress sutures 2–3 mm apart with 2–3 mm between halves of each stitch, 1–2 mm into healthy skin from the skin border. Pull all sutures tight; do not leave room for swelling. Do not include any subcutaneous fat in the everted lip of the closure as it may

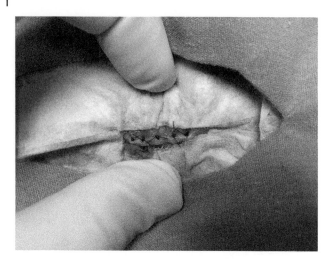

Figure 19.6 Typical closure of lacerations and keel repairs in highly aquatic birds. Use tightly spaced snug horizontal mattress sutures spaced 1–2 mm from skin edge with knots 5 mm part.

weep lipids into plumage. In birds with subcutaneous fat, run the needle 2 mm from the skin edge to the visceral side of the cut edge so that subcutaneous fat is not exposed in the lip, just the cut skin edge. To avoid mismatches and puckers when fitting the two sides together, place the first suture in the middle, then in quarters, then close each quadrant. This can also help control bleeding by applying general tension. Blot any blood promptly to avoid contaminating plumage. Extend the sutures at each end at least half a stitch past the end of the lesion – do not leave even a tiny area of unsutured lip at the ends. Inspect the closure and add additional horizontal mattress sutures if needed to close any gaps (Figure 19.6).

Open Keel Repair, Complicated

The keel itself is involved in these lesions. Using rongeurs, remove the ventral edge of affected keel. If the bone edge appears lytic or disorganized, trim deeper. If osteomyelitis is suspected, collect culture samples prior to closure. Infusion with antibiotic or placement of antibiotic-impregnated beads may be useful. Palpate the new edge and remove any sharp areas, leaving a smooth edge. Trimming the bone margin releases the ventral pectoral fascia from attachment at the keel. Close this fascia across the keel with a simple continuous pattern, pulling the pectoral muscle together to make a soft tissue pad between keel and skin. Close the skin as previously described.

In grade 4 lesions, necrotic skin may remain adhered to the keel while the pectoral muscle rips open parallel to the keel during flapping (e.g., during capture from a pool). These lesions are often highly contaminated but may heal well. Thoroughly lavage after surgical debridement. Gently appose tissues into as normal a position as possible prior to closure. Torn pectoral muscle is often friable but associated fascia, even if torn, may hold sutures well.

Postsurgical waterproofing recovery time for diving ducks and grebes is typically 24–48 hours. Birds that have had laceration or keel repairs will likely require a haul-out available for at least 24 hours while they reestablish waterproofing. Postoperative birds preoccupied with preening may require supplemental feedings.

Despite using absorbable sutures, remove sutures in 7–14 days to facilitate inspection of all areas of each lesion. Some sutures may show a deep scab that indicates need for a second surgery.

Internal Fish Hook Removal Techniques

Take radiographs of any bird displaying evidence of fishing gear injury to rule out hooks or tackle inside. If fishing line protrudes from the mouth, secure it by tying an extension to the line and fastening it to a tape necklace. Taping line to the bill often fails.

If two orthogonal radiographs do not indicate a hook is engaged in GI tract walls, "cotton balling" may be effective for gulls, cormorants, and herons. Cotton balling involves gutting several food fish, liberally packing the abdomens with cotton cast padding, and force feeding to the patient once it has been stabilized. The cotton will increase the amount of indigestible material in the stomach and the bird may regurgitate the hook and cotton. A potential disadvantage is that if the bird does not regurgitate within a few days and a surgical approach is needed, the cotton wadding may obscure the hook visually.

Internal hook removal techniques vary somewhat by species and the equipment of the clinic. In some species such as gulls, if the line is still available, a thick-walled tube such as ¾" external diameter, ½" internal diameter with rounded edges on one end may be advanced over the line down to the hook, and then the tube used to push the hook out of the flesh while the thick wall collects the bulk of the hook's curvature and prevents reembedment on the way out. In herons and cormorants, the gastrointestinal tract is very distensible and this method does not work well. Endoscopy is an option, or esophagostomy at the right caudal neck just cranial to the thoracic inlet.

A common nonsurgical method of hook removal from pelicans is the "human endoscope" where someone with small hands gloves using a rectal sleeve and disposable glove, lubricates the hand, and reaches into the bird's proventriculus for manual removal. If the hook is engaged internally, gently back the hook out following its curve. Despite the embedded barb, this often causes minimal trauma and avoids a proventriculotomy. Sedation or anesthesia is necessary.

Surgical approach for a proventriculotomy is from the ventral midline due to the presence of an apteria in most species. A left lateral approach may be used as well. Consider the radiographic location of the hook tip in choosing the approach. These species tend to have a larger, thinner-walled, more caudally located proventriculus and minimal ventriculus compared to chickens; hence, entering these structures is relatively simple. Bear in mind the surgeon will not be able to flush blood or GI contents from the coelom due to unavoidable air sac involvement. Use laparotomy pads and stay sutures to hold the incised proventriculus and suction or swab any liquid (or verminous) contents. Blot any bleeding that occurs without letting it run into the air sacs. Close the proventriculus or ventriculus with a double layer of 4-0 Monocryl or PDS in a Cushing pattern.

If the hook tip is located in a difficult position, such as in the esophagus at the heart or on the dorsal side of the viscera, it may be easiest to allow the bird to dissolve the luminal portion of the hook (over several weeks), then remove it when the tip has been encapsulated and is strictly located on the serosal side of the GI tract. This is also an option for birds in poor condition; remove the hook tip later after other health issues such as entanglement wounds have been resolved. Leaving the hook permanently is an option, but the author prefers to remove all internal metal whenever possible.

Close the body wall with a simple continuous pattern and hyperinflate the air sacs to check for leakage before closing the skin.

Fishing Hook/Line Injuries and Other Wounds

Remove fish hooks by advancing the tip until the barb exits the skin, clip the tip off and back the remainder out. Rescuers sometimes remove gear and may leave hook fragments in the bird, or not communicate exactly where hooks were embedded, which complicates monitoring for abscess development. Fish hook punctures appear innocuous at first but often develop into severe infections and abscesses. Punctures into joints, tendons, or bones, and hock and patagium constrictions are common. Only consider immediate release when the hook is known to have hooked superficial skin only, and the animal does not have skin damage from line constriction. Skin that has been constricted often becomes necrotic; assessment of necrosis depth is difficult until time passes. The presence of edema is not a perfect predictor of damage severity, as avian tissue does not become edematous as easily as mammalian tissue. Whether affected structures will cause loss of function is also difficult to predict. Some losses of structures may still result in a

releasable bird if the bird is able to do what it needs to do with the limb after healing. The patagium can take a lot of damage and still result in a releasable bird (see Scott 2010). Physical therapy techniques can be a helpful adjunct during recovery.

Pelican fishing hook- or line-related skin lacerations often dehisce when promptly surgically repaired due to continued necrosis of affected skin, and often must be managed as open wounds that heal by second intention. Delayed primary closure after a week or more of open wound care is more likely to be successful than immediate primary closure. Partially close wounds if necessary to cover bone; surgical staples may be efficacious. Pelicans begin to granulate in approximately one week. Healing of extremely large wounds in pelicans occurs routinely. Opening subcutaneous pockets of debris to facilitate debridement is helpful. Once large wounds begin granulating, closure occurs quickly and granulation tissue is often exuberant. Scar formation is transitory.

Pelican hock entanglements often lead to knuckling of digit #1 (hallux), folding it under the foot and causing damage to the toe which may lead to amputation. All pelicans with hock entanglements should be monitored for knuckling and stiff shoes applied to keep the toe in normal position while the hock injury heals. Control of the toe often returns once the tissue has healed.

Fresh, minimally contaminated skin lacerations may sometimes be closed with tissue glue or skin staples. Razor wire injuries heal well with staples, fish hook injuries do not. Use water-based topical gels, creams, and hydrogel dressings when tissues need to be kept moist as oil-based topicals cause plumage contamination. Wet-to-dry dressings are useful in debridement of necrotic material. Sugar/honey wraps have been used to reduce bacterial contamination and foster granulation in wounds. These species commonly heal skin over pockets of infected material that may be a continual source of inflammation and worsening infection. Consequently, scabs cannot be assessed as being "healthy" unless they have been removed to assess whether necrotic debris penetrates deeper into tissues. Wounds healing by second intention should be debrided regularly until a full granulation bed is present deep to the defect.

Micropore paper tape and Tegaderm™ (3M, St Paul, MN, USA) adhesive materials may be used on aquatic bird plumage as part of wound treatments, but any adhesive may leave a sticky residue if the material contacts feathers for several days. Use great care when applying and removing tape from small birds such as rails or plovers. Fractures may be managed as in other avian species, although pelicans require modified pinning techniques (Duerr and Purdin 2017).

Clinically Relevant Anatomy and Physiology

Anatomical adaptations for swimming are common in these species, and this diversity is beyond the scope of this chapter. Loons, grebes, and tubenoses have plantar foot surfaces easily injured when exposed to hard surfaces. These species do not have thickened fat pads and other weight-bearing structures on the plantar aspects of the toes, only skin covering the digit's tendons and ligaments. Lesions are often acutely ischemic or traumatically ulcerating injuries. Focal ischemic necrosis with adherence to deeper tissues is common. Chronic pododermatitis is a potential problem if an aquatic bird is housed out of water long term, but this is less common than acute lesions in these species. Once nutritional condition and waterproofing have been corrected, lesions may granulate well but removal of devitalized tissue may be necessary, as is management to minimize osteomyelitis of affected joints. Granulation rarely occurs over exposed tendon; tendonectomy is generally indicated. Loss of toe tendons does not result in perceptible differences in swimming or diving competence. Leaving inflamed tendons in place often results in ascending tendinitis.

Severe anemia and hypoproteinemia are common concerns. Species vary in how predictive severe anemia is for eventual release: brown pelicans generally recover packed cell volume (PCV) quickly with supportive care and IBR routinely releases birds that entered care with PCV <10%. Conversely, common murres with extreme anemia are not likely to survive to release (Duerr et al. 2016). Hypoproteinemic birds may benefit from IV colloids; transfusions are rarely feasible or necessary.

Infectious or Parasitic Diseases of Concern

See Chapter 2 for information on zoonotic diseases in aquatic birds; only those of clinical importance will be discussed here. Double-crested cormorants are affected by endemic Newcastle disease at several geographic areas including the Salton Sea in California (Kuiken 1999), Gulf of Mexico (Farley et al. 2001; Allison et al. 2005), and the Great Lakes (Meteyer et al. 1997). Clinical signs include hemorrhagic diarrhea and neurological dysfunction including ataxia and unilateral or bilateral paralysis (Kuiken 1999). West Nile virus was the cause of a mass mortality of eared grebes in Utah (Ip et al. 2014). *Mycobacterium avium* causes vague chronic signs of illness and is usually diagnosed on necropsy by immunohistochemistry of granulomatous lesions (Converse 2007).

Aspergillus fumigatus infection is a frequent cause of death in aquatic birds. Birds may enter care with active infections or acquire infection within the facility. Diagnosis in individual wild birds is complicated by vague clinical signs and expensive nondefinitive diagnostic tests (Burco et al. 2012, 2014). Radiography of anesthetized birds during maximal inflation is the most useful diagnostic tool in the opinion of the author. Although nonspecific, this method easily visualizes filling defects in air sacs and visceral adhesions; almost all possible etiologies hold a poor prognosis. Endoscopy is useful but limited by locations of entry. Diagnosis of aspergillosis carries a grave prognosis because long-term drug therapy is not usually feasible in these species. Susceptible species such as gulls, alcids, cormorants, and tubenoses are prophylactically given trizoles such as itraconazole and voriconazole until no longer handled regularly (Bunting et al. 2009). Sporonox™ (Janssen Pharmaeuticals, Inc. Titusville, NJ, USA) has best efficacy but is prohibitively expensive for most wildlife caregivers. Compounded preparations have poor efficacy (Hawkins et al. 2013). Brown pelicans are also susceptible to aspergillosis, but not commonly enough for prophylactic treatment (RD unpublished data).

Shorebirds are vulnerable to avian botulism; with intensive supportive care, these birds have a good prognosis for rapid recovery. Brevetoxin from the dinoflagellate *Karenia brevis* can cause stranding of numerous seabird species. With treatment, 33–54% of birds survive to release (Barron et al. 2013; Fauquier et al. 2013). Seabirds are regularly affected by domoic acid toxicity from blooms of the diatom *Pseudoneitzschia australis*, especially off southern California. Clinical signs range from mild obtundation to confusion to seizures or death prior to admission. Brown pelicans may be seen in large numbers exhibiting head-weaving and other neurological behaviors. Research is needed on effective treatment protocols for seabirds. Other harmful algal blooms may produce surfactants that affect waterproofing and birds may require washing (Phillips et al. 2011) while others may produce toxins such as microcystins (Miller et al. 2010).

Many seabird species have heavy parasite burdens and may excrete or regurgitate impressive quantities of worms when treated with praziquantel. A variety of trematodes affect the GI and respiratory tracts of aquatic birds, and most are responsive to fenbendazole. Pelicans with brown mucus at the glottis often have trematode eggs found in smears of the mucus and numerous flukes in trachea and air sacs. Herons and egrets may present with severe cases of several nematode worms, including *Avioserpens* spp., which present as spaghetti-like masses of worms within the floor of the mouth, and *Eustrongylides ignotus*, which is a relatively large nematode that is found in the proventriculus or body cavity. *Eustrongylides* can cause verminous coelomitis with sometimes extremely large debilitating abscesses of externalized GI contents and intestinal adhesions that impair peristalsis. These worms are often palpable as abnormal ridges on the ventral abdominal organs. Severe infestations of *Eustrongylides* carry a poor prognosis. Other nematodes may be found in soft tissue swellings anywhere on the body, particularly in herons, egrets, and grebes. Persistent focal swellings may benefit from surgical lancing to physically remove worms. *Cyathostoma* spp. nematodes have been found in the respiratory tract of cormorants. Piscivorous birds often have large numbers of *Contracaecum* in their proventriculus.

Pre-release Considerations

Plunge-diving species must be able to fly athletically to avoid starvation after release, including actively taking flight from a floating position, symmetrical and powerful flapping, and excellent plumage quality to facilitate flight. Long-distance migrants face similar requirements for athleticism on release. Anemia must resolve prior to release; at IBR, release criteria include a PCV >40%. Pre-release conditioning through physical therapy techniques is recommended prior to release for any bird which has recovered from a wing injury. Passive range of motion stretching, active exercise stimulation, and assisted active range of motion exercise all have a role in recovery to a releasable state for birds recovering from musculoskeletal injuries. Aviaries or net-enclosed pools of sufficient size must be available for pre-release conditioning. Birds must have access to clean water pools in pre-release housing to assure plumage is in optimal condition.

Acknowledgments

Endless thanks to those who have taught me about these species and their needs: Julie Skoglund, Michelle Bellizzi, Hayden Nevill, Greg Massey, Duane Tom, Jay Holcomb, Mike Ziccardi, Nancy Anderson, Kirk Klasing, and Flo Tseng.

References

Allison, A.B., Gottdenker, N.L., and Stallknecht, D.E. (2005). Wintering of neurotropic velogenic Newcastle disease virus and West Nile virus an double-crested cormorants (*Phalacrocorax auritus*) from the Florida keys. *Avian Diseases* 49: 292–297.

Barron, H.W., Bartleson, R.D., Mcinnis, K.B., et al. (2013). Hematologic and Biochemical Parameters in Seabirds with Brevetoxicosis. 7th Symposium on Harmful Algae in the US, Sarasota, FL (27–31 October 2013).

Bunting, E.M., Abou-Madi, N., Cox, S. et al. (2009). Evaluation of oral itraconazole administration in captive Humboldt penguins (*Spheniscus Humboldti*). *Journal of Zoo and Wildlife Medicine* 40 (3): 508–518.

Burco, J.D., Ziccardi, M.H., Clemons, K.V. et al. (2012). Evaluation of plasma (1–>3) beta-d-glucan concentrations in birds naturally and experimentally infected with *Aspergillus fumigatus*. *Avian Diseases* 56 (1): 183–191.

Burco, J.D., Massey, J.G., Byrne, B.A. et al. (2014). Monitoring of fungal loads in seabird rehabilitation centers with comparisons to natural seabird environments in northern California. *Journal of Zoo and Wildlife Medicine* 45 (1): 29–40.

Converse, K.A. (2007). Avian tuberculosis. In: *Infectious Diseases of Wild Birds* (ed. N.J. Thomas, D.B. Hunter and C.T. Atkinson), 289–302. Ames, IA: Wiley.

Duerr, R.S. and Klasing, K.C. (2015). Tissue component and organ mass changes associated with declines in body mass in three seabird species received for rehabilitation in California. *Marine Ornithology* 43: 11–18.

Duerr, R.S. and Klasing, K.C. (2017). Effects of added lipids on digestibility and nitrogen balance in oiled Common Murres (*Uria aalge*) and Western Grebes (*Aechmophorus occidentalis*) fed four formulations of a critical care diet. *Journal of Avian Medicine and Surgery* 31(2): 132–141.

Duerr, R.S. and Purdin, G.J. (eds.) (2017). *Topics in Wildlife Medicine; Orthopedics*, vol. 4. St Cloud, MN: National Wildlife Rehabilitators Association.

Duerr, R.S., Ziccardi, M.H., and Massey, J.G. (2016). Investigation into mortalities during treatment: Factors affecting oiled Common Murre (*Uria aalge*) survival to release through rehabilitation. *Journal of Wildlife Diseases* 52(3): 495–505.

Farley, J.M., Romero, C.H., Spalding, M.G. et al. (2001). Newcastle disease virus in double-crested cormorants in Alabama, Florida, and Mississippi. *Journal of Wildlife Diseases* 37: 808–812.

Fauquier, D.A., Flewelling, L.J., Maucher, J.M. et al. (2013). Brevetoxicosis in seabirds naturally exposed to *Karenia brevis* blooms along the central west coast of Florida. *Journal of Wildlife Diseases* 49 (2): 246–260.

Frankfurter, G., Ziccardi, M., and Massey, J.G. (2012). Effects of freshwater housing and fluid types on aquatic bird serum electrolyte concentrations. *Journal of Zoo And Wildlife Medicine* 43 (4): 852–857.

Goldstein, D. and Skadhauge, E. (2000). Renal and extrarenal regulation of body fluid composition. In: *Sturkie's Avian Physiology*, 5e (ed. G.C. Whittow), 265–297. San Diego, CA: Academic Press.

Greenacre, C.B. and Lusby, A.L. (2004). Physiologic responses of Amazon parrots (*Amazona* species) to manual restraint. *Journal of Avian Medicine and Surgery* 18 (1): 19–22.

Hawkins, M.G., Barron, H.W., Speer, B.L. et al. (2013). Birds. In: *Exotic Animal Formulary*, 4e (ed. J.W. Carpenter and C.J. Marion), 183–437. St Louis, MO: Elsevier Saunders.

Herzberg, G.R., Brosnan, J.T., Hall, B. et al. (1988). Gluconeogenesis in liver and kidney of common Murre (*Uria Aalge*). *American Journal of Physiology* 254: R903–R907.

Holcomb, J. (1988). Net bottom caging for waterfowl. *Wildlife Journal* 11 (1): 3–4.

Ip, H.S., van Wettere, A.J., Mcfarlane, L. et al. (2014). West Nile virus transmission in winter: the 2013 Great Salt Lake bald eagle and eared grebes mortality event. *Plos Currents* 6: ii.

Jeffrey, D.A., Peakall, D.B., Miller, D.S. et al. (1985). Blood chemistry changes in food-deprived herring gulls. *Comparative Biochemistry and Physiology* 81a: 911–913.

Kuiken, T. (1999). Review of Newcastle disease in cormorants. *Waterbirds: The International Journal of Waterbird Biology* 22 (3): 333–347.

Meteyer, C.U., Docherty, D.E., Glaser, L.C. et al. (1997). Diagnostic findings in the 1992 epornitic of neurotropic velogenic Newcastle disease in double-crested cormorants from the upper Midwestern United States. *Avian Diseases* 41: 171–180.

Meyers, M.R. and Klasing, K.C. (1999). Low glucokinase and high rates of gluconeogenesis contribute to hyperglycemia in barn owls (*Tyto Alba*) after a glucose challenge. *Journal of Nutrition* 129: 1896–1999.

Migliorini, R.H., Linder, C., Moura, J.L. et al. (1973). Gluconeogenesis in a carnivorous bird (black vulture). *American Journal of Physiology* 225 (6): 1389–1392.

Miller, E.A. (ed.) (2012). *Minimum Standards for Wildlife Rehabilitation*, 4e. St Cloud, MN: National Wildlife Rehabilitators Association.

Miller, M.A., Kudela, R.M., Mekebri, A. et al. (2010). Evidence for a novel marine harmful algal bloom: cyanotoxin (microcystin) transfer from land to sea otters. *PLoS One* 5 (9): e12576.

Padilla, L.R. (2015). Gaviiformes, podicipediformes, and procellariiformes. In: *Fowler's Zoo and Wild Animal Medicine*, vol. 8 (ed. R.E. Miller and M. Fowler), 89–95. St Louis, MO: Elsevier Saunders.

Pham, H.N. (2004). Carbohydrate digestibility in the American kestrel (Falco sparverius). Master's thesis. University of California, Davis.

Phillips, E.M., Zamon, J.E., Nevins, H.M. et al. (2011). Summary of birds killed by a harmful algal bloom along South Washington and North Oregon coasts during October 2009. *Northwestern Naturalist* 92 (2): 120–126.

Scott, D. (2010). *Handbook of Raptor Rehabilitation*. Raleigh, NC: Lulu Press Inc.

Shapiro, C.J. and Weathers, W.W. (1981). Metabolic and behavioral responses of American kestrels to food deprivation. *Journal of Comparative Biochemistry and Physiology* 68a: 111–114.

William, T.D., Gawlawski, P.Q., Strickland, D.M. et al. (1988). Surgical repair of the gular sac of the brown pelican (*Pelecanus Occidentalis*). *Journal of Zoo Animal Medicine* 19 (3): 122–125.

20

Medical and Surgical Management of Deer and Relatives

Kelli Knight[1] and Peach van Wick[2]

[1] *Southwest Virginia Wildlife Center of Roanoke, Roanoke, VA, USA*
[2] *Wildlife Center of Virginia, Waynesboro, VA, USA*

Introduction

Deer is the common name for the various ungulate ruminant mammals in the family Cervidae. Although cervid taxonomy is still evolving, the deer family Cervidae consists of 53 living species placed in 18 genera (Mattioli 2011). There are two living subfamilies: Cervinae (Old World plesiometacarpal deer) largely inhabit Eurasia, while Capriolinae (New World telemetecarpal deer) are found primarily in North and South America (Groves and Grubb 2011). Five deer species are found in North America: white-tailed deer (*Odocoileus virginianus*), mule deer (*Odocoileus hemionus*) including the subspecies black-tailed deer, caribou (*Rangifer tarandus*), elk or wapiti (*Cervus canadensis*), and moose (*Alces alces*) (Cronin 1992; Polziehn and Strobeck 2002). White-tailed deer are the most widespread cervid in North America, with 2010 population estimates exceeding 30 million in the United States alone (Rooney 2010). Hence, white-tailed deer will be the focus of this chapter but much of the information can be applied to other cervid species.

Many states prohibit rehabilitation of white-tailed deer fawns and adults, with the most common reason being as a precaution against the spread of diseases. Some states allow rehabilitation of fawns but not adults. Currently, in Virginia, adult white-tailed deer (a fawn becomes an adult on December 31 of the year of birth) may not be housed, rehabilitated or reared in any facility (VDGIF 2014). Some states require special permission to rehabilitate deer. For example, Indiana limits the number of deer that can be rehabilitated by allowing each licensed rehabilitator to rehabilitate 20 white-tailed per calendar year (Indiana Administrative Code 2011). The state's Department of Natural Resources or Department of Fish and Game should be contacted before initiating medical care.

Natural History

Range/Habitat

White-tailed deer inhabit southern Canada, all but two or three southwestern states of the mainland United States, Mexico, Central America, and the northern aspect of South America (Smith 1991; Dewey 2003). The 38 subspecies of white-tailed deer thrive in a wide range of terrestrial habitats from deciduous and coniferous forests, wetlands, grasslands, desserts, rainforests, farmlands, and suburban neighborhoods. Deer adapt easily to environmental change and flourish in close proximity to humans.

White-tailed deer and mule deer have overlapping ranges in 17 western states and three Canadian provinces while white-tailed deer and moose are sympatric in three states and parts of Canada.

Diet/Food Habits

Deer are herbivores and feed on a variety of foliage. White-tailed deer select the most nutritious vegetation that is available in their habitat, which can vary with each season. Farm crops, orchards, and nurseries are favorite food sources and can be heavily damaged. Deer spend more time foraging than any other activity and are typically crepuscular. Hay, deer pellets, and local flora can provide short-term feed during medical care.

Reproduction

Mating season for white-tailed deer is from October to December. A doe generally has one fawn in her first year of breeding; twins, or occasionally three or four fawns, are born in subsequent years. Gestation ranges from 187

Medical Management of Wildlife Species: A Guide for Practitioners, First Edition. Edited by Sonia M. Hernandez,
Heather W. Barron, Erica A. Miller, Roberto F. Aguilar and Michael J. Yabsley.
© 2020 John Wiley & Sons, Inc. Published 2020 by John Wiley & Sons, Inc.

to 222 days depending on subspecies. Parturition is in the spring and neonates are precocious. Birth weight averages between 2.5–4.0 kg (5.5–17.6 lb). Fawns triple their weight in their first month and are weaned between 8 and 12 weeks of age. Their spotted hair coat remains until autumn when their first molt occurs.

Doe–Fawn Behavior

When foraging, a doe leaves her fawn(s) unaccompanied for extended periods and visits periodically during the day (Hirth 1985). A newborn fawn remains hidden in foliage for camouflage. Good Samaritans often find fawns by themselves, assume they are abandoned, and present them for rehabilitation. True rejection is indicated by frequent, loud neonatal vocalization (Chitwood et al. 2014). Simply finding a solitary fawn is not an indication of neglect and efforts should be made to return the fawn to the doe (Connell 1996).

Aging of Fawns

A newborn fawn's coat will be reddish brown all over. If the fawn is less than a week old, you may feel a scab on its abdomen from the umbilical cord. They will have a series of white spots in two rows running lateral to the spine. As the fawn matures, the white spots will gradually disappear. Most fawns lose their spots at about 3–4 months of age. Male fawns will start to develop antler pedicles at around four months and these will be much more visible by seven months. Fawns weigh less than 10 lb (4.5 kg) at birth and steadily gain weight after birth. At around six months they will weigh closer to 75–85 pounds (34–38.5 kg) and by one year of age, most fawns will weigh over 90 pounds (41 kg). Fawns have four teeth when born. After two months, they will grow premolars and incisors and by 1.5 years they will have a full set of adult teeth.

Housing in Captivity

At admission, sick or injured fawns may be housed in airline-style crates placed in a holding room (Papageorgiou et al. 2002). For deer, the minimum recommended size for crates is 4 ft wide by 4 ft long by 2 ft high (1.2 × 1.2 × 0.6 m) (Miller 2012). These cage standards also apply to pronghorn and bighorn sheep infants but increase to 6 ft wide by 6 ft long by 2 ft high (1.8 × 1.8 × 0.6 m) for elk infants (Miller 2012). Line the crate with blankets and provide a thermo-gradient by placing a heating pad externally under half of the crate. Minimize stress by reducing visual and auditory stimuli: cover crates, provide visual barriers, place in low traffic areas, refrain from talking, and minimize human exposure (Miller 2012).

Healthy fawns should be individually quarantined indoors in airline-style crates if the umbilicus is still present or within an outdoor cage after the umbilicus sloughs off. Unrelated fawns that arrive within a short time period may be managed as a "cohort." Cohorts are housed in individual crates grouped together in a location separate from other cohorts. Each cohort is quarantined for a minimum of six days until three fecal exams have been performed on each fawn every other day and all are negative for intestinal parasites.

Once a fawn clears quarantine, they can move to outdoor runs or stalls and be placed with conspecifics (Papageorgiou et al. 2002). Runs for nursing/preweaned deer, pronghorns or bighorn sheep should measure a minimum of 10 ft wide by 15 ft long by 6 ft high (3 × 4.6 × 1.8 m); 12 ft wide by 20 ft long by 6 ft high (3.6 × 6 × 1.8 m) for elk (Miller 2012). Wooden stalls are superior to chainlink fencing which, if used, should be covered by plywood or shade cloth to avoid injury (Miller 2012). Each run should have a double door system and latches or locks on all gates to prevent escapes (Papageorgiou et al. 2002). Natural flooring is less damaging to hooves while concrete is easier to disinfect. If housed on concrete, bedding such as shavings or straw should be used. Shelter and protection from the elements should be provided using doorless dog houses/igloos or lean-tos. Each stall should contain a bottle rack which can be mounted at an appropriate height or a free-standing sawhorse-style rack (Figure 20.1) (Papageorgiou et al. 2002). No more than three or four fawns should be housed per stall to prevent overcrowding.

As fawns grow and are rack trained, they are moved to large outdoor yards or paddocks. Fencing must be at least 8 ft (2.4 m) high to prevent escapes and should encompass a minimum area of 1500 square feet (139 m²) for deer, pronghorns, and bighorn sheep juveniles; 4000 square feet (372 m²) for elk (Miller 2012). The interior of the paddock should attempt to replicate natural habitat as much as possible by providing a dirt or grass floor, native trees and foliage appropriate for deer browsing (Miller 2012; Papageorgiou et al. 2002). If no part of the paddock is roofed, shelter is provided in the form of a shed or overhang with straw bedding and a hay rack. The bottle rack is accessible from the outside via a panel which allows feeding without entering the enclosure (Papageorgiou et al. 2002). Additional access panels can be provided to place supplemental browse, food, and water in the paddock from the exterior. Access panels help minimize human exposure during weaning and discourage taming. Electric fencing may be used to keep out predators. A maximum of 15–20 fawns are housing per 30 ft by 50 ft (9.1 m × 15.2 m) deer yard.

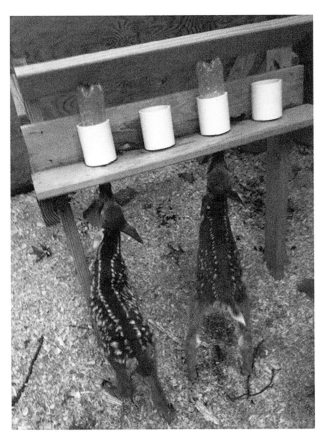

Figure 20.1 Free-standing sawhorse-style bottle rack for feeding fawns. *Source:* Courtesy Wildlife Center of Virginia.

In those jurisdictions which allow the rehabilitation of adult cervids, outdoor wooden paddocks are recommended at a minimum size of 30 ft wide by 50 ft long by 8 ft high (9.1 m × 15.2 m × 2.4 m) for deer and bighorn sheep; 50 ft wide by 80 ft long by 8 ft high for elk (15.2 m × 24.4 m × 2.4 m). Most cervid enclosures are square or rectangular but circular pens encourage animals to run along walls rather than corner themselves, which can lead to injury. Species differences should be considered in housing plans; for example, pronghorn are capable of leaping long distances while bighorn sheep are not long jumpers but can bound great heights. In order to prevent injury, it is advised to release deer and pronghorn directly from adult caging (Miller 2012).

Restraint and Handling

The goal of proper restraint is to prevent stress or injury to the animal while ensuring human safety. Before handling cervids, personal protective equipment, consisting of disposable gloves, gowns, and shoe covers, is recommended to reduce the risk of zoonotic disease transmission. White-tailed deer can shed *Giardia* and *Crystosporidium* spp. in their feces or have cutaneous infections with dermatophytes or *Dermatophilus congolensis* (causative agents of ringworm and dermatophilosis, respectively). They are also hosts for ticks, which may transmit bacterial or viral pathogens to humans and some animals (Campbell and VerCauteren 2011).

Physical Restraint

A fawn's main defense mechanism is escape. Newborn fawns will exhibit "freeze behavior" which may assist in restraint but they can still squirm, kick, and vocalize. Fawns over seven days old will demonstrate "flight behavior" and will run and jump when approached (Ruth 2012). The defenses for yearling and adult deer include striking and kicking with sharp hooves, gouging with antlers, and evading capture (Bewig and Mitchell 2009). Deer of any age should never be chased, as this can result in hyperthermia, capture myopathy or trauma (Papageorgiou et al. 2002).

Most infants and nursing fawns can be examined using only physical restraint. To pick up a fawn, squat down and pin the fawn between one hip and elbow. Place the same arm under the fawn's body and grip its front legs by placing a finger between each leg. Hold the fawn's head with your other arm to prevent head rearing. Lift off the ground and hold upright while making sure the fawn's back legs are behind you so that it doesn't kick you (Papageorgiou et al. 2002). If necessary, a second person can control the rear legs. Covering the fawn's eyes with a hood or mask will greatly reduce stress and resistance (Figure 20.2) (Papageorgiou et al. 2002). Most fawns will settle down and allow physical and ocular examinations,

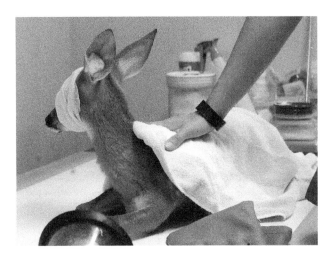

Figure 20.2 Fawns can be physically restrained and can be kept calm by reducing auditory and visual stimuli with a blindfold and gauze in the ears. At this age, they are relatively easy to pick up and handle. *Source:* Courtesy Heather Barron.

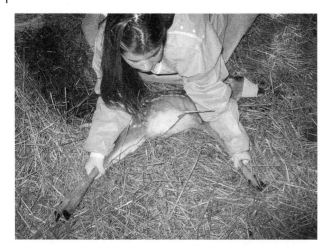

Figure 20.3 As fawns get older, or if they are anxious, additional physical restraining is needed. Fawns should be restrained in left lateral recumbency to decrease the chance of pressure on the rumen and subsequent bloat: the fawn's spine is held against the handler's body, forelegs are grasped with one hand and hindlegs with the other, placing one finger between the legs. Be careful not to lean on the fawn's throat and suffocate it. *Source:* Papageorgiou et al. (2002). *Source:* Courtesy Wildlife Center of Virginia.

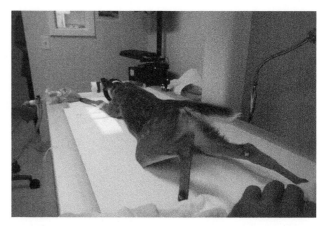

Figure 20.4 Juvenile deer can be masked down with inhalant anesthetics for routine procedures such as radiography. *Source:* Courtesy of Heather Barron.

medication administration, nonpainful procedures, and carrying in this position.

For routine procedures, such as subcutaneous fluids and phlebotomy, lateral recumbency is preferred. Lay the fawn on its left side to decrease the chance of bloat, with the fawn's spine against the front of your body (Figure 20.3) (Papageorgiou et al. 2002). Grasp the forelegs with one hand, the hindlegs with your other hand and secure both grips by placing one finger between the legs. Use your elbows to apply pressure to the fawn's pelvis and base of the neck while being careful not to lean on the fawn's throat. If this position is used for examination, do not roll fawns onto their backs when flipping to the other side to reduce the risk of regurgitation (Papageorgiou et al. 2002).

Chemical Restraint

If physical restraint is not sufficient, fawns can be masked down using isoflurane and oxygen (Figure 20.4) (Masters and Flach 2015). Larger fawns may require injectable immobilization which should only be administered after the patient is stabile. Fawns can be immobilized for radiographs or minor procedures using several chemical immobilization protocols, some of which are reversible (see Appendix II: Formulary) (Papageorgiou et al. 2002). For more information on anesthesia/analgesia, see Chapter 5. The jugular, cephalic, and lateral saphenous veins provide easy venous access (Caulkett and Haigh 2007). To help prevent aspiration of rumen contents during anesthesia, sternal recumbency is recommended; support the head up with nose down (Masters and Flach 2015).

If inhalation anesthesia is needed for more invasive procedures, fawns can be induced with chemical agents (Caulkett and Haigh 2007). Airway protective reflexes are absent under inhalational anesthesia so deer should be intubated and given supplemental oxygen (Caulkett and Haigh 2007). Intubation can be difficult in cervids due to a deep larynx and mobile epiglottis, so a laryngoscope with a long, flat blade and endotracheal tube stylet are recommended (Masters and Flach 2015). To intubate, place the fawn in sternal recumbency, extend the head and neck, and depress the epiglottis ventrally with the laryngoscope to allow visualization of the glottis opening and intubate (Caulkett and Haigh 2007). Attach the endotracheal tube to an anesthetic machine with a 3–6 L rebreathing bag and use a flow rate of 10–20 mL/kg/min. (Caulkett and Haigh 2007). Fawns can be maintained on inhalant anesthetics. Hypoventilation and hypoxemia are common anesthetic complications corrected by intermittent positive pressure ventilation. Hyperthermia or hypothermia can also occur during anesthesia so rectal temperature should be monitored every 5–10 minutes (Caulkett and Haigh 2007). Normal body temperature for a fawn is 37–38.3 °C (99–101 °F) (Papageorgiou et al. 2002). Cooling for hyperthermia or rewarming for hypothermia should be started and can be passive to aggressive, and may include other therapies depending on the severity of the condition.

Yearlings and Adults

Injured yearling and adult cervids can be dangerous in captivity and should be handled with vigilance and caution. Use extreme care when approaching an injured adult deer with antlers. Severely hurt adults may present recumbent or appear tame if in shock but they are unpredictable and can quickly arouse without warning (Bewig and Mitchell 2009). Chemical immobilization drugs and euthanasia solution should be prepared and accessible before attempting to handle. In most cases, chemical restraint is necessary to examine an injured adult deer and ensure human safety and prevent the animal from self-trauma (Bewig and Mitchell 2009). Numerous chemical immobilization drugs, some of which are available in premixed high concentrations or lyophilized to avoid large volumes, can be administered via pole syringes or dart gun. One combination used by these authors is xylazine and tiletamine HCl/zolazepam HCl (Telazol, Zoetis, Parsippany, NJ, USA). This dosage provides safety and reversibility with an induction time of approximately 1–6 minutes depending on the extent of the injury, excitement level, and dosage (Amass et al. 2013). Hyperthermia, self-trauma, and capture myopathy are common potential complications of anesthesia in deer (Caulkett and Haigh 2007).

Because of the inherent risk involved with treating injured adult deer, euthanasia may be considered more humane than treatment (Bewig and Mitchell 2009). In states where rehabilitation of adult deer is not permitted, regulations may require humane euthanasia of injured adult deer.

Common Presentations

Cervids admitted to practitioners by Good Samaritans are most commonly white-tailed deer fawns and can typically be divided into two categories: injured or orphaned, though some of these animals may also be clinically ill with or carrying infectious diseases of concern.

Injuries

Traumatic injuries occur when deer are involved in animal interactions (frequently with domestic dogs) or automobile collisions, or become entangled or entrapped (often in fencing). The resulting injuries can include fractures, lacerations, open wounds, etc. Limb, pelvis, rib, and facial fractures are most common (Bewig and Mitchell 2009). Light sedation (see section 20.4.2 and Chapter 5) is typically required to obtain quality radiographs and minimize patient stress. The type and extent of the fracture(s) will determine if it is repairable or if euthanasia is indicated (Papageorgiou et al. 2002). Lacerations can be sutured under anesthesia while wounds can be managed using standard wound care protocols.

Even if the animal survives the initial trauma and could be successfully treated, it may develop capture myopathy hours to weeks after handling. The stress of capture and transport by Good Samaritans, or the examination, diagnostics, and treatment can also result in capture myopathy. See Chapter 4 for more details on this topic.

The decision whether to treat or euthanize injured wildlife should always be based on the likelihood of full recovery resulting in release back to the wild. Deer must have adequate vision to forage for food and locomotive skills to escape predators. Even if the wounds heal, wildlife must demonstrate a fight or flight behavioral response and proper species behavior, including a wariness of humans, as minimum standards for release (Miller 2012). Fawns habituated to humans are not releasable because they can become dangerous and unpredictably violent adults, especially male deer (Bewig and Mitchell 2009). Animals who are poor candidates for release should be euthanized (Bewig and Mitchell 2009).

Infectious and Noninfectious Disease Concerns

This section presents common diseases and captive-associated conditions observed in deer in North America, treatment options, and zoonotic potential.

Bacterial Diseases

Dermatophilosis is a zoonotic disease of deer caused by *D. congolensis*. Infection can cause crusty, scabbed lesions on the skin often associated with patches of hair loss. Lesions can occur anywhere on the skin but commonly affect the muzzle, ears, periocular region, and distal extremities (Davidson and Nettles 2006; Nemeth et al. 2014). Transmission is by direct contact and, potentially, arthropod vectors. Diagnosis consists of examining stained exudate or an impression smear from the underside of a scab. Both topical and systemic antibiotics have been used in treatment, but have not provided consistent results (Williams and Barker 2001). Controlling ectoparasites and limiting interaction of infected animals with noninfected animals are recommended management practices (Williams and Barker 2001). If an animal is severely infected and poses a health risk to other animals or caretakers, humane euthanasia may be considered.

Deer, as well as other species, can serve as the reservoir for the zoonotic bacterium *Leptospira interrogans*, which usually resides in the urinary tract (Davidson and Nettles 2006). Transmission is typically from direct or indirect contact with the mucous membranes or urine. Infected deer may present with jaundice, fever, death, or no clinical signs at all (Williams and Barker 2001; Davidson and Nettles 2006).

Other zoonotic bacterial diseases that should be taken into consideration when treating deer include tuberculosis (*Mycobacterium bovis*), brucellosis (*Brucella abortus*), and anthrax (*Bacillus anthracis*). Tuberculosis and brucellosis are typically only found in specific geographic regions but because they could occur in new areas and because all three diseases are reportable, rehabilitators and veterinarians triaging wildlife should have knowledge of their signs and consider their presence. Concerns regarding these diseases can be directed to individual state agencies or to the USDA APHIS website for current information.

Blackleg (*Clostridium chauvoei*), lumpy jaw (*Actinomyces bovis*), and tetanus (*Clostridium tetani*) also may occur in deer.

Viral Diseases

Epizootic hemorrhagic disease (EHD) and bluetongue disease (BT) viruses cause similar clinical signs in deer. Signs may vary depending on the stage of the disease but generally include depression, fever, respiratory disease, and loss of appetite, and affected deer are often found near water (Davidson and Nettles 2006). Common ante- and postmortem lesions include hemorrhagic ulcerations of the dental pad and gastrointestinal tract, edema of the head, neck, and lungs, and defects in or complete sloughing of the hoof walls (Williams and Barker 2001; Davidson and Nettles 2006). Death can occur in acutely affected deer or the animal may survive the initial effects of the virus but eventually succumb to secondary conditions such as lameness and/or poor body condition (due to rumen scarring). Biting midges in the *Culicoides* genus transmit the virus; therefore, there is a seasonal pattern of infection, typically in the late summer and early fall. Vector control methods should be implemented to prevent the spread of these viruses. EHD or BT viruses are no direct threat to humans but both can be transmitted to/from domestic sheep and cattle (Williams and Barker 2001).

Papillomavirus, or cutaneous fibroma, is commonly observed and causes irregular hairless growths, or warts, on the skin and mucous membranes. The virus is spread by biting insects and by contact either directly with an abraded lesion or indirectly with a contaminated object. The disease is usually self-limiting and typically only becomes a concern when lesions interfere with eyesight, mastication, copulation, etc. or when secondary bacterial infections occur (Williams and Barker 2001). In those cases, systemic antibiotics may be used or in severe cases affecting quality of life, humane euthanasia may be considered. Papillomaviruses of deer are not zoonotic and cutaneous fibromas usually do not affect the quality of the meat for consumption unless accompanied by a secondary bacterial infection (Davidson and Nettles 2006).

Other zoonotic and nonzoonotic viral diseases of deer include rabies virus and vesicular diseases such as vesicular stomatitis. Rabies is rare in deer but the virus can affect any warm-blooded mammal and should not be dismissed in cases of neurological patients (Monroe et al. 2016). Vesicular diseases include those that cause blister-like lesions or erosions in and around the mouth and nose, tongue, coronary bands, and teats. In deer, these signs may be seen in animals affected with EHDV, BTV, vesicular stomatitis, malignant catarrhal fever, and foot-and-mouth disease. Due to the similarities in clinical signs between these domestic and reportable foreign animal diseases, any animal with vesicular lesions should be quarantined, tested, and reported.

Parasitic Diseases

Ectoparasites

Demodicosis, or demodectic mange, is caused by *Demodex* spp. mites and is a common occurrence in deer older than two years of age but can also affect younger fawns (Nemeth et al. 2014). This condition presents very similarly in deer as it does in other species, such as areas of alopecia with skin thickening and crusting lesions (Jacques et al. 2001; Davidson and Nettles 2006). Diagnosis can be made with skin scraping and microscopic evaluation and identification of mites, and treatment with ivermectin may be efficacious. Demodicosis in deer is considered to be species specific and although transmission to other deer is possible, this mite is a commensal organism and does not typically cause disease in otherwise healthy individuals (Jacques et al. 2001). The lesions associated with this disease tend to be superficial and do not affect the meat for human consumption (Davidson and Nettles 2006).

Recent screwworm infestations of Florida Key deer (*Odocoileus virginianus clavium*) were reported but have now been eradicated. Screwworms are the larvae of a fly (*Cochliomya hominivorax*) that feeds on the living flesh of warm-blooded mammals, including humans. Control methods have historically targeted the fly population by releasing sterile male flies into affected areas but manual removal of larvae and treatment with antiparasitics can be used (USDA APHIS 2016).

Deer can serve as the host for many tick species that can transmit causative agents of Lyme disease, anaplasmosis, babesiosis, and ehrlichiosis in people and/or animals. Manual removal of ticks, and treating the deer with ivermectin, topical permethrin, or other acaricides are effective ways to manage the parasites (Pound et al. 1996; Solberg et al. 2003). Deer may also have infestations with lice, mites, or keds (louse flies) which are rarely clinically relevant but can be managed similar to ticks.

Endoparasites

The meningeal worm *Parelaphostrongylus tenuis* is a nematode parasite that usually does not cause clinical signs in its typical host, the white-tailed deer. However, serious neurological disease has been observed in other wild and domestic species (Samuel et al. 2001; Davidson and Nettles 2006). For that reason, careful management of white-tailed deer should be considered prior to intermingling species in captivity or selecting locations for release. Diagnosis of *P. tenuis* in white-tailed deer can only be confirmed via examination of adult worms from the meninges during postmortem examination or by genetic testing of larvae passed in feces as these larvae are morphologically similar to other nematode larvae (Samuel et al. 2001).

Another parasite commonly found in white-tailed deer is the liver fluke, *Fascioloides magna*, often found within fibrous capsules in the liver. Clinical signs are typically not seen in deer but serious disease and death may occur in domestic sheep and other livestock (Samuel et al. 2001). *F. magna* infection in cattle may lead to condemnation of the liver (Davidson and Nettles 2006). Therefore, liver flukes are yet another important consideration when selecting a release site for white-tailed deer.

Other endoparasites may cause clinical signs while others are usually incidental findings at necrospy. However, none of the following deer parasites pose a risk to human health or consumption: lung worm (*Dictyocaulus viviparous*), stomach worm (*Haemonchus contortus*), abdominal worm (*Setaria yehi*), and nasal bots (*Cephenemyia* spp.) (Davidson and Nettles 2006). Some gastrointestinal parasites of deer, especially fawns, can pose a risk to humans, other deer, and other species (see section 20.7.3).

Fungal Diseases

Dermatophytosis, or ringworm, is not commonly reported in adult deer but there have been cases reported in fawns (Hall et al. 2011). Ringworm in deer can be transmitted to other species, including humans. Diagnosis is made by skin scraping or collection of a hair sample and observation of growth or color change in a dermatophyte test medium (DTM) plate. Treatment and prevention of transmission consist of systemic antifungals and topical therapies similar to those used in domestic species, along with quarantine and time (Williams and Barker 2001). If the infection is severe and results in a poor quality of life, or if the infected individual cannot adequately be quarantined, humane euthanasia may be considered.

Prion Diseases

Chronic wasting disease (CWD) is a transmissible spongiform encephalopathy (TSE) disease caused by a prion that leads to neurological abnormalities and death. CWD causes spongiform lesions in the brain that can be confirmed on postmortem exam. Clinical signs may include a loss of body condition, abnormal behavior, changes in mentation, and ataxia, so these animals should also be suspected of hemorrhagic disease or rabies. Antemortem diagnostics are still being studied for various species but generally require rectal and/or retropharyngeal lymph node biopsies. Postmortem diagnosis is most commonly made via histopathological evaluation of the medulla oblongata at the obex (Williams and Barker 2001). Transmission mainly occurs via the fecal–oral route and the infectious prion is capable of persisting in the environment for years (Masters and Flach 2015; Pritzkow et al. 2015). At this time, CWD has not been shown to be transmissible to domestic animals or humans. This disease has raised serious management considerations, especially concerning relocating cervids, as CWD is not endemic in many areas of North America (Masters and Flach 2015).

Captive-Related Conditions

Exertional rhabdomyolosis (capture myopathy) is commonly seen in captive deer as a result of the stress of being in captivity, handled, medicated, etc. and may result in death. Therefore, it is important to consider the risk versus benefit of handling wild deer in captivity (Masters and Flach 2015). Since handling and treatment of certain diseases or wounds are sometimes necessary, all precautions should be taken to minimize capture myopathy, including minimizing audio and visual stimuli, avoiding the need to chase the animal, and avoiding high temperatures.

Abomasal or ruminal bloat may occur in deer in captivity as a result of inappropriate diet, sudden change in diet, stress of weaning, or other similar circumstances. Treatment is similar to domestic ruminants but it is important to minimize the stress of treatment and the risk of capture myopathy. One option for a minimally invasive procedure to alleviate a bloated rumen is inserting a large-bore catheter as a trocar in the left paralumbar fossa and removing the stylet. The catheter can be left in place in an attempt to prevent the build-up of excess gas.

Orphans

When a fawn is presented for rehabilitation, it is important to determine if the fawn is a true orphan or a kidnapped healthy animal (Bewig and Mitchell 2009). True orphans are those that are rejected by a doe or the doe has died. Unless a fawn is lying next to a dead doe, it is often difficult to confirm whether a fawn is orphaned or temporarily unattended while the doe is off foraging. Vocalizing, dehydration, and presence of fly eggs are indicators of a true orphan. Truly orphaned fawns should be medically evaluated, rehydrated, and transferred to an experienced wildlife rehabilitator for fostering or continued care once stable.

If a fawn is found alone but is quiet, well hydrated, in good body condition and free of ectoparasites, it is likely a healthy fawn that was temporarily unattended. Citizens should be educated on natural history and instructed to return the fawn to where they found it within 24 hours (Bewig and Mitchell 2009). It is a common myth that the smell of humans on the fawn will prevent the doe from taking the fawn back. Citizens may want to wait around to see the reunion but should be aware that a doe will never approach the fawn while people are in the area. Rarely, the fawn will still be in the same spot the next day; if this is the case, it needs to be admitted for care.

Intake and Stabilization

Examination

Perform a complete physical exam and be sure to check the umbilical cord. Observe the cervid standing and walking on a nonslip surface for splay leg or lameness. Record the body temperature, pulse, and respiratory rate (TPR). For white-tailed deer, normal heart rate varies with activity level and was found to be 65, 74, and 106 beats per minute for laying, standing/walking, and running, respectively (Mautz and Fair 1980). Obtain an accurate intake weight with a scale or use a goat weight tape to obtain a reasonable estimate. Collect blood for a minimum of a packed cell volume (PCV), total protein (TP), and blood glucose (BG), and collect a fecal sample for parasite analysis (Papageorgiou et al. 2002). If more than one animal of the same species is admitted, individuals should be identified with shaving, livestock markers, or ear tags.

Fluid Therapy

Fluid therapy in cervids follows the same basic principles as domestic animal medicine (Bewig and Mitchell 2009). Dehydration can be assessed by observing skin tenting and capillary refill time. Calculate the volume of replacement fluids needed using the dehydration percentage and the daily maintenance rate. Recommended maintenance fluid rates for wildlife mammals vary from 60 mL/kg/day (McRuer and Hall 2013) to 100 mL/kg/day (Bewig and Mitchell 2009). The deficit can be corrected over 24–36 hours. Any isotonic fluid is appropriate, with lactated Ringer's solution (LRS) used most commonly.

Fluids should be warmed to body temperature before administration. Acceptable methods of administration include *per os*, subcutaneous, or intravenous. The method chosen depends on the degree of dehydration and whether the gastrointestinal tract is functional.

Healthy orphans admitted for care are assumed to be at least 5% dehydrated based on history of capture and transport. Each receives an initial bolus of lactated Ringer's solution at a dose of 60 mL/kg divided into several subcutaneous locations. A few hours later, their first feeding consists of 8–16 oz of an oral electrolyte solution such as Bounce Back (Manna Pro, Chesterfield, MO, USA), HydroPet (PetAg, Hampshire, IL, USA) or an isotonic fluid. Additional details are in Chapter 12.

Fecal Analysis

Fecal samples can be obtained from deer by voluntary defecation, manual extraction, or using a fecal loop. Individuals should be tested using both sugar (sucrose) centrifugation and zinc sulfate centrifugation according to the fecal examination procedures recommended by the Companion Animal Parasite Council (www.capcvet.org). Sugar centrifugation is a common screening test for coccidia and *Cryptosporidium* sp.; zinc sulfate centrifugation is used preferentially to detect *Giardia*. Regardless of the etiology, clinical symptoms of intestinal parasitism in deer can include diarrhea, hematochezia, fever, weight loss, anorexia, dehydration, emaciation, and/or weakness.

Eimeria spp. are the most common endoparasites in young deer (Papageorgiou et al. 2002; Dubey et al. 2009). Although commonly found in clinically normal deer, these parasites can cause diarrhea if present in large numbers. Asymptomatic or mild cases do not require treatment. Deer can be treated with sulfadimethoxine or amprolium if clinical signs are severe or if they are passing large numbers of oocysts, even if asymptomatic. Prevention involves sanitation, preventing contamination of feed/water, and coccidiostats.

Giardia and *Cryptosporidium* spp. are periodically detected and the latter may also cause diarrhea (Rickard et al. 1999). Both are potentially zoonotic and immediately infectious so personal protective equipment should be used when handling infected patients.

Both are diagnosed by fecal floatation, ideally centrifugal flotation. Sugar centrifugation (specific gravity 1.25) is preferred for *Cryptosporidium* detection while zinc sulfate (specific gravity 1.18) is preferred for *Giardia*. *Cryptosporidium* oocysts are very small and may be easily missed. Addition of Lugol's iodine stain can help visualize both parasites.

There is no widely accepted medication for the treatment of *Cryptosporidium* so the mainstay of therapy is supportive care until the immune system can mount an effective response (Ramsay 1986). Even after clinical signs have resolved and fecal analysis is repeatedly negative, patients may occasionally shed *Cryptosporidium*, which makes housing with conspecifics controversial. *Giardia* is generally treated with fenbendazole; metronidazole should not be used as use in food animals is illegal in the US (Payne et al. 1999). After the treatment regimen and if clinical signs have resolved, repeat three zinc sulfate centrifugations 48 hours apart. Only after three negative fecal tests are obtained should the individual join or be reunited with the cohort or herd.

After clearing initial quarantine, monitoring fecal samples once a week using both sugar and zinc sulfate centrifugation analysis is recommended for all cervids undergoing rehabilitation.

Hypoglycemia

Neonatal cervids are susceptible to hypoglycemia which can be secondary to diarrhea, sepsis, or malnutrition. Treatment for hypoglycemia is recommended when blood glucose levels are less than 3.3 mmol/L or 60 mg/dL in white-tailed deer or black tailed deer (Papageorgiou et al. 2002). Hypoglycemia in neonatal elk or wapiti is defined as a blood or serum glucose concentration less than or equal to 4.2 mmol/l or 76 mg/dl) (Klein et al. 2002). Although not formally evaluated, hand-held glucometers appear accurate in assessing the glucose status of wildlife.

Glucose can be supplemented by applying Karo syrup (ACH Food Companies Inc., Oakbrook Terrace, IL, USA) to the gums, gavaging 20% dextrose orally via stomach tube, administering 2.5% dextrose with an isotonic solution subcutaneously, or placing an intravenous (IV) catheter for delivery of 50% dextrose (Papageorgiou et al. 2002). If blood glucose is less than 3 mmol/L or 54 mg/dL), an IV bolus of 50% dextrose can be administered. Treatment method should be catered to the degree of hypoglycemia, symptoms, and stress induced to the patient.

Nutrition

Digestive System

Deer are ruminants so they regurgitate their cud and have a four-chambered stomach consisting of the rumen, where storage and mixing occurs, reticulum, where microorganisms facilitate fermentation, omasum, where water is absorbed, and abomasum, which is the glandular stomach. Deer have a small reticulorumen in relation to body size, making them concentrate selectors that selectively browse trees and shrubs. Fawns do not become fully functioning ruminants until they are two months old, but will begin grazing at a few weeks of age (Smith 1991).

Formula

Colostrum can be administered orally to fawns less than 12–24 hours of age to provide them with absorbable immunoglobulins. Frozen bovine or caprine colostrum, or a powdered colostrum supplement like Colostrx® (AgriLabs, St Joseph, MO, USA), are recommended.

Fawns should be gradually weaned onto a milk replacer in order to prevent gastroenteritis secondary to a rapid change in diet. The first meal can be an oral electrolyte solution or an isotonic fluid administered orally. Subsequent feedings should transition to formula gradually; for example, 25% formula mixed with 75% water, then 50% formula mixed with 50% water, then 70% formula mixed with 25% water, until feeding 100% formula.

Lamb or kid nipples like Pritchard or Rhinehart nipples mimic the doe's teat more closely than human baby bottle nipples. Sod bottles, lamb/kid bottles, noncollapsible bottles, regular baby bottles, or glass bottles are appropriate. All nipples and bottles should be washed after each feeding and sterilized at the end of the day.

Bottle Feeding

A quiet location and a no talking policy will minimize patient stress during feedings. Stand the fawn on a non-slip surface such as a piece of carpet. Kneel down and straddle the fawn between your legs since it may back up in an attempt to escape. Place the nipple into the fawn's mouth while squirting out a small amount of formula. Sometimes encouraging the fawn to suckle on a gloved finger can kickstart the suckling reflex. New fawns may struggle or vocalize until the feeding process becomes familiar.

During bottle feeding, hold the bottle at a 45° angle to prevent aerophagia. The fawn's neck should be outstretched, and head raised to ensure formula flows down the esophageal groove. Do not bottle feed fawns while they are lying down.

Neonatal deer need to be manually stimulated to urinate and defecate at each feeding using a warm wet cloth. Without stimulation, constipation or urine retention may result. Stimulation should continue until voluntary elimination is consistently observed.

Fawns may suckle on prepuces of conspecifics, which can lead to penile inflammation, hernia, etc. Providing additional enrichment, adding surrogate mothers or alternative items to suckle, use of anxiolytics, or application of nonappetizing material (e.g., bitter apple), and physical barriers on the prepuce may decrease this behavior, but are unlikely to be as effective as environmental enrichment.

Volume and Frequency

Various feeding schedules are used by wildlife rehabilitators for fawns but the consensus is to start with frequent feedings for neonates and gradually decrease the frequency while increasing the volume as the deer grows. The amount of formula per feeding should not exceed 50–66 mL/kg, which is stomach capacity for most mammals. For newborns, feedings can be evenly spread out over a 16–18-hour day. Enough time needs to pass between each feeding to allow gastric emptying. Middle of the night feedings are not typically required with healthy orphans.

One regime recommends feeding 4 ounces (30 mL) of formula four times daily for the first 1–2 weeks of age. Increase the amount as the fawn grows until feeding 16 oz (480 mL) of formula per feeding. By four weeks of age, cut back to three feedings per day. A week later, reduce to two feedings per day at dusk and dawn. Weaning starts once feeding is reduced to once per day (Cherney and Nieves 1992).

More precise feeding amounts can be based on body weight instead of age by using an allometric food calculator to estimate the 24-hour energy requirement (kcals) needed for growth. Use the kcal/mL of a milk replacer formula from the manufacturer to accurately estimate daily volume requirement to meet energy demands.

The best way to assess growth and development is to regularly monitor body weight. Weigh first thing in the morning before feeding, at least twice weekly until three weeks old, then at least once a week as long as the patient can be safely handled.

Rack Training

Once fawns are feeding well from hand-held bottles and housed outside, a bottle rack can be introduced. To begin rack training, let the fawn start suckling on the bottle then slowly move the bottle into the rack. Optimally, the fawn will reattach to the nipple but it is a process that will require repetition. Rack training decreases human contact and reduces the association of food with people. Monitor for dominant individuals that may limit access of some fawns to nipples.

As herd animals, deer should preferentially not be raised alone. Conspecifics can be introduced as soon as an individual clears quarantine. Bottle racks allow the simultaneous feeding of more than one fawn at a time, greatly reducing the time required to feed a small herd.

Weaning

By the time fawns are 1–2 weeks old, they should begin sampling solid food. Provide daily fresh foliage and natural browsing foods that are indigenous to your location. Use a field guide to determine what tree, shrubs, and grasses to browse and identify potentially toxic plants. In the mid-Atlantic region, sassafras, blueberry, dogwood, willow, and wintergreen are considered best browse for white-tailed deer. The key to browse is providing variety and volume. By the time fawns are consuming 16 oz of formula per feeding, they should also be eating an average of 15–20 lb (6.8–9 kg) of fresh roughage including another 3 lb of wild fruit and berries (Cherney and Nieves 1992).

In additional to browse, offer a commercial deer diet like Wild Herbivore (Mazuri, St Louis, MO, USA), AntlerMax (Purina, Shoreview, MN, USA), or Calf Manna (Manna Pro) in low-sided pans. In limited quantities, apples, acorns, and corn can be added to the diet. Free choice alfalfa or grass hay can also be accessible to supplement the diet. Fresh clean water should also be available at all times.

Once fawns are eating solid food along with their bottles and continuing to gain weight (around six weeks of age), gradually reduce the volume of milk replacer and frequency of bottle feedings. During this time, human contact should be minimized because a healthy fear of humans is required for success in the wild. Formula is typically discontinued between eight and 12 weeks of age, which is the natural weaning age for white-tailed deer. Fawns should forage exclusively on natural browse for at least three weeks after weaning and prior to considering release.

Release

Deer should be evaluated for minimum criteria to assess readiness for release, including physical health, recovery from injury, normal body condition score, adequate pelage, appropriate flight or fight response in reaction to humans/noise/vehicles and be weaned and demonstrating proper foraging behavior (Miller 2012). Groups of fawns raised together should be released together (Cherney and Nieves 1992).

Check with wildlife officials in your area before planning a release. Some state agencies require the release of rehabilitated deer in specific areas. Others may prevent release after a certain date because fawns would then be considered adults. Additionally, Wisconsin requires rehabilitated fawns to be ear-tagged before release while New Jersey prohibits tagging of released wildlife.

There are several philosophies regarding the best time to release fawns. One common choice is an autumn release when fawns are approximately four months old and losing their spots. Foliage is typically plentiful, and the weather is often mild in September and October. Another option is to release fawns as soon as they are weaned (some at six weeks) and able to fend for themselves. This quicker return to the wild may promote more natural behaviors than fawns kept longer in captivity. A disadvantage of early release is that young fawns on their own may be more susceptible to predators and unable to provide for themselves. In areas where there is concern about releasing fawns during the hunting season, a third option is to release them in winter after the hunting season has ended. The advantage is that fawns are bigger and stronger while the disadvantage is a potential lack of adequate natural food sources. A final option is to release them the following spring, consistent with the natural dispersal period. However, holding deer in captivity until spring may contribute to taming and dependence on humans.

Regardless of when fawns are released, the release process can be hard or soft. In a soft release, the door to the outdoor area is opened to allow the herd to come and go. Supplemental food continues to be provided and eventually as fawns establish their own territory and find wild food sources, visits to the cage become less frequent (Diehl and Stokhaug 1991). A hard release involves capture and transport to the release site with no postrelease support provided.

Depending on the size of the fawns, capture for transport can be done during a round-up where a human wall or chute is used to corral fawns, manually restrain them, and move them onto a horse or livestock trailer. Use of experienced handlers, covering the fawn's eyes with a hood or mask, or using dark crates can help minimize stress to the animals. Fawns up to six months of age are surprisingly calm, often lying down during transport. For older or larger fawns, chemical immobilization may be required (see sections 20.4.2 and 20.4.3 and Chapter 5).

Choosing an appropriate release site is critical to the success of any reintroduced animal. The location should be an appropriate habitat with plenty of natural browse, a water source nearby, and far away from humans, farms, roads, and hunters. Releasing fawns early in the day during good weather will give them the best chance to return to life in the wild (Diehl and Stokhaug 1991).

References

Amass, K.D., Drew, M., Waldrup, K. et al. (2013). *Chemical Immobilization of Animals. Technical Field Notes: 2013*. Mt Horeb, WI: Safe-Capture International, Inc.

Bewig, M. and Mitchell, M.A. (2009). Wildlife. In: *Manual of Exotic Pet Practice* (ed. M.A. Mitchell and T.N. Tully), 493–529. St Louis, MO: Saunders.

Campbell, T.A. and VerCauteren, K.C. (2011). Diseases and parasites [of white-tailed deer]. In: *Biology and Management of White-Tailed Deer* (ed. D.G. Hewitt), 219–249. Boca Raton, FL: CRC Press.

Caulkett, N. and Haigh, J.C. (2007). Deer (Cervids). In: *Zoo Animal & Wildlife Immobilization and Anesthesia* (ed. G. West, D. Heard and N. Caulkett), 607–612. Ames, IA: Wiley.

Cherney, L. and Nieves, M.A. (1992). How to care for orphaned wild mammals part II. *Iowa State University Veterinarian* 54 (1): 6.

Chitwood, M.C., Lashley, M.A., Moorman, C.E. et al. (2014). Vocalization observed in starving white-tailed deer neonates. *Southeastern Naturalist* 3 (2): N6–N8.

Connell, A. (1996). When to return white-tailed deer (*Odocoileus virginianus*) fawns to their mothers. *Wildlife Rehabilitation* 14: 127–141.

Cronin, M.A. (1992). Intraspecific variation in mitochondrial DNA of north American cervids. *Journal of Mammalogy* 73 (1): 70–82.

Davidson, W.R. and Nettles, V.F. (2006). *Field Manual of Wildlife Diseases in the Southeastern United States*, 3e. Athens, GA: Southeastern Cooperative Wildlife Disease Study.

Dewey, T. (2003). *Odocoileus virginianus*. Animal Diversity Web. http://animaldiversity.org/accounts/Odocoileus_virginianus

Diehl, S. and Stokhaug, C. (1991). Release criteria for rehabilitated wild animals. In: *Wildlife Rehabilitation*, vol. 9 (ed. D.R. Ludwig), 159–181. St Cloud, MN: National Wildlife Rehabilitators Association.

Dubey, J.P., Jenkins, M.C., Kwok, O.C. et al. (2009). Seroprevalence of *Neospora caninum* and *Toxoplasma gondii* antibodies in white-tailed deer (*Odocoileus virginianus*) from Iowa and Minnesota using four serologic tests. *Veterinary Parasitology* 161: 330–334.

Groves, C.P. and Grubb, P. (2011). *Ungulate taxonomy*. Baltimore, MD: Johns Hopkins University Press.

Hall, N., Swinford, A., McRuer, D. et al. (2011). Survey of haircoat fungal flora for the presence of dermatophytes ina population of white-tailed deer (*Odocoileus virginianus*) in Virginia. *Journal of Wildlife Diseases* 47 (3): 713–716.

Hirth, D.H. (1985). Mother-young behavior in white-tailed deer, *Odocoileus virginianus*. *Southwestern Naturalist* 30 (2): 297–302.

Indiana Administrative Code. (2011). Title 312. Natural Resources Commission. Article 9. Fish and Wildlife. Rule 10. Special Licenses; Permits and Standards. 312 IAC 9–10-9 Wild Animal Rehabilitation Permit.

Jacques, C., Jenks, J., Hildreth, M. et al. (2001). Demodicosis in a white-tailed deer (*Odocoileus virginianus*) in South Dakota. *Prairie Naturalist* 33 (4): 221–226.

Klein, K.A., Clark, C., and Allen, A.L. (2002). Hypoglycemia in sick and moribund farmed elk calves. *Canadian Veterinary Journal* 43 (10): 778–781.

Masters, N.J. and Flach, E. (2015). Tragulidae, Moschidae and Cervidae. In: *Zoo and Wild Animal Medicine*, vol. 8 (ed. R.E. Miller and M.E. Fowler), 611–625. St Louis, MO: Saunders.

Mattioli, S. (2011). Family Cervidae (deer). In: *Handbook of the Mammals of the World. Volume 2. Hoofed Mammals* (ed. D.E. Wilson and R.A. Mittermeier), 350–443. Barcelona: Lynx Edicions.

Mautz, W.W. and Fair, J. (1980). Energy expenditures and heart rate for activities of white-tailed deer. *Journal of Wildlife Management* 44 (2): 333–342.

McRuer, D.L. and Hall, N.H. (2013). Wildlife. In: *Exotic Animal Formulary*, 4e (ed. J.W. Carpenter and C.J. Marion), 663–683. St Louis, MO: Elsevier Saunders.

Miller, E.A. (2012). *Minimum Standards for Wildlife Rehabilitation*, 4e. St Cloud, MN: National Wildlife Rehabilitators Association.

Monroe, B., Yagar, P., Blanton, J. et al. (2016). Rabies surveillance in the United States during 2014. *Journal of the American Veterinary Medical Association* 248 (7): 777–788.

Nemeth, N., Ruder, M., Gerhold, R. et al. (2014). Demodectic mange, dermatophilosis, and other parasitic and bacterial dermatologic diseases in free-ranging white-tailed deer (*Odocoileus virginianus*) in the United States from 1975 to 2012. *Veterinary Pathology* 51 (3): 633–640.

Papageorgiou, S., DeGhetto, D., and Convy, J. (2002). Black-tailed and white-tailed deer. In: *Hand-Rearing Wild and Domestic Mammals* (ed. L.J. Gage), 244–255. Ames, IA: Iowa State University Press.

Payne, M.A., Baynes, R.E., Sundlof, S.E. et al. (1999). Drugs prohibited from extralabel use in food animals. *Journal of the American Veterinary Medical Association* 215 (1): 28.

Polziehn, R.O. and Strobeck, C. (2002). A phylogenetic comparison of red deer and wapiti using mitochondrial DNA. *Molecular Phylogenetics and Evolution* 22 (3): 342–356.

Pound, J., Miller, J., George, J. et al. (1996). Systemic treatment of white-tailed deer with ivermectin-medicated bait to control free-living populations of lone star ticks (*Acari: Ixodidae*). *Journal of Medical Entomology* 33 (3): 385–394.

Pritzkow, S., Morales, R., Moda, F. et al. (2015). Grass plants bind, retain, uptake, and transport infectious prions. *Cell Reports* 11: 1168–1175.

Ramsay, E.C. (1986). Management of cryptosporidiosis in a hoofstock contact area. In: *Fowler's Zoo and Wild Animal Medicine Current Therapy*, vol. 7 (ed. R.E. Miller and M. Fowler), 570–572. St Louis, MO: Saunders.

Rickard, L.G., Siefker, C., Boyle, C.R. et al. (1999). The prevalence of *Cryptosporidium* and *Giardia* spp. in fecal samples from free-ranging white-tailed deer (*Odocoileus virginianus*) in the southeastern United States. *Journal of Veterinary Diagnostic Investigation* 11: 65–72.

Rooney, T.P. (2010). What do we do with too many white-tailed deer? Action Bioscience. www.actionbioscience. org/biodiversity/rooney.html

Ruth, I. (2012). *Wildlife Care Basics for Veterinary Hospitals: Before the Rehabilitator Arrives*. Washington, DC: Humane Society of the United States.

Samuel, W.M., Pybus, M.J., and Kocan, A.A. (2001). *Parasitic Diseases of Wild Mammals*, 2e. Ames, IA: Iowa State University Press.

Smith, W.P. (1991). *Odocoileus virginianus*. *Mammalian Species* 388: 1–13.

Solberg, V., Miller, J., Hadfield, T. et al. (2003). Control of *Ixodes scapularis* (*Acari: Ixodidae*) with topical self-application of permethrin by white-tailed deer inhabiting NASA, Beltsville, Maryland. *Journal of Vector Ecology* 28: 117–134.

USDA APHIS Stakeholder Announcements (2016). USDA Confirms New World Screwworm in Big Pine Key, Florida. www.aphis.usda.gov

VDGIF (2014). *Wildlife Rehabilitation Permit Conditions*. Richmond, VA: Virginia Department of Game & Inland Fisheries.

Williams, E.A. and Barker, I.K. (2001). *Infectious Diseases of Wild Mammals*, 3e. Ames, IA: Iowa State University Press.

21

Natural History and Medical Management of Procyonids

Emphasis on Raccoons

Renée Schott

Wildlife Rehabilitation Center of Minnesota, Roseville, MN, USA

Introduction

The family Procyonidae includes 14 living species in six genera which are found throughout the New World (Kurta 2001). Although procyonids are in the order Carnivora, they are mostly omnivorous. All are small to medium sized and are generally good climbers (Kurta 2001).

In North America, the most common procyonid that presents for rehabilitation is the northern raccoon, *Procyon lotor*, also called the common raccoon. The only other procyonids found in the United States are the ringtail (*Bassariscus astutus*) and the white-nosed coati (*Nasua narica*). Remaining procyonid species are found in Mexico, Central, or South America.

Natural History

Species Identification, Habitat, and Conservation Status

The northern raccoon is a medium-sized (6–20 kg) mammal with brown to black fur, a distinctive black mask across a white face, and a striped tail. Raccoons have acute hearing and smell (Zollman and Winkelmann 1962; Kurta 2001). They have increased range of motion in their forelimb joints and are able to rotate their hind feet 180° at the subtalar joint (Iwaniuk and Whishaw 1999). Raccoon forepaws have sensory innervation similar to primates and these extremely dexterous and sensitive forepaws are used to manipulate and palpate almost everything (Welker et al. 1964; Turnbull and Rasmusson 1986).

The raccoon has an extensive natural range in North and Central America and is listed as a Species of Least Concern with the International Union for the Conservation of Nature. Through translocation and release, raccoons are now considered invasive in many countries of Europe and Asia (Inoue et al. 2011; García et al. 2012; Davidson et al. 2013; Biedrzycka et al. 2014). The other *Procyon* species are the Cozumel raccoon (*Procyon pygmaeus*), a critically endangered species only found on Cozumel Island off the coast of Mexico, and the crab-eating raccoon (*Procyon cancrivorus*) which is widely distributed throughout Central and South America and is a Species of Least Concern.

The northern raccoon is highly adaptable and utilizes a wide range of habitat types, ranging from natural forested areas to highly urbanized environments (Bozek et al. 2007). Raccoon home ranges can vary greatly based on many variables including land-use type and location (Kurta 2001; Prange et al. 2003; Bozek et al. 2007; Graser et al. 2012; Rodewald and Gehrt 2014). One study in northeastern Illinois found that raccoons in rural areas had larger home ranges (216–243 ha) compared with those in urban areas (127–129 ha); however, no difference was found when comparing suburban and urban raccoons (Bozek et al. 2007).

Similar to home ranges, densities of raccoons can vary considerably between habitats and land-use types. Some studies have found higher densities of raccoons in urban parks or in urban/suburban areas compared with rural areas (Riley et al. 1998; Smith and Engeman 2002; Prange et al. 2003). However, one study found that urban open (i.e., urban parks, open vegetation) areas had the highest density of raccoons followed by rural areas whereas urbanized residential areas had the lowest density (Graser et al. 2012). In general, the presence of trees is one of the most important factors in predicting raccoons density; however, other variables, such as access to anthropogenic food sources, are also important (Pedlar et al. 1997; Byrne and Chamberlain 2011). Because of the complex interaction of variables, it can be difficult to

Medical Management of Wildlife Species: A Guide for Practitioners, First Edition. Edited by Sonia M. Hernandez, Heather W. Barron, Erica A. Miller, Roberto F. Aguilar and Michael J. Yabsley.

generalize what raccoon density or carrying capacity is for a particular area.

Behavior and Sociality

Raccoons are nocturnal and are active from dusk until after sunrise (Kurta 2001). Raccoons do not hibernate, but during the winter they may remain inactive in their dens for weeks; however, heart rate and body temperature do not decrease. They may den communally to conserve energy. During harsh, cold winters, raccoons have been reported to lose 10–50% of their body mass (Prange et al. 2003). In southern climates raccoon may remain active throughout the winter.

Raccoons are generally solitary but often form social affiliations, with older individuals usually having hierarchy (Hauver et al. 2013), and may become social when raising young. Raccoons often have large and elaborate social networks that are very interconnected, increasing the risk for disease transmission (Hirsch et al. 2013; Robert et al. 2013; Reynolds et al. 2015). Additionally, contact among raccoons increases during the winter and mating season (Prange et al. 2003; Hirsch et al. 2013).

Reproduction and Development

Raccoons typically mate January through March, although in southern regions mating can extend into August and very northern region raccoons may delay mating until June. Raccoons typically have one litter of 1–8 kits per year with a gestation period of approximately 63 days (Kurta 2001). If the first litter is lost, the female may come into estrus again.

Raccoons are born altricial with eyes and ears closed. Kits can be aged using several characteristics including tooth eruption, weight, and other factors (Table 21.1). Raccoon young will usually den with their mother during the first winter and disperse at the start of the next breeding season (Kurta 2001). The lifespan of free-ranging raccoons is 2–13 years (Kurta 2001).

Dietary Habits

Raccoons are adaptable omnivores with a simple digestive tract lacking a cecum. Diet varies with food availability and taste preference, with a large part typically being plant items in the summer and animal items in the fall and winter (Schoonover and Marshall 1951; Rivest and

Table 21.1 Characteristics used to determine the approximate age of young raccoons.

Approximate age (weeks)	Tooth eruption[a]	Approximate weight (grams)	Other notes
Birth		45–85[b–d]	Altricial, sparse back hairs, eyes/ears closed
1			Well-covered back hair[d]
2		200[c]	
3	i1 (L), i2 (U), i3 (U)	450[c]	Eyes open[c,d]
4	i1 (U, L), i3 (L), c (U, L)	320–570[b,d]	Eyes open, start walking[d]
5	i1 (U), i2 (L), i3 (L)		Start walking[d]
6	p2 (U, L)	410–680[b,d]	Guard hairs appear, start walking[d]
7	p3 (U, L), p4 (U, L)		
8	p1 (L)	900[b]	
9	p1 (U), I1 (U, L)		
10	I2 (U, L)	1000[b]	
11	M1 (U, L)		
12	I3 (L)		
13	I3 (U)	1500[b]	
14	I3 (U), C (L)		
15	C (U, L)		

L, lower; U, upper.
Sources:
[a] Montgomery (1964).
[b] Sanderson (1961).
[c] Kurta (2001).
[d] Zeveloff (2002).

Bergeron 1981; Parsons et al. 2013). Examples of plant items include acorns and other nuts/seeds, corn and other grains, and fleshy fruits and typical animal items include frogs, crayfish, grasshoppers, minnows, large insects, and small vertebrates (e.g., muskrats, rabbits, and eggs) (Schoonover and Marshall 1951; Rivest and Bergeron 1981; Greenwood 1982; Parsons et al. 2013).

Urbanized raccoons have adapted to utilize a wide range of anthropogenic resources (Parsons et al. 2013). However, this may have negative effects on their health as raccoons from human-inhabited areas have higher rates of dental caries and human–wildlife conflicts (Hungerford et al. 1999). Furthermore, congregations of raccoons around supplemental food resources could lead to intra- and interspecific aggression with other carnivores and pathogen transmission (Wright and Gompper 2005; Monello and Gompper 2010).

Captive Husbandry Guidelines

Housing Guidelines

For all ages of raccoons, cages made of nonporous surfaces are necessary for cleaning and disinfecting. Ideally, caging would be all metal to allow flaming or boiling between patients or litters as this is the only way to kill *Baylisascaris procyonis* (raccoon roundworm) eggs. Additionally, any cage items that cannot be flamed/boiled (i.e., food dishes, cloth, nonmetal enclosures, etc.) should be submerged in boiling water or dedicated to raccoons only to prevent nontarget species from ingesting *B. procyonis* eggs. Caging size and structure should increase with age to match activity requirements (Table 21.2).

Because raccoons are born altricial, neonates need supplemental heat and humidity (detailed care is covered

Table 21.2 General guidelines for the feeding and housing of young raccoons.

Weight (grams)	Formula per feeding (ml)/number feedings per day[a]		Housing guidelines with minimum recommended dimensions
	Option 1	Option 2	
100	5.0/6		Incubator temperature 90 °F (32 °C) at birth
150	7.7/5	6.5/6	and wean down to 70 °F (21 °C) by 500 grams[c]
200	10/5		Humidity 55–65%
250	13/5		10–20 gallon-sized enclosure per litter[b]
300	15/5		
350	17.5/5		
400	20/4	17/5	_____
450	22.5/4	18/5	size-appropriate crate with hammock
500	25/4		heating pad under ½ of crate[b]
550	27.5/3	27/4	
600	30/3	28.5/4	For a litter of 3: 3 ft × 3 ft × 3 ft[b]
650	32.5/3	30.5/4	
700	35/3	32/4	Begin adding enrichment
750	37.5/3	34/4	
800	40/3	36/4	
850	42.5/2	37/3	_____
900	45/2	39/3	
950	47.5/2	40.5/3	Once weaned, house outside (weather permitting)
1000	50/1	42/2	10 ft W × 12 ft L × 6 ft H[b]
1050	52.5/1	43/2	30 square feet per animal[b]
1100	self-feeding	44/1	See self-feeding diet
1200	should be fully weaned		

[a] Adapted from DeGhetto et al. (2002) and the Wildlife Rehabilitation Center of Minnesota Raccoon Care Manual (unpublished).
[b] Miller (2012).
[c] Peterson and Kutzler (2011).

in the orphaned section below). Neonates should be housed together whenever possible to reduce stress. If this is not possible, single animals should have a stuffed animal for comfort. Bedding should consist of nonwoven cloth (e.g., fleece) as toes can get caught in frays, strings, etc. Multiple layers of cloth will allow the neonate to burrow. Visual barriers, white noise or natural sounds playing in the room and rack feeding can minimize chances of habituation.

Once mobile, raccoon kits are extremely messy. Caging should include a hammock or other elevated sleeping area; nontip water and food bowls; a litter pan (either empty or with paper-based litter) to encourage latrine use; daily rotation of enrichment items; and cage size should increase with age (Table 21.2) so that kits can learn to climb, forage, den, etc. Juveniles, like neonates, should always be housed with similar-aged conspecifics; however, gradual supervised introductions are important as older kits may haze.

Raccoons will quickly learn how to open doors or unlatch cages so secure latches with a mechanism that cannot be opened from the inside must be used. If housed outside, locks are encouraged to prevent the public from entering cages.

Ideally adults should be housed in a self-shifting cage/room to facilitate cleaning and feeding. Also, adults should be housed alone as they can become aggressive.

Outdoor caging for weaned juveniles or adults should include the following.

- Cage sides: Should be able to be climbed to facilitate juvenile learning and enrichment for adults. However, keep in mind hazards that might entrap individuals. For example, if using chainlink panels, the corners are rounded so where they come to a corner, the gap at the top is larger than the gap at the bottom. Raccoons who climb the corner to the top and fall can get their leg trapped in the narrowing space. Half inch wire hardware cloth works well for outdoor cage sides.
- Latrine area: Raccoons prefer to defecate/urinate in the same area. To facilitate efficient cleaning, place a shallow pan in that area. The pan can be empty or filled with a paper-based litter. To encourage latrine use of the pan, place the patient's feces in the pan for a few days.
- Den area: Raccoons prefer to sleep in an elevated enclosed area. An enclosed shelf or a hanging plastic barrel work well. This den should be positioned in the cage as to provide shelter from inclement weather. If applicable, the den should be adequately insulated.
- Floor: The bottom of the cage should either be concrete or have wire buried under the substrate to prevent digging. If using a substrate like gravel or dirt, the substrate should be removed and replaced between animals/groups. Spread

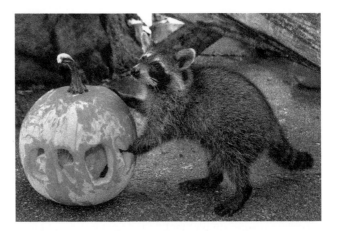

Figure 21.1 Enrichment is important for wildlife in rehabilitation for many reasons. A raccoon enjoys a frozen pumpkin with treats hidden inside that provides sensory enrichment (e.g., tactile, olfactory, visual, and gustatory stimuli) and nutritional enrichment (e.g., encourages foraging behaviors and problem-solving strategies). *Source:* Courtesy of CROW.

natural items (branches, leaves, clean dirt) on the floor for enrichment and stress reduction. These items should be completely removed between animals/groups.
- Food/water: Should be on the ground, especially for juveniles so they can practice foraging. For example, scatter dry food items under leaves, put insects and other food items in a container of clean dirt, offer live minnows in a dish of dechlorinated water, etc.
- Double-door system: All outdoor caging should have a double-door system to prevent escape.

Enrichment

Raccoons are highly intelligent and need enrichment that is frequently alternated (Davis 1907; Pettit 2010). Raccoons who become bored are susceptible to stereotypic behavior, self-mutilation, and chronic stress. Stress, especially chronic stress, can lead to death or several other negative health sequelae such as impaired growth, impaired metabolism, impaired immune system, and slowed wound healing (Blecha 2000; Guo and Dipietro 2010). For kits, enrichment should be provided once eyes open as it decreases stress and helps them learn skills.

Enrichment can consist of natural items (leaves, acorns, branches, live minnows, sounds of the forest soundtracks) or unnatural items such as dog treat toys (such as the Kong [Kong Company, Golden, CO, USA]), dog puzzle toys, toddler toys, and other home-made items (Figure 21.1). Rotate enrichment at least daily and vary items to target all five senses (hearing, touch, eyesight, smell, and taste). Items should be solid (unbreakable), large enough that they cannot be ingested, with no strings/loops/frays that can entangle limbs or digits, and able to be disinfected.

All enrichment items should be for raccoons only (not used with other species) and porous items should be single-use as they cannot be sterilized. It is not known if any plants are potentially toxic to raccoons; however, avoiding plants that are toxic to canids and felids (e.g., avocado, chocolate, onion, etc.) is advised. However, grapes do not cause any health problems in raccoons in the author's experience.

Diet in Captivity

In the wild, raccoon kits are weaned by 16 weeks old but begin to feed on solid foods around eight weeks. Several different feeding schedules have been proposed and details are provided below in the orphan section and in Table 21.1. Several commercial formulas have been used with good success (see Chapter 12) (Shibley 2005; Taylor 2008).

Juveniles and adult diets should be balanced and carefully monitored because obesity is common in captive raccoons, especially if they are housed for an extended period of time. For an adult in captive care, an example daily diet may include: ½ cup dry dog food, ½ cup dry cat food, ½ cup moist dog/cat food, ¾ cup chopped fruit and vegetables, five minnows (live or freshly dead), cracked raw/scrambled egg (once per week). A variety of fruits, vegetables, and insects should also be offered. Amounts should be monitored and adjusted as necessary if the animal becomes overweight or loses weight. Amounts will likely need to be increased in the fall/winter months if housed outdoors.

Handling, Restraint, and Clinical Techniques

Handling and Restraint

Personal protective equipment (PPE) is not optional when working with rabies vector species such as raccoons. Personnel working with raccoons should have received a preexposure rabies prophylaxis vaccination series and have biennial titer levels monitored. However, if bitten or saliva enters broken skin, check with your local state department of public health and/or physician to discuss the need for a rabies vaccine booster or postexposure treatment. If an animal bites a handler, health officials will normally recommend or require euthanasia so that the animal can be tested for rabies, even if the raccoon is very young or is not displaying any neurological abnormalities.

For handling of kits with eyes still closed, latex gloves should be sufficient. If eyes are open, assume they can bite and you should wear leather welder's gloves or other bite-resistant gloves (e.g., BiteBuster gloves, Bitebuster, Gilbert, AZ, USA). Long sleeves are ideal to prevent accidental bites or scratches when young are feeding. To facilitate handling, young raccoons can be scruffed and/or wrapped in a towel.

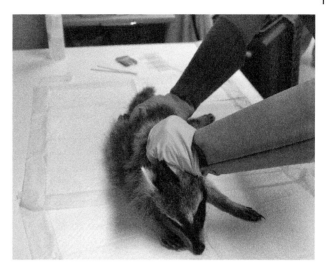

Figure 21.2 Raccoons can be physically restrained, with caution and proper protective equipment. Note the exam gloves over the leather gloves to prevent contamination.

For older juveniles/adults, leather gloves, a large bath towel or blanket, and a net or catch pole are recommended (Figure 21.2). If the animal is free in a room or large cage, first capture it with a long-handled net, step on the handle, throw the bath towel or blanket over the animal, and then pin the neck/shoulders and hips to the ground while wearing thick welder's gloves. An assistant can then inject an appropriate sedative/anesthetic agent (Table 21.3). A squeeze cage is useful and animals may enter on their own because it is dark or it can be baited with food items placed inside. Once they enter, the door can be closed and injections given through a side screen. Alternatively, a catch pole with noose can be used. After the patient is adequately sedated, masking down with inhalant agents to facilitate the exam/procedures is preferable.

Clinical Techniques

Phlebotomy locations are similar to cats and dogs, with common sites being the jugular, cephalic, and saphenous veins (Figure 21.3). The cranial vena cava can also be used. Blood collection should only be performed under anesthesia. Body condition is an important consideration for site selection as peripheral veins may be inaccessible or difficult to visualize when there is abundant subcutaneous fat.

Infectious and Parasitic Diseases of Concern

Baylisascaris procyonis (Raccoon Roundworm)

This parasite is a common intestinal roundworm of raccoons in many regions of the United States. It is zoonotic

Table 21.3 Recommended anesthetic protocols for chemical restraint of healthy adult (>12 weeks) raccoon (IM).[a,b]

Agents (mg/kg)	Reversal doses (mg/kg)	Induction time (min)	Recovery time (min)[c]	Comments (doses, citations)
Dexmeditomidine (0.015–0.02) + Butorphanol (0.3–0.4) + Midazolam (0.2–0.5)	Atipamezole (same volume as dexmed.) Flumazenil	5–15	5–30	[d] Patient may be slightly sedated for 1–3 hours
Tiletamine/zolazepam (3–3.5)	---	4–7	30–60	[e]
Tiletamine/zolazepam (3) + Xylazine (2)	---	2–12	55–231	[f]
Medetomidine (0.16–0.26)	Atipamezole (0.4)	10–23	1–5	[g]
Ketamine (5–5.5) + Dexmedetomidine (0.05) or Medetomidine (0.05–0.055)	Atipamezole (0.025–0.0375)	3–11	10–30	[h, i]
			30–60	[j] Chemical immobilization
Ketamine (10) + Xylazine (2)	Yohimbine (0.1–0.2)	3–4	3–11	[k]
Alfaxalone (12–15)		3–36	3–45	[l] Doses are likely low

[a] After IM injection, allow animal to rest in quiet dark room until sedated; always allow animal to recover in a quiet dark environment.
[b] Analgesia may not be adequate for painful procedures.
[c] Recovery time is minutes after reversal is given, or time after induction medication is given (if no reversal is given).
[d] Author's experience.
[e] Pitt et al. (2015).
[f] Belant (2004).
[g] Baldwin et al. (2008).
[h] Allan (2015).
[i] Robert et al. (2012).
[j] Norment et al. (1994).
[k] Deresienski and Rupprecht (1989) and Clutton and Duggan (1986).
[l] Clutton and Duggan (1986).

and transmitted by ingestion of eggs passed in the feces of raccoons. This parasite also causes severe or fatal larva migrans in a large range of bird and mammal species. Because raccoons as young as eight weeks of age can pass *B. procyonis* eggs in their feces, it is recommended that all raccoons in captivity be prophylactically treated with appropriate anthelmintics (see Appendix II: Formulary) (Bauer and Gey 1995). Since the prepatent period is 50–76 days (Bauer 2013), treatment should be repeated every 14 days for a minimum of 50 days. Additional details are given in Chapter 2.

Parvoviral Enteritis

Parvoviruses are highly infectious and can spread quickly. There are at least two strains of parvovirus that can infect and cause clinical disease in raccoons: canine parvovirus and feline parvovirus (feline panleukopenia virus). These viruses were once separate species but were classified as a single species, carnivore protoparvovirus I, by the International Committee on Taxonomy of Viruses (Allison et al. 2012, 2013). Clinical signs may include diarrhea and vomiting but the first clinical sign often observed is mild

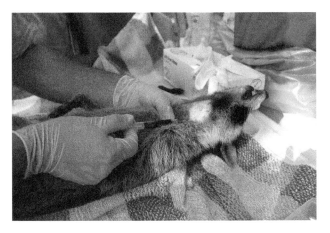

Figure 21.3 Jugular venipuncture in an anesthetized adult raccoon. Shaving the neck is helpful for visualizing the vessel, but wetting the neck with alcohol is sufficient in some animals. *Source:* Courtesy of Sonia Hernandez.

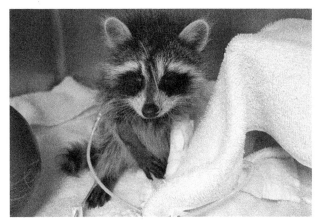

Figure 21.4 Juvenile raccoon undergoing treatment for infection with parvovirus with total parenteral diet and fluid therapy.

weight loss and lethargy. Some raccoons die before they develop diarrhea and/or vomiting. Cross-species transmission of these viruses is common so comprehensive biosecurity practices should be utilized by establishments that house other carnivores (Allison et al. 2013). Disinfectants capable of killing parvoviruses (e.g., 10% bleach solution, accelerated hydrogen peroxide [Accel, Virox Technologies, Oakville, ON, Canada], potassium peroxymonosulfate [Virkon S, Dupont, Willmington, DE, USA]) should be used to maintain a clean environment and to minimize intracenter transmission (Eleraky et al. 2002).

Even with aggressive treatment, prognosis is poor and many individuals will die or be euthanized. If the condition suspected or diagnosed early, treatment may be successful but even then, survival rates may be low (e.g., 3.7% survival in one study) (Blandford 2008). Management is similar to puppies with parvovirus and includes antibiotics, gastroprotectants, fluids, interferon, and early nutritional intervention (Bird and Tappin 2013) (Figure 21.4). Although off-label use of oseltamivir occurs, improved survival was not noted in one study (Savigny and Macintire 2010). An important consideration for treatment is the housing and density of other young raccoons in the rehabilitation center as intracenter transmission is a high risk.

If treatment is attempted, sick individuals should be isolated and the facility should stop admissions of new raccoon patients. Vaccination can be used to minimize risk of clinical disease but efficacy is unknown (see Chapter 7).

Canine Distemper Virus (CDV)

This virus is highly infectious and can spread quickly. Numerous species in the order Carnivora are susceptible. Clinical signs vary considerably and may include depression, mucopurulent oculonasal discharge, cough,

fever, depression, anorexia, vomiting, and diarrhea. In addition, central nervous system signs may or may not be present. These may include general abnormal behavior, seizures, paresis, or paralysis. Hyperkeratosis may also be observed. The virus is killed with common disinfectants. Vaccines are commonly used in captive animals to prevent disease (see Chapter 7).

Rabies Virus

Rabies is an important viral disease of many mammal species, including raccoons. Any raccoon with unusual behavior or neurological signs should be considered a rabies suspect. If a person is bitten, the state department of public health should be notified and they will likely recommend euthanasia of the animal for testing. See Chapters 2 and 7 for more information.

Common Reasons for Presentation

Orphaned Young

Assess Status
Many raccoon kits are admitted after being found and presumed to be orphaned. The mother raccoon may move her neonatal kits to a different den and can drop one along the way and if the kit is left undisturbed, even for several hours, she will likely return. Older kits (>5 weeks) are often caught during the day exploring, which is normal behavior. Young kits who are clearly weak or sick (dehydrated, with ocular discharge, lethargic) should be admitted for care. Luther (2010) provides additional details on navigating different rescue scenarios.

It is incredibly important to understand the prognosis of your patient and to make euthanasia decisions on admission when appropriate (e.g., will injuries prevent release?). Also, there are a finite group of licensed wildlife rehabilitators and funds for them to care for orphaned wildlife, so it is possible that not all apparently healthy orphaned raccoons can be placed for care.

One useful measure for a decision to admit or euthanize is admission weight. Younger kits take much more time and resources to care for than older kits. Euthanizing those of a low body weight or maturity level may seem cruel but the natural survival of nestling raccoons (includes birth to first emergence from den) is 45–75% (Gehrt and Fritzell 1999) so resources should be focused on those with the greatest chance of surviving, thriving, and being releasable.

Orphan Health and Care

A general intake protocol for kits is detailed in Box 21.1. If any signs of disease (diarrhea, dehydration, low body weight, ocular discharge) are noted on the physical exam, a full diagnostic work-up is warranted, especially in a private practice setting as many infectious diseases of raccoons are transmissible to cats and dogs.

Some common diagnostics that may be available include complete blood counts or serum biochemistry assays to assess the general patient health. If a raccoon presents with diarrhea, an in-house Parvo Snap Test (IDEXX Laboratories, Westbrook, ME, USA) can be used to detect parvoviruses; however, false negatives are extremely common (R. Schott, personal experience, H. Barron, unpublished data). Fecal floats may be done to detect intestinal parasites but kits should be treated for *B. procyonis* even if the fecal exams are negative.

After a patient is examined, thermoregulation should be addressed first, then hydration, and finally feeding. The patient should then be transitioned to formula over several feedings (see Box 21.1).

Ideally, raccoons would be quarantined for 14 days prior to introduction to other raccoons. However, kits are extremely stressed when isolated, so singletons should be placed with other singletons and the litter then quarantined.

In the last several years, the production of milk replacers has changed to a single-step spray-dry method which reduces the solubility of these products, resulting in some powder not dissolving (Casey and Casey 2010). This causes diarrhea in many mammals, so to fully mix

---

Box 21.1 Young Raccoon Kit Intake Protocol

- First, determine if the kit needs to be in rehabilitation? Can a reunion be attempted? (Luther 2010).
- Perform a full physical exam (anesthesia usually not indicated unless patient >3 months old).
  - Weigh with digital scale accurate to 1 g increments.
  - Mark patients to tell litter mates apart (nail polish on the pinnae works well).
  - Remove ectoparasites and treat for endoparasites (in general, products that are safe for felines are safe for raccoons).
- Perform any necessary diagnostics based on findings of the physical exam (e.g., complete blood count [CBC], radiographs, infectious disease testing, etc.).
- Address any immediate health concerns.
  - Thermoregulation: Neonates cannot thermoregulate when young. Incubators work well to provide warmth. It is imperative that neonates have a normal body temperature before rehydration.
  - Hydration should be assessed as described in Chapter 4. The patient must be hydrated before starting formula. For rehydration, neonatal maintenance is 120–180 mL/kg/day.
- In general, assume a kit is admitted with at least 5% dehydration and give subcutaneous fluids. One option is lactated Ringer's solution (LRS) with 30 mEq/L KCl with 1 mL vitamin B complex added.
- If clinical signs of hypoglycemia (severe lethargy, hypothermia, dehydration) are present, can give 2.5% dextrose subcutaneously (one part LRS, one part 5% dextrose) and a small amount of sugar (e.g., corn syrup) on gums.
- Assess hydration at every feeding and give subcutaneous fluids as needed, up to 20% dehydration deficit per day.
- Nutrition: Provide 100% electrolytes orally for the first feeding. If the patient is stable (normohydrated, normothermic, active), weaning onto formula can begin using the following protocol (ratios are X% formula: X% rehydration solution).
  - First feeding: 0:100 or if stable/hydrated can start at 25:75.
  - Second feeding (once hydrated): 25:75.
  - Third feeding: 50:50.
  - Fourth feeding: 75:25.
  - Fifth feeding: full strength.
  - If older kit, can wean them onto formula faster (25:75, 50:50, 100:0).

and improve palatability, formula should be made with hot water (>52 °C, >125 °F) followed by a rest period of ~4 hours in the refrigerator. Alternatively, using 80 °C (175 °F) water and an immersion blender can render milk replacer ready for use immediately after cooling. See Chapter 12 for formula, feeding, and schedule options.

Once eyes have opened, offer the litter ½ C moist puppy chow with formula poured over plus 2–3 pieces fruit or vegetables per kit. Once kits are around 900 grams, add in dry puppy chow and pieces of minnows. Once kits are weaned, offer the captive diet previously described. Initially, very young neonates (<3–4 weeks) cannot urinate or defecate on their own and must be stimulated after each feeding (DeGhetto et al. 2002). Gently rub a moist, warm cloth or cotton ball over genital/rectal areas.

Older Juvenile or Adults

Healthy older juvenile or adult raccoons should not be easily captured unless they are sick or injured. Older juveniles and adults generally present with an acute injury (vehicle collision, gunshot), chronic injury (old, infected, open fracture, emaciation) or an infectious disease (canine distemper, rabies, etc.). Sarcoptic or demodectic mange is a common presentation for juvenile or adult

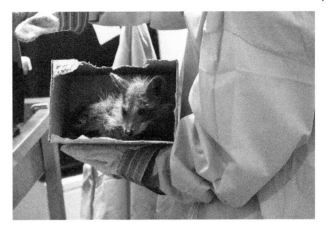

Figure 21.5 Mange is a common presentation for raccoons. *Source:* Courtesy of Heather Barron.

raccoons in some areas of the country (Figure 21.5). Raccoons present with crusty alopecia and pruritus. Mange responds well to standard treatment doses with avermectins (Revolution® or Ivomec®) or isoxazolines, such as afoxolaner (NexGard®).

In some cases of infectious disease, especially if animals are neurological, euthanasia is indicated. Rehabilitation of adult raccoons is challenging so it is important to

---

Box 21.2 Older Juvenile/Adult Raccoon Intake Protocol

- Observe patient in crate/carrier, and in an empty, closed room (if possible/indicated). Observe mentation, temperament, ambulation and for any other neurological clinical signs.
- Anesthetize.
  - Unstable: Physical restraint, gas mask or chamber induction.
  - Stable or active/aggressive: Chemical immobilization (see Appendix II: Formulary).
- Full physical exam.
  - Normal heart rate: 94–134 bpm (Heatley 2009)
  - Normal body temperature: 38.1 °C
  - Normal CBC and serum chemistries; see Appendix I.
  - Eosinophilia of spinal fluid has been reported to be a normal finding (Hanlon et al. 1989).
- Diagnostics.
  - Draw blood for CBC and other testing that might be available.
  - Parvovirus Snap Test if indicated; however, note lack of sensitivity.
  - Radiographs: *At least one* radiographic view because it can be difficult to fully palpate areas like the pelvis.
- Obtain accurate body weight.
- If needed, give all fluids/medications as injectables before patient wakes up.
- This author euthanizes on admission in the following circumstances.
  - Seizures of any time (grand mal or focal).
  - A human or domestic animal was bitten by the raccoon.
  - Positive Parvovirus Snap Test.
  - White blood cell <4000 WBC/μL with abnormal neurological signs.
  - "Tame" or "less aggressive than normal" older juveniles/adults with no other injuries and not a juvenile during a hard winter. Usually behaviors as above are due to distemper infection. An older juvenile during the fall/winter may become so thin and weak that it affects behavior.
- Have patient wake up in a quiet enclosure (preferably in the dark).

objectively develop a list of conditions on which to euthanize new admissions prior to admitting wildlife to help remain objective. See Box 21.2 for this author's intake protocol for older juvenile and adult raccoons.

Release

In the wild, raccoon kits may be on their own as early as 16 weeks of age but usually remain with their mother for the first winter. For captive raised kits, release should be no sooner than 16 weeks of age, with some rehabilitators releasing at 20–24 weeks. Soft releases are preferred (compared to hard releases) in areas that are scarcely populated by humans but still have good raccoon habitat. Whenever possible, raccoons should be released in the vicinity of where they were found.

Relocating animals a great distance from where they are found is controversial for several reasons, including legality (some counties/states limit the distance that animals can be moved), movement of pathogens is possible, and individuals may be unfamiliar with food and shelter sources at the new site (Clark 1994). One study indicated that relocating raccoons can cause up to 50% mortality of adults during the first three months following release (Rosatte and MacInnes 1989) whereas a study in Illinois found survival rates of resident raccoons and translocated raccoons were similar (Mosillo et al. 1999). However, when compared with reported natural mortality rates (47–60%) of resident raccoons (Chamberlain et al. 1999), the mortality of relocated raccoons may not be higher than normal. However, movements of relocated animals are much greater than for native individuals (Rosatte and MacInnes 1989), suggesting that there are territorial conflicts and/or animals have difficulty in finding sufficient food/shelter. Controlled studies are needed to better understand the survival and long-term health of raccoons that are released and/or relocated.

Importantly, relocating animals may facilitate the transmission of pathogens, which is one of the reasons the American Veterinary Medical Association and the National Association of State Public Health Veterinarians recommend against the translocation of wildlife (Nettles et al. 1979; Schaffer et al. 1981; Griffith et al. 1993; Woodford and Rossiter 1994; AVMA 2009; Giovanna et al. 2010).

Finally, two additional considerations regarding the release of raccoons are that the local genetics of the raccoons in an area may be altered by the introduction of animals from a different region and this may have unknown consequences. Also, the existing density of raccoons in an area is often unknown. The release of large numbers of new animals may cause the raccoon population to exceed the natural carrying capacity. Because so many variables may determine the carrying capacity for an area, it may be difficult to take this into consideration.

Postrelease Monitoring

Unfortunately, few data are available on the short-term and long-term survival or fitness of rehabilitated raccoons. Two postrelease studies performed with kits raised in wildlife rehabilitation showed similar survival compared to their wild counterparts; however, the sample sizes were small so additional studies are needed (Rosatte et al. 2010; McWilliams and Wilson 2014).

References

Allan, M.R. (2015). The use of ketamine-xylazine and ketamine-medetomidine with and without their antagonists yohimbine and atipamezole hydrochloride to immobilize raccoons (*Procyon lotor*) in Ontario, Canada. *Canadian Field-Naturalist* 129 (1): 84–89.

Allison, A.B., Harbison, C.E., Pagan, I. et al. (2012). Role of multiple hosts in the cross-species transmission and emergence of a pandemic parvovirus. *Journal of Virology* 86 (2): 865–872.

Allison, A.B., Kohler, D.J., Fox, K.A. et al. (2013). Frequent cross-species transmission of parvoviruses among diverse carnivore hosts. *Journal of Virology* 87 (4): 2342–2347.

AVMA. 2009). Rabies. www.avma.org/Events/pethealth/Pages/world-rabies-day.aspx

Baldwin, J., Winstead, J., Hayden-Wing, L. et al. (2008). Field sedation of coyotes, red foxes, and raccoons with medetomidine and atipamezole. *Journal of Wildlife Management* 72 (5): 1267–1271.

Bauer, C. (2013). Baylisascariosis-infections of animals and humans with 'unusual' roundworms. *Veterinary Parasitology* 193 (4): 404–412.

Bauer, C. and Gey, A. (1995). Efficacy of six anthelmintics against luminal stages of *Baylisascaris procyonis* in naturally infected raccoons (*Procyon lotor*). *Veterinary Parasitology* 60 (1–2): 155–159.

Belant, J.L. (2004). Field immobilization of raccoons (*Procyon lotor*) with Telazol and Xylazine. *Journal of Wildlife Diseases* 40 (4): 787–790.

Biedrzycka, A., Zalewski, A., Bartoszewicz, M. et al. (2014). The genetic structure of raccoon introduced in Central Europe reflects multiple invasion pathways. *Biological Invasions* 16 (8): 1611–1625.

Bird, L. and Tappin, S. (2013). Canine parvovirus: where are we in the 21st century? *Companion Animal* 18 (4): 142–146.

Blandford, M. (2008). Parvovirus outbreak in raccoons (*Procyon lotor*) being rehabilitated at wildcat wildlife Center. *Wildlife Rehabilitation Bulletin* 26 (1): 41–43.

Blecha, F. (2000). Immune response to stress. In: *The Biology of Animal Stress: Basic Principals and Implications for Animal Welfare* (eds. G.P. Moberg and J.A. Mench), 111–121. New York: CABI Publishing.

Bozek, C.K., Prange, S., and Gehrt, S.D. (2007). The influence of anthropogenic resources on multi-scale habitat selection by raccoons. *Urban Ecosystems* 10 (4): 413–425.

Byrne, M.E. and Chamberlain, M.J. (2011). Seasonal space use and habitat selection of adult raccoons (*Procyon lotor*) in a Louisiana bottomland hardwood forest. *American Midland Naturalist* 166 (2): 426–434.

Casey, Allan M., and Casey, Shirley J. 2010). Manufacturing changes for Esbilac powder affect wildlife rehabilitators. www.researchgate.net/publication/242459712_Manufacturing_Changes_for_EsbilacR_Powder_Affect_Wildlife_Rehabilitators

Chamberlain, M.J., Hodges, K.M., Leopold, B.D. et al. (1999). Survival and cause-specific mortality of adult raccoons in Central Mississippi. *Journal of Wildlife Management* 63 (3): 880–888.

Clark, K.D. (1994). Managing Raccoons, Skunks, and Opossums in Urban Settings. Proceedings of the Sixteenth Vertebrate Pest Conference, Santa Clara, CA, pp. 317–319.

Clutton, R.E. and Duggan, L.B. (1986). Saffan anesthesia in the raccoon: a preliminary report. *Journal of Zoo Animal Medicine* 17: 91–99.

Davidson, R.K., Øines, Ø., Hamnes, I.S. et al. (2013). Illegal wildlife imports more than just animals – *Baylisascaris procyonis* in raccoons (*Procyon lotor*) in Norway. *Journal of Wildlife Diseases* 49 (4): 986–990.

Davis, H.B. (1907). The raccoon: a study in animal intelligence. *American Journal of Psychology* 18 (4): 447–489.

DeGhetto, D., Papageorgiou, S., and Convy, J. (2002). Raccoons. In: *Hand-Rearing Wild and Domestic Mammals*, 1e (ed. L.J. Gage), 191–202. Ames, IA: Blackwell.

Deresienski, D.T. and Rupprecht, C.E. (1989). Yohimbine reversal of ketamine-xylazine immobilization of Raccoons (*Procyon lotor*). *Journal of Wildlife Diseases* 25 (2): 169–174.

Eleraky, N.Z., Potgieter, L.N.D., and Kennedy, M.A. (2002). Virucidal efficacy of four new disinfectants. *Journal of the American Animal Hospital Association* 38 (3): 231–234.

García, J.T., García, F.J., Alda, F. et al. (2012). Recent invasion and status of the raccoon (*Procyon lotor*) in Spain. *Biological Invasions* 14 (7): 1305–1310.

Gehrt, S.D. and Fritzell, E.K. (1999). Survivorship of a nonharvested raccoon population in South Texas. *Journal of Wildlife Management* 63 (3): 889–894.

Giovanna, M., Quy, R.J., Gurney, J. et al. (2010). Can translocations be used to mitigate human–wildlife conflicts? *Wildlife Research* 37: 428–439.

Graser, W.H., Gehrt, S.D., Hungerford, L.L. et al. (2012). Variation in demographic patterns and population structure of raccoons across an urban landscape. *Journal of Wildlife Management* 76 (5): 976–986.

Greenwood, R.J. (1982). Nocturnal activity and foraging of prairie raccoons (*Procyon lotor*) in North Dakota. *American Midland Naturalist* 107 (2): 238–243.

Griffith, B., Scott, J.M., Carpenter, J.W. et al. (1993). Animal translocations and potential disease transmission. *Journal of Zoo and Wildlife Medicine* 24 (3): 231–236.

Guo, S. and Dipietro, L.A. (2010). Factors affecting wound healing. *Journal of Dental Research* 89 (3): 219–229.

Hanlon, C.A., Ziemer, E.L., Hamir, A.N. et al. (1989). Cerebrospinal fluid analysis of rabid and vaccinia-rabies glycoprotein recombinant, orally vaccinated raccoons (*Procyon lotor*). *American Journal of Veterinary Research* 50: 364–367.

Hauver, S., Hirsch, B.T., Prange, S. et al. (2013). Age, but not sex or genetic relatedness, shapes raccoon dominance patterns. *Ethology* 119 (9): 769–778.

Heatley, J.J. (2009). Cardiovascular anatomy, physiology, and disease of rodents and small exotic mammals. *Veterinary Clinics of North America. Exotic Animal Practice* 12 (1): 99–113.

Hirsch, B.T., Prange, S., Hauver, S.A. et al. (2013). Raccoon social networks and the potential for disease transmission. *PLoS One* 8 (10): e75830.

Hungerford, L.L., Mitchell, M.A., Nixon, C.M. et al. (1999). Periodontal and dental lesions in raccoons from a farming and a recreational area in Illinois. *Journal of Wildlife Diseases* 35 (4): 728–734.

Inoue, K., Kabeya, J., Fujita, H. et al. (2011). Serological survey of five zoonoses, scrub typhus, japanese spotted fever, tularemia, Lyme disease, and Q fever, in feral raccoons (*Procyon lotor*) in Japan. *Vector Borne and Zoonotic Diseases* 11 (1): 15–19.

Iwaniuk, A.N. and Whishaw, I.Q. (1999). How skilled are the limb movements of the raccoon (*Procyon lotor*)? *Behavioural Brain Research* 99 (1): 35–44.

Kurta, A. (2001). Raccoons and their allies (family Procyonidae). In: *Mammals of the Great Lakes Region*, 218–222. Ann Arbor, MI: University of Michigan Press.

Luther, E. (2010). *Answering the Call of the Wild*, 1e. St Cloud, MN: National Wildlife Rehabilitators Association.

McWilliams, M. and Wilson, J.A. (2014). Home range, body condition, and survival of rehabilitated raccoons (*Procyon lotor*) during their first winter. *Journal of Applied Animal Welfare Science* 18 (2): 133–152.

Miller, E. (ed.) (2012). *Minimum Standards for Wildlife Rehabilitation*, 4e. St Cloud, MN: National Wildlife Rehabilitators Association and International Wildlife Rehabilitation Council.

Monello, R.J. and Gompper, M.E. (2010). Differential effects of experimental increases in sociality on ectoparasites of free-ranging raccoons. *Journal of Animal Ecology* 79 (3): 602–609.

Montgomery, G.G. (1964). Tooth eruption in preweaned raccoons. *Journal of Wildlife Management* 28 (3): 582–584.

Mosillo, M., Heske, E.J., and Thompson, J.D. (1999). Survival and movements of translocated raccoons in northcentral Illinois. *Journal of Wildlife Management* 63 (1): 278–286.

Nettles, V.F., Shaddock, J.H., Sikes, R.K. et al. (1979). Rabies in translocated raccoons. *American Journal of Public Health* 69 (6): 601–602.

Norment, J.L., Elliott, C.L., and Costello, P.S. (1994). Another look at chemical immobilization of raccoons (*Procyon Lotor*) with ketamine hydrochloride. *Journal of Wildlife Diseases* 30 (4): 541–544.

Parsons, A.W., Simons, T.R., O'Connell, A.F. et al. (2013). Demographics, diet, movements, and survival of an isolated, unmanaged raccoon *Procyon lotor* (Procyonidae, Carnivora) population on the outer banks of North Carolina. *Mammalia* 77 (1): 21–30.

Pedlar, J.N., Fahrig, L., and Merriam, H.G. (1997). Raccoon habitat use at 2 spatial scales. *Journal of Wildlife Management* 61 (1): 102–112.

Pettit, M. (2010). The problem of raccoon intelligence in behaviourist America. *British Journal for the History of Science* 43 (3): 391–421.

Pitt, J., Larivi, S., Source, M. et al. (2015). Efficacy of Zoletil for field immobilization of raccoons. *Wildlife Society Bulletin* 34 (4): 1045–1048.

Prange, S., Gehrt, S.D., and Wiggers, E.P. (2003). Demographic factors contributing to high raccoon densities in urban landscapes. *Journal of Wildlife Management* 67 (2): 324–333.

Reynolds, J.J., Hirsch, B.T., Gehrt, S.D. et al. (2015). Raccoon contact networks predict seasonal susceptibility to rabies outbreaks and limitations of vaccination. *Journal of Animal Ecology* 84 (6): 1720–1731.

Riley, S.P.D., Hadidian, J., and Manski, D.A. (1998). Population density, survival, and rabies in raccons in an urban national park. *Canadian Journal of Zoology* 76: 1153–1164.

Rivest, P. and Bergeron, J.M. (1981). Density, food habits, and economic imortance of racoons (*Procyon lotor*) in Quebec agrosystems. *Canadian Journal of Zoology* 59: 1755–1762.

Robert, K., Garant, D., and Pelletier, F. (2012). Chemical immobilization of raccoons (*Procyon Lotor*) with ketamine-Medetomidine mixture and reversal with atipamezole. *Journal of Wildlife Diseases* 48 (1): 122–130.

Robert, K., Garant, D., Vander Wal, E. et al. (2013). Context-dependent social behaviour: testing the interplay between season and kinship with raccoons. *Journal of Zoology* 290 (3): 199–207.

Rodewald, A.D. and Gehrt, S.D. (2014). Wildlife population dynamics in urban landscapes. In: *Urban Wildlife Conservation: Theory and Practice*, 1e (eds. R.A. McCleery, C.E. Moorman and M.N. Peterson), 117–145. New York: Springer.

Rosatte, R., & MacInnes, C. (1989). Relocation of City Raccoons. Great Plains Wildlife Damage Control Workshop Proceedings, pp. 87–92.

Rosatte, R., Ryckman, M., Meech, S. et al. (2010). Home range, movements, and survival of rehabilitated raccoons (*Procyon lotor*) in Ontario, Canada. *Journal of Wildlife Rehabilitation* 30 (1): 7–14.

Sanderson, G.C. (1961). Techniques for determining age of raccoons. *Illinois Natural History Survey, Biological Notes* 45: 1–16.

Savigny, M.R. and Macintire, D.K. (2010). Use of oseltamivir in the treatment of canine parvoviral enteritis. *Journal of Veterinary Emergency and Critical Care* 20 (1): 132–142.

Schaffer, G.D., Davidson, W.R., and Nettles, V.F. (1981). Helminth parasites of translocated raccoons (*Procyon lotor*) in the southeastern United States. *Journal of Wildlife Diseases* 17 (2): 217–227.

Schoonover, L.J. and Marshall, W.H. (1951). Food habits of the raccoon (*Procyon lotor* Hirtus) in north-Central Minnesota. *Journal of Mammology* 32 (4): 422–428.

Shibley, S. (2005). Orphan raccoon (*Procyon lotor*) rehabilitation – born to be free. *Wildlife Rehabilitation* 23: 73–90.

Smith, H.T. and Engeman, R.M. (2002). An extraordinary racoon, *Procyon lotor*, density at an urban park. *Canadian Field-Naturalist* 116 (4): 636–639.

Taylor, J. (2008). *WildCare Foster Care Program: Raccoons Captive Rearing Protocol*. San Rafael, CA: WildCare.

Turnbull, B.G. and Rasmusson, D.D. (1986). Sensory innervation of the raccoon forepaw: 1. Receptor types in glabrous and hairy skin and deep tissue. *Somatosensory Research* 4 (1): 43–62.

Welker, W.I., Johnson, J.I., and Pubols, B.H. (1964). Some morphological and physiological characteristics of the somatic sensory system in raccoons. *American Zoologist* 4 (1): 75–94.

Woodford, M.H. and Rossiter, P.B. (1994). Disease risks associated with wildlife translocation projects. In: *Creative Conservation*, 1e (eds. P.J.S. Olney, G.M. Mace and A.T.C. Feistner), 178–200. Dordrecht, The Netherlands: Springer Science.

Wright, A.N. and Gompper, M.E. (2005). Altered parasite assemblages in raccoons in response to manipulated resource availability. *Oecologia* 144 (1): 148–156.

Zeveloff, S.I. (2002). *Raccoons: A Natural History*. Washington, DC: Smithsonian Institution Press.

Zollman, P.E. and Winkelmann, R.K. (1962). The sensory innervation of the common north american raccoon (*Procyon lotor*). *Journal of Comparative Neurology* 119: 149–157.

22

Natural History and Medical Management of Mustelids

Noha Abou-Madi

Section of Zoological Medicine, Cornell University, Ithaca, NY, USA

Members of the Musteloidea superfamily attract attention, polarize public opinion, and help raise public awareness on conservation and emerging disease concerns. Working with wild mustelids poses interesting challenges but can be tremendously rewarding.

Taxonomy

Composed of 25 genera and 67 species, the Musteloidea represent the largest and most diverse group of carnivores, with vastly different habitat and dietary preferences. Mustelids are adapted to fossorial, semiarboreal, semiaquatic, or fully aquatic environments and are found on every continent except Australia and Antarctica (Table 22.1). Currently, the superfamily Musteloidea has four families: Ailuridae (red pandas), Procyonidae (raccoons and relatives), Mephitidae (skunks), and Mustelidae (otters, badgers, weasels, and relatives) (Dragoo and Honeycutt 1997). However, within these families, the phylogenetic relationships are generally poorly resolved (Sato et al. 2003; Koepfli et al. 2008; Simeone et al. 2015).

Estimation of age in mustelids is difficult. As there are large gender and geographic differences in sizes, their size during the growth phase and the presence of deciduous teeth and macroscopic teeth wear may help in differentiating between immature and adult animals and estimating aging (Baitchman and Kollias 2000). Although more invasive, cementum annuli layer analysis from a canine tooth will provide accurate estimation of age in adults. This procedure requires a fair amount of experience (Baitchman and Kollias 2000; Ansorge and Suchentrunk 2001).

Natural History

The vast majority of mustelids are solitary, with males and females converging only during the breeding season. Many species will aggressively defend their territory (including sea otters). Striped and spotted skunks share a communal den while hog-nosed skunks are more solitary (Burnie and Wilson 2005; Reed-Smith 2012). Most are nocturnal with a few species engaging in crepuscular activities (e.g., striped skunk). Male and female sea otters are territorial, sedentary, and solitary but can congregate in rafts or pods when resting. North American river otters display social plasticity (particularly males), forming groups of 8–15 individuals when food resources are abundant (Reed-Smith 2012). Thus, when a female and her pups are brought in for medical care, provisions must be made to keep the family unit together. However, it is recommended to keep adults individually housed and to maintain a safe distance between them, especially between males. Knowing the normal comportment for each species is particularly important for this group of animals in order to rule out abnormal behaviors, or, for example, a gait that may be indicative of neurological diseases.

Mustelids are usually seasonal breeders and the length of their breeding season varies among species and with geographic distribution. Their mating strategy has been described as polygynous or polygynandrous. In all species, ovulation is induced following prolonged copulation. In only a few species (American mink, Eurasian badger), conception during pregnancy or superfetation has been confirmed to play an important role in their reproductive strategy. Because many species experience delayed implantation, gestation periods are often difficult to estimate. The duration of embryonic diapause is variable and has been reported to last between 1.5 and 12 months depending on the species. Parturition usually occurs 22–65 days following embryonic implantation, resulting in births in March–April or April–May. If a female is captured around that time, late-term pregnancy or pups should be suspected and finders should search for a potential litter in hiding. Females display

Medical Management of Wildlife Species: A Guide for Practitioners, First Edition. Edited by Sonia M. Hernandez,
Heather W. Barron, Erica A. Miller, Roberto F. Aguilar and Michael J. Yabsley.

Table 22.1 Summary of geographic distribution and biological data of North American species of Mustelidae and Mephitidae.

Species	Natural range	Dental formula I C PM M (upper) I C PM M (lower)	Life expectancy Weight range (males (M) and females (F) when available)	Notes on development
American badger	Southern Canada and Midwestern USA to Central Mexico	3 1 3 1 3 1 3 2 Total 34	16 years 5–12 kg	Weaning 2–3 months, independent 5–6 months
Wolverine	Alaska, northern Canada, mountainous regions along Pacific coast, and northern Eurasia	3 1 4 1 3 1 4 2 Total 38	18 years 8–20 kg	Weaning 8–10 weeks
American marten	Across Canada and northern USA (Alaska, New York, Michigan, Minnesota, Maine, Wisconsin)	3 2 4 1 3 1 4 2 Total: 40	17 years F: 400–775 g M: 700–1300 g	Weaning 42 days Staying with mother through first summer
Fisher	Across North America but not in prairie or southern regions of the USA	3 1 4 1 3 1 4 2 Total: 38	2.0–5.5 kg (males twice as large as females)	Weaning 6–16 weeks Independence around 5 months
North American river otter	Throughout Canada and the USA except in the Mojave desert, and areas in southern California, New Mexico, and Texas	3 1 4 1 3 1 3 2 Total 36	14 years 4–15 kg	Otter pups weigh 128 g at birth Weaning 3–4 months
Sea otter	Coast of north Pacific Ocean, California to South Alaska	3 1 3 1 2 1 3 2 Total 36	15 (M)–22 (F) years F: 16–36 kg M: 45 kg	Weaning 6 months
Weasel, least	Circumboreal species, from Alaska south throughout Canada and northern USA	3 1 3 1 3 1 3 2 Total 34	Approx. 1 year F: 30–120 g M: 36–250 g	Weaning 9–12 wks
Weasel, short-tailed ermine	North temperate regions of North America, and Eurasia (absent from Great Plains)	3 1 3 1 3 1 3 2 Total 34	Approx. 1 year F: 47–80 g M: 70–200 g	Weaning 3 months
Weasel, long-tailed	Most of North America	3 1 3 1 3 1 3 2 Total 34	F: 85–115 g M: 140–280 g	Weaning 3 months
Black-footed ferret	Wild populations only found in northeastern Montana, eastern South Dakota, southeastern Wyoming	3 1 3 1 3 1 3 2 Total 34	12 years F: 400–780 g M: 650–1000 g	Weaning 42 days Independence after first summer
American mink	Across most of North America north of Mexico (except Arizona)	3 1 3 1 3 1 3 2 Total 34	8–10 years F: 0.5–1.58 kg M: 0.7–2 kg	Weaning 5–6 wks
Hooded skunk	Southern United States, Mexico, and Central America. South Arizona to western Texas, South to southwest Costa Rica	3 1 3 1 3 1 3 2 Total 34	0.5–2.0 kg	

Table 22.1 (Continued)

Species	Natural range	Dental formula I C PM M (upper) I C PM M (lower)	Life expectancy Weight range (males (M) and females (F) when available)	Notes on development
White-backed hog-nosed skunk	Found only in south Arizona, New Mexico to Texas, and from Mexico to Nicaragua	3 1 3 1 3 1 3 2 Total 34	1.1–4.5 kg	Weaning 2 months
Striped skunk	Most of North America, continental USA, southern Canada, and northern Mexico	3 1 3 1 3 1 3 2 Total 34	10 years 1.0–6.6 kg (larger in north than south)	Weaning 8–12 weeks
Eastern spotted skunk	Much of east and midwest USA, Florida and Mexico	3 1 3 1 3 1 3 2 Total 34	0.25–1.0 kg	
Western spotted skunk	Southwestern British Colombia to Colorado, western Texas and north Mexico	3 1 3 1 3 1 3 2 Total 34	200–900 g	

Sources: Burnie and Wilson (2005), Reid (2006), Kollias and Fernandez-Moran (2015), and Encyclopaedia Britannica (2015).

denning behavior, give birth and raise their offspring in quiet and secluded dens (Lindenfors et al. 2003; Melquist et al. 2003; Thom et al. 2004; Yamaguchi et al. 2004; Persson et al. 2006; Yamaguchi et al. 2006; AZA 2009, 2010).

In preparation for cold winter months in temperate regions, mustelids will deposit a heavy layer of fat that may compromise our ability to accurately administer intramuscular injections. They do not truly hibernate but will spend most of the cold winter months in protected dens, undergoing cycles of deep sleep or torpor. Mustelids periodically arouse when the temperature warms up and their metabolism increases, feed, and then return to their den.

Many species such as the striped skunk have adapted well to urbanized areas and are regularly found in cities. With ever-increasing human activities encroaching into natural habitats, human–mustelid conflicts are inevitable. These animals have become habituated to the presence of food and shelter near human homes, resulting in potentially dangerous interactions with domestic pets, yard damage (skunk digging), and fear of attacks on humans with disease (rabies) transmission (Lucherini and Merino 2008). This is exacerbated when an animal is approached or cornered. Unwelcomed interactions can be reduced or even corrected by eliminating open food sources, blocking access to shelters (garages, areas under decks), creating exclusion devices near domestic poultry,

and using deterrents (e.g., Pine-Sol® original scent soaked rags around problem areas; Barbara Hollands, personal communication).

Housing in Captivity

When hospitalizing sick or injured mustelids and mephitids, a balance between safe housing, ability to restrain, and to provide proper medical care must be kept in mind. A clinic committed to treating wild mustelids must have isolation rooms with a flexible caging system. In the context of a small animal practice, veterinarians must seriously consider the dangers of pathogen transmission between domestic animals and wild mustelids (e.g., parvovirus, canine distemper virus, etc.) as well as zoonotic threats (e.g., rabies virus, *Salmonella*, *Yersinia*, *Francisella tularensis*, *Leptospira*, *Baylisascaris*, *Cryptosporidium*, etc.) (Appel and Summers 1995; Rosatte 2011; Siembieda et al. 2011; Steinel et al. 2001). Regardless of the situation, biosecurity is always warranted and should include isolation of mustelid patients into assigned wards and compulsory personal protection equipment for all involved. In the right conditions, euthanasia of rabies-suspect animals can be performed outdoors in a contained and secured area that can be easily disinfected and is free from regular human and pet traffic.

Most species of mustelids are highly strung and most are aggressive. If cornered into a confined space, individual animals will often pace incessantly and attempt to escape until they self-inflict severe injuries or escape from their cage. This is particularly important when an animal is brought in captivity following injuries (trap injuries), with a normal mental status. Depressed animals may show similar behavior once their condition improves. Providing hiding boxes, covering cages with sheets or towels, darkening the room, and keeping the environment quiet and free of unnecessary human activities and noises (including vibrations) will help prevent some of this distress (Kollias and Fernandez-Moran 2015). Exertional myopathy and clostridial enteritis are well-documented complications following capture of North American river otters, badgers, black-footed ferrets, and sea otters (Hartup et al. 1999; Williams and van Blaricom 1989; Kollias and Fernandez-Moran 2015). Limiting procedures to short handling periods performed by well-trained handlers will help alleviate some of these complications.

Nets and capture material must be available at all times and assigned to these species. Most mustelids dig powerfully and many are skilled climbers and/or swimmers, requiring enclosed thick-gauge fencing for outdoor pens and sturdy caging for indoor facilities. Cage design should allow for thorough cleaning and safe administration of food and oral medication as would be obtained by using large squeeze cages with wire bottoms, or by providing a connection between a holding and a squeeze cage (Figure 22.1). Because these animals are scent oriented, disinfectants must be thoroughly rinsed to remove residues (AZA 2009, 2010).

Environmental temperatures in captivity should match the range to which each species is habituated. With the exception of hypothermic or sick animals, cooler environments are usually preferred. North American river otters tolerate a wide range of temperatures. Indoor housing should provide a thermal gradient ranging between 10 °C and 24 °C (50–75 °F), with a relative humidity of 30–70% (Stoskopf et al. 1997; AZA 2009), preferably under a natural photoperiod. Outdoor housing should provide shelters against the sun and inclement weather, sufficient dry land ideally with natural substrate, and a pool if long-term housing is considered (3.5:1 to 4:1 land to water ratio).

Fresh water sources must be available at all times. North American river otters are semiaquatic, often defecating in water, and thus multiple sources of clean, fresh water are essential. Chlorine should be below detectable levels. Deep pools of fresh water should be provided if long-term housing or rehabilitation for release are considered.

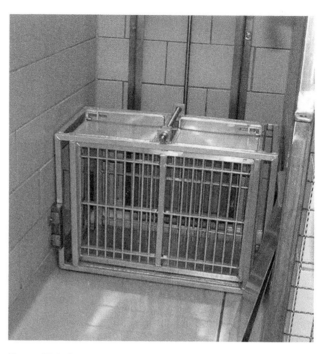

Figure 22.1 Squeeze cage strategically placed between holdings allowing the animal to be captured for injection.

Bedding material and/or towels for drying and grooming of hair coat will help maintain proper fur and feet condition. Cement floors are easy to clean and disinfect but are abrasive to the footpads and are too cold, especially for sick and young animals. Nest/hiding boxes and dens will provide shelter and warmth (in winter) and must be designed to allow for proper ventilation.

Crates and cages used to transport, anesthetize, and recover these animals must be sturdy and designed to evenly squeeze the animal for injections, and equipped with door opening systems to safely transfer the patient from one area/cage to another. Cage design should take into consideration proper ventilation and prevention of oral and dental injuries if the animal bites at the wire (Figure 22.2). Covering windows and exposed doors will help calm down the animals. To transfer the animal from one cage to another, it is useful to keep the receiving cage covered and expose the cage containing the animal to light, encouraging the animal to transfer from one cage into another (Kollias 1999).

Diets in Captivity

The variety of natural diet underlines the importance of knowing the natural history of each species. The short-tailed weasel will eat birds, eggs, frog, fish, insects, and small rodents; skunks are omnivores (insects, rats, mice, moles, worms, snakes, bird eggs, grubs, slugs, berries,

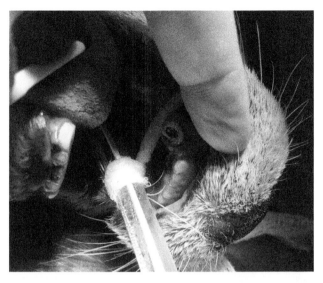

Figure 22.2 Oral examination of a geriatric North American river otter showing severe dental disease, wear, fractured canine with exposure of the pulp cavity.

nuts, grasses, roots, grains, frogs, carrion) and North American river otters primarily piscivorous (Malanska et al. 2012). Diets used during the medical phase of rehabilitation should reflect individual species adaptations, be analyzed for content and monitored for quality, particularly in selecting freshness of fish. The amount can be based on calculation of metabolic rates and tailored to the current condition of each animal. Monitoring of the patient's body weight then allows for adjustment of caloric intake.

Feeding skunks commercial dog and cat diets could potentially habituate individuals to these diets and may predispose them to seeking/recognizing food around houses. With that in mind, a varied diet consisting of good-quality commercial dog or cat diet, small rodents (mice, rats), eggs, with invertebrates, vegetables, and fruits representing a smaller percentage of the total, constitutes a balanced diet for omnivore species (Dragoo 2009). North American river otters are offered a variety of frozen fish (herring, smelt, trout) supplemented with vitamin E (100 IU/kg of fish fed, if the fish has been stored frozen for more than four months), thiamine (25 mg/kg of fish fed) and carnivore commercial diet. Given their high metabolic rate and fast intestinal transit time, meals should be provided at least 2–3 times a day. Of note, otters consume 25% of their body weight daily (Worthy 2001).

For critical animals and emaciated patients, liquid enteric diets available for small domestic animals provide a palatable and easily digestible food source (e.g., Carnivore Critical Care, Oxbow, Murdock, NE or A/D Hills Prescription diet, Hills Pet Nutrition, Topeka, KS, USA). Volumes are calculated based on daily caloric

needs and gastric capacity of each animal and the frequency of meals is adjusted in consequence.

In captivity, common nutritional problems include obesity, thiamine deficiency, steatitis, gingivitis, and dental disease. Ingestion of tainted rodents or fish may cause severe gastroenteritis with resulting vomiting, diarrhea, clostridial overgrowth, hepatitis, etc. (Kollias and Fernandez-Moran 2015). Metabolic bone disease in young animals continues to be a common problem if diets are not carefully balanced for growth. Urolithiasis has been documented in captive and wild otters, including the North American river otter, emphasizing the importance of thorough examinations and respect for natural diet adaptations (Grove et al. 2003; Niemuth et al. 2014).

Capture, Restraint, Anesthesia, and Clinical Techniques

All mustelids are capable of inflicting severe bite wounds. In addition, skunks can severely incapacitate their opponent with the spraying of anal gland secretions. Skunks will show a series of cautionary and threatening behaviors before spraying but they can also spray with little warning if startled. Moving slowly around them will help prevent some of the spraying behavior. With the added threat of rabies, handlers are urged to use caution and to always wear personal protective gear.

As with domestic species, preanesthetic preparation is essential. Preanesthetic bloodwork is unlikely to be available, but sick animals should be stabilized before anesthesia. Obtaining an accurate body weight will permit calculation of correct doses. Overnight fasting is recommended for larger species whereas fasting for 2–4 hours is recommended for smaller species.

Small species may be manually restrained (with the aid of heavy gloves and towels) for short treatments but should be anesthetized for more involved procedures such as radiographs and blood collection. General anesthesia can be induced by either placing the animal in an induction chamber and vaporizing isoflurane or sevoflurane, or by administration of parenteral anesthetic drugs.

Parenteral anesthetics can be administered intramuscularly using a squeeze cage or a sturdy plexiglass shield. The efficacy of various combinations of alpha-2 adrenergic agonists, benzodiazepine, and dissociative agents has been described; they provide short (15–30 up to 45 minutes) anesthetic episodes. Improved quality of induction is obtained by leaving the injected animal in a quiet and dark environment until the drugs have taken effect. Subcutaneous administration of anesthetic drugs often results in erratic effects, excitement and poor quality of induction, requiring further dosing until inhalant anesthetic can be administered.

Ketamine is often preferred and has been used alone (10 mg/kg IM). More efficiently, ketamine (15–20 mg/kg) is combined with midazolam (0.3 mg/kg), or medetomidine (0.04–0.06 mg/kg) is combined with ketamine (2–4 mg/kg). The reported range of doses for tiletamine/zolazepam is very large (2.2–22 mg/kg); the high doses are associated with very long recoveries and should be avoided so using the lower doses and titrating them on a case-by-case basis is recommended. Supplemental oxygen should be provided via facemask or flow-by delivery (Kollias and Abou-Madi 2014; Kollias and Fernandez-Moran 2015).

For longer procedures, supplementation with inhalation anesthesia is recommended. Tracheal intubation is straightforward as long as the animal has achieved an adequate plane of anesthesia. Routine and attentive monitoring is recommended, with particular attention to fluctuations in body temperatures. The use of antagonists (atipamezole) will accelerate and improve the quality of recovery. Recovery in a dark, quiet, and warm environment is essential with close monitoring of the animal's condition to prevent hypo- or hyperthermia and apnea during emergence (Kollias and Abou-Madi 2014; Mortenson and Moriarty 2015).

Analgesics used in small domestic animals and specifically in ferrets are effective in mustelids. Meloxicam (0.2 mg/kg SID) and tramadol (5 mg/kg PO BID) are effective (Morrisey 2013). Butorphanol (0.05–0.5 mg/kg) and buprenorphine (0.01–0.03 mg/kg) are used postoperatively and may at higher doses cause sedation. In all cases, careful monitoring of renal and gastrointestinal functions is recommended and these doses should be tapered down to effect.

Clinical techniques in mustelids are very similar to those used in domestic ferrets. Blood is collected from jugular, cephalic, saphenous, femoral, anterior vena cava, and ventral caudal veins, depending on the species and individual preferences (Figure 22.3). The short limbs and thick and loose skin may create challenges to placing intravenous catheters and for blood collection. By far, jugular phlebotomy will yield the largest volume of blood. In most mustelids (as in ferrets), the jugular veins are located more laterally than the anticipated position in dog and cats. Radiographs are obtained under general anesthesia or heavy sedation in debilitated animals. The position of the heart is normally more caudal in the thoracic cavity than seen in dogs and cats (Baitchman and Kollias 2000).

Oral medications can be hidden in preferred food items and fed alternatively with unmedicated pieces of food. Compliance is improved when the medicated pieces are presented close to the animal's mouth (e.g., using a blunt-tipped wooden dowel for otters).

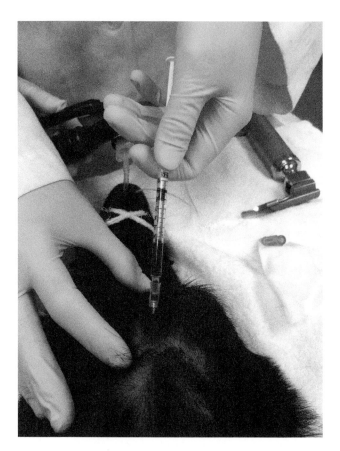

Figure 22.3 Blood collection in an anesthetized striped skunk using the jugular vein/anterior vena cava. Please note the appropriate personal protective gear.

Anatomy and Physiology

Mustelidae and Mephitidae have an elongated body with short legs, except for wolverines and skunks that tend to be stockier. They are very active, aggressive, and seem to "roll in their skin," making manual restraint very difficult and risky. The smallest member of this group is the least weasel (114 mm, 25 g) and the largest is the sea otter (1 m, 45 kg). Body weights vary with gender and season but in general, males are about 25–30% larger than females, and sometimes up to 50% larger. Their stomach is simple and the intestinal tract is short, being adapted for digestion of protein and fat versus diets high in fiber and carbohydrates. Transit time is fast, often 2–4 hours in smaller species. Otters benefit from a very dense pelage that ensures protection against the cold and insulates them in water so subcutaneous fat stores are minimal and usually limited to the tail (Baitchman and Kollias 2000).

Some species are digitigrade while others are plantigrade, and with the exception of wolverines that can partially retract their claws, most have sharp claws that do not retract. Mustelidae lack clavicles (vestigial) and a cecum and all have a baculum. For females, the os clitoris should not be confused with abnormal calcifications or a foreign body in radiographs.

All mustelids have well-developed anal scent glands that are used for marking territories and other chemical communications. In skunks, these glands are particularly well developed, powered by muscles for accurate spraying of a powerful combination of acrid-smelling chemicals that may cause severe irritation and temporary blindness, a very effective self-defense. The chemicals in the musk include several thiol compounds (Wood et al. 2002). Several commercial products are available to help remove the resulting acrid smell. A simple recipe consists of mixing 1 quart of hydrogen peroxide (3%), 1 teaspoon of liquid dish detergent, and ¼ cup of baking soda.

Common Infectious or Parasitic Diseases of Concern

Mustelidae and Mephitidae share many infectious and parasitic diseases with small domestic animals and several are important zoonoses. A comprehensive review of diseases affecting mustelids can be found in Kollias and Fernandez-Moran (2015). Although exposure to numerous viruses and bacteria found in domestic dogs and cats has been detected serologically (Kimber et al. 2000; Kimber and Kollias 2000), these animals were clinically healthy at the time of sampling. Trauma and infectious diseases represent the most common presenting problems affecting wild Mustelidae and Mephitidae. Orphans (true or kidnapped) in various states of health may be brought to rehabilitation centers for hand rearing.

Infection with canine distemper virus and rabies virus can cause severe clinical signs. Manifestations for both viruses are primarily neurological and are not really distinguishable clinically. In a 2009 survey, about 24% of animal rabies cases were found in skunks (Green et al. 2011). In exposed canines, the skunk variants tend to cause the paralytic clinical presentation (Green et al. 2011). Euthanasia of animals displaying neurological signs followed by necropsy and diagnostic testing is often indicated.

Outbreaks of canine distemper regularly occur in wild mephitids and mustelids. The virus has severely compromised the sustainability of captive and wild populations of black-footed ferrets. Clinical signs relate to infections of the respiratory, gastrointestinal, and nervous systems. Susceptibility of each species to this virus is variable but in general is high. Mustelids affected by this disease often present with severe neurological signs. Canine distemper is highly contagious and usually fatal, and treatment

is not recommended (Deem et al. 2000). In the presence of a potential outbreak in a rehabilitation facility, isolation of the animals and biosecurity are essential. Vaccination may be warranted but must be used with caution. However, there are multiple reports of fatal vaccine-induced canine distemper virus infection indicating that most modified-live vaccines are insufficiently attenuated to be safe (Carpenter et al. 1976). When available, the canarypox recombinant canine distemper virus (Merial Inc., Athens, GA, USA) seems to provide an acceptable alternative (Lamberski 2012; Wimsatt et al. 2003). See Chapter 7 for more details.

Infection with the rabies virus will result in neurological disease often difficult to differentiate from canine distemper virus infection. All members of the two families are susceptible to rabies virus and skunks are hosts to three variants of the rabies virus found in three distinct areas (California, north central and south central USA); however, spillover cases of rabies from other hosts may occur anywhere within the range of skunks (Green et al. 2011). Skunks are considered the primary terrestrial rabies vector species in several states. Attacks on humans by confirmed rabid North American otters are also reported sporadically (Potter et al. 2007). Any human exposure (confirmed or suspected) to neurological Mustelidae or Mephitidae should be reported to public health authorities immediately. There is scant information on the exact pathogenesis of this disease and presumptively a large variation is expected between species and viral variant. For example, clinical illness in rabid skunks has been reported to last between one and 18 days (Charleton et al. 1991; Balachandran and Charlton 1994; Green et al. 2011). Oral rabies vaccines have been used successfully in the field in striped skunks to help with management of rabies outbreaks (Pommerening et al. 2002; Fehlner-Gardiner et al. 2012).

Although skunks may be resistant to feline parvovirus, mink and ferrets are susceptible to infections. Mustelids appear to be susceptible to canine parvovirus-2 and Aleutian mink disease virus (both reclassified in the genus Amdoparvovirus) and canine adenovirus-1 (Karstad et al. 1975; Steinel et al. 2001; Allison et al. 2013; Kollias and Fernandez-Moran 2015; Canuti et al. 2017). A novel herpesvirus was discovered associated with oral ulceration and plaques in sea otters (Tseng et al. 2012) and a novel adenovirus (adenovirus-1) causing acute hepatitis was recently isolated in skunks (Kozak et al. 2015).

A serosurvey in Connecticut showed that 13% of 30 sampled skunks were positive for antibodies to *Leptospira grippotyphosa*; skunks are considered as reservoirs for leptospirosis, including *Leptospira interrogans* (Richardson and Gauthier 2003). Many other bacteria have been identified to cause infections in mustelids (Orloski and Lathrop 2003; Kollias and Fernandez-Moran 2015), including *Yersinia pestis* (particularly important in black-footed ferrets), *Salmonella, Brucella, Francisella tularensis,* and *Campylobacter jejuni.* A thorough work-up of each case with appropriate diagnostic testing will help identify the primary and/or secondary causes of illness.

North American river otters are often infected with the lungworm *Crenosoma.* These infections may be asymptomatic but may also cause focal pneumonia and nasal discharge, especially in stressed animals.

Several *Baylisascaris* spp. occur in mustelidsm including *Baylisascaris columnaris* in skunks, *B. melis* in badgers, and *B. devosi* in fishers and martens, all of which can cause larva migrans in the tissues of susceptible intermediate hosts. Eggs are very resistant in the environment and environments may remain contaminated for years. Treatment of definitive hosts is recommended to prevent further spread of the parasites to other hosts and to prevent environmental contamination. Pyrantel, fenbendazole, albendazole, and ivermectin are all likely to be effective for treatment of mustelids (Stringfield 2008). Skunks and minks are definitive hosts to *Skrjabingylus nasicola,* a sinus nematode (Carreno et al. 2005). The ingested larva of this parasite molts and the worms migrate through the gastrointestinal wall into the spinal column and into sinuses. Infections have been proven to reduce braincase size in adult male minks and anecdotally in skunks (Bowman and Tamlin 2007). Mustelids (skunks and otters) are susceptible to *Toxoplasma gondii* and can develop fatal clinical disease. Additionally, sea otters have succumbed to infections with *Sarcocystis neurona* and *Isospora* (Charleton et al. 1991; Cheadle et al. 2001; Burns et al. 2003; Dabritz et al. 2007; Jessup et al. 2007; Miller et al. 2008; Larkin et al. 2011; Duncan et al. 2015).

Common Reasons for Presentations

Injured or sick wild Mustelidae and Mephitidae are brought to veterinary clinics and wildlife centers following vehicular trauma, weakness or disability from infectious diseases, hypothermia/exposure, emaciation, and/or orphaned animals. Furthermore, negative interactions with the public may result in head trauma, trap injuries, deliberate nefarious or accidental poisoning (including to anticoagulants used as rodent bait) (Ruder et al. 2011; Quinn et al. 2012). Medical and surgical care recommended in small animal practice is directly applicable, but the need for each procedure should be evaluated and adjusted in the context of wildlife practice. For example, an intravenous catheter may be placed during the initial treatment of a sick mustelid (either comatose or under anesthesia) but long-term maintenance of this catheter may not be an option in many of these patients.

Veterinarians and biologists may also be involved as part of cooperative capture and release projects, during mortality events, or to help at times of increased incidence of sick animals found around a community. Mustelidae and Mephitidae share many infectious and parasitic diseases with small domestic animals and several are important zoonoses. Biosafety precautions are again of utmost importance and veterinarians should consult with their local health organizations on how to proceed.

Veterinarians who are called to provide medical care to rehabilitation centers housing Mustelidae and Mephitidae must emphasize the importance of a comprehensive preventive medicine program. All staff should have undergone special training to receive and care for rabies vector species. Veterinarians can help monitor the proper application of biosecurity measures. Complete and up-to-date medical records and provision for necropsies and rabies testing must be in place. Routine examination, including body score evaluation, dental examination and prophylaxis, blood testing (complete blood count [CBC], chemistry panel), urinalysis, heartworm testing and prophylaxis in endemic areas, and vaccination as indicated, is recommended yearly and fecal analysis for parasite detection quarterly. Preventive medicine also includes careful evaluation of diets, hand-rearing protocols, and release programs.

At times, immediate euthanasia is warranted (neurological condition, trauma that would preclude release to the wild or good-quality life in captivity). In these cases, the animal is anesthetized (either in an induction chamber or with parenteral administration of injectable drugs) and, if indicated, euthanasia is performed following proper biosafety measures.

Medical Management

Basic triage evaluation is performed upon receiving an injured or sick mustelid. This can be limited to a visual assessment and administration of supportive care (using a squeeze cage or carefully chosen manual restraint) until the animal can be safely restrained or anesthetized. Daily maintenance fluid rate is estimated to be 50–70 mL/kg depending on the species, possibly higher in the smallest species. Veterinarians will have to judge the need to immediately anesthetize an animal to further stabilize it against providing supportive care to the awake patient and delaying diagnostic testing. In order to decrease stress, veterinarians and staff should strive to handle and interact with these species as little as possible.

In general, blood is collected for a CBC, chemistry panel, and serum/plasma banking. Whole-body radiographs are recommended after a thorough physical examination to identify fractures (head, spine, extremities, pelvis), thoracic injuries or disease, diaphragmatic hernia, or foreign bodies (Krista et al. 2003). If available, ultrasound examination of the abdomen may rule out enteritis, foreign bodies, or a ruptured bladder, spleen, or liver in trauma cases.

As indicated, the application of warmth, supplemental oxygen, dextrose (especially for small and emaciated animals) and fluids (SQ or IV as indicated by the animal's condition) are the usual first treatments to consider. Heart and respiratory rates can be falsely elevated during handling. Body temperatures average 38.8–39.4 °C (101.9–102.9 °F), but may vary from 37.7 °C to 40 °C (99.9–104 °F) (Kollias and Fernandez-Moran 2015). Wound care, antibiotics, and analgesics are provided as indicated by the animal's condition.

Once life-threatening emergency conditions have been controlled and the animal is stabilized, further work-up is performed. Working up traumatic injuries should include ruling out underlying causes that may have weakened the animal and predisposed them to vehicular trauma or an attack by wild or domestic animals. Therapeutic options can be extrapolated from recommendations in domestic ferrets, dogs, and cats as deemed appropriate.

The high incidence of fatal postcapture myopathy and stress-related clostridial disease observed in translocation projects of North American river otters has led to the development of a preventive therapeutic protocol (Kollias 1999). Key modifications in handling or specific procedures have resulted in reduced mortality. When these animals were captured, they were transported directly (<12–24 hours post capture) to a healthcare center where they were immediately given vitamin E (40 IU/kg SQ repeated in seven days), thiamine (10 mg/kg SQ in fluid pocket, repeated in five days), and antibiotics as indicated by condition and important in the prevention of clostridial enteritis (Figure 22.4) (Kollias 1999). To treat endoparasites and, more specifically, lungworms, ivermectin (0.4 mg/kg SQ repeated in 14 days) and fenbendazole (50 mg/kg PO, SID, once a day for 3 days) were given. See Appendix I for reference ranges for hematological and biochemistry parameters.

Surgery

Surgical techniques used for small domestic animals can be applied to Mustelidae and Mephitidae. Special considerations include minimizing clipping of the fur in otters since they rely completely on their pelage for

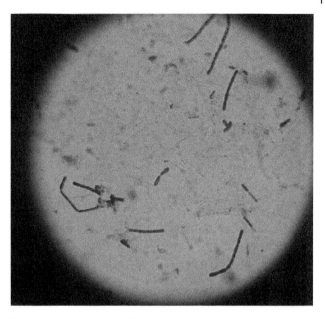

Figure 22.4 Gram stain of feces from a North American river otter with diarrhea. Many spore-forming clostridium-like organisms can be seen.

thermal insulation, and placement of intradermal sutures to reduce self-trauma to surgical wounds.

Long bone fracture surgical repair using plates will allow the animal to return to normal activities (especially swimming in otters) but is costly. External fixators with intramedullary pins are an option if the device can be protected from getting trapped and damaged in the caging material. Bandages may or may not be tolerated depending on species and individuals.

Anal sacculectomy has been described in skunks that are kept as pets or in education programs. Since this procedure is done under clean but not sterile conditions, many veterinarians opt to perform it outdoors in case one or both glands rupture (Capello 2006). The openings of the glands are located at 3 and 9 o'clock cranial to the anal sphincter and appear at the tip of a papilla. With the animal in dorsal or sternal (preferred) recumbency and under general anesthesia, the tail is bandaged away from the site and the area is surgically prepared. Digital eversion of the rectal mucosa will help locate the papillae (Figure 22.5). The tip of the papilla is carefully clamped and ligated, avoiding damage to the rectal mucosa. A circumferential incision is made around the papilla, and the mucosa is gently reflected away from the gland. When the gland is completely exteriorized, the caudal end is excised, and the integrity of the rectal wall is assessed using a cotton-tip applicator. Any damage to the rectal wall should be immediately repaired. Incisions are left to heal by second intention, and the site is monitored for abscess formation. In addition, postoperative broad-spectrum antibiotics and analgesics are prescribed.

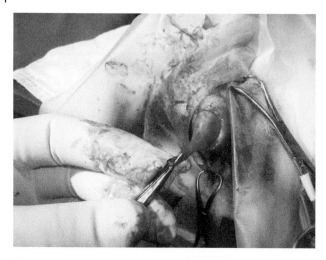

Figure 22.5 Anal sacculectomy in a male striped skunk. The papilla has been clamped and the gland is gently dissected out.

Vaccinations

Many rehabilitators vaccinate mustelids to protect them against diseases during captivity. The consideration about vaccinating animals presented for rehabilitation comes up frequently. There are no FDA-approved vaccines for these species and any use would be considered off-label vaccination (see Chapter 7).

It is important to remember that despite being vaccinated against rabies, any wild mammal that bites a human (or a domestic animal) should be euthanized and submitted for rabies testing.

Care for Orphans

Babies are born with eyes and ears closed, covered with a very fine hair coat and are totally dependent on their mother for care. Trauma to the mother, accidental separation (by domestic pets), or disease can cause the babies to become orphaned. Once it has been determined that an orphaned mustelid cannot be reintegrated to its family, provisions must be made to transfer it to a rehabilitation facility for continued care and rehabilitation. Every effort should be made during treatment and rehabilitation to prevent imprinting of these animals to humans and domestic animals (Gode and Ruth 2010; Haire 2011a,b).

Upon presentation, young animals should be warmed up immediately as they undergo physical examination. Bradycardia is often the result of hypoglycemia and/or hypothermia (and, of course, terminal shock). Once warmed, the babies are rehydrated parenterally (the SQ route is most often used but intraosseous catheters may also be placed in the femur or ileum). If possible, a small blood sample should be obtained (in the hub of a needle) and quick assessment tests performed (packed cell volume, total solids, glucose, blood urea nitrogen, blood smears). If blood cannot be collected, a skinprick and hand-held glucometer can be helpful, although these readings are only an approximation of the actual blood level.

Once normal transit and function of the gastrointestinal tract is confirmed, oral electrolytes are first administered and then the formula is introduced at low concentration. As long as the formula is tolerated (no bloating and no diarrhea), the concentration is progressively increased (about 25% every 2–3 feedings, highly dependent upon the species) (Figure 22.6). Several commercial formulas are available and have been used successfully. Two companies, Fox Valley Animal Nutrition, Inc. (Lake Zurich, IL, USA) and Zoologic® Milk Matrix (PetAg, Hampshire, IL, USA), offer several milk replacer lines that can be adapted to the specific needs of the species. Kitten and puppy milk replacers have been used but may provide incomplete nutrition in many species. Other publications provide details for species-specific needs (AZA 2009, 2010; Haire 2011a) and also see Chapter 12 for selected species.

Feeding schedules will depend on the animal and its condition. The estimated gastric capacity is 5–7%. It would be advisable to start with smaller volumes and increase slowly. For the striped skunk, the formula is fed every 2–3 hours from birth to day 7 of age (with one night feeding), every 2–3 hours from day 8 to day 14 of age (eliminating the night feeding), every 3–4 hours from day 15 to day 21 of age (adding a dish of water), three times a day during the fourth week of age (and adding weaning and natural food), then at five weeks of age, the formula is fed twice a day; they are offered soft food after six weeks of age, and weaned and offered a variety of natural food at 8–10 weeks of age (Gode and Ruth 2010). One acceptable soft diet includes ¼ cup soaked dog food, 1 tsp canned dog food, ¼ chopped hard-boiled egg, 1 tsp

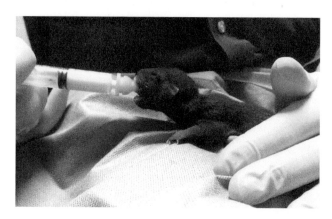

Figure 22.6 Hand-rearing a neonatal North American river otter.

yogurt, 1 tbsp mixed vegetables (no corn or asparagus), 2 tbsp mixed dark greens, 1 tsp berries, 200 mg taurine, and one pinkie mouse or 10 mealworms or five crickets placed in bowl together. This should be supplemented with chewable taurine tablets (250 mg juveniles, 500 mg adults/per day).

Otters less than seven weeks of age should be stimulated to urinate/defecate prior to each feed. Unweaned juveniles should not go more than 6–8 hours between feedings. One protocol that has been frequently used with success is to feed neonates with Fox Valley Beaver milk replacer (30/50) at 30–40% body weight per day. The stomach capacity is 50 mL/kg, so volume and number of feeds can be determined from these parameters. Formula should be made a minimum of 4–8 hours prior to feeding, or the previous night, to allow the powder to go fully into solution. Reconstituted formula should be discarded after 24 hours. Warm the formula in a water bath to ~100 °F prior to feeding. The following feeding schedule can be used for otters:

- 0–2 weeks: feed every 2–3 hours (including overnight)
- 3–4 weeks: feed 5–6 times per day, every 3 hours (no overnight feeds)
- 5–6 weeks: feed 5 times per day, every 3–4 hours
- 7–8 weeks: feed 4–5 times per day, every 4 hours (introduce fish)
- 9–10 weeks: feed 4 times per day (decreasing formula with weaning)

Start pups less than four weeks of age on nipple/bottle feeding. Human baby bottles with preemie nipples can be used for otters older than four weeks. Caretakers can help otter pups to adjust to bottle feeding by covering the pup's eyes and holding the mouth closed over the nipple to prevent chewing and then gently squeezing a small amount of formula into the mouth to acclimate to taste. Pups older than six weeks can be offered milk in a heavy ceramic bowl. Monitor for diarrhea and bloating at each feed. Once eyes are fully open at seven weeks, the weaning diet should be offered. Formula feedings should *not* be skipped until consistently eating the weaning diet. This diet may consist of chopped smelt and kitten chow soaked in formula when first introduced. New food items should only be introduced every few days and may include crickets, mealworms, chopped mice, chicks, and a variety of fish and crabs. Complete weaning occurs after 16 weeks. Approximately 90% of the postweaning diet should be whole fish and kitten chow. Wild otters eat 15–20% of their body weight per day as adults. Older juvenile or adult captive otters need to be fed 3–4 times per day due to their high metabolism.

Diets with high carbohydrate content, rapid changes in diet, concentrations of formula too elevated, and overfeeding are common causes of dysbiosis, diarrhea, and eventually clostridial enteritis. A granular appearance of the feces (presence of bird seed-like material) is an abnormal finding and may indicate malabsorption and should be investigated (Figure 22.7). Establishing a baseline normal fecal gram stain profile will help monitor changes and interpretation of findings. Probiotics can be used to help reestablish normal gut flora and products used in dogs and cats are available (Bene-Bac®, PetAg, Hampshire, IL; FortiFlora®, Nestlé Purina PetCare Co., St Louis, MO, USA). Proper positioning of the babies during hand rearing and controlling the flow of milk delivery during nursing will prevent aspiration pneumonia. Coughing and/or choking events during suckling should be monitored and radiographs will help document the occurrence of pneumonia, leading to early intervention.

See Appendix I for reference ranges for hematological and biochemistry parameters.

Pre-release Conditioning or Postrelease Monitoring

At all times during the process of medical care and rehabilitation of mustelids, precautions must be taken to avoid habituation of the animals to humans or domestic pets, commercial food and shelters near human homes. Skunks must remain shy around humans and dogs and exhibit proper warning when approached. Proper

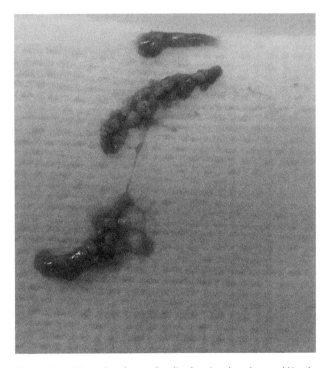

Figure 22.7 Mucoid and granular diarrhea in a hand-reared North American river otter due to dysbiosis and intolerance to formula.

socialization of the young animals should be targeted so they are capable of interacting normally with conspecifics and avoiding contact with domestic animals.

In captivity, adequate biosecurity measures are essential to avoid transmission of diseases from mustelids to pets and humans and from pets to mustelids. The candidates for release should be in excellent physical and psychological health, and with a strong chance of competing for survival and propagation. Consultation with governmental natural resource agencies is necessary to insure that release sites are legal, safe, and proper habitats with sufficient carrying capacity. Special provisions must be made for rabies vector species (skunk) and the appropriate state governmental agency should be consulted.

Monitoring of released animal is possible via radiotelemetry (Kollias 1999; Hernandez-Divers et al. 2001). Data from these studies will help determine the challenges and successes of reintroduction programs and promote future conservation efforts.

References

Allison, A.B., Kohler, D.J., Fox, A.K. et al. (2013). Frequent cross-species transmission of parvoviruses among diverse carnivore hosts. *Journal of Virology* 87 (4): 2342–2347.

Ansorge, H. and Suchentrunk, F. (2001). Aging steppe polecats (*Mustela eversmannii*) and polecats (*Mustela putorius*) by canine cementum layers and skull characters. *Wissenschaftliche Mitteilungen aus dem Niederosterreichischen Landesmuseum* 14: 79–106.

Appel, M.J.G. and Summers, B.A. (1995). Pathogenicity of morbilliviruses for terrestrial carnivores. *Veterinary Microbiology* 44: 187–191.

AZA Small Carnivore TAG. (2009). *Otter (Lutrinae) Care Manual*. Silver Spring, MD: Association of Zoos and Aquariums.

AZA Small Carnivore TAG. (2010). *Mustelid (Mustelidae) Care Manual*. Silver Spring, MD: Association of Zoos and Aquariums.

Baitchman, E.J. and Kollias, G.V. (2000). Clinical anatomy of the north American river otter (*Lontra canadensis*). *Journal of Zoo and Wildlife Medicine* 31 (4): 473–483.

Balachandran, A. and Charlton, K. (1994). Experimental rabies infection of non-nervous tissues in skunks (Mephitis mephitis) and foxes (Vulpes vulpes). *Vet Pathol.* 31 (1): 93–102.

Bowman, J. and Tamlin, A.L. (2007). The effect of sinus nematode infection on braincase volume and cranium shape in the mink. *Journal of Mammalogy* 88 (4): 946–950.

Burnie, D. and Wilson, D.E. (2005). *Smithsonian Institution. Animal: The Definitive Visual Guide to the World's Wildlife*, 196–203. New York: DK Publishing, Inc.

Burns, R., Williams, E.S., O'Toole, D. et al. (2003). *Toxoplasma gondii* infections in captive black-footed ferrets (*Mustela nigripes*), 1992–1998: clinical signs, serology, pathology, and prevention. *Journal of Wildlife Diseases* 39 (4): 787–797.

Canuti, D.M.H.E., Britton, A.P., and Lang, A.S. (2017). Full genetic characterization and epidemiology of a novel amdoparvovirus in striped skunk (Mephitis mephitis). *Emerging Microbes & Infections* 6: e30.

Capello, V. (2006). Sacculectomy in the pet ferret and skunk. *Exotic DVM* 8 (2): 16–24.

Carpenter, J.W., Appel, M.J., Erickson, R.C. et al. (1976). Fatal vaccine-induced canine distemper virus infection in black-footed ferrets. *Journal of the American Veterinary Medical Association* 169 (9): 961–964.

Carreno, R.A., Reif, K.E., and Nadler, S.A. (2005). A new species of *Skrjabingylus* Petrov, 1927 (Nematoda: Metastrongyloidea) from the frontal sinuses of the hooded skunk, *Mephitis macroura* (Mustelidae). *Journal of Parasitology* 91 (1): 102–107.

Charleton, K.M., Webster, W.A., and Casey, G.A. (1991). Skunk rabies. In: *The Natural History of Rabies*, 2e (ed. G.M. Baer), 307–324. Boca Raton, FL: CRC Press,.

Cheadle, M.A., Yowell, C.A., Sellon, D.C. et al. (2001). The striped skunk (*Mephitis mephitis*) is an intermediate host for *Sarcocystis neurona*. *International Journal for Parasitology* 31: 843–849.

Dabritz, H.A., Miller, M.A., Atwill, E.R. et al. (2007). Detection of *Toxoplasma gondii* oocysts in cat feces and estimates of the environmental oocyst burden. *Journal of the American Veterinary Medical Association* 231 (11): 1676–1684.

Deem, S.L., Spelman, L.H., Yates, R.A. et al. (2000). Canine distemper in terrestrial carnivores: a review. *Journal of Zoo and Wildlife Medicine* 31 (4): 441–451.

Dragoo, J.W. (2009). Nutrition and behavior of striped skunk. *Veterinary Clinics of North America: Exotic Animal Practice* 12 (2): 313–326.

Dragoo, J.W. and Honeycutt, R.L. (1997). Systematics of mustelid-like carnivores. *Journal of Mammalogy* 78 (2): 426–443.

Duncan, C., Gill, V.A., Worman, K. et al. (2015). *Coxiella burnetii* exposure in northern sea otters *Enhydra lutris kenyoni*. *Diseases of Aquatic Organisms* 114: 83–87.

Fehlner-Gardiner, C., Rudd, R., Donovan, D. et al. (2012). Comparing ONRAB® and RABORAL V-RG® oral rabies vaccine field performance in raccoons and striped skunks, New Brunswick, Canada, and Maine, USA. *Journal of Wildlife Diseases* 48 (1): 157–167.

Gode, D. and Ruth, I. (2010). *Wild Mammal Babies: The First 48 Hours and Beyond*, 2e. 357–360 and 369–374. Published by the authors.

Green, A.L., Carpenter, L.R., and Dunn, J.R. (2011). Rabies epidemiology, risk assessment, and pre- and post-exposure vaccination. *Veterinary Clinics of North America: Exotic Animal Practice* 14: 507–518.

Grove, R.A., Bildfell, R., Henny, C.J. et al. (2003). Bilateral uric acid nephrolithiasis and ureteral hypertrophy in a free-ranging river otter (*Lontra canadensis*). *Journal of Wildlife Diseases* 39 (4): 914–917.

Haire, M. (2011a). *Successful Hand-Rearing and Rehabilitation of North American River Otter (Lontra canadensis): When to Rehabilitate, Young Pup Care, Formula Feeding, and Weaning*. OZ Task Force, IUCN/SCC Otter Specialist Group.

Haire, M. (2011b). *Successful Hand-Rearing and Rehabilitation of North American River Otter (Lontra canadensis): Hand-Rearing and Release Techniques to Maximize Change of Success*. OZ Task Force, IUCN/SCC Otter Specialist Group www.otterspecialistgroup.org/osg-newsite/.

Hartup, B.K., Kollias, G.K., Jacobsen, M.C. et al. (1999). Exertional myopathy in translocated river otters from New York. *Journal of Wildlife Diseases* 35 (3): 542–547.

Hernandez-Divers, S.M., Kollias, G.V., Abou-Madi, N. et al. (2001). Surgical technique for intra-abdominal radiotransmitter placement in north American river otters (*Lontra canadensis*). *Journal of Zoo and Wildlife Medicine* 32 (2): 202–205.

Jessup, D.A., Miller, M.A., Kreuder-Johnson, C. et al. (2007). Sea otters in a dirty ocean. *Journal of the American Veterinary Medical Association* 231 (11): 1648–1652.

Karstad, L., Ramsden, R., Berry, T.J. et al. (1975). Hepatitis in skunks caused by the virus of infectious canine hepatitis. *Journal of Wildlife Diseases* 11 (4): 494–496.

Kimber, K.R. and Kollias, G.V. (2000). Infectious and parasitic diseases and contaminant-related problems of north American river otters (*Lontra canadensis*): a review. *Journal of Zoo and Wildlife Medicine* 31 (4): 452–472.

Kimber, K.R., Kollias, G.V., and Dubovi, E.J. (2000). Serologic survey of selected viral agents in recently captured wild north American river otters (*Lontra canadensis*). *Journal of Zoo and Wildlife Medicine* 31 (2): 168–175.

Koepfli, K.P., Deere, K.A., Slater, G.J. et al. (2008). Phylogeny of the Mustelidae: resolving relationships, tempo and biogeographic history of a mammalian adaptive radiation. *BMC Biology* 6 (10).

Kollias, G.V. (1999). Health assessment, medical management, and prerelease conditioning of translocated north American river otters. In: *Zoo and Wild Animal Medicine. Current Therapy*, vol. 4 (ed. E.M. Miller and M. Fowler), 443–448. Philadelphia, PA: W.B. Saunders.

Kollias, G.V. and Abou-Madi, N. (2014). Procyonids and mustelids. In: *Zoo Animal and Wildlife Immobilization and Anesthesia*, 2e (ed. G. West, D. Heard and N. Caulkett), 607–618. Ames, IA: Wiley.

Kollias, G.V. and Fernandez-Moran, J. (2015). Mustelidae. In: *Fowler's Zoo and Wild Animal Medicine*, vol. 8 (ed. R.E. Miller and M.E. Fowler), 476–491. St Louis, MO: Elsevier Saunders.

Kozak, R.A., Ackford, J.G., and Slaine, P. (2015). Characterization of a novel adenovirus isolated from a skunk. *Virology* 485: 16–24.

Krista, D., Hanni, K.D., Jonna, A.K. et al. (2003). Clinical pathology and assessment of pathogen exposure in southern and Alaskan sea otters. *Journal of Wildlife Diseases* 39 (4): 837–850.

Lamberski, N. (2012). Updated vaccination recommendations for carnivores. In: *Zoo and Wild Animal Medicine Current Therapy*, vol. 7 (ed. R.E. Miller and M.E. Fowler), 442–450. St Louis, MO: Elsevier Saunders.

Larkin, J.L., Gabriel, M., Gerhold, R.W. et al. (2011). Prevalence to *Toxoplasma gondii* and *Sarcocystis* spp. in a reintroduced fisher (*Martes pennanti*) population in Pennsylvania. *Journal of Parasitology* 97 (3): 425–429.

Lindenfors, P., Dalèn, L., and Angerbjörn, A. (2003). The monophyletic origin of delayed implantation in carnivores and its implications. *Evolution* 57 (8): 1952–1956.

Lucherini, M. and Merino, M.J. (2008). Perceptions of human-carnivore conflicts in the high Andes of Argentina. *Mountain Research and Development* 28 (1): 81–85.

Malanska, B.H.M., Heuer, K., Reed-Smith, J. et al. (2012). *Summary of Nutrition Guidelines for Otters in Zoos, Aquaria, Rehabilitation, and Wildlife Sanctuaries*. OZ Task Force, IUCN/SCC Otter Specialist Group www.otterspecialistgroup.org/osg-newsite/.

Melquist, W.E., Polechla, P.R. Jr., and Toweill, D. (2003). River otter (*Lontra canadensis*). In: *Wild Mammals of North America: Biology, Management, and Conservation*, 2e (ed. G.A. Feldhamer, B.C. Thompson and J.A. Chapman), 708–734. Baltimore, MD: Johns Hopkins University Press.

Miller, M., Conrad, P., James, E.R. et al. (2008). Transplacental toxoplasmosis in a wild sea otter (*Enhydra lutris nereis*). *Veterinary Parasitology* 153: 12–18.

Morrisey, J.K. (2013). Ferrets. In: *Exotic Animal Formulary*, 4e (ed. J.W. Carpenter), 560–592. St Louis, MO: Elsevier Saunders.

Mortenson, J.A. and Moriarty, K.M. (2015). Ketamine and midazolam anesthesia in Pacific martens (*Martes caurina*). *Journal of Wildlife Diseases* 51 (1): 250–254.

Mustelid. (2015). Encyclopædia Britannica Online. www.britannica.com/animal/mustelid

Niemuth, J.N., Sanders, C.W., Mooney, C.B. et al. (2014). Nephrolithiasis in free-ranging North American river otter (*Lontra canadensis*) in North Carolina, USA. *Journal of Zoo and Wildlife Medicine* 45 (1): 110–117.

Orloski, K.A. and Lathrop, S.L. (2003). Plague: a veterinary perspective. *Journal of the American Veterinary Medical Association* 222 (4): 444–448.

Persson, J., Landa, A., Andersen, R. et al. (2006). Reproductive characteristics of female wolverines (*Gulo gulo*) in Scandinavia. *Journal of Mammalogy* 87 (1): 75–79.

Pommerening, A.V.E., Neubert, L., Kachel, S. et al. (2002). Safety studies of the oral rabies vaccine SAD B19 in striped skunk (*Mephitis mephitis*). *Journal of Wildlife Diseases* 38 (2): 428–431.

Potter, T.M., Hanna, J.A., and Freer, L. (2007). Human north American river otter (*Lontra canadensis*) attack. *Wilderness & Environmental Medicine* 18 (1): 41–44.

Quinn, J.H., Girard, Y.A., Gilardi, K. et al. (2012). Pathogen and rodenticide exposure in American badgers (*Taxidea taxus*) in California. *Journal of Wildlife Diseases* 48 (2): 467–472.

Reed-Smith, J. (ed.) (2012). *The North American River Otter (Lontra canadensis) Husbandry Notebook*. Grand Rapids, MI: John Ball Zoological Garden and Core Gorsuch Foundation/AZA Small Carnivore Taxon Advisory Group.

Reid, F.A. (2006). *Mammals of North America Peterson Field Guides*, 4e. Boston, MA: Houghton Mufflin.

Richardson, J. and Gauthier, J.L. (2003). A serosurvey of leptospirosis in Connecticut peridomestic wildlife. *Vector Borne and Zoonotic Diseases* 3 (4): 187–193.

Rosatte, R. (2011). Evolution of wildlife rabies – control tactics. *Advances in Virus Research* 79: 398–419.

Ruder, M.G., Poppenga, R.H., Bryan, J.A. et al. (2011). Intoxication of nontarget wildlife with rodenticides in northwestern Kansas. *Journal of Wildlife Diseases* 47 (1): 212–216.

Sato, J.J., Hosoda, T., Wolsan, M. et al. (2003). Phylogenic relationships and divergence times among mustelids (Mammalia: Carnivora) based on nucleotide sequences of nuclear interphotoreceptor retinoid binding protein and mitochondrial cytochrome *b* genes. *Zoological Science* 20: 243–264.

Siembieda, J.L., Miller, W.A., Byrne, B.A. et al. (2011). Zoonotic pathogens isolated from wild animals and environmental samples at two California wildlife hospitals. *Journal of the American Veterinary Medical Association* 238 (6): 773–783.

Simeone, C.A., Gulland, F.M.D., Norris, T. et al. (2015). A systematic review of changes in marine mammal health in North America, 1972–2012: the need for a novel integrated approach. *PLoS One* 10 (11).

Steinel, A., Parrish, C.R., Bloom, M.E. et al. (2001). Parvovirus infections in wild carnivores. *Journal of Wildlife Diseases* 37 (3): 594–607.

Stoskopf, M.K., Spelman, L.H., Sumner, P.W. et al. (1997). The impact of water temperature on core body temperature of North American river otters (*Lutra canadensis*) during simulated oil spill recovery washing protocols. *Journal of Zoo and Wildlife Medicine* 28 (4): 407–412.

Stringfield, C. (2008). *Baylisascaris* neuronal larva migrans in zoo animals. In: *Zoo and Wild Animal Medicine Current Therapy*, vol. 6 (ed. M.E. Fowler and R.E. Miller), 284–288. St Louis, MO: Elsevier Saunders.

Thom, M.D., Johnson, D.D.P., and Macdonald, D.W. (2004). The evolution and maintenance of delayed implantation in the Mustelidae (Mammalia: Carnivora). *Evolution* 58 (1): 175–183.

Tseng, M., Fleetwood, M., Reed, A. et al. (2012). Mustelid herpesvirus-2, a novel herpes infection in northern sea otters (*Enhydra lutris kenyoni*). *Journal of Wildlife Diseases* 48 (1): 181–185.

Williams, T.D., and van Blaricom, G.R. (1989). Rates of Capture Myopathy in Translocated Sea Otters, with Implications for Management of Sea Otter Rescue Following Oil Spills. Proceedings of the Eighth Biennial Conference on the Biology of Marine Mammals, Pacific Grove, CA, p. 72.

Wimsatt, J., Biggins, D., Innes, K. et al. (2003). Evaluation of oral and subcutaneous delivery of an experimental canarypox recombinant canine distemper vaccine in the Siberian polecat (*Mustela eversmanii*). *Journal of Zoo and Wildlife Medicine* 34 (1): 25–35.

Wood, W.F., Sollers, B.G., Dragoo, G.A. et al. (2002). Volatile components in defensive spray of the hooded skunk, *Mephitis macroura*. *Journal of Chemical Ecology* 28 (9): 1865–1870.

Worthy, G.A.J. (2001). Nutrition and energetics. In: *CRC Handbook of Marine Mammal Medicine*, 2e (ed. L.A. Dierauf and F.M.D. Gulland), 791–828. Boca Raton, FL: CRC Press.

Yamaguchi, N., Dugale, H., and Macdonald, D.W. (2006). Female receptivity, embryonic diapause, and superfetation in the European badger (meles meles): implications for the reproductive tactics of males and females. *Quaterly Review of Biology* 81 (1): 33–48.

Yamaguchi, N., Sarno, R.J., Johnson, W.E. et al. (2004). Multiple paternity and reproductive tactics of free-ranging American minks, *Mustela vison*. *Journal of Mammalogy* 85 (3): 432–439.

23

Natural History and Medical Management of Opossums

Antonia Gardner

South Florida Wildlife Center (SFWC), Fort Lauderdale, FL, USA

Natural History

Description

The Virginia opossum, *Didelphis virginiana*, is the only marsupial native to North America. It is a member of the order Didelphimorphia of the subclass Marsupialia. Four subspecies of *D. virginiana* are recognized. They are found throughout the eastern United States, in parts of California and the Pacific Northwest, portions of Mexico, and the Yucatan Peninsula. The species is a heavy-bodied animal; females on average weigh 1.9 kg (4.2 lb), males 2.8 kg (6.2 lb), but weight is widely varied and can range from 1.8 to 5.5 kg (4–12 lbs). They have dense white underfur, sometimes with darker tips, and dark guard hairs, giving them an overall mottled gray coloration. Southern populations have less dense underfur and an overall darker appearance. The opossum has a hairless, somewhat scaly tail that is prehensile. Contrary to popular belief, adult opossums do not suspend themselves by their tails, although they do use them for stability while climbing and to gather materials for nest building. Ears, feet, and tail are usually pink with some dark gray pigment. The hind feet have opposable thumbs, which are the only digits without claws (McManus 1974; Krause and Krause 2006).

Reproduction

The hallmark of the marsupial subclass is the presence of a pouch, or marsupium, in which extremely altricial young are raised. The marsupial female reproductive tract has two completely separate uteri and cervices, and two separate lateral vaginas separated by a median septum (Holtz 2003). Male opossums have a forked glans penis and a stalked scrotal sac cranial to the penis. Despite a relatively low sperm count, opossums have extremely efficient sperm due to an adaptation where sperm pairs in the epididymis prior to ejaculation. The paired sperm have higher motility and a large percentage of them reach the oviduct, where they separate and conception takes place. This adaptation is not found in eutherian mammals or Australian marsupials (Krause and Krause 2006). The reproductive tract empties in the common opening for the digestive and urinary tract, or cloaca, a common anatomical feature of all marsupials.

All marsupials are born blind and naked with partially developed hindlimbs; Virginia opossums weigh about 0.16 g (0.005 oz) at birth. Around 13 days after conception, the altricial young make their way into the pouch using their relatively well-developed forelimbs and attach to one of the 13 nipples. Although litters may contain from 18 to 21 young at birth, on average only 7–9 survive (McManus 1974). The babies remain in the pouch attached to the nipple until around 60 days post parturition, when they begin to venture out of the pouch and eat solid food. Weaning occurs around 95 days of age. The month after weaning, juvenile opossums start to venture out from the den and begin foraging. After this they gradually start to disperse from the denning site and slowly expand their home range over the next three months. One study showed that at the time of weaning, female opossums moved to denning sites with denser brush, which would provide more protection for young foraging juveniles (Hossler et al. 1994).

Opossums usually produce two litters a year and females usually breed during the first season following birth (McManus 1974). However, in the northern parts of their range, females may not breed their first year and have only one larger litter a year (Hossler et al. 1994). Mating season begins around January and generally extends through July (McManus 1974). In a very temperate environment such as southern Florida, breeding may occur nearly year round.

Medical Management of Wildlife Species: A Guide for Practitioners, First Edition. Edited by Sonia M. Hernandez, Heather W. Barron, Erica A. Miller, Roberto F. Aguilar and Michael J. Yabsley.
© 2020 John Wiley & Sons, Inc. Published 2020 by John Wiley & Sons, Inc.

Virginia opossums are short-lived. Of those that survive past weaning, fewer than 10% survive their first year. Wild opossums generally live less than two years, although in captivity the life span may be 3–4 years, with the occasional captive opossum living 8–10 years. Anthropogenic causes (e.g., automobiles, hunting, etc.) are the primary reasons for mortality. Also, high numbers of parasites can cause general debilitation and a higher susceptibility to disease and malnutrition. Juvenile opossums are specifically prone to predation by owls and canids. Opossums in their second year may show typical aging changes, such as cataracts, muscle wasting, generalized weakness, and dental disease (Hossler et al. 1994; Krause and Krause 2006; McRuer and Jones 2009).

Diet

During lactation, the composition of opossum milk changes to adjust to the needs of the growing joeys. Milk solids steadily increase throughout lactation, until their peak of 34% at 11 weeks. Milk solids then decrease to 27% until the end of lactation at 15 weeks. Protein concentration shows a similar increase to a peak of 10% at 11 weeks. Carbohydrates, mainly hexose, increase to a maximum of 7% at seven weeks, and lipids increase rapidly from week 9 to 11 from 8% to 17%. This peak of lipid concentration is stable for two weeks, until it declines to 11% at 13 weeks. For most of the time, lipids provide the major component of milk solids. Electrolyte and mineral concentrations also fluctuate, as the growing joeys' needs change (Green et al. 1996; McRuer and Jones 2009).

There are several formula recipes for this species as well as commercial marsupial formulas available for various stages. The rehabilitator may choose to mimic the changes in opossum milk or use a single formula throughout. Additional information on raising orphan opossums is given in Chapter 12.

Because they are so underdeveloped at birth, very young opossums cannot be successfully hand-reared. In the author's experience babies under the weight of 25 g have a very poor prognosis, and those between 25 and 40 g have a guarded prognosis and a lower chance of release. Babies must be warm and hydrated prior to feeding. Warmed lactated Ringer's solution or Pedialyte® work as a hydrating solution. They can also be used to dilute the chosen formula when first introducing to new orphans. Babies under 35 g (1.2 oz) do not have a suckle reflex and usually must be gavage fed every 3–4 hours 24 hours a day with a 5 Fr red rubber tube, as they receive constant nutrition in the pouch. As they age, syringe feeding may also be employed, although this method is much more time-consuming with large litters (Taylor 2002).

As opossums age, a variety of foods may be introduced into their diets. In the wild, Virginia opossums are omnivorous and very opportunistic, eating insects, small vertebrates, fruits, nuts, and vegetation. Although they begin to wean around 12 weeks postpartum, at a size of around 165 g (5.8 oz), some wildlife centers have success introducing food to young opossums at a much younger age, at around 50 g (1.8 oz) size. Young opossums may start to lap at a tray of formula at this age, and nibble or suck at small pieces of fruit. As they grow, other foods are introduced gradually, such as small chunks of soft cooked vegetables (sweet potatoes, broccoli, cauliflower, squash), and softened high-quality dog or cat food. Once opossums reach juvenile status, around 200 g (7 oz), they may be switched to an adult opossum diet.

A suitable adult opossum diet consists of high-quality dry and canned dog or cat food, egg (with shell), mealworms or crickets, and mouse pieces. Although weanling opossums under 200 g should be offered food twice daily, adult opossums usually will not eat during the day and should be offered food in the evening. Adult opossums are prone to obesity and have a metabolism about 30% that of comparably sized placental mammals. If an opossum is in rehabilitation for an extended amount of time, the amount of food offered should be limited and the amount of dog or cat food in the diet reduced to avoid obesity (McRuer and Jones 2009). At the author's center, daily, we offer ¾ cup moistened dog food, ¾ cup bite-sized vegetables, ½ cup bite-sized fruits, and one source of animal protein (e.g., canned salmon, eggs, cooked chicken livers, cottage cheese, etc.). Twice a week we offer a prey item, such as a mouse or chick. Examples of diets for various life stages are shown in Table 23.2.

Opossums are nocturnal, so they are very efficient at producing vitamin D3 in the skin without sunlight and require little UV light or vitamin D supplementation. However, they are susceptible to nutritional secondary hyperparathyroidism if fed a diet with an inappropriate Ca:P ratio such as excessive fruits and vegetables, too much protein, or an incorrect infant formula (McRuer and Jones 2009).

In a larger rehabilitation facility raising a large number of orphans, a phase system may be used to standardize the care for growing infants (see Chapter 12 for the author's protocol).

Housing and Husbandry

Baby and juvenile opossums show some activity during daylight hours, but older juvenile and adult opossums are extremely somnolent, at times even difficult to rouse during the day. This species should be housed in an area where there is less noise and daytime traffic. While recuperating indoors, sick or injured juveniles or adults do well in dog kennels, stainless steel cages, or carriers lined with sheets or fleece blankets. The latter is preferable in extremely debilitated animals or those who have neurological signs, as they tend to abrade their paws.

Housing baby opossums must take into consideration the unique environment the mother's pouch would normally provide. Opossums less than 55 days old have no ability to thermoregulate. They also tend to dehydrate easily, as the pouch is very moist. Thus opossums under 40 g (1.4 oz) do best in a very warm, moist container. At the South Florida Wildlife Center, a plastic container lined with towels on a heating pad is used for smaller babies. Moist, warmed cloths are placed within to maintain a higher relative humidity. Although these containers work well to keep small orphans warm and moist, bacterial and mold contamination is a constant concern and the container must be cleaned and disinfected 2–3 times daily. Aquariums also work well for a humidified enclosure. Damp towels placed under the bedding and over the top of the aquarium keep the enclosure moist (Taylor 2002). Soft pouches or nests, similar to those for ferrets or sugar gliders, should be provided. Towels and washcloths are not good bedding as small babies tend to catch their claws in the loops. Family groups should be kept together, and babies from different groups can be combined if they are the same size.

Young opossums need to be stimulated to urinate and defecate. A damp cotton ball or tissue may be used to gently rub the cloaca from front to back until the bladder is empty and the baby is no longer defecating. As they grow older, signs that stimulation is no longer necessary include urine and feces in the enclosure and the baby being restless during the stimulation process (Taylor 2002).

Once babies become a little larger, over 40 g (1.4 oz), they can be moved to a bigger but still very warm container. A pediatric incubator or a larger plastic container on top of a heating pad with good ventilation is perfect for this. The South Florida Wildlife Center uses stackable drawers in a walk-in incubator (Figure 23.1). At this point, they will start to move around more and may even begin to lap. If they are offered trays of formula, they get very messy and must be cleaned several times daily.

Once they have begun to regulate their own body temperature, around 80–100 g (2.8–3.5 oz), they may be moved to indoor caging. Large rodent cages or other wire cages can be used for this; cages with levels such as a ferret cage can provide opportunities for early climbing (Johnson-Delaney 2014). It is important to ensure that the cage bars are narrow enough that the babies cannot escape or get stuck. They take well to wire wheels for exercise (Figure 23.2). Plastic igloos, extra bedding, or boxes should be provided for hiding during the day. A heat lamp may be added. A UV light may be beneficial but is not necessary.

At around 150 g (5.3 oz), depending on the outdoor climate, the babies may be ready to move to an outdoor habitat. At this point, they should have some opportunities to climb and forage. Ramps or cleaned branches with

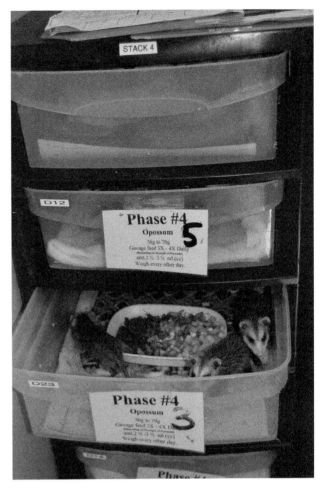

Figure 23.1 Baby opossums in drawers in a walk-in incubator (South Florida Wildlife Center). These babies are under 70 g, somewhat ambulatory, lapping formula, and eating a small diet.

no sharp points can be provided for climbing. Food can be scattered or hidden in boxes to provide opportunities to forage. Trays of cultivated wheat grass or piles of branches or leaf litter can also be provided to simulate a more natural environment and provide enrichment. These older babies can be placed in habitats suitable for adults in groups of no more than six. At this point, smaller groups or single animals may still be combined successfully into larger groups, although at times even these smaller juveniles fight and mutilate each other's tails to the point of requiring amputation. It is important that these outdoor enclosures are monitored closely, and that they are rodent- and predator-proof, as young opossums are very susceptible to predation and can have tails and limbs bitten through larger mesh wire.

Outdoor habitats for juvenile opossums and adults should be secure and provide plenty of room for moving around and climbing. Areas for hiding should be provided. The top half of an old carrier will suffice, as will purpose-made boxes filled with straw or old cardboard

(a)

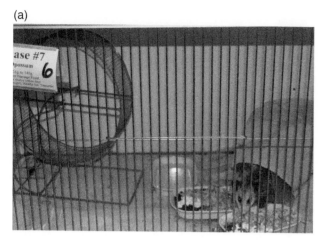

(b)

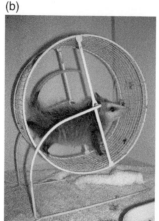

Figure 23.2 (a,b) Baby opossums in a cage bank (South Florida Wildlife Center). They are being prepared for an outdoor cage. They are eating on their own and exercising on a wire wheel. The wheel is a safe way for them to exercise in a smaller space. *Source:* (b) Courtesy of Jessica Sayre.

boxes (Figure 23.3). At the South Florida Wildlife Center, wire runs (5′W × 10′L × 8′H) lined on the outside with rodent-proof mesh have been constructed as outdoor opossum habitats. The floors are poured concrete for easy cleaning and disinfection.

Housing for adult opossums in rehabilitation can also be retrofitted to evaluate fitness for release (Figure 23.4). Often, it is difficult to fully assess an adult's ability to function without putting it in an outdoor habitat. It is advantageous to have a camera with night vision installed in these habitats, since opossums are more active at night. Food should be hidden and plenty of obstacles, hiding areas, and climbing substrates provided. With nighttime video from these convalescent enclosures, it is often easier to evaluate neurological status, vision, and overall fitness in recovering adults, as well as orphans' readiness for release.

Mature opossums have been described as solitary creatures, except during mating, although there are studies that suggest opossums may form nonsexual relationships at times (Kimble 1997). However, adult and unrelated juvenile opossums over 150–200 g (5.3–7 oz) at presentation should be housed alone or in small groups in very large habitats with a lot of hide spaces.

Through every stage of opossum rehabilitation, housing must be easy to clean and disinfect. Opossums are messy, with smelly feces, and can have high parasite loads, so habitats should be thoroughly disinfected between individuals or groups of animals. They tend to defecate outside their nests or dens, so hide areas do not

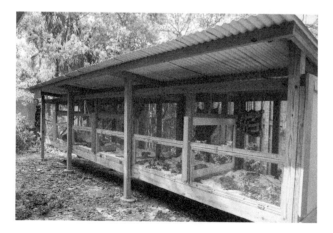

Figure 23.3 Juvenile opossums in outdoor enclosures with environmental enrichment items and hammocks. *Source:* Courtesy of Heather Barron.

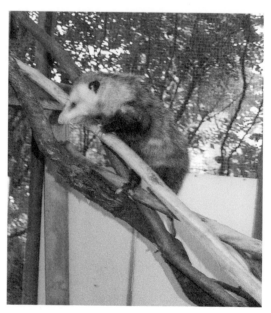

Figure 23.4 An adult opossum that was treated for a fractured scapula exhibiting normal climbing skills after being placed in an outdoor habitat.

have to be cleaned as often. The minimum size requirements for housing Virginia opossum at all life stages are given in Table 23.1.

Release

Generally, opossums are ready for release around 400–500 g (14.1–17.6 oz) but some wait until 700 g (24.7 oz) (McRuer and Jones 2009; Taylor 2002). Opossums in warmer climates are generally smaller, so are more mature at a smaller size. Insect prey and food items are also more readily available year-round. Regardless of size, readiness for release should be evaluated by the opossum's ability to forage sufficiently and exhibition of normal behavior (nocturnal activity, fear, and aggression toward humans).

Virginia opossums are nocturnal, opportunistic, and omnivorous. This, along with their high reproductive rate, contributes to their success in establishing populations in both rural and urban environments (Kanda et al. 2006). Opossums utilize various dens during the day, then at night move around for foraging and mating. During extreme weather, they may stay denned but do not hibernate. Studies on home range find that male opossums utilize a home range roughly twice as large as that of females. Home ranges in urban environments are about half those of opossums in rural environments, due to the ready availability of food sources and suitable habitat for denning (Meier 1983).

Although it is always desirable to release an opossum at or near where it was found, it is acceptable to release opossums anywhere safe with suitable denning. Dens may just be an area of tangled underbrush or a hidden hollow. If extra protection is desired, one may also put an old carrier without a door in the release area. When possible, release sites should be away from busy roads or areas with high human traffic. Juvenile release sites should have dense underbrush and plentiful areas for foraging.

Medical Management

Handling and Restraint

Baby opossums may be held in the palm of the hand until they become more active. As they start to move more, gentle restraint at the base of the tail may help, along with gently holding the head. Another method of restraining young opossums is to wrap a towel around the neck and suspend the body gently, which is calming (McRuer and Jones 2009). Very young opossums become hypothermic very easily, so it is advisable to perform physical exams and treatment in steps, keeping them in a heated container in between.

Older juvenile and adult opossums may act slow, but can deliver a painful bite that can puncture the skin. Heavy gloves are often necessary to prevent injury. Often, one can hold a larger opossum by the base of the tail, then slowly move the hand under the opossum's chest to support the body. Because of their short necks, opossums cannot reach the hand under the chest and usually do not seem to be alarmed by this method of restraint. Alternatively, for a close exam or treatments, the opossum should be held by the base of the tail then at the upper neck or base of the jaw to control the head.

An interesting behavioral adaptation in the Virginia opossum is feigning death, or "playing possum." In this behavior, the opossum lies on its side with its tail curved ventrally, mouth and eyes open, and salivates, urinates, or defecates. This freezing behavior does not normally occur with human handling, rather during very severe threats such as those from a larger predator (e.g., dogs). Although the opossum appears catatonic during this behavior and heart and respiratory rates may drop, electroencephalogram (EEG) studies show that the animal is fully conscious (Kimble 1997).

Venipuncture

In adult animals, the skin is thick and many of the accessory vessels are easily collapsible. The jugular vein is usually visible at any age, and in young animals it is the most reliable site for obtaining any significant amount of blood. This site requires sedation in all but young and extremely moribund animals. Opossums have short necks and the vessel is positioned relatively laterally.

Table 23.1 Housing size recommendations.

Life stage	Minimum housing size
Infant (litter)	10 gal 38 L
Nursing (litter)	3 ft × 3 ft × 3 ft 0.9 m × 0.9 m × 0.9 m
Juvenile outside (litter)[a]	10 ft W × 12 ft L × 8 ft H 3.0 m × 3.7 m × 2.4 m
Restricted/ injured adult	2 ft × 2 ft × 2 ft 0.6 m × 0.6 m × 0.6 m
Adult outside	10 ft W × 12 ft L × 8 ft H 3.0 m × 3.7 m × 2.4 m

Source: Miller (2012).

[a] In most instances number housed outdoors together should not exceed six.

The cephalic and medial saphenous veins are accessible, but the veins are small and easily collapsible in most animals. The skin is thick in adults and must usually be shaved in order to visualize the vessel. In females, the vessels feeding the pouch are often quite large and may be used for euthanasia in a sedated animal, but the walls are collapsible and it is usually not possible to obtain a substantial amount of blood from these vessels.

There are two sites in the tail. One is the lateral tail vein, which looks quite large and robust but often collapses. It is usually best visualized by shaving the hair that extends over the proximal tail, then placing pressure at the sides of the tail base. The other site is on the ventral tail, where the coccygeal vein is located. It can be accessed blindly by inserting a needle at midline perpendicular to the tail, in the fleshy depression palpated between caudal vertebrae 5 and 6, until bone is contacted, then aspirating while withdrawing the needle (Williams-Newkirk et al. 2013). A good amount of blood can be collected from adults using this vein, and it is also a good site for injecting euthanasia drugs. In deeply sedated and anesthetized animals, cardiac puncture may also be used to administer euthanasia drugs, but is not recommended for blood collection.

Catheter Placement

Intravenous catheter placement is difficult in opossums. The cephalic and medial saphenous veins are both sites where placement can be attempted. The cephalic vessel is rather tortuous and both can be difficult to visualize due to thick skin. Even in large opossums it is sometimes necessary to use 24-gauge catheters. In these cases, the author pierces the skin first with a 22-gauge needle to prevent burring of the small-gauge catheter. IV catheter placement in the lateral tail vein has been described (McRuer and Jones 2009) but in the author's experience, this can lead to superficial necrosis of the skin at the site. Another potential catheter site in very moribund patients is the jugular vein. Interosseous catheters may also be placed in the tibia or the femur (Johnson-Delaney 2014).

Sedation, Anesthesia, and Analgesia

Sedation or anesthesia may be necessary for thorough exam and diagnostic testing on older juvenile and adult opossums. Tiletamine-zolazepam (Telazol®, Zoetis, Parsippany, NJ, USA) is the medication most often described for sedation in marsupials. It is fairly safe and easily dosed and injected. A dose of 3–5 mg/kg intramuscularly usually provides adequate sedation for many procedures or premedication for general anesthesia (Gamble 2004). The author has also used tiletamine-zolazepam/ketamine/xylazine (TKX) using the intramuscular route at doses listed for felines.

For more debilitated animals, a combination of midazolam at 0.5–1.0 mg/kg and butorphanol at 0.3–0.5 mg/kg is preferred. The combination can be given intramuscularly and is especially useful in cases of head trauma, as this combination does not increase intracranial pressure at higher doses; or when the patient is especially unstable. The sedation is lighter with this combination and isoflurane via mask is often also needed for good radiographic positioning. Dexmedetomidine in combination with other drugs, such as ketamine, at cat doses may also be used for many cases, and has the advantage of being reversible.

The most common nonsteroidal antiinflammatory drug (NSAID) used in opossums is meloxicam. Although safe dosages have not been evaluated, 0.2 mg/kg is recommended (Johnson-Delaney 2000). This author recommends a loading dose of 0.2 mg/kg, followed by maintenance doses of 0.1 mg/kg every 24 hours. Patients should be well hydrated for use of this medication. Buprenorphine or tramadol are the opiates of choice for opossums at dosages recommended for domestic cats.

Anesthesia

Isoflurane anesthesia is commonly used for opossums and is relatively safe. Young animals can easily be restrained and anesthetized via mask, but most adult animals are strong enough to require presedation. Masked induction is contraindicated in cases of head trauma because of the potential for increased intracranial pressure, and because of severe cranial and jaw fracture concerns. Intubation is easy, although a laryngoscope is helpful because the opossum's low glossopharyngeal arch tends to partially obscure the pharyngeal opening. Although not commonly utilized, propofol is safe to use for anesthetic induction if IV or IO access is available at published canine and feline doses. Recently, the author has used Alfaxalone (Alfaxan™ Multi-dose, Jurox Inc., North Kansas City, MO, USA) at doses ranging from 5–10 mg/kg intravenously or intramuscularly for anesthetic induction. If given intravenously the lower doses are extremely quick-acting and effective and appear to be very safe.

Other Medications

Antibiotics that are commonly prescribed for domestic small mammals are appropriate for Virginia opossums. Although marsupials generally are considered to have a lower metabolism than eutherian mammals, the few pharmacological studies that have been done support the dosage of common pharmaceuticals in ranges prescribed for commonly treated domestic mammals (Johnson-Delaney 2000).

Clinically Relevant Anatomy and Physiology

The Pouch

The marsupial pouch is the most unique feature of the Virginia opossum, but certainly not the only unusual thing about their anatomy and physiology. There are several unique features the clinician should be aware of when evaluating this species. The pouch should always be evaluated during the physical exam, as well as periodically during care. It is quite common for a female to present without babies, and then give birth several days later. Without close examination, and pulling the pouch open, it is very easy to miss tiny bumble bee-sized newborns.

It is normal for the opossum pouch to be yellowish, sticky, and moist. These secretions serve to keep the delicate newborns moist and protected.

Opossums are born immunologically naive, as no prenatal transfer of antibodies has been found in the species. Antibodies are secreted in maternal milk for most of their lactation, as are antimicrobial peptides (AMPs), molecules that provide defense against a broad spectrum of bacteria and fungi; in some marsupials the pouch epithelium also secretes AMPs (Peel et al. 2013).

The pouch is quite expandable; in nonreproductive females it can appear quite shallow and insubstantial, although it has the ability to stretch to accommodate 8–10 large babies. The pouch has developed as an invagination of the skin through the panniculus muscle and the animal has voluntary control of the opening (Krause and Krause 2006). In a mother with pouch young, this muscle can close the pouch quite tightly. The epipubic bones are a cranial extension of the pelvis in marsupials and are present in males as well as females. They are commonly fractured in trauma cases but this does not seem to affect pouch function.

Urogenital Anatomy

All marsupials have a cloaca that serves as a common exit for the urogenital and digestive tracts. Opossums have a cloacal gland that secretes a strong-smelling greenish fluid, especially during handling (Johnson-Delaney 2014). The opening to the male urinary tract is at the base of the bifid penis. Male opossums are very difficult if not impossible to catheterize. During gross necropsy, this author has found that the bladder is pulled to one side by the round ligament of the bladder, causing an acute flexure just proximal to the bladder, as the urethra passes through the prostate (Figure 23.5). During dissection, if the ligament is broken down, the catheter can be passed but *in vivo* passage of a catheter into the bladder is very unlikely to be successful.

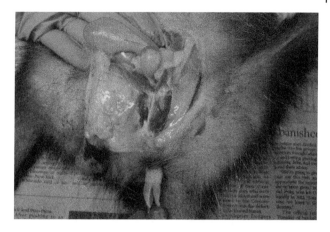

Figure 23.5 A dissection of the male opossum urogenital organs showing acute flexure of the urethra just proximal to the bladder, which makes urinary catheterization extremely difficult. *Source:* Courtesy of Christopher Drolet.

Special Senses

As they are nocturnal, and often do not have a predictable menace response, opossums are thought to have poor vision. However, they do have fairly accurate near visual acuity, and are able to distinguish small insects quite accurately during foraging. *Didelphis* species are also able to maneuver along tree branches quite adeptly. They are myopic and see mostly in black and white, although they do appear to have some limited color vision. Some sources incorrectly state that Virginia opossums have dilated pupils; in the author's experience the normal opossum has extremely miotic pupils under daylight conditions, so much so that the pupils are often hard to distinguish from the dark brown iris. The lid aperture is somewhat small and the species is prone to microphthalmia; it is not uncommon to see cases in which one globe is completely underdeveloped and not functional. Blind opossums can often navigate relatively well using their sensitive and extensive vibrissae, which can complicate evaluation of vision. Their hearing appears to be quite acute. It is usually considered acceptable to release an opossum with only unilateral vision, as long as they act normally otherwise and can forage and climb (McManus 1974; Volchan et al. 2004; Krause and Krause 2006).

Resistance to Venom

One fascinating adaptation of the Virginia opossum is its resistance to crotalid snake venom. There is very little measurable physiological response to either a direct bite or injection of venom, and a bite causes no tissue damage aside from the trauma caused by the fangs (Kilmon 1976). This resistance is not present for bites from elapid snakes, sea snakes, or puff adders, although opossums do show resistance to venom from the Malayan pit viper. The agent of resistance is a metalloproteinase inhibitor that neutralizes the hemorrhagic and proteolytic effects of the venom shortly after absorption into the opossum's serum. These proteins are being investigated for possible use in human envenomation cases (Werner and Vick 1977; Pornmanee et al. 2008).

Parasitic and Infectious Diseases of Interest

Parasites

In healthy adult opossums, many parasite burdens are generally low and clinically irrelevant. However, even normal parasite loads can become clinically relevant during times of injury or illness, or in young orphans.

Gastrointestinal Parasites

Only a few gastrointestinal parasites are considered clinically relevant. *Turgida* (=*Physaloptera*) *turgida* is a common stomach nematode that is off-white in color, robust, and coiled. This parasite can cause ulcerative stomach lesions along the greater curvature of the fundus, which may lead to secondary bacterial infection. Clinical signs include melena, weight loss, anorexia, anemia, general debilitation, and death (Alden 1995; Jones 2013). *Gnathostoma turgidum*, another gastric nematode, is found deeply embedded in the stomach mucosa, causing ulceration and occasionally perforation; the immature form is found in the liver and causes cirrhotic lesions (Potkay 1970).

Although rarely noted in the literature, at the South Florida Wildlife Center the author commonly sees young or debilitated opossums with coccidian infections, possibly *Eimeria indianensis*. Clinical signs include diarrhea, inappetance, and lethargy, which vastly improve with treatment. *Sarcocystis neurona* infects the intestine of opossums but does not cause disease, although it may cause debilitating disease in intermediate host species. *Sarcocystis* sporocysts are commonly detected in opossum feces during routine fecal flotation (Dubey et al. 2001).

The suggested treatment for the most common nematode parasites is Fenbendazole at 50 mg/kg for up the 14 days. One author suggests concomitant treatment with Ivermectin at 0.1–0.2 mg/kg, as it seems to have a synergistic effect on Fenbendazole (Jones 2013). Gastrointestinal coccidia can be treated with a course of sulfadimethoxine (Albon) at published cat doses, or in the case of young or debilitated opossums, or cases that do not respond to Albon, Ponazuril at 25 mg/kg for 3–5 days. Supportive care is very important for debilitated animals, and they often respond well to subcutaneous fluids and small animal recovery diets added to their regular diets. Liquitinic or another similar vitamin and mineral supplement should be administered for anemia.

Pulmonary Parasites

Didelphostrongylus hayesi and *Capillaria didelphis* are the most commonly detected lung parasites (Alden 1995). *Capillaria* causes an extensive inflammatory reaction in the pulmonary parenchyma, with granulomatous and necrotic foci and dilated bronchioles with nematode eggs filling the lumen (Snyder et al. 1991). Similar lesions are observed with *D. hayesi* except for larvae being present instead of eggs (Lamberski et al. 2002; Jones 2013). Opossums with lungworm infections may be clinically normal, or they may have chronic weight loss, hair loss, dyspnea, aerophagia, and other clinical signs. Radiographic lesions include increased interstitial and peribronchial patterns of varying severity (Lamberski et al. 2002).

One suggested treatment for *D. hayesi* is fenbendazole at 50 mg/kg daily for 3–14 days; adjunctive treatment with dexamethasone at 0.25 mg/kg q12h can be used to decrease the inflammatory reaction caused by dying worms and larvae (Lamberski et al. 2002). The suggested treatment for the most common nematode parasites is Fenbendazole at 50 mg/kg for up the 14 days. One author suggests concomitant treatment with Ivermectin at 0.1–0.2 mg/kg, as it seems to have a synergistic effect on Fenbendazole (Jones 2013). These options are also suggested for *Capillaria* infections. Antibiotics should be considered for secondary bacterial infections and this author generally uses amoxicillin-clavulanic acid (Clavamox®, Zoetis) or trimethoprim-sulfa (TMS) at small animal doses. As always, supportive care is important; extremely dyspneic animals may require oxygen supplementation.

Systemic Parasites

Besnoitia darlingi, a protozoan parasite, uses domestic cats as definitive hosts and opossums as intermediate hosts. Severely infected opossums will have multiple round, firm, white cysts in the ear pinnae, lips, tongue, retinal and iridal tissue, and throughout the myocardium, liver, kidneys and other organs (Figure 23.6) (Dubey et al. 2002; Elsheikha et al. 2004; Ellis et al. 2012). The author has seen radiographically evident bony lesions caused by *Besnoitia* cysts in the periosteum. Although initially considered to be nonpathogenic, morbidity and mortality have been reported. Numerous cysts in vital organs or the eye can predispose animals to predation or hinder foraging. Young age, immunosuppression, and stress may contribute to an individual's predilection for a pathogenic infection of *Besnoitia*,

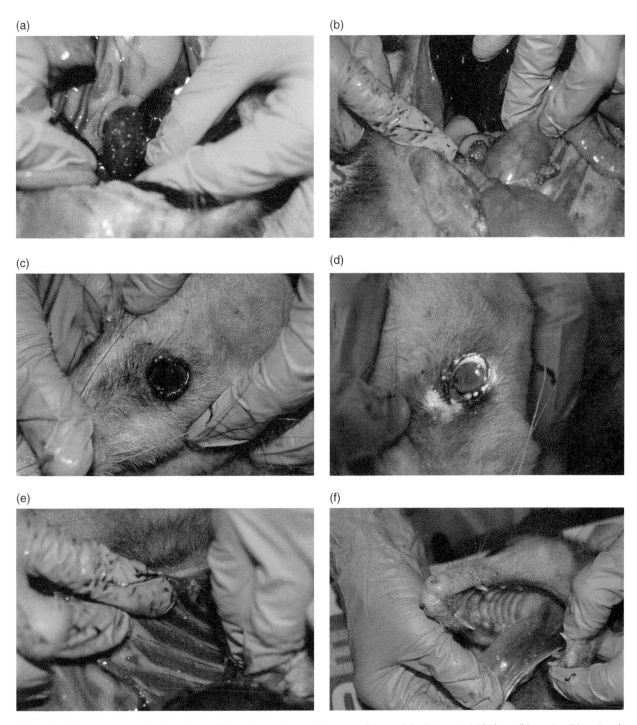

Figure 23.6 An opossum with disseminated besnoitiosis shows glistening white nodular lesions in (a) kidney; (b) ovaries; (c) periocular tissues; (d) anterior chamber; (e) thoracic wall; (f) tongue and lip.

although these mechanisms are not completely understood (Ellis et al. 2012). Treatment is generally not recommended because efficacy appears to be poor and may lead to additional damage associated with inflammation around dead parasites (Ellis et al. 2012 and this author's experience).

Zoonotic Diseases

Rabies

Opossums are generally considered to be low risk for rabies virus infection but they are not immune. The few reported cases tend to present with paralysis and anorexia ("dumb rabies"), making them very unlikely to attack and bite. However, a bite from a wild opossum should be taken seriously and at minimum the animal should be observed closely for neurological signs (Barr 1963; Potkay 1970).

Other Zoonotic Pathogens

Other zoonoses reported in Virginia opossum include the agents for salmonellosis, leptospirosis, Chagas disease, tularemia, relapsing fever, ringworm, toxoplasmosis, and histoplasmosis. Further details can be found in Chapter 2; however, opossums have tested positive for a variety of pathogenic leptospira serovars, and in South America are considered one of the most potent wildlife vectors of the disease because of their close proximity to human establishments. Opossums are an important wildlife reservoir for *Trypanosoma cruzi* in Latin America. Chagas disease is thought to be underdiagnosed; in the USA, and people can have asymptomatic infection and may not seek medical attention for mild, acute cases. Recent prevalence studies in the USA have indicated that the Virginia opossum is one of the most important wildlife reservoirs. Infected animals can suffer subacute myocarditis, and inflammatory lesions in other tissues have also been found. Evidence of *T. cruzi* infection in opossums has been found in all the southern states and as far north as Maryland (Roellig et al. 2008; Houk et al. 2010).

Common Reasons for Presentation

Vehicular Trauma

The most common cause for adult Virginia opossums to present for care is vehicular trauma, especially in areas where there is a dense human population. Unfortunately, the results are often severe with a poor prognosis as there is almost always severe head trauma. Commonly, the animals have multiple fractures of the skull bones, including the mandible, maxilla, zygomatic arches, occipital, nasal, and palatal bones. Fractures of the mandible and palate are often open. These patients present moribund and extremely obtunded. They are often extremely dyspneic from nasal bone fractures and bleeding from the nares, ears, and/or mouth. Proptosis of one or both eyes is common. Limb, rib, and/or pelvic fractures are also relatively common.

The neurological status of these patients should be evaluated prior to sedation. The evaluator should allow the patient to stand and walk if able, and assess whether ataxia or vestibular signs are present. The pupils should also be evaluated before sedation. As opossum pupils are normally extremely miotic, severely dilated pupils are a poor prognosis for vision. The jaw and skull should be thoroughly palpated and the oral cavity examined. The limbs should be palpated for dislocations or fractures and any abrasions or wounds noted. The pouch of female opossums should always be checked for young; whether the mother is going to be treated or euthanized, the presence of young is an important consideration. If the mother is euthanized, the young will need to be evaluated separately. If the mother is treated, medications should be chosen that would not adversely affect any pouch young through passage in the milk.

Patients with open skull fractures, bilateral blindness, jaw fractures that are segmental or affect the temporomandibular joint, severe mental depression or coma, cerebral spinal fluid from the ears, or limb fractures in addition to head trauma should be euthanized. In theory, blindness due to trauma where a retinal detachment is not evident could resolve with antiinflammatory medication, although in practice these cases rarely resolve.

Sedation is usually necessary for complete evaluation and to prevent spikes in intracranial pressure due to the stress of handling. A combination of butorphanol and midazolam is recommended in cases of severe head trauma; in other cases Telazol alone or in combination may be sufficient. Isoflurane should be avoided or used sparingly in cases of head trauma. Administering supplemental oxygen is helpful as long as it is not too stressful.

In any trauma cases, complete radiographs should be taken initially if sedation is adequate or once the patient is stable. It is easy to miss orthopedic injury on initial exam because these animals are usually not ambulatory. Wounds should be cleaned and cared for immediately. Broken teeth should be noted, as they may need to be extracted at a later time.

Patients with closed jaw fractures that do not interfere with jaw alignment may be managed with long-term pain management and a slurry diet. Although uncomplicated jaw fractures may be surgically repaired, in the author's experience those that are easily accessible for surgery are either open or associated with multiple fractures, worsening the overall prognosis.

The most important factor in the successful treatment of head trauma is nursing care. Pain medication and wound care are also important, but brain swelling is most likely to resolve on its own if the animal is kept quiet and comfortable. If the mental status of a patient is deteriorating and intravenous or intraosseous access is an option, mannitol, hetastarch, or hypertonic saline may be used in an attempt to reduce brain swelling. Doses suggested for small animals are appropriate. Supportive care such as intravenous, intraosseous, or subcutaneous fluid administration and hand feeding should be administered as needed for inappetent animals. Antibiotics are usually indicated with severe nasal bone trauma or intraoral trauma. Any animal that is treated long term with severe head trauma should be closely evaluated in an outdoor habitat for residual neurological damage prior to release.

Limb fractures unaccompanied by severe head trauma are uncommon; if present, these may be treated by pinning or plating. Casting or splinting alone is rarely successful in this species because their legs are so short and thick. Uncomplicated pelvic and scapula injuries can resolve with cage rest alone.

Interspecies Attacks

It is not uncommon to see opossums present with injuries from domestic animals. Dogs are usually the culprits in attacks on adults, while cats are often responsible for attacks on infants and juveniles. Dog bites can be quite extensive but with proper care and antibiotics, most otherwise healthy adults recover well. Bite wound treatment is similar to that in other mammals. Affected areas should be shaved under sedation and punctures thoroughly flushed. Large pockets in affected areas are common, and in these cases Penrose drains should be placed. Sizeable lacerations should be sutured. A good first-line antibiotic for bite wound is amoxicillin-clavulanic acid. Meloxicam and tramadol are good pain management options. Open wounds should be flushed daily and treated with an antimicrobial gel or cream such as silver sulfadiazine.

When stable, patients with extensive wounds should have full-body radiographs. Pelvic, scapular, and rib fractures are commonly seen in dog attacks. Even with multiple fractures, these animals usually do well with cage rest. In fact, these types of healed fractures are found often in road-killed opossums, indicating that many opossums survive severe predator attacks without any human intervention (Mead and Patterson 2009).

Opossum skin is somewhat thick with a subcutaneous fatty layer. Small defects may simply be closed with skin sutures, while larger lacerations may require a subcutaneous layer. It is extremely rare for an opossum to traumatize sutures or drains, so there is no need to attempt to place an Elizabethan collar to protect the wounds.

There is a common misconception that opossums are more prone to infection from wounds than other species. However, with the appropriate topical therapy and antibiotics, severe wounds can heal quite well and with little scarring (Figure 23.7).

Nonhealing puncture wounds with persistent purulent discharge should be cultured for a second-line antibiotic choice. The author has cultured a variety of pathogens as well as atypical *Mycobacterium* from nonhealing bite wounds. This pathogen can have a very guarded prognosis in domestic mammals but the affected opossums responded to long-term treatment with the appropriate antibiotic (Gunn-Moore 2014; Lloret et al. 2013).

Chronic Debilitation

Virginia opossums sometimes present with nonspecific signs in a debilitated condition (i.e., emaciated, weak, dehydrated, exhibiting neurological signs, chronic wounds, etc.). As with many wild animals, sick or injured opossums tend to evade capture until they are too weak to do so. It can be difficult to diagnose the primary cause. As they have short lifespans, it is common for them to present with geriatric conditions such as cataracts, severe tartar and gingivitis, and multiple old scars to the body may be indications of advanced age. An opossums's age should be a major consideration when deciding whether

(a)

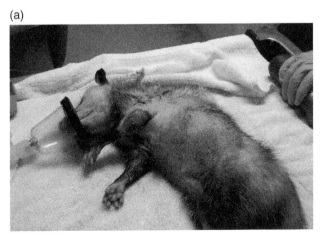

(b)

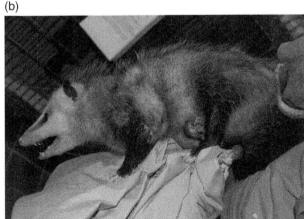

Figure 23.7 (a,b) Before and after pictures of a large wound on an opossum's elbow; treated with bandaging and antibiotics, the wound healed with minimal scarring and normal range of motion in one month. Note the pouch young present in the after picture. They were born while in treatment.

or not to rehabilitate a wild patient. Parasites are common and may or may not be the primary problem.

Both hypertrophic and dilated cardiomyopathy have been reported for aging captive opossums. Cardiomyopathy was also detected histologically in a rehabilitated opossum that died due to lungworm infection. Cardiac disease found in captive opossums may be related to obesity or nutrition, but cardiomyopathy should not be overlooked as a differential for chronic disease (Lamberski et al. 2002; Heatley 2009; Johnson-Delaney 2014).

Neurological Disease

Debilitated opossums may present with neurological signs without apparent cause, especially in older animals. Diagnosis and treatment of these cases can be challenging, as poor condition from inability to feed is usually present, confounding diagnosis of the underlying illness. A thorough physical exam, including a good neurological exam and vision assessment, is very important. Bloodwork and radiographs are often unrewarding. Differential diagnoses include trauma, migrating parasitic larvae, infectious meningitis/encephalitis, and neoplasia. Treatment often consists of "shotgun" therapy of antiinflammatories, antibiotics, and antiparasitic drugs. The author usually initially uses meloxicam and TMS (as it penetrates the meninges and has some antiparasitic activity), and may add an antiparasitic drug such as ponazuril or fenbendazole.

Mastitis

Moribund female opossums with infections of the mammary glands are encountered periodically. There are usually no babies in the pouch or dying newborn joeys. At times, it appears that the mastitis is secondary to another condition, but often the jill's condition greatly improves once her mastitis is successfully treated. Hot-packing the mammary glands and expressing some of the milk will give temporary relief. Culturing milk from the affected nipples can help with antibiotic selection. Pain medications and supportive care are also important.

Nutritional Diseases

These issues are usually easily avoided with the appropriate diet, but occasionally an animal will come to a rehabilitation center from a third party that has fed it improperly. Opossums fed diets lacking in calcium or with an inappropriate Ca:P ratio may suffer from secondary nutritional hyperparathyroidism. Treatment may be successful if the deficiency is caught and corrected early and usually involves careful correction of diet. Calcium supplementation may be necessary but must be done judiciously. If there are noticeable changes to limb conformation or hindlimb paresis, prognosis is poor (McRuer and Jones 2009).

Dental Disease

Severe gingival recession and dental tartar are not uncommon in opossums. These animals are usually thought to be geriatric and often are thin, weak, and have other signs of generalized debilitation. Often flushing of the gumline and appropriate antibiotic treatment, such as amoxicillin-clavulanic acid or clindamycin, along with supportive care, results in improvement of the animal's overall condition, suggesting that dental disease may contribute to some debilitation. Before release is attempted, it is wise to perform some degree of dental scaling and polishing to stave off the worsening of periodontal disease.

Tooth fracture is a common injury in trauma cases. The canines are long and especially prone to injury. Initially, the broken teeth should be examined for pulp exposure. If it is present, antibiotics and pain medications should be given until the patient is stable for extraction. Nerve blocks may be administered using the same landmarks as in small animals. The opossum canine has a long root and a mucoperiosteal flap should be created to allow access to the full root and adequate room to break down the periodontal ligament. Patience and gentle force are required, as it is easy to break off the tip of the root. The alveolar bone must be smoothed with a dental burr or rongeurs before the flap is sutured to cover the socket. Postoperatively, daily flushing with a dilute chlorhexidine solution is recommended for 5–7 days. Because of their opportunistic, foraging lifestyle, opossums do well with one or more missing canines so tooth extraction should not preclude release.

A common cause of dental injury is entrapment of an opossum in a humane trap, such as a Havaheart trap. In an attempt to escape, opossum will often severely damage the mandible with the bars of the cage, causing erosive lesions of the lower jaw gingiva and skin, as well as fractures and root exposure of the associated teeth. These lesions often become progressively necrotic and require long-term care. The author has used periodontal filler gels (i.e Clindoral Clindamycin HCl, TriLogic Pharma, Tallahassee, AL, USA) along with surgery and systemic antibiotics for resolution of these injuries.

Medical Care of Orphaned Infants

Most Virginia opossums presented for care are orphaned young. Evaluation of orphans generally should be done with long-term prognosis in mind, and taking into

Table 23.2 Diet by phase or life stage.

Phase 1	Weight range 25–35 g	Gavage feed diluted formula[a] ½–1 mL 6× daily
Phase 2	Weight range 36–45 g	Gavage feed 1.5–2 mL formula 5× daily
Phase 3	Weight range 46–55 g	Gavage feed 2–2.5 mL formula 4× daily. Start offering lapping tray
Phase 4	Weight range 56–70 g	Gavage feed 2.5–3.5 mL formula 3× daily. PLUS offer tray of 1 tbsp each soft cat food (moistened hard food or canned), finely chopped soft vegetables, finely chopped soft fruit or apple sauce, ½ tbsp yogurt
Phase 5	Weight range 71–100 g	Gavage feed 3.5–5 mL formula 2× daily PLUS offer tray of 1 tbsp soft cat food (moistened hard food or canned), 1½ tbsp finely chopped soft vegetables, 1 tbsp finely chopped soft fruit or apple sauce, ½ tbsp yogurt, ½ tbsp protein[b]
Phase 6	Weight range 101–120 g	ONLY if not eating well, gavage feed 5–6 mL daily PLUS 2 tbsp each moistened cat food and coarse chopped vegetables, 1½ tbsp coarse chopped fruit, ½ tbsp yogurt, ½ tbsp protein
Phase 7	Weight range 121–145 g	2 tbsp each lightly moistened cat food and coarse chopped vegetables (nickel-sized), 2 tbsp coarse chopped fruit (nickel-sized), 1 tbsp yogurt, 1 tbsp protein
Juvenile	125–200 g (indoor)[c]	2 tbsp lightly moistened dog food, ¼ cup each coarse chopped vegetables and fruit (nickel-sized), 1 tbsp yogurt, 1 tbsp protein; twice a week offer pieces of whole prey animal protein
Adult	>200 g	¾ cup moistened dog food, ¾ cup bite-sized vegetables, ½ cup bite-sized fruits, 1 protein from list; twice a week offer a prey item

Source: South Florida Wildlife Center diet book and nursery phase sheets.
[a] Formula recipe: 1 part Esbilac to ½ part Zoologic 30/52 to 2 parts water. Add 5 mL live cultured yogurt to every 100 mL.
[b] Proteins include canned salmon, eggs, cooked chicken livers, fish, cottage cheese, mice, and chicks. Proteins should be alternated on a daily basis.
[c] These are juveniles that present to care at a larger size, not nursery raised.

account all variables that contribute to prognosis helps this endeavor. For example, an opossum that is small and hypothermic on presentation has a poorer prognosis than a larger warm orphan. A more objective method of evaluation is a scoring system, which adds together all

Table 23.3 A score system to assess prognosis for orphaned opossums.

– The higher the total score is, the better prognosis the orphan has.
– Temperature, age, and condition scores are added together for a total.
– A score of 7 or greater carries the best prognosis for survival.
   1) **T = Assign a value according to the temperature of the animal**
   The score reflects the number value of temperature on arrival.
      0 = very cold to touch
      1 = cool or abnormally warm to touch
      2 = room temperature
      3 = just below human temperature (slightly cooler than the human hand)
      4 = normal temperature for the animal (the same temperature or slightly warmer than the human hand)
   2) **A = Assign a value according to the age of the animal**
      0 = <30 g
      1 = 31–80 g
      2 = 81–160 g
      3 = 160–300 g
      4 = >300 g
   3) **C = Assign a value according to the condition of the animal**
      0 = paresis/paralysis, severe emaciation, open fracture, extensive degloving wounds, missing body parts, incomplete umbilical closure, blind
      1 = closed fracture, very thin, neurological signs, extreme pallor, maggot-infested wounds, mandibular fractures, severe dyspnea, extensive necrosis
      2 = severe parasitism, weakness, dyspnea, severe dehydration, closed fractures midshaft, mild dehydration
      3 = minor wounds, abrasions, bruising, mild external parasitism, mild pallor, slightly thin
      4 = no significant findings on physical exam
      Note: being attached to a dead jill subtracts 1–2 condition points, depending on how long ago she died

Source: South Florida Wildlife Center's neonatal scoring system.

variables in an attempt to come up with an overall score as a prognostic indicator. An example of such a scoring system is given in Table 23.3. Refer to Chapter 12 for additional information on formula and feeding options.

Opossums are generally orphaned in groups and should be kept together for comfort and warmth. A soft pouch similar to those marketed for pet sugar gliders provides a place for the babies to find comfort and warmth.

Orphaned opossums are often found in a dead jill's pouch still suckling on her teats, and are considered prone to systemic infection due to their underdeveloped immune system and bacterial contamination of the milk. Because of this, orphans under 80 g (this is our current protocol) found on a dead mother should be treated with antibiotics – amoxicillin is typically appropriate. Internal and external parasites can often be a serious problem. Pyrantel (10 mg/kg) is a safe empirical choice for a dewormer, although fecal testing of any baby presenting with diarrhea or anemia is recommended to definitively identify intestinal parasites. Fleas are often a serious problem, causing life-threatening anemia in older haired babies. Selemectin (6–10 mg/kg) is safe for haired babies over 50 g (1.8 oz) and is often used prophylactically on initial presentation. This roughly works out to 1 drop/100 g for the least concentrated version of the drug (e.g., Revolution® for cats and kittens). Young that are undernourished may also benefit from a multivitamin supplement (e.g., Liqui-tinic™, PRN Pharmacal, Pensacola, FL, USA).

Dermatological Conditions

Skin problems are common in orphaned opossums. They also have very delicate skin that is easily abraded, torn, or subject to drying. A humid environment is best to imitate the conditions in the pouch. Using a damp towel in a very warm plastic container should provide enough moisture, although even then the skin can dry out. Vitamin E oil may be used to moisturize body parts prone to drying, such as the legs and tail, but must be used sparingly to avoid toxicity if ingested. Alternatively, oil-free humectant sprays, such as Humilac (Virbac, Carros, France) can be used as directed for domestic animals with no adverse effects.

A fairly common syndrome in young opossums is dermal septic necrosis, also known as "crispy-ear syndrome." This is likely caused by vasculitis secondary to systemic yeast or bacterial infection (McRuer and Jones 2009). It is at times responsive to antibiotics and amoxicillin-clavulanic acid or TMS are good empirical choices. Orphans are also prone to multiple dermal abscesses, most likely

from sepsis. These are also treated with antibiotics, but often have a poor prognosis. Prompt culturing of the lesions gives the veterinarian the best chance of successful treatment. Flaking of the skin on the legs and tail may be due to poor nutrition, lack of environmental humidity, or cutaneous fungal infections usually caused by an environmental dermatophyte (*Trichophyton* spp. or a nonpathogenic *Microsporum* spp.) which respond to topical treatment. Systemic antifungal medications are usually not necessary but griseofulvin has been shown to be efficacious (Johnson-Delaney 2014).

Diarrhea

Young opossums often develop diarrhea while in care. The list of differential diagnoses for this problem includes internal parasites, dietary intolerance, bacterial or fungal overgrowth, or antibiotic-induced diarrhea. If fecal examination is negative for parasites, an empirical course of metronidazole may be attempted. If the animal continues to decline, a fecal culture is recommended, as *Salmonella* is capable of causing serious illness. Supportive care such as fluid therapy and dietary modification are also important in restoring gastrointestinal health.

Conclusion

Although a common patient in wildlife rehabilitation settings, there is relatively little research on the Virginia opossum. Much of the literature about the species is research based, with clinical literature focusing on the more charismatic members of the marsupial family, such as macropods. However, the opossum, North America's only marsupial, is a resilient and fascinating animal and can be very rewarding to rehabilitate.

References

Alden, K.J. (1995). Helminths of the opossum, *Didelphis virginiana*, in southern Illinois, with a compilation of all helminths reported from this host in North America. *Journal of the Helminthological Society of Washington* 62 (2): 197–208.

Barr, T.R.B. (1963). Infectious diseases in the opossum: a review. *Journal of Wildlife Management* 27 (1): 53–71.

Dubey, J.P., Lindsay, D.S., Saville, W.J.A. et al. (2001). A review of *Sarcocystis neurona* and equine protozoal myeloencephalitis (EPM). *Veterinary Parasitology* 95: 89–131.

Dubey, J.P., Lindsay, D.S., Rosenthal, B.M. et al. (2002). Establishment of *Besnoitia darlingi* from opossums

(*Didelphis virginiana*) in experimental intermediate and definitive hosts, propagation in cell culture, and description of ultrastructural and genetic characteristics. *International Journal for Parasitology* 32: 1053–1064.

Ellis, A.E., Mackey, E., Moore, P.A. et al. (2012). Debilitation and mortality associated with besnoitiosis in four Virginia opossums (*Didelphis virginiana*). *Journal of Zoo and Wildlife Medicine* 43 (2): 367–374.

Elsheikha, H.M., Fitzgerald, B.M., Rosenthal, L.S., and Mansfield, L.S. (2004). Concurrent presence of *Sarcocystis neurona* sporocyts, *Besnoitia darlingi* tissue cysts, and *Sarcocystis inghami* sarcocysts in naturally infected opossums (*Didelphis virginiana*). *Journal of Veterinary Diagnostic Investigation* 16: 352–356.

Gamble, K.C. (2004). Marsupial care and husbandry. *Veterinary Clinics: Exotic Animal Practice* 7: 283–298.

Green, B., Krause, W.J., and Newgrain, K. (1996). Milk composition in the North American opossum (*Didelphis virginiana*). *Comparative Biochemistry and Physiology* 113B (3): 619–623.

Gunn-Moore, D.A. (2014). Feline mycobacterial infections. *Vet J* 201 (2): 230–238.

Heatley, J.J. (2009). Cardiovascular anatomy, physiology, and disease of rodents and small exotic mammals. *Veterinary Clinics of North America: Exotic Animal Practice* 12: 99–113.

Holtz, P. (2003). Marsupialia (Marsupials). In: *Fowler's Zoo and Wild Animal Medicine*, 5e (ed. M.E. Fowler and R.E. Miller), 288–303. St Louis, MO: Elsevier.

Hossler, R.J., McAninch, J.B., and Harder, J.D. (1994). Maternal denning behavior and survival of juveniles in opossums in southeastern New York. *Journal of Mammology* 75 (1): 60–70.

Houk, A.E., Goodwin, D.G., Zajac, A.M. et al. (2010). Prevalence of antibodies to Trypanosoma cruzi, Toxoplasma gondii, Encephalitozoon cuniculi, Sarcocystis neurona, Besnoitia darlingi, and Neospora caninum in North American opossums, Didelphis virginiana, from southern Louisiana. *Journal of Parasitology* 96 (6): 1119–1122.

Johnson-Delaney, C.A. (2000). Therapeutics of companion exotic marsupials. *Veterinary Clinics of North America: Exotic Animal Practice* 3 (1): 173–181.

Johnson-Delaney, C. (2014). Pet Virginia opossums and skunks. *Journal of Exotic Pet Medicine* 23: 317–326.

Jones, K.D. (2013). Opossum nematodiasis: diagnosis and treatment of stomach, intestine, and lung nematodes in the virginia opossum (*Didelphis virginiana*). *Journal of Exotic Pet Medicine* 22: 375–382.

Kanda, L.L., Fuller, T.K., and Sievert, P.R. (2006). Landscape associations of road-killed Virginia opossum (*Didelphis virginiana*) in central Massachusetts. *American Midland Naturalist* 156: 128–134.

Kilmon, J.A. Sr. (1976). High tolerance to snake venom by the Virginia opossum, *Didelphis virginiana*. *Toxicon* 14: 337–340.

Kimble, D.P. (1997). Didelphid behavior. *Neuroscience and Biobehavioral Reviews* 21 (3): 361–369.

Krause, W.J. and Krause, W.A. (2006). *The Opossum: Its Amazing Story*. Columbia, MO: Department of Pathology and Anatomical Sciences, School of Medicine, University of Missouri (e-book).

Lamberski, N., Reader, J.R., Cook, L.F. et al. (2002). A retrospective study of 11 cases of lungworm (*Didelphostrongylus hayesi*) infection in opossums (*Didelphis virginiana*). *Journal of Zoo and Wildlife Medicine* 33 (2): 151–156.

Lloret, A., Hartmann, K., Pennisi, M.G. et al. (2013). Mycobacteriosis in cats: ABCD guidelines on prevention and management. *Journal of Feline Medicine and Surgery* 15: 591–597.

McManus, J.J. (1974). *Didelphis virginiana*. *Mammalian Species* 40: 1–6.

McRuer, D.L. and Jones, K. (2009). Behavioral and nutritional aspects of the Virginia opossum. *Veterinary Clinics of North America: Exotic Animal Practice* 12: 217–236.

Mead, A.J. and Patterson, D.B. (2009). Skeletal lesions in a population of Virginia opossums (*Didelphis virginiana*) from Baldwin County, Georgia. *Journal of Wildlife Diseases* 45 (2): 325–332.

Meier, E. K. (1983). Habitat use by opossums in an urban environment. MS thesis. Oregon State University.

Miller, E.A. (ed.) (2012). *Minimum Standards for Wildlife Rehabilitation*, 4e. St Cloud, MN: National Wildlife Rehabilitators Association.

Peel, E., Jones, E., Belov, K., and Cheng, Y. (2013). Protection in the pouch: antimicrobial peptides in marsupials and monotremes. In: *Microbial Pathogens and Strategies for Combatting Them: Science, Technology, and Education*, vol. 2 (ed. A. Méndez-Diaz), 1247–1256. Badajoz, Spain: Formatex Research Center.

Pornmanee, P., Sánchez, E.E., López, G. et al. (2008). Neutralization of lethality and proteolytic activities of Malayan pit viper (*Calloselasma rhodostoma*) venom with North America Virginia opossum (*Didelphis virginiana*) serum. *Toxicon* 52: 186–189.

Potkay, S. (1970). Diseases of the opossum (*Didelphis marsupialis*): a review. *Laboratory Animal Care* 20 (3): 502–509.

Roellig, D.M., Brown, E.L., Barnabé, C. et al. (2008). Molecular typing of *Trypanosoma cruzi* isolates, United States. *Emerging Infectious Diseases* 14 (7): 1123–1125.

Synder, D.E., Hamir, A.N., Hanlon, C.A., and Rupprecht, C.E. (1991). Lung lesions in an opossum (*Didelphis viginiana*) associated with *Capillaria didelphis*. *Journal of Wildlife Diseases* 27 (1): 175–177.

Taylor, P. (2002). Opossums. In: *Hand-rearing Wild and Domestic Mammals* (ed. L. Gage), 45–54. Ames, IA: Iowa State Press.

Volchan, E., Vargas, C.D., da Franca, J.G. et al. (2004). Tooled for the task: vision in the opossum. *BioScience* 54 (3): 189–194.

Werner, R.M. and Vick, J.A. (1977). Resistance of the opossum (*Didelphis viginiana*) to envenomation by snakes of the family Crotalidae. *Toxicon* 15: 29–33.

Williams-Newkirk, A.J., Salzer, J.S., Carroll, D.S. et al. (2013). Simple method for locating a suitable venipuncture site on the tail of the Virginia opossum (*Didelphis virginiana*). *European Journal of Wildlife Research* 59: 455–457.

24

Natural History and Medical Management of Canids

Emphasis on Coyotes and Foxes

Jeannie Lord[1] and Erica A. Miller[2]

[1] *Pine View Wildlife Rehabilitation and Education Center, Fredonia, WI, USA*
[2] *Wildlife Medicine, Department of Clinic Studies, University of Pennsylvania School of Veterinary Medicine, Philadelphia, PA, USA*

Introduction

The red fox (*Vulpes vulpes*) and gray fox (*Urocyon cin-eroargenteus*) are two of 21 species of fox found on four continents and are the most common fox species in North America (Henry 1996b). Other fox species found in lesser numbers in North America include the swift fox (*Vulpes velox*), found in the western grassland habitats of Colorado, Oklahoma, New Mexico and Texas; the kit fox (*Vulpes macrotis*) closely related to the swift fox (possibly the same species), found in the southwestern US and northern and central Mexico, and listed as endangered in the US; and the arctic fox (*Alopex lagopus*), found in parts of Alaska and Canada.

The coyote (*Canis latrans*) has 19 different subspecies that vary in physical attributes and survival methods depending on geographical location (Grady 1994).

Three species of wolves are also native to North America but are encountered less frequently in rehabilitation. The red wolf (*Canis rufus*) is endangered, with only about 50 individuals remaining in the wild. Reintroduction programs and natural spread have contributed to a growing gray wolf (*Canis lupus*) population in Alaska, Canada, and north central and northwestern US. The eastern timber wolf (*Canis lycaon*) is found in the northeast US.

Networking with rehabilitators experienced with these species is encouraged. Collaborative efforts can help in developing protocols for treatment and isolation of the wild canid patient for the safety of domestic animals in the clinic. As they are the most commonly presented species, the emphasis of this chapter is on the natural history and appropriate techniques and management of red and gray foxes and coyotes.

Natural History

Male canids are typically larger than females, and wild canids can easily hybridize with domestic canids as well as other wild canid species.

Red Fox

An adult red fox's head and body measure from 18 to 34 in. (46–86.5 cm), plus a tail of 12–22 in. (30.5–56 cm). The red fox is larger and heavier than the gray fox, weighing from 2.9 to 10.9 kg (Henry 1996b). Red foxes live an average of 2–4 years in the wild and up to 14 years in captivity (MacDonald 2000; Gosselink et al. 2010).

The red fox typically has a russet-colored coat with distinct black "stocking" markings on the lower legs and a full, bushy tail with a distinct white tip. Red foxes can also have golden, reddish-brown, silver, or black coats.

The supracaudal gland of all wild canids is located midway along the dorsal surface of the tail from the seventh to ninth caudal vertebrae and is composed of both apocrine and sebaceous glands. This gland is twice as large in red foxes as in other foxes, and secretes a mixture of volatile terpenes, creating a musky odor used in intraspecies signaling and scent marking.

The average range of a red fox is 1–2 mi² (2.6–5.2 km²); weather and habitat will influence this range. The size of a red fox's defended territory can be as small as an acre (0.4 hectare) in an urban area, and as much as 25 acres (10.1 hectare) in more remote areas; the preferred habitat consists of fields bounded by forest. Though often thought nocturnal, the red fox may be crepuscular; the availability of food sources often determines their activity. Red foxes are excellent scavengers, foragers, and

Medical Management of Wildlife Species: A Guide for Practitioners, First Edition. Edited by Sonia M. Hernandez,
Heather W. Barron, Erica A. Miller, Roberto F. Aguilar and Michael J. Yabsley.
© 2020 John Wiley & Sons, Inc. Published 2020 by John Wiley & Sons, Inc.

hunters. They are known for being cunning and quick, and can reach speeds of over 48 km/h (30 mi/h) (Henry 1993).

Red foxes are primarily monogamous. The mating season begins in the middle of January. The den used by the male (dog) and female (vixen) is a burrow or hole, which is frequently located on a slope or hillside and may be more than 15–40 ft (5–12 m) deep. Dens are located in open areas, as opposed to deep woods. Litters average 4–6 kits, but may be as large as 12–13. The vixen may move the kits (also called pups) to a different den more than once during their care in response to perceived threats (Storm et al. 1976).

Gray Fox

The gray fox is smaller than the red fox, and weighs an average of 2.7–6.3 kg (Henry 1996a). It has a shorter body and muzzle, with shorter legs and smaller feet; the claws are sharper and recurved on the forefeet. Lifespan for wild gray foxes averages 6–10 years (Davis and Schmidly 1994).

The gray fox "salt-and-pepper" colored coat is coarser than that of the red fox. The gray fox can have reddish patches behind the ears and on the front of the legs, and a white throat and belly. The tail is shorter proportionately than the red fox and has a black stripe running along the dorsal midline from the tip of the tail.

From the top of the cranium, the temporal ridges on a red fox skull form a "V"-shaped pattern, while the skull of the gray is "U"-shaped, providing the useful mnemonic of "V" for *Vulpes* and "U" for *Urocyon* (Jackson 1961; Henry 1993).

Gray foxes usually have a smaller litter of pups, averaging four kits (Jackson 1961). Dens can be located in hollow logs, cavities of trees, or beneath boulders or rock piles. Gray foxes also tend to inhabit forest or deep woodlands. Proximity to humans is a contributing factor to selection of den site (Lesmeister et al. 2015).

In general, when escaping pursuit, the red fox runs at full speed and may suddenly change directions, whereas the gray fox will climb a tree or search for a hole in the ground.

Coyotes

Coyotes are found throughout North America; individual territories average 26 km^2 (10 mi^2). Their preferred territories are thick brush areas, borders of forests, and dense woodlands. Habitat loss and human encroachment have required versatility and adaptability for their survival, making it more common for coyotes to establish territories in urban areas. Average life expectancy for a coyote in the wild is approximately five years, compared to 12 years in captivity (Wilkinson 1995; Beckoff 2001).

The coyote has marked variation in color, with most being a shade of brown. The mantle may contain black, reddish-blond, gray, or light blond tints. Adult weight ranges from 9 to 22 kg, depending on geographic location (Wilkinson 1995). The coyote can run 40–64 km/h (25–40 mi/h) and leap up to 14 ft (4.3 m). Their two anal glands may release a musky odor (Grady 1994).

Coyotes tend to be crepuscular and have well-developed senses, especially sight. Hunting techniques vary with available prey and coyote age. While coyotes chase rabbits, they tend to pounce on small rodents. Hunting typically results in a successful kill approximately 25% of the time.

Their vocalization is one of the coyote's distinguishing characteristics. As opposed to the call of the fox, which usually consists of a few short yaps or barking followed by a shrill shriek, the coyote call is a howl followed by yipping noises (Grady 1994).

Diet

Fox

Over 85% of the red fox diet is composed of small mammals, although deviations occur depending on habitat and region. Gray foxes have expanded second upper molars that provide additional crushing surfaces for a diet that includes plants, fruits, nuts, insects, eggs, and reptiles indigenous to their habitat. Depending on the season, an assortment of small birds and mammals is also consumed by both species. Diets in captivity should be primarily meat-based, but include a variety of fruits, eggs, and insects. Suggested diets for weaning are discussed in Section 24.9.

Coyotes

Coyotes are omnivores and opportunists. The main staple of their diet is mammals, including mice, voles, chipmunks, woodchucks, and rabbits or larger prey, depending on the territory. They will also consume birds, fruit, and insects, and in urban areas, coyotes will forage in human garbage. As opportunists, coyotes will select prey that is easily obtainable and plentiful.

Handling and Restraint

When handling or restraining a canid, experience, planning, and appropriate equipment are necessary to limit trauma, stress, and potential exacerbation of an existing injury. Preestablished handling criteria are necessary for the safety of the handler and the animal. Age, size,

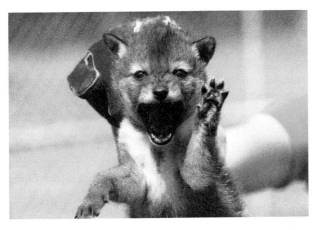

Figure 24.1 Using a gloved hand to scruff and carry a pup as the parent would naturally carry it by the nape.

and condition of the animal determine the handling protocol.

At 3–6 weeks of age, young pups are often transported to alternate dens by the parent mouthing the pups by the nape and trotting with the pup dangling. This technique has proven to be a safe and effective handling method; use one gloved hand to grasp the pup by the back of the neck, while the other gloved hand supports the pup's rear (Figure 24.1). While transporting or moving the pup for purposes of examination, cover the animal's eyes to minimize stress. The pups are developing teeth at this age, so use protective gloves and a firm grip.

The physical restraint of an older, injured fox requires different capture and handling technique and equipment. Hoop nets, squeeze boxes, plastic shields, crowding boards, and quality handling gloves are commonly used to handle older foxes and juvenile coyotes. Once restrained, most will calm down quickly with a placed towel over the head. Soft roll gauze tied around the snout or commercial dog muzzles can be used to prevent biting, but the animal should be closely monitored for overheating or signs of respiratory distress. The use of blindfolds and placement of cotton in the ears will reduce stress.

Snare poles are not recommended for juvenile/immature canids, unless the user is experienced operating them. Snare poles should be placed over the head and one front leg; improper use may place constricting forces on the neck, resulting in damage to the trachea, vasculature, and/or cervical spinal cord if the animal struggles (Munoz-Igualada et al. 2008). Chemical restraint may be necessary for older juveniles and adult canids. Commonly used immobilization drugs are given in Appendix II: Formulary. Animals may then be intubated and maintained on isoflurane for longer procedures (see Chapter 5).

Young

Young wild canids should never be raised alone: they are highly social and it is essential they be raised with conspecifics. Lack of peer or sibling role models increases the possibility of habituation through human socialization and decreases the likelihood of a successful return to the wild. When confronted with a single pup, the practitioner should immediately contact other rehabilitators and arrange its transfer to be raised with conspecifics.

Red Fox

The gestation period is approximately 53 days with an average litter size of 5–6 kits, though 11 kits have been documented (Jackson 1961; Saunders 1988). Red fox pups weigh about 85–110 g at birth and measure 6–8 in. in length (15–20 cm) (Grambo 1994; Henry 1993). They usually produce one litter per year. The pups are dark brown with a dab of white on the very tip of the tail. The vixen remains in the den with the pups, whose eyes open by the eighth or ninth day. During this time, the family is dependent on the dog for food and protection.

Milk teeth appear in the second week followed by canines, incisors, and then molars (Gingerich and Winkler 1979). High human activity, lack of food sources or predation may cause the vixen to move the pups to a new den at this time (Storm et al. 1976). At 3–4 weeks of age, the pups are still in the den, but sibling fighting does occur and vicious disputes can be fatal (Henry 1996a). This behavior establishes the social hierarchy that will exist until the young leave the den. It is essential that pups in rehabilitation have the opportunity to engage in this type of challenge behavior as it not only establishes the "pecking order," but fosters and promotes skills which will be needed in hunting. Careful monitoring is necessary to avoid serious injuries or fatalities.

Pups are weaned at about five weeks of age, and the food provided should replicate what is available in the wild (see Section 24.3). At weaning, they will weigh an average of 600 g and their appearance changes to the familiar reddish-orange coloration of the coat and the black stockings on the legs. As the maturation process occurs, both parents will leave the den to satisfy the pups' hunger. It is during this time that healthy pups may be assumed to be "abandoned" and presented for rehabilitation.

At three months, the pups begin to accompany a parent on hunting expeditions. By 4–5 months, the familial structure of the den has begun to erode (Gosselink et al. 2010). Young males are usually the first to leave the den, followed by the next oldest sibling. At this time, the pups weigh about 3 kg.

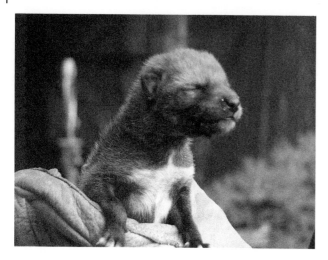

Figure 24.2 Approximately two-week-old coyote pups with eyes just opened; ears are still down and muzzles are short.

Gray Fox

Depending on the region, 3–5 pups are born between late March and early April, after a 51-day gestation period. The pups are altricial and average 85 g at birth, with a body length of 3–5 in. (8–13 cm). At birth, the neonates do not appear fox-like. Their ears are round and lie flat to the head, which is round with a short nose. The hair is short and dark. By the fourth to fifth day, identifiable rust-colored markings become visible behind the ears. Pups' eyes open within two weeks, and the coat develops density and a deeper color (Figure 24.2).

The vixen will remain with the neonates for the first three weeks while the dog brings food to the den. By three weeks of age, the young pups are active in the den and canines and incisors are replacing milk teeth. By the fifth or sixth week, the pups weigh between 450 and 800 g and become active outside the den (Grambo 1994). This is the age when a pup is most likely to be presented for care.

Gray fox pups are weaned at 7–8 weeks of age, when they weigh on average 1 kg. Food brought to the den at this time is provided through regurgitation or by dropping food items on the ground, including berries and fruits, small mammals, insects, and plant material. Food may be consumed or cached. Soon after weaning, the pups will begin to hunt and forage with their parents. The pups are hunting on their own at three months, and the family disperses in the autumn (Grambo 1994).

Coyote

The coyote gestation period is 60 days. Depending on geographic location, pups may be born in February to April. Natural dens, excavated by the parents, are usually located in an area not easily approached by predators. However, reports of coyotes using dog houses,

abandoned trailers, and old refrigerators for dens are becoming more common.

The average litter for a coyote is 6–7 pups, although 9–11 have been reported. The mortality rate of coyote young due to disease and anthropogenic factors can be high, often with only two pups surviving to November (Grady 1994; Wilkinson 1995).

Newborn coyotes weigh approximately 300–350 g (Beckoff 2001). At birth, the young are brownish or gray in color with short rough hair. The pups have white chests and darkish muzzles and may have a faint black stripe traveling from the neck to the tip of the tail, which can be dark gray to black. The ears are dark, distinctively rounded, and lie back almost flat to the head.

When the pups are about three weeks of age, they begin to interact socially with their peers and initiate a variety of body displays referred to as "motor patterns." It is at this age that the canine teeth appear (Beckoff 2001). Pups are fed by regurgitation and often assisted by the betas in the familial structure (Wilkinson 1995). By four weeks of age, after weaning has occurred, the social hierarchy has been established. Agonistic behaviors, such as biting, wrestling, chasing, body posturing and vocalizations, will continue among the siblings for another 4–5 weeks, with the alpha dominance established for eating and control (Beckoff 2001). By 10–12 weeks, juveniles begin to disperse as a result of hostile behavior or aggression from the adults.

Initial Housing

Pups

Depending on age and condition, external heat sources may be necessary to maintain body temperature. An incubator can be used for intensive care or for very young, altricial pups, but for pups requiring less intense heat, the use of a pet carrier on a heating pad is appropriate.

The carrier can be set up with three layers, the bottom being two layers of newspaper covered by a layer of paper towel to absorb moisture and provide a degree of stability for feet and paws, followed by a top cover of a towel or blanket for bedding (Figure 24.3). Towels and blankets used inside the kennel must not have holes or strings which could cause the young pup to become entangled. The outside of the carrier should be draped to limit visual stimuli.

If a heating pad is used, use the lowest setting and place the pad underneath the back half of the carrier. This allows the pups to move away from the heat source if they become too warm. The ideal temperature for newborn to two-week-old pups is 26.7–29.4 °C (80–85 °F). By 4–5 weeks of age, the pups should not need supplemental heat if

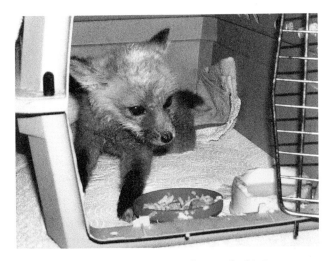

Figure 24.3 A kennel carrier set up to house a fox kit. Paper towels cover newspaper lining, and a heating pad set on low is under the back half of the carrier.

they are housed indoors. As soon as weather conditions allow, the young should be moved permanently to outside housing.

Adults

Injured subadult and adult canids initially should be housed individually in restricted caging 0.9 m × 0.9 m × 0.9 m (Miller 2012). Ideal hospital caging allows for shifting to a second cage without having to handle the animal (Figure 24.4). As soon as the subadult or adult canid is stable and the nature of its injuries no longer requires limited activity, it should be moved into an outdoor cage or transferred to a rehabilitator with appropriate outdoor caging (see Section 24.10).

Infant Feeding

The importance of preventing human socialization and habituation in infant mammals cannot be overemphasized. The caretaker must limit vocalizations and overhandling during feeding times to avoid the risk of taming the animal.

Amounts fed should be carefully monitored, as overfeeding can result in diarrhea. Neonates should be fed using a small syringe or a baby bottle fitted with an infant-sized nipple.

The pup's ability to swallow does not fully develop until about three weeks of age. To prevent the pup sucking formula too quickly, risking aspiration, the size of the slit in the nipple should be adjusted to provide an easy but safe flow. Unless the pup is severely dehydrated and intravenous or gavage-feeding methods are necessary, nursing is the preferred feeding method as it invokes normal suckling behavior. Pups should be fed lying on their stomachs, not on their backs.

After each feeding, the urogenital area must be stimulated for urination and defecation. This may be done using a soft cloth moistened with warm water to massage the urogenital area gently until urination or defecation

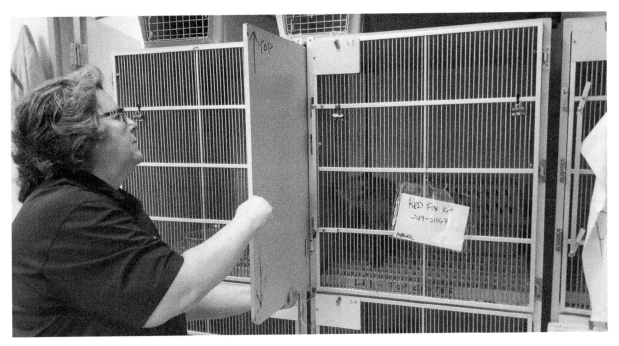

Figure 24.4 A hospital shift cage, allowing the animal to be moved to one side while providing access to safely clean the other side.
Source: Courtesy of Diane Nickerson.

Table 24.1 Sample orphan formula dilution for dehydrated animals.

Feeding schedule	Electrolyte replacement	Amount of formula prepared as directed	Amount of bottled water to be added to prepared formula	Total amount to be provided at each feeding
Feeding 1	6 mL	—	—	6 mL
Feeding 2	—	2 mL	4 mL	6 mL
Feeding 3	—	3 mL	3 mL	6 mL
Feeding 4	—	4 mL	2 mL	6 mL
Feeding 5	—	5 mL	1 mL	6 mL

occurs. Stimulation after feeding is discontinued once the pup's eyes are open.

Monitoring of feces and body temperatures at this age is important so that diet and housing can be adjusted as needed.

Red and Gray Fox

Immature fox pups should be fed warm-to-the-wrist (38.9–40.5 °C, 102–105 °F) Esbilac® (PetAg, Inc., Hampshire, IL) as replacement formula, mixed according to package instructions. For slightly dehydrated pups, dilute the formula for the first day or two to increase hydration (Table 24.1).

Although feeding frequency may vary, the general schedule listed in Table 24.2 should be adequate.

Coyote

Coyote pups should be bottle-fed every four hours initially, providing approximately 5% of the body weight (BW) by volume per feeding (e.g., 1500 g BW × 0.05 = 75 mL). This feeding schedule should be maintained until the pups' eyes open. Warm-to-the-wrist liquid Esbilac is the recommended formula for coyote.

Habituation

If the practitioner is to raise a properly socialized animal, exposure to human voices must be limited. Association with the human voice and other human-related noise,

Table 24.2 Orphan formula dosage.

Weight	Amount of formula fed	Frequency
100 g	5–6 mL	q3.5h
200 g	10–12 mL	q4h
350 g	20–25 mL	q4.75h
500 g	25–30 mL	q6h

together with unnecessary handling or "petting," can result in tameness or habituation. Because the pup will habituate to specific human-related sounds, such as doors, phones, or footsteps, these sounds must be minimized as well. While limiting human interaction with the pup, interactions with their conspecifics are essential. Pups should never be raised alone.

Weaning

Red and Gray Fox

The authors use a good grade of kitten and cat food for both fox patients and those in permanent captive care. Some permanent resident foxes have lived 14–18 years on this diet.

Once the eyes are open, weaning should begin with the introduction of solid foods. A base diet of soaked kitten chow (enough water to just cover the chow to soften it, with approximately 30–45 mL Esbilac formula poured on top); thumb-sized bits of cut-up mice, birds, or venison; one to three mealworms or cut-up earthworms, or one or two small pieces of chicken or beef; and one or two small pieces of berries or fruit indigenous to the region. This is supplemented with cooked egg and live-culture plain yogurt. The egg can be hard-boiled and then minced or scrambled. Eggs are only provided three times per week.

As the pups mature, the Esbilac is reduced and finally eliminated and soaking the kitten chow is discontinued. This should occur by the time the pups are 5–6 weeks old. Discreet observation of the pups, as they consume their food, will assist in making the change to dry kitten chow at the appropriate time.

Once the pups have transitioned to dry kitten chow, whole mice, whole eggs, small birds, and small mammals should be added to the diet. After 2–2.5 weeks, regular cat food should replace the kitten chow. Use of chow should be gradually reduced and eliminated by seven weeks of age. By 6–7 weeks, live prey should be introduced as described below.

Small rats, mice, chicks, quail, rabbit, and worms simulate the natural diet of the red fox. Indigenous fruits should be continued as a supplement, as should native nuts and other foraged food items: small insects, worms, grubs, fallen fruit, seeds, and fresh carrion.

The interactions and behaviors of the pups should be monitored for the first few feedings. As the alpha dominant fox pup may have a tendency to monopolize the best portions, the youngest pup may not get enough food and become compromised. Supplying multiple food bowls may reduce this problem.

Coyote

The weaning diet should be introduced a few days after the eyes of the young have opened at 4–5 weeks and is usually composed of previously water-softened, premium dry puppy food with 45–60 mL of warm Esbilac. Small amounts of meat or chopped mice may be added, as well as 3.5 mL of plain, unsweetened, live-culture yogurt, to aid digestion. As part of the weaning process, the introduction of other food items will replace the Esbilac and yogurt, which are gradually reduced.

Pieces of chicken, venison, beef, and egg should be added to the diet of one-quarter cup (~60 g) commercial dry dog food. Insects, including mealworms, crickets and wax worms, and cooked vegetables, such as carrots, peas, and squash can be given. A maximum of 10% of the total diet should be fruit native to the area.

Weaning diets should be fed to the pups three times a day until they reach juvenile status at 7–8 weeks of age. At this time, the dry dog food should be discontinued and natural foods increased, including live prey. A natural diet consists of mice, chicks, quail, venison, pheasant, apples, berries, nuts, seeds, raw carrots or other vegetables. Fresh road kill can also be a part of this diet. Carrion should be used cautiously, and only if the practitioner can be sure the food item does not contain any poison, foreign bodies, parasites, or pathogens that could jeopardize the patient. Carrion must be frozen to reduce the transfer of ecto- and endoparasites, and then thawed before feeding; it should be radiographed to ensure the absence of gunshot/foreign bodies. Fresh water should be available at all times.

Concurrent with the weaning process is the establishment of the social structure among the pups. When raising pups together, the same interactions will occur as in the wild, including aggressive biting, nipping, wrestling, and vocalizations. Vocalizations and dominance over the food supply will accelerate as the pups age. The carrier or cage used to house the pups at this age must be large enough to allow for normal activity until the pups can be transferred outdoors.

Live prey

The introduction of live prey at the time canid pups are moved to an outdoor enclosure promotes their hunting instincts and assists in the development of behaviors associated with stalking prey. Live mice, chicks, quail, and rats are available from a variety of commercial sources. Practitioners who find it difficult to facilitate this feeding process should make arrangements for pre-release conditioning by a rehabilitation facility equipped to offer live prey.

Outdoor Housing

Depending on weather conditions, pups should have as much opportunity to be outdoors as possible during the weaning period. Permanent outdoor facilities are the best option but an extra-large pet carrier (40″ L by 27″ W by 30″ H, 101 × 69 × 76 cm) inside a fenced area can serve as a good den-like enclosure for a few limited daylight hours. The outdoor enclosure should replicate the wild as much as possible, allowing exposure to sunlight while providing protection from the rain. Cages should be large enough for active and energetic pups to explore, climb, and romp. Practitioners can refer to the *NWRA/IWRC Minimum Standards* (Miller 2012) for caging specifications for canid species of all ages.

Enclosures should be constructed of chainlink material as the foundation to prevent escapes. This foundation must extend 1 ft outside the vertical walls of the enclosure, and the vertical walls should be secured to the foundation. The foundation is then covered with a sand/dirt mix followed by a top layer of sand. This layering and combination of substrates allows for drainage, facilitates waste removal, and minimizes pathogen accumulation. The corners and one side of the enclosure should be covered to provide a visual block from humans and create privacy.

The pet carrier used by the pups or injured adults while indoors should be moved to the outdoor caging to provide them with a familiar, protected area. Additional large pet carrier tops, placed open side down on the sand, make excellent den-like hiding areas where they can engage in play behaviors, seek shelter, and cache objects. Large logs or flat pieces of wood provide additional places for the animals to sit or exercise.

Natural objects such as feathers, pine cones, leaves, tree stumps, bark, branches, small twigs, old bones, and large stones provide natural stimulation and promote interaction and "play" between the young as they acquire future survival skills prerequisite to hunting.

Fox

For gray foxes, large branches or tree-like structures must be provided to encourage their natural inclination to climb. Wooden platforms, covered with artificial turf such as AstroTurf, will promote jumping and leaping. Hollow logs are beneficial for exercise and caching of food items. Creating enrichment to simulate natural environments is essential in helping foxes acquire or regain skills needed for survival (Figure 24.5).

Coyote

Coyotes require a larger area than foxes for exploration and exercise. Minimum enclosures should measure 12 ft long, 6 ft high and 8 ft wide ($3.6 \times 1.8 \times 2.4$ m) (Miller 2012).

Coyotes are excellent escape artists and will dig tenaciously. The use of chainlink fencing minimizes injury and withstands constant pressure and possible escape. As coyotes are crepuscular, feedings in outdoor caging should be in the early morning and at dusk.

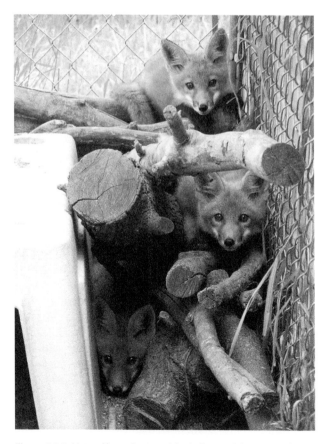

Figure 24.5 Natural branches provide shelter, enrichment, and exercise for fox kits housed outdoors. A kennel carrier top is provided as a den, but the branches are often preferred by the young.

Reasons for Presentation

The most common reasons for presentation of a fox or coyote to a rehabilitation facility or clinic include vehicular trauma, steel leg-hold trap injury, wild, or domestic animal attack, direct or indirect consumption of toxins, gunshot wounds, emaciation, disease, and found orphaned or abandoned.

Triage and Initial Exam

Triage and Euthanasia

An immediate physical assessment determines appropriate protocols and procedures. The initial exam will determine if the patient's condition indicates euthanasia. Examples of this include irreparable compound fractures to limbs; certain infectious diseases including rabies, advanced distemper, or disseminated mange in an adult; seizures associated with severe head trauma; and other injuries resulting in debilitating damage.

A key tenet guiding the practitioner's choice to euthanize is to determine if the patient could survive if released back to the wild. The decision to continue care must include an assessment of the animal's quality of life or evidence from previous studies. As an example, severe compound fractures of a leg may result in inability to survive in the wild. In a study in Arizona, coyotes with severe fractures that were surgically repaired and monitored post release were frequently victims of vehicular trauma (Hernandez, personal communication). Knowledge of the natural history of canid species suggests that coyotes that are missing legs will struggle for survival as a result of the inability to catch prey, dig a den or escape predation.

Physical Exam

Initial exam should include a rectal temperature, assessment of hydration status, and addressing any immediate needs (hemorrhage, seizure, hypothermia, etc.). Normal temperature for foxes and coyotes is 37.8–39.4 °C (100–103 °F); however, vital signs are often above normal due to stress. A thorough examination should include age/size (Table 24.3), weight, color of mucous membranes, fundic exam, check for ectoparasites, and limb palpation. Assessment of limb use, sensitivity to touch, and any fractures, bruising, lacerations, or other injuries should be recorded. As soon as possible after admitting a fox or coyote pup into care, a fecal sample should be examined, as young pups are usually infected with intestinal parasites.

If rehydration is necessary, this should be done orally unless the animal is severely dehydrated. Oral rehydration

Table 24.3 Age determination in wild canids.

Species	Age	Description
Coyote	Neonate	Eyes/ears closed, brown-gray, wooly fur, ~300–350 g
	8–12 days	Eyes open
Fox, gray	Neonate	Dark skin, naked, ~85–100 g
	9 days	Eyes open, fuzzy fur
	4 wks	Hair growth
	16 wks	Milk teeth lost
Fox, red	Neonate	Naked, ~100 g
	9 days	Eyes open, fuzzy fur
	7 wks	Pale yellowish-brown
	8–9 wks	Pale reddish-brown
	16–20 wks	Reddish, milk teeth lost
Fox and coyote	18–19 wks	Adult upper canines appear
	19–21 wks	Adult 3rd lower premolars appear
	24–27 wks	(Last) 3rd lower molar appears
	6 months	Full adult dentition

Source: Szuma (1997), Maher (2002), and Miller (2007).

for the young pup can be accomplished using a syringe or a bottle. If using a bottle, only a very small slit should be made in the nipple to avoid aspiration. Fluid replacement guidelines can be found in Chapter 4 and in the NWRA *Quick Reference* (Miller 2007). Pedialyte® (Abbot Laboratories, Abbott Park, IL) or other crystalloids may be used but human liquid nutrition formulas are not recommended. Parenteral hydration can be administered following the same guidelines and routes used for domestic dogs.

Diseases

Foxes and coyotes are commonly afflicted with the same diseases and parasites and diagnosis and treatment are similar.

Parasites

Wild canids are host to a variety of endoparasites and ectoparasites. Prevalence and distribution of various diseases and parasites vary geographically so local knowledge is important.

Endoparasites
Numerous trematodes, cestodes, and nematodes have been reported from wild canids (Samuel et al. 2008). Isolation of canid patients is recommended to prevent transmission of zoonotic parasites, such as *Echinococcus* spp., to other animals or humans.

Endoparasites commonly associated with coyotes include *Dirofilaria immitis*, *Paragonimus kellicotti*, *Echinococcus* spp., *Ancylostoma caninum*, *Trichuris vulpis*, *Sarcocystis* spp., *Capillaria* spp., *Toxoplasma gondii*, and *Leishmania* spp. (Davidson et al. 1992; Gates et al. 2014; Chitwood et al. 2015).

Heartworm (*Dirofilaria immitis*) and lungworms (*P. kellicotti*) occur commonly in wild canids and may impact the health of rehabilitating patients (Stuht and Youatt 1972; Nelson et al. 2003). Canid patients older than six months should be tested for heartworm before treating with ivermectin and related products in order to minimize the risk of thromboemboli. Wild canids with heartworm may exhibit abdominal swelling (ascites) or signs of caval syndrome (right heart enlargement, labored respiration, coughing, anemia, pale mucous membranes, poor stamina, and hematuria). *Paragonimus* lung flukes often are only diagnosed on necropsy, though affected animals may show an array of respiratory signs including coughing, dyspnea, and hemoptysis. Thoracic radiographs or transtracheal washes and fecal sedimentation to check for ova may help to confirm the antemortem diagnosis. Treatment with fenbendazole or praziquantel in domestic canids has been successful (Bowman 2009; Saini et al. 2012). The pancreatic fluke, *Eurytrema procyonis*, may cause maldigestion, weight loss and loose stools in foxes, but is rarely reported.

Intestinal nematodes are common in wild canids, but may be particularly detrimental to orphaned pups. *Ancylostoma* and *Uncinaria* hookworms, *Physaloptera* stomach worms, and *Trichuris* whipworms are most common and may cause diarrhea, poor weight gain, and anemia in young animals, but are generally not associated with clinical illness in adults (Davidson et al. 1992; Padilla and Hilton 2015). Coccidia (*Isospora* spp.) are also common in wild canids and may cause rapid onset of diarrhea and death in pups (Dubey 1980; Davidson et al. 1992; Gates et al. 2014). Deworming is essential in the successful rearing of wild canids and should be initiated at four weeks of age, though treatment may begin as early as two weeks of age (Grant 2011). In the authors' experience, sulfamethoxazole/trimethoprim oral suspension has been used in combination with sulfadimethoxine for successful treatment of coccidia, and both ivermectin and albendazole have been used separately for treatment of gastrointestinal parasites. Others recommend routine treatment every 2–3 weeks with pyrantel pamoate or fenbendazole for nematodes and ponazuril for coccidia (Grant 2011; Hays 2014) (see Appendix II: Formulary).

The red fox and coyote are both definitive hosts for *Taenia* spp. and *E. multilocularis*; although neither generally cause clinical illness in adults, both may cause poor weight gain in young (Padilla and Hilton 2015). *Echinococcus* spp. have the zoonotic potential of causing hydatid disease in humans. Importantly, the eggs of these two genera cannot be morphologically distinguished. Praziquantel can be used for treatment.

Ectoparasites

Common ectoparasites associated with the red fox include fleas, ticks, the louse *Felicola vulpis*, the ear mite *Otodectes cynotis*, and the mange mite *Sarcoptes scabiei*. On admission, young foxes should be treated for ectoparasites to prevent transmission to other animals in care. Topical parasitides include selamectin (Revolution®, Pfizer, New York, USA; the cat formulation is used for foxes) to treat mange and ivermectin for most external parasites including mange. See Appendix II: Formulary for additional treatments.

Mange

The most common signs of mange include hyperkeratosis and crusting of the skin, emaciation, dehydration, loss of fur on the tail and extremities, watery eyes, excessive scratching and licking, and a distinct musky odor. A skin scraping can provide definitive diagnosis and differentiate the etiology of fur loss from dermatophytoses, poor nutrition or other causes.

Mange can be very severe in the red fox and is rare in the gray fox. The life cycle is 10–14 days, so even very young animals may be affected. When presented with a fox pup with mange, the extent of damage to the pup will determine the protocol for treatment. If the pup is alert, fairly active, clear-eyed, and the amount of crusty skin is minimal, treatment should begin immediately with an avermectin. If the animal is debilitated, dehydrated, or otherwise weakened, supportive care (especially fluids and appropriate nutrition) should be provided for several days before treating mange.

The mange debris can be removed gently with a light brush or comb or alternatively with a medicated shampoo/bath. The crusty yellowish accumulations that occur at the onset of mange are usually located at the tail and head.

Mange patients should be kept isolated from other patients until at least two negative skin scrapings 10–14 days apart. Treatment should continue until two weeks after a negative skin scrape.

Immature and adult foxes with advanced cases of mange often have underlying concurrent disease and may be candidates for euthanasia if they exhibit the following symptoms: severe dehydration and emaciation; extremities, head, eyes and body covered by extensive thick layer of mange debris; and an inability to stand, react, or focus.

Bacterial Diseases

Several species of *Brucella* have been reported in serosurveys of wild canids, most commonly as a result of scavenging infected fetuses and placentae, or ingesting infected rodents (Davidson and Nettles 2006; Padilla and Hilton 2015). Significant clinical illness has not been reported.

Leptospira antibodies are frequently detected in wild canids (Davidson and Nettles 2006). Little is known regarding illness in wild canids, but infection most likely mimics that in domestic canids, ranging from no signs to severe illness and death. When present, signs in domestic dogs include fever, muscle tenderness, polyuria/polydipsia, vomiting, diarrhea, and icterus (see Chapter 2).

Francisella tularensis, the causative agent of tularemia, has been detected in wild fox and coyote, but little is known regarding clinical signs or the significance for wild canids (McKeever et al. 1958). Experimental infection in red foxes caused anorexia, diarrhea, and labored breathing (Lillie and Francis 1936).

Natural infection with *Neorickettsia helminthoeca*, the causative agent of salmon poisoning transmitted by the intestinal fluke *Nanophyetus salmincola*, is common in red fox and coyote in the northwestern US (Headley et al. 2011; Padilla and Hilton 2015). Disease presents as disseminated lymphadenopathy, diarrhea, and eventual death. Treatment in domestic dogs consists of oxytetracycline or doxycycline for 3–5 days and a single dose of praziquantel to control the flukes (Headley et al. 2011).

Fungal Diseases

Dermatophytosis caused by *Trichophyton mentagrophytes* has been described in wild red foxes (Knudtson et al. 1980). The lesions consist of alopecia and crusty foci, similar to mange. Treatment with griseofulvin was effective.

Viral Diseases

Rabies is of great zoonotic concern in wild canids. Unusual behavior, including lack of fear of humans, aggression, disorientation, circling or unusual diurnal activity, is the key presentation of rabies in foxes (Hanes 1991). See Chapter 2 for more information. Wild canids suffering from rabies and distemper may exhibit many of the same signs including lethargy, emaciation, ataxia, or incoordination, photosensitivity, seizures, nasal discharge, and dyspnea (Hanes 1991; Davidson and Nettles 2006). Diarrhea may also be present in cases of distemper or canine parvovirus (CPV), which need to be distinguished. Coyotes with CPV may present with vomiting, depression, lethargy, fever, anorexia, and/or diarrhea with or without blood.

Distemper is seen most frequently in gray foxes, but regional outbreaks in coyotes may also occur (Deem et al. 2000). Distemper is rare in red foxes. In order to avoid possible cross-transmission of these viruses to other wild or domestic canids, foxes or coyotes suspected of having either canine distemper or parvovirus should be quarantined for a minimum of 30 days, with strict biosecurity and appropriate supportive therapy provided during that time. Because prognosis for full recovery is poor, treatment is prolonged, and risk of transmission is high, euthanasia should be considered for wild canids confirmed to have distemper.

Oral papillomas, most likely caused by a canine papillomavirus, have been reported in coyotes and wolves in Canada and Texas (Trainer et al. 1968; Samuel et al. 1978). These wart-like growths are found on the lips and tongue and may extend into the throat. No effective treatment has been reported, but the lesions most likely resolve with time as do similar lesions in domestic dogs.

Other viral diseases of concern include infectious canine hepatitis (ICH) and pseudorabies. ICH, caused by a canine adenovirus, can cause diarrhea, conjunctivitis and rhinitis, seizures, and disseminated coagulopathies in foxes, coyotes, and wolves, but is rarely reported (Cabasso 1981). Pseudorabies, caused by a herpes virus (Suid herpesvirus 1), has been reported to cause pruritus, anorexia, salivation, and convulsions in both wild and captive foxes (Trainer 1981). Infection is most likely from ingesting infected swine. It is not commonly reported but should be considered as a differential in animals exhibiting pruritus and/or neurological signs.

Vaccination

Vaccination of free-roaming wildlife is a controversial subject, but may be necessary for controlling disease outbreaks in wildlife centers where large numbers of young animals are raised in close proximity to one another. Vaccines and vaccination protocols are addressed in detail in Chapter 7.

Trauma

Traumatic injuries are common causes for presentation of wild canids, especially older juveniles and adults. Vehicular collisions, trap-related injuries, bite wounds from domestic canids and conspecifics, and gunshot wounds account for the majority of trauma cases. See Chapter 11 for more information on wound management.

Collisions with vehicles often result in fractures and degloving injuries, as well as internal injuries (hemorrhage, diaphragmatic hernia, contusions, etc.) common with those seen in domestic canids. Full body radiographs should be performed on any animal struck by a vehicle to assess these possible injuries. Pain medications used in domestic canids are appropriate for use in wild canids with traumatic injuries.

Wild canids with trap-related injuries may have had the traps removed in the field by the finder or may present with the trap still on the limb. In the latter case, the animal should be assessed quickly and sedated prior to trap removal as the trapped animal is usually frightened and in pain. Sedation also allows for more thorough evaluation and treatment of injuries after the trap is removed. Common injuries related to both padded and unpadded leg-hold traps include skin laceration, edema, hemorrhage, tendon, and ligament laceration, bone fractures, and joint luxations (Englund 1982; Olsen et al. 1986). Such compression injuries may result in ischemic injuries and subsequent loss of the limb distal to the trap location. Self-mutilation, before or after trap removal, may occur so the affected limb may need extended monitoring. Furthermore, canids with trapping injuries should also be examined closely for dental injuries, as most will incur tooth fractures and/or gingival lacerations from chewing at the traps (Englund 1982).

Release Conditioning and Considerations

Red and Gray Fox

The young leave the den in late summer or early fall, following the natural depletion of food in the natal area, and allowing time for juveniles to locate and establish a territory that can support them through the winter. The practitioner must consider the availability of natural local food items and attempt to provide similar items in preparation for release.

As foxes mature, key behavioral mannerisms indicate readiness for release. As one approaches the cage, the fox should run to hide. Fox-like body language and behaviors indicating maturity include food caching or burying, digging holes, alertness to approaching sounds, displaying food envy to siblings (bared teeth with ears back), placing the backside and tail toward peers, elevating tail and moving hindquarters while eating, growling or yipping, and successfully killing and consuming assorted prey.

Coyote

In the wild, pups usually leave the den at the onset of fall. Release of a coyote is dependent on a variety of criteria including age, health, psychological maturity, and ability to hunt, kill, and cache. In addition, the coyote must show avoidance, distrust or fear of humans, as demonstrated by running and hiding, seeking cover, and lowering the head and pulling the front lip back when approached by humans. These skills signal the viability of release.

Release

The actual release occurs rapidly; soft release methods are not applicable. When returned to the wild, the rehabilitated coyote or fox will usually bolt immediately from the transport carrier although some may linger briefly.

Red and Gray Fox

It is best to release a fox in preferred habitat (meadows and fields, with woods nearby) that can support the animal. Avoid an area inhabited by coyotes as they prey on foxes, especially the young, and compete for similar food sources (Farias et al. 2006; Henry 1996a). A site with ample supplies of food and water is preferable, as is a site distant from humans and their recreational areas, where hunting and trapping may occur. When possible, release in sync with the fox's circadian rhythm: early morning, late afternoon or dusk.

Coyote

Releasing a captive-raised coyote into an area already occupied by another coyote can be dangerous and potentially fatal to the incoming animal. Identify an appropriate environment based on the preferred habitat, food supply, water, and distance from humans, livestock, and pets. Coyotes may be transported to the release site in an extra-large pet carrier with a large sheet draped over the outside to reduce stress.

Acknowledgement

The authors would like to thank Yvonne Wallace Blane for her assistance with reviewing and editing various stages of this chapter.

References

Beckoff, M. (2001). *Coyotes: Biology, Behaviors, and Management*. Caldwell, NJ: Blackburn Press.

Bowman, D.D. (2009). *Georgis' Parasitology for Veterinarians*, 9e. St Louis, MO: Elsevier Saunders.

Cabasso, V.J. (1981). Infectious canine hepatitis. In: *Infectious Diseases of Wild Mammals*, 2e (ed. J.W. Davis, L.H. Karstad and D.O. Trainer), 191–195. Ames, IA: Iowa State Press.

Chitwood, M.C., Swingen, M.B., and Lashley, M.A. (2015). Parasitology and serology of free-ranging coyotes (*Canis latrans*) in North Carolina. *Journal of Wildlife Diseases* 51 (3): 664–669.

Davidson, W.R. and Nettles, V.F. (2006). *Field Manual of Wildlife Diseases in the Southeastern United States*, 3e. Athens, GA: Southeastern Wildlife Disease Cooperative Study.

Davidson, W.R., Appel, M.J., Doster, G.L. et al. (1992). Diseases and parasites of red foxes, gray foxes, and coyotes from commercial sources selling to fox-chasing enclosures. *Journal of Wildlife Diseases* 28 (4): 581–589.

Davis, W.B. & Schmidly, D.J. (1994). Common gray fox. *The Mammals of Texas*. www.nsrl.ttu.edu/tmot1/uroccine.htm.

Deem, S., Spelman, L., Yates, R., and Montali, R. (2000). Canine distemper in terrestrial carnivores: a review. *Journal of Zoo and Wildlife Medicine* 13 (4): 441–451.

Dubey, J.P. (1980). Coyote as a final host for *Sarcocystis* species of goats, sheep, cattle, elk, bison, and moose in Montana. *American Journal of Veterinary Research* 41 (8): 1227–1229.

Englund, J. (1982). A comparison of injuries to leg-hold trapped and foot-snared red foxes. *Journal of Wildlife Management* 46 (4): 1113–1117.

Farias, V., Fuller, T., Wayne, R., and Sauvajot, R. (2006). Survival and cause-specific mortality of gray foxes (*Urocyon cinereoargenteus*) in southern California. *Journal of Zoology* 266: 249–254.

Gates, M., Gerhold, R.W., Wilkes, R.P. et al. (2014). Parasitology, virology, and serology of free-ranging coyotes (*Canis latrans*) from central Georgia, USA. *Journal of Wildlife Diseases* 50 (4): 896–901.

Gingerich, P.D. and Winkler, D.A. (1979). Patterns of variation and correlation in the dentition of the red fox, *Vulpes vulpes*. *Journal of Mammalogy*. 60 (4): 691–704.

Gosselink, T., Piccolo, K., van Deelen, T. et al. (2010). Natal dispersal and philopatry of red foxes in urban and agricultural areas of Illinois. *Journal of Wildlife Management* 74: 1204–1217.

Grady, W. (1994). *The World of the Coyote*. San Francisco, CA: Sierra Club Books.

Grambo, R. (1994). *The World of the Fox*. Vancouver, BC: Sierra Club Books.

Grant, K. (2011). Hand-rearing gray fox (*Urocyon cinereoargenteus*). *Wildlife Rehabilitation Bulletin* 29 (2): 19–32.

Hanes, P.C. (1991). Red fox (*Vulpes vulpes fulva*) and gray fox (*Urocyon cinereoargenteus*). *Wildlife Journal* 14 (2): 9–16.

Hays, D.L. (2014). Raising coyotes: not your average pup. *Wildlife Rehabilitation Bulletin* 32 (1): 1–8.

Headley, S.A., Scorpio, D.G., Vidotto, O., and Dumler, J.S. (2011). *Neorickettsia helminthoeca* and salmon poisoning disease: a review. *Veterinary Journal* 187: 165–173.

Henry, J.D. (1993). *How To Spot a Fox*. Shelburne, VT: Chapter Publishing.

Henry, J.D. (1996a). *Living on the Edge: Foxes*. Minocqua, WI: Northwood Press.

Henry, J.D. (1996b). *Red Fox: The Catlike Canine*. Washington, DC: Smithsonian Institution Press.

Jackson, H. (1961). *Mammals of Wisconsin*. Madison, WI: University of Wisconsin Press.

Knudtson, W.U., Gates, C.E., Ruthleanor, G.K. et al. (1980). *Trichophyton mentagrophytes* dermatophytosis in wild fox. *Journal of Wildlife Diseases* 16 (4): 465–468.

Lesmeister, D., Nielsen, C., Schauber, E., and Hellgren, E. (2015). Spatial and temporal structure of a mesocarnivore guild in midwestern North America. *Wildlife Monographs* 191: 1–61.

Lillie, R.D. and Francis, E. (1936). The pathology of tularemia. *National Institute of Health Bulletin* 167: 1–217.

MacDonald, D.W. (2000). *Foxes*. Stillwater, MN: Voyageur Press.

Maher, M. (2002). Aging Coyotes Using Dental Characteristics. Masters Theses. Paper 1510. https://thekeep.eiu.edu/theses/1510/

McKeever, S., Schubert, J.H., Moody, M.D. et al. (1958). Natural occurrence of tularemia in marsupials, carnivores, lagomorphs, and large rodents in southwestern Georgia and northwestern Florida. *Journal of Infectious Diseases* 103 (2): 120–126.

Miller, E.A. (2012). *Minimum Standards for Wildlife Rehabilitation*, 4e. St Cloud, MN: National Wildlife Rehabilitators Association.

Miller, E.A. (ed.) (2007). *Quick Reference*, 3e. National Wildlife Rehabilitation Association: St Cloud, MN.

Munoz-Igualada, J., Shivik, J., Dominguez, F. et al. (2008). Evaluation of cage-traps and cable restraint devices to capture red foxes in Spain. *Journal of Wildlife Management* 72 (3): 830–836.

Nelson, T.A., Gregory, D.G., and Laursen, J.R. (2003). Canine heartworms in coyotes in Illinois. *Journal of Wildlife Diseases.* 39 (3): 593–599.

Olsen, G.H., Linhart, S.B., Holmes, R.A. et al. (1986). Injuries to coyotes caught in padded and unpadded steel foothold traps. *Wildlife Society Bulletin* 14 (3): 219–222.

Padilla, L.R. and Hilton, C.D. (2015). Canidae. In: *Fowler's Zoo and Wild Animal Medicine*, vol. 8 (ed. R.E. Miller and M.E. Fowler), 457–467. St Louis, MO: Elsevier Saunders.

Saini, N., Ranjan, R.L., Singla, L.D. et al. (2012). Successful treatment of pulmonary paragonimiasis in a German shepherd dog with fenbendazole. *Journal of Parasitic Diseases* 36 (2): 171–174.

Samuel, W.M., Chalmers, G.A., and Gunson, J.R. (1978). Oral papillomatosis in coyotes (*Canis latrans*) and wolves (*Canis lupus*) of Alberta. *Journal of Wildlife Diseases* 14 (2): 165–169.

Samuel, W.M., Pybus, M.J., and Kocan, A.A. (eds.) (2008). *Parasitic Diseases of Wild Mammals*, 2e. Ames, IA.: Iowa State University Press.

Saunders, D.A. (1988). *Adirondack Mammals*. Syracuse, NY: State University of New York, College of Environmental Science and Forestry.

Storm, G., Andrews, R., Phillips, R. et al. (1976). Morphology, reproduction, dispersal, and mortality of midwestern red fox. *Wildlife Monographs* 49: 3–82.

Stuht, J.N. and Youatt, W.G. (1972). Heartworms and lung flukes from red foxes in Michigan. *Journal of Wildlife Management* 36 (1): 166–170.

Szuma, E. (1997). Partial eruption of teeth in the red fox *Vulpes vulpes*. *Acta Theriologica* 42: 253–258.

Trainer, D.O. (1981). Pseudorabies. In: *Infectious Diseases of Wild Mammals*, 2e (ed. J.W. Davis, L.H. Karstad and D.O. Trainer), 102–107. Ames, IA: Iowa State Press.

Trainer, D.O., Knowlton, F.F., and Karstad, L.H. (1968). Oral papillomatosis in the coyote. *Bulletin of the Wildlife Disease Association* 4: 52–54.

Wilkinson, T. (1995). *Track of the Coyote*. Minocqua, WI: Northland Press.

25

Natural History and Medical Management of Ursids

Dave McRuer[1] and Helen Ingraham[2]

[1] *Parks Canada Agency, Charlottetown, PEI, Canada*
[2] *Veterinary Emergency & Critical Care, Las Vegas, NV, USA*

Introduction

There are eight recognized species of bears worldwide, of which three, the American black bear (*Ursus americanus*), the brown bear, including the Grizzly bear (*Ursus arctos*), and the polar bear (*Ursus maritimus*), are native to North America. The American black bear (hereafter referred to as black bear) has the largest range of the three species and can be found in all Canadian provinces and territories except Prince Edward Island, in Alaska and 40 of the 48 contiguous United States, and in mountainous areas of northern Mexico. Black bears are the most likely species to present for rehabilitation in North America due to their abundance and distribution compared to the limited range of brown bears (Canada: British Columbia, Alberta, Yukon, Northwest Territories, Nunavut, Manitoba; United States: Alaska, Idaho, Wyoming, Montana, Washington) and polar bears (Canada: Yukon, Northwest Territories, Nunavut, Manitoba, Ontario, Quebec, Newfoundland, and Labrador; United States: Alaska). This chapter will focus entirely on black bears and practitioners are encouraged to consult with brown bear and polar bears experts if working with these species.

It is important to recognize the long-term goal before initiating treatment. Black bears that are destined to become part of a permanent zoo or sanctuary collection will have access to ongoing medical and supportive care and therefore may be able to achieve an adequate quality of life despite compromised form or function. Wild bears destined for release must meet established minimum criteria to give them the best opportunity to survive (Miller 2012).

Before working with wild bears, veterinarians should ensure that state laws permit veterinary care and rehabilitation. In many states, there are designated black bear rehabilitation facilities that have experience and approved protocols, equipment, and enclosures. State wildlife agencies will be able to provide this information and often assist with capture, transfer, and release of black bears. Coordinating with these agencies for release is especially important as knowledge of local bear populations, habitat quality, and sites of potential human conflict must be considered.

Black bears may present for veterinary care throughout the year. However, they may enter dormancy as cold weather approaches and are less likely to be injured or orphaned at that time. Bears may require veterinary and rehabilitation assistance for a variety of reasons. The most common causes of admission include orphaning, regulated and nonregulated hunting, weather events, vehicular collisions, dog interactions, and nuisance events (Beecham 2006). In addition, younger cubs and yearlings may also present after abandonment or emaciation as a result of food shortage or as a result of inappropriate human possession.

General Natural History

There are 16 recognized subspecies of black bear in North America and while most are black with brown muzzles, several color morphs exist including brown, cinnamon, blonde, and creamy white or bluish-gray (Wilson and Reeder 2005). The average lifespan of a black bear is 3–5 years for males and 5–8 years for females; however, the occasional animal will survive to 15–20 years in the wild (Pelton 1982).

American black bears are sexually dimorphic. The average weight range for adult males is 60–140 kg, whereas adult females typically weigh 40–70 kg. Occasionally adult males may exceed 250–300 kg (Pelton 1982). Sows are seasonally monoestrus and are induced ovulators. Mating occurs during the summer months but through the process of delayed implantation, the fertilized egg lies

Medical Management of Wildlife Species: A Guide for Practitioners, First Edition. Edited by Sonia M. Hernandez, Heather W. Barron, Erica A. Miller, Roberto F. Aguilar and Michael J. Yabsley.

dormant in the uterus until the fall when it implants in the uterine wall. At northern latitudes, sows will begin to den during the late fall or early winter and will stay in the same location for 5–7 months unless disturbed. Bears in the southern United States may be active throughout the year. One to six cubs (average 2–3) weighing approximately 200–450 g are born in January or early February. The eyes are initially closed and open around day 25 (Nowak 1999). The sows and cubs emerge from the den in April or May when the cubs weigh approximately 2–5 kg.

Black bears are members of the Carnivora, but are essentially omnivorous and the diet varies by season and habitat type. Early spring diet might typically consist of tender leaves and shoots and deciduous mast (e.g., acorns, walnuts, hickory nuts) from the previous fall. During the summer and autumn, bears consume fruit and nuts which make up the vast proportion of their diet. They will eat a variety of insects, fish, frogs, small rodents and rabbits, fawns, bird's eggs, and carrion but these represent only a small part of their diet (Nowak 1999).

It is important to understand black bear defensive behavior before working with this species. Defensive behaviors are reactions to stress and may be directed toward humans or other bears if the overt reaction distance is breached (Herrero et al. 2005). If room allows, black bears will choose to run from stressful situations but if they feel cornered, they may exhibit both physical and auditory defensive behaviors (Herrero et al. 2011). Physical defensive behaviors may include swatting at the ground with one or both paws, bluff charges that stop just short of contact, slow and deliberate approaches, and clacking of the teeth by opening and closing the jaws. Auditory defensive noises include huffing, snorting, gurgling, and loud growling. These behaviors are often observed in wild black bears held in captivity and caution is necessary when procedures need to be performed (Jordan 1976; Eager and Pelton 1979; Herrero 1983).

Captive Management

Safety

Due to their strength and size, handling and restraint of black bears often require special equipment, chemical immobilization, and training. Bears use their teeth and claws to defend themselves and have extremely powerful jaw muscles. While clumsy in appearance, bears can be fast and agile and one should always be aware of a bear's location and behavior when working in close proximity (Fowler 1995).

It is important to establish safety protocols before capturing and working with bears. All equipment required for a procedure should be prepared prior to capture (stretcher, blanket, nets, etc.) and all personnel should wear protective clothing, including coveralls, leather gloves, and proper footwear (Convy 2002). It is recommended to always wear a primary layer of latex or vinyl gloves when working with any wildlife regardless of any other protective gloves worn. The handler is advised to wear heavy gloves to prevent puncture wounds but crushing injuries are still possible. Bears of all ages can be unpredictable and there should be at least two people for any procedure that requires capture and restraint (Convy 2002).

Handling

Short procedures like physical examinations on cubs under 7.5 kg may be performed without chemical immobilization or gas anesthesia. However, sedation is required for all lengthy procedures, on fractious bears, or on bears over 7.5 kg.

Young cubs that weigh <7.5 kg can be restrained manually by scruffing the skin over the shoulders and securing the body by wrapping them in a blanket like a burrito with the head sticking out one end. If sedation is necessary, isoflurane inhalant anesthesia via mask is usually adequate with or without subsequent intubation. Cubs undergoing lengthy anesthetic procedures require general supportive care and supplemental crystalloid fluids (lactated Ringer's solution or Normasol-R [Abbott Laboratories, Abbott Park, IL, USA] with 2.5% dextrose) given at 10 mL/kg/h (Papageorgiou et al. 2002). Catheters may be placed in the cephalic, femoral, or jugular veins to facilitate fluid therapy or given as a subcutaneous bolus between the shoulders for shorter procedures. Cubs that weigh between 7.5 and 18 kg can usually be restrained using a strong net or rabies catchpole within the enclosure or carrier and then hand injected with a sedative through the grates with a syringe, syringe pole, or dart gun. Chemical immobilization will be discussed in a subsequent section.

Once the cub is sedated, it should be supported with oxygen or isoflurane inhalant anesthesia via facemask or intubation to maintain the depth of anesthesia. Juvenile and adult bears over 18 kg require chemical immobilization under the supervision of a veterinarian. Bears presenting after a vehicular collision may be unconscious and thus not stable enough for general anesthesia or chemical immobilization. These bears should be examined in a secured room by experienced staff with a veterinarian prepared to chemically immobilize the animal should it regain consciousness (Convy 2002).

A physical examination should be performed shortly after admission, usually on sedated, stable bears. The examination is similar to that performed on a domestic dog. However, the clinician should check for injuries

Table 25.1 Aging black bears by dentition.[a]

Age	
Cub of the year (<10 mo)	No permanent teeth. All incisors on bottom jaw have not erupted, "puppy" canines are present
Yearling	All permanent teeth are present, canines are not fully grown. Small space between upper canine and upper third incisor
2 years	All permanent teeth are present, canines are fully grown. Increasing space between upper canine and upper third incisor as bear ages and head lengthens, no wear on incisors
2–4 years	Begin to see minor wear on upper incisor cusps but the 1st and 2nd upper incisors are not rounded or flat and no dentin is showing
4–7 years	1st and 2nd upper incisors are rounded to flat and there is exposed dentin, no wear on upper canines
7–15 years	Moderate wear and staining on all teeth
16+	All teeth show extreme wear and staining. Two or more canines are broken and/or worn smooth

Source: LeCount (1986), Beausoleil and Lackey (2015), and Sajecki (2016).

[a] Black bear dental formula: I3/3, C1/1, PM 2–4/2–4, M 2/3 = 34–42.

associated with trauma and exposure, which are two of the most common reasons for admission. Common diagnostics performed during the examination include venipuncture for a complete blood cell count (CBC) and serum biochemistry, radiographs (including dental films if warranted), fecal and urine examination, and skin scrapes for ectoparasites. The most common sites for venipuncture are the femoral and jugular veins. Bears can be aged through dentition (Table 25.1 and Figure 25.1).

Housing

Bears that are <12 weeks old may be housed in a large airline kennel, preferably one that locks (e.g., Zinger® Aluminum Dog Crates, Zinger Winger Inc., Niagara Falls, NY, USA). The kennel should be lined with soft blankets to simulate a den and supplemental heat may need to be initially provided by placing a heating board or pad under half of the crate or having a heat lamp placed outside the kennel but shining inside over half of the space. It is important to provide a heat gradient within the kennel to allow the cub to thermoregulate on its own.

Bear cubs should initially be housed indoors in a room away from other animals and have minimal human contact. Visual barriers should be erected between the kennel and human caretakers, cleaning and feeding should be done as quickly as possible, eye contact should be avoided, and human voices should be kept to a minimum in order to decrease human exposure and interaction. While black bear cubs are dependent on their caretakers at this age, excessive human interaction may lead to habituation, rendering them nonreleasable (Convy 2002). For this reason, bear cubs should never be raised alone. Efforts should be made to place solo bear cubs with conspecifics close in size. Introductions should be done slowly over a 24–48-hour period in a manner that allows the cubs to see and smell each other prior to allowing direct contact. In the author's experience, bear cubs of different sizes are rarely aggressive to one another, although rough play may give this appearance. If housing two bear cubs together is not possible (not available, one requires extensive medical care, etc.), providing a large stuffed toy (especially ones that have "beating hearts") similar in appearance to a bear may help decrease habituation and decrease psychological stress on a solo cub.

It is recommended that cubs larger than infants but still not weaned be housed in a minimum space of 3′ W × 6′ L × 3′ H. After the cubs are weaned from the bottle, they should be moved outside into an enclosure at least 20′ W × 36′ L × 16′ H (Miller 2012). As most veterinary facilities lack such an enclosure, it is important to research appropriate rehabilitation facilities permitted to accept bear cubs as early as possible. Appropriate housing for older juvenile and adult bears is beyond scope of this chapter and readers are referred to Convy (2002) and Papageorgiou et al. (2002).

Diets

Black bears are omnivores, with most of their diet consisting of natural vegetation (~75%) supplemented with insects, honey, small to medium sized mammals or fish, and occasional scavenging on carcasses. Bear milk contains high concentrations of protein, fat, and minerals but low concentrations of carbohydrates. Milk from American black bears consists of approximately 44.5% total solids, 24.5% fat, 0.4% lactose, 8.8% casein, 5.7% whey protein, 1.8% ash, 0.41% calcium, and 0.28% phosphorus (Jenness et al. 1972).

Many milk formulas have been used successfully to rear infant bear cubs but in most cases success is based on stable health, weight gain, and absence of gastrointestinal issues rather than objective research. Most bear rehabilitators use commercial formulas but it is possible to formulate an appropriate diet using products commonly found in small animal practice or local agricultural stores (Table 25.2).

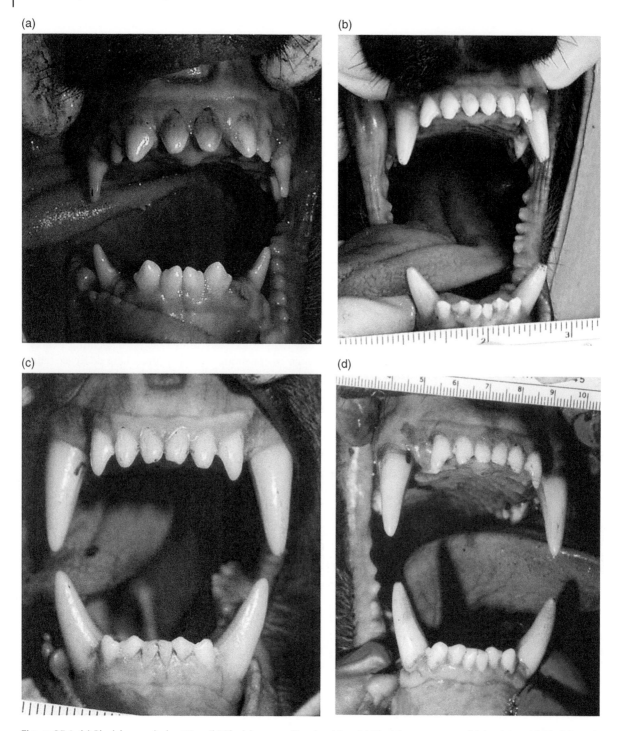

Figure 25.1 (a) Black bear cub dentition. (b) Black bear yearling dentition. (c) Black bear two year old dentition. (d) Black bear four year old dentition. (e) Black bear five year old dentition. (f) Black bear six year old dentition. (g) Black bear seven year old dentition. (h) Black bear eight–ten year old dentition. (i) Black bear 12 year old dentition. *Source* (a–i): Reproduced with permission from Sajecki (2016).

Multiple methods of introducing milk formulas to infant cubs have been used but it is universally agreed that the first "meal" or all meals served on the first day consist of a hypertonic (high dextrose content) oral rehydrating/electrolyte solution (~600 mOsm/kg).

Following rehydration, some bear care facilities choose to start feeding full-strength formula while others gradually increase the percentage of formula to rehydrating solution in stepwise daily increments (e.g., day 1 – rehydrating solution; day 2 – two-thirds rehydrating

(e)

(f)

(g)

(h)

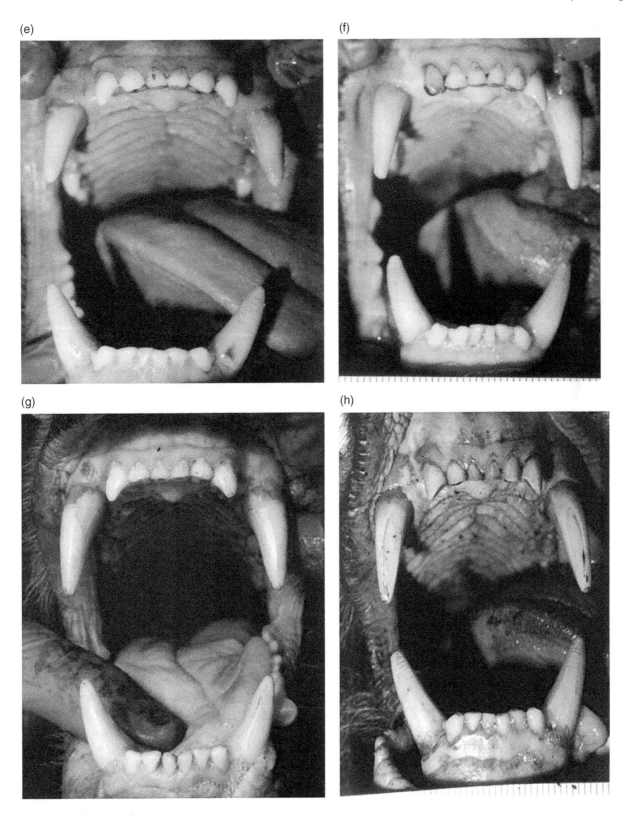

Figure 25.1 (Continued)

(i)

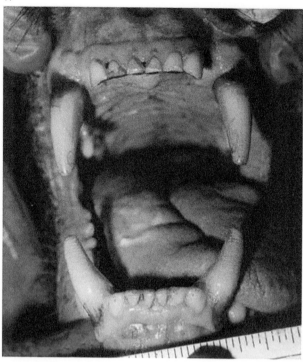

Figure 25.1 (Continued)

Table 25.2 Infant black bear diets used successfully during rehabilitation.

Diet source	Ingredients and mixing instructions
Fox Valley (2016)	Two parts Fox Valley 30/50® milk powder to three parts warm water
Maughan (2014)	Mix 75% Multi-Milk® (PetAg) powder and 25% Esbilac (PetAg) powder. Mix one part powder to two parts water
Beecham (2006)	Make puppy milk replacer powder and water as directed. Add 1 tbsp plain yogurt, 1 tsp multivitamin powder, and 1 tsp vegetable oil
Convy (2002)	One part Esbilac powder to two parts water

solution, one-third formula; day 3 – one-third rehydrating solution, two-thirds formula; day 4 – 100% formula) (Convy 2002).

Bear cubs that present with their eyes still closed need to be bottle fed (Figure 25.2). Each infant cub may have a different preference for nipple shape, bottle color, or feeding position and it is important to stick to a routine once it is determined how a cub feeds best (Beecham 2006). Commercial nipples to try include different shaped human nipples, calf nipples, and lamb nipples. It is important that the nipple opening not be too large as this may lead to aspiration. In addition, feeding too quickly may lead to

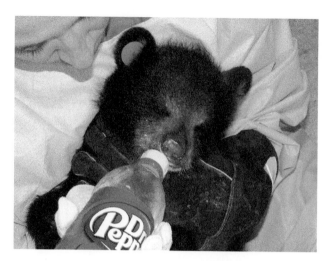

Figure 25.2 Bottle feeding a black bear cub. A selection of artificial nipples may need to be tried to determine individual cub preferences.

displaced suckling on ears and other body parts as sucking behavior is genetically driven. While it is important to limit human contact time with bear cubs, spending too little time feeding cubs less than eight weeks of age may lead to dependence on the caregiver and subsequent separation anxiety (Beecham 2006).

The amount of food offered at each meal depends on the cub's weight and its stomach capacity. In order to compensate for growth, cubs should be fed 2–3 times the basal metabolic rate (BMR) on a daily basis where:

$$BMR = (K) \times (\text{body weight in kg})^{0.75}$$
$$\text{where } K = 70 \text{ for placental mammals}$$

The volume of food delivered at each meal is approximately 10% of the bear's body weight divided into 2–6 feedings per day depending on age: roughly 100 mL/kg body weight (Papageorgiou et al. 2002).

It is preferable to switch from bottle feeding to feeding from a bowl shortly after the cub's eyes open (~25 days) in order to decrease human interaction (Figure 25.3). Some bears take to this transition quickly while others may need to be directed and redirected to the bowl until they learn to drink. Bowls should be fastened securely to the floor or wall as cubs are messy eaters and will easily tip the contents, decreasing the amount of food available. Try to feed older cubs directly from bowls on presentation, resorting to bottles only if they cannot figure it out. Once the cub is eating, slowing try to transition it to a bowl for meals. If more than one cub is being housed together, each should have its own bowl. Once cubs are bowl feeding, they should be housed in a larger enclosure, preferably one connected to a separate enclosure so that they can be safely shifted to allow cleaning and food delivery (Convy 2002).

Captive weaning occurs far faster than in wild conditions which take place between six and eight months of age

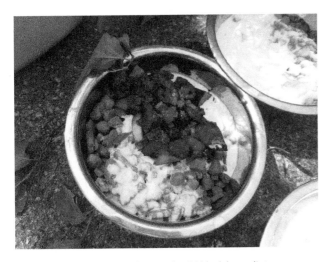

Figure 25.3 Appropriate six-month-old black bear diet.

Table 25.3 Feeding guide for black bear cubs.

Age	Food items
Newborn to 10 weeks	Infant formula via baby bottle and nipple
25+ days	Bear mush and formula, mixed together – dish feed
10–12 weeks	Formula and bear mush, mixed together, include a few fruits – dish feed
14 weeks	Fruits, soaked puppy chow, and natural vegetation are introduced
18 weeks	Hard puppy chow and omnivore diet are introduced, natural vegetation, fruits
6 months	Weaned diet: Mazuri® Omnivore diet, a good-quality puppy chow, mealworms, fruits, fish, berries, and natural vegetation

Source: Reprinted from Convy (2002) with permission from NWRA.

(Nowak 1999). Once the cub is consistently lapping milk from a bowl, "bear mush" can be added to the formula to make it thicker. Bear mush consists of one half cup of ground, kibbled puppy chow, one half cup of baby cereal, one tablespoon of Esbilac® powder (PetAg, Hampshire, IL, USA), mixed with one cup of warm water to give it the consistency of oatmeal. Three tablespoons of cottage cheese are mixed in to create the final product (Convy 2002). As the cubs age, bear mush replaces formula, fruit and soaked puppy kibble are added to the diet, and by six months the diet is made of a good-quality puppy chow, fruits, garden vegetables, natural vegetation, insects, berries, and fish (Table 25.3).

Enrichment

Environmental enrichment is particularly important for captive bears. Cubs housed together will play and wrestle, which is necessary to develop appropriate social behaviors. As soon as cubs can be moved to a larger space, climbing features such as logs, hammocks, and straw bales should be added to allow for natural behaviors. Toys that can be sterilized, including bowling balls and large Kong® balls (Long Company, Golden CO, USA), can be added to the enclosure in a rotating schedule to ensure there is always something novel to investigate. When bears are on a solid diet, puppy kibble, insects, fruits, and other food items can be hidden in the enclosure to create foraging opportunities that will be necessary once released. Food enrichment can also take the form of novel food presentation including fruits frozen in large blocks of ice or melons hung from ropes in the enclosure (Figure 25.4).

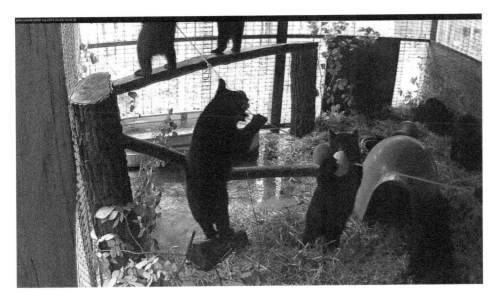

Figure 25.4 An enrichment program should be established for captive black bears that includes novel food presentation.

Preventive Medicine

Annual preventive medicine protocols are normally restricted to bears held in zoos and sanctuaries and are beyond the scope of this chapter. Few vaccines are recommended for captive bears but routine anthelmintics may be necessary for ascarid infections, and facilities in heartworm-endemic areas may consider testing and prevention.

Clinical Techniques

Common diagnostic procedures for bears include a through physical exam (Figure 25.5), CBCs, serum biochemistry, radiographs (including dental films if warranted), fecal and urine examination, skin scrapes, ultrasound, etc (Figure 25.6). The jugular and cephalic veins are most

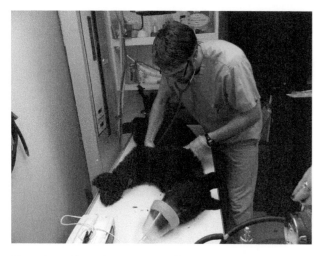

Figure 25.5 Physical examination of a black bear cub.

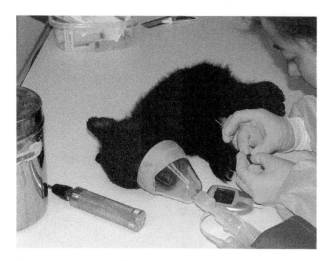

Figure 25.6 A range of diagnostic tests, similar to canine medicine, may be performed on black bears.

commonly used for venipuncture and the femoral may be used to obtain large volumes of blood (Collins 2015).

Few pharmacokinetic studies have been performed on bears and those that exist tend to focus on immobilization drugs (White et al. 1996; Wolfe et al. 2008; Ryan et al. 2009). As such, drugs and dosages are typically extrapolated from domestic dogs and delivered by similar routes of administration.

The placement of intramuscular injections, including darts, may vary by the time of year. During the late fall and winter, bears develop a thick layer of fat over their hindquarters which may prevent injection into the muscle and interfere with drug metabolism. During these times of year, the practitioner should administer intramuscular injections in the shoulder or neck.

Medical Conditions

Hypoglycemia, hypothermia, and emaciation/poor condition secondary to starvation and exposure are common findings in cubs separated from the sow. Supportive care should be initiated immediately and include nutritional, thermal, and fluid support.

In suspected hypoglycemia, the practitioner should consider obtaining a blood glucose (BG) sample during the initial physical examination. If the BG is determined to be low (in small animal medicine, hypoglycemia is typically considered to be a BG of <60 g/dL), serial BGs should be obtained until values are consistently above normal. It should be noted that in dogs with hemodilution or hemoconcentration, point-of-care glucometers are inaccurate compared to clinical laboratory biochemical analyzers (Lane et al. 2015). The same may hold true for bears.

It is not uncommon to have emaciated bears present in the spring in need of supportive care. These are typically yearlings or subadults which have not acquired enough food the previous fall, usually due to abandonment, injury, inability to acquire food, or mast failure (hard mast: acorns and wild nuts; soft mast: berries, fruit). Typically, these bears have a good prognosis but need to be given supportive care and slow reintroduction to calories.

Refeeding syndrome describes multiple metabolic disturbances that occur during the reinstatement of nutrition in malnourished or starved patients if calories are introduced too quickly (Lippo and Byers 2008). The hallmark and most significant biochemical change of this syndrome is hypophosphatemia which may result in hemolytic anemia. Multiple other concurrent biochemical imbalances may be present.

Clinical signs of refeeding syndrome, as documented in domestic animals, may include lethargy, anorexia, weight loss, weakness, nausea, vomiting, diarrhea, pigmenturia, restlessness, seizures, coma, and death. Serum biochemistry abnormalities can include hypophosphatemia, hypokalemia, hypomagnesemia, hyperglycemia, hyperbilirubinemia, hypoproteinemia, and possibly elevated liver enzymes. CBC abnormalities may include anemia, Heinz bodies in cats, and possible spherocytosis in dogs (Lippo and Byers 2008).

The practitioner should extrapolate refeeding protocols from domestic animal medicine since bear-specific research has not been conducted. Initial food introduction should be delivered slowly and at a fraction of the calculated resting energy requirements (RERs). Alimentation should be started at 25–30% of calculated RER for the first 24 hours and then slowly increased over 3–5 days until RERs are met. Routes of alimentation may include oral, enteral, and parenteral (Lippo and Byers 2008).

Calculations for the RER are as follows:

Weight 3–25 kg:
$$(30 \times \text{current body weight in kg}) + 70 = \text{kcal/day}$$

Weight < 3 kg or > 25 kg:
$$70 \times (\text{current body weight in kg})^{0.75} = \text{kcal/day}$$

Depending on the patient's biochemical abnormalities, other initial treatments may include supplementation of phosphate, potassium, magnesium, thiamine, blood transfusions, and insulin therapy (Lippo and Byers 2008)

Patient monitoring should include monitoring the body weight and body condition daily, packed cell volume (PCV) for evidence of anemia, and serum for evidence of hemolysis in animals with hypophosphatemia. Serum phosphate, glucose, potassium, and magnesium levels should be obtained at least daily during the initial five days of the refeeding period. These should be obtained more frequently in patients receiving potassium, magnesium, or insulin supplementation. For patients receiving IV phosphates, serum phosphorus and serum calcium levels should be obtained every 6–12 hours. Food intake or administration of nutritional support should be reviewed at least once daily (Lippo and Byers 2008).

Infectious Diseases

Black bears are an important keystone species and as such can serve as important sentinels for environmental health. Healthy bears rarely succumb to disease or parasites and diagnostic efforts and serosurveys may provide valuable information on regional pathogen and parasite exposure and potential zoonotic diseases (Dunbar et al. 1998; Chambers et al. 2012; Bronson et al. 2014).

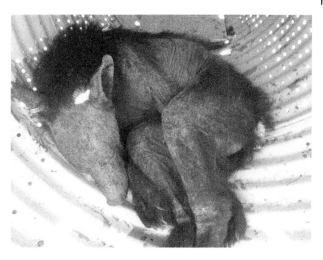

Figure 25.7 Sarcoptic mange (*Sarcoptes scabiei*) and audycoptic mange (*Ursicoptes americanus*) may be diagnosed in black bears and may present as localized to full-body alopecia. Courtesy of Pennsylvania Game Commission.

Ectoparasites rarely cause pathological effects in black bears, the exception being mites (Yunker et al. 1980). Sarcoptic mange (*Sarcoptes scabiei*), audycoptic mange (*Ursicoptes americanus*), and demodectic mange (*Demodex ursi*) may be common depending on region and result in a variety of skin conditions, including alopecia, crusting and/or thickening of the skin, pustular dermatitis, and pruritus (Figure 25.7). Sarcoptic mange may be treated with ivermectin or one of its derivatives. The recommended treatment of audycoptic mange is amitraz (as a spray or sponge-on dip) since ivermectin treatment does not appear to be efficacious (Collins 2015).

Over 30 species of endoparasites have been reported from black bears (Zimmerman and Mitchell 2006). *Baylisascaris transfuga* and *Dirofilaria ursi* are ubiquitous and common in black bears (Pence et al. 1983). Although *B. transfuga* has never been reported to cause larva migrans in humans, unlike the closely related *B. procyonis* (see Chapters 2 and 21), experimental studies indicate larval migrans can occur in mice (Papini et al. 1996), gerbils (Sato et al. 2004), and guinea pigs (Matoff and Komandarev 1965) and natural infection occurred in a colony of Japanese macaques (*Macaca fuscata fuscata*) housed next to a black bear enclosure in a zoo (Sato et al. 2005).

Although most endoparasitic infections are asymptomatic, treatment may be considered in a captive setting where stress and immunosuppression may lead to shedding and environmental contamination. Fenbendazole (50 mg/kg PO for three consecutive days) is usually effective (Ramsay 2003; Collins 2015). Importantly, *Baylisascaris* ova can remain infective for several years in the environment and are not destroyed by routine disinfection and cleaning (Collins 2015).

Historically, black bears were shown to produce antibodies against canine distemper, yet were thought not to develop clinical disease (Deem et al. 2000). However, several recent reports of clinical canine distemper cases have now surfaced and clinicians should consider it as a differential diagnosis when bears present with neurological signs, hyperkeratotic foot pads or other clinical signs commonly noted in canids (Cottrell et al. 2013).

Noninfectious Diseases

Similar to domestic animals, bears can be affected by toxins. Clinical signs may be toxin and dose dependent and practitioners are encouraged to obtain a thorough history and perform diagnostic tests if safe and appropriate. In most cases, the cause of the toxicity cannot be determined antemortem.

Nutritional secondary hyperparathyroidism (NSH) is a concern in young cubs fed an inappropriate diet for a prolonged period of time, sometimes by the rescuer. Inappropriate diets are typically deficient in calcium (Ca), most often all-meat diets or improperly formulated milk. It is crucial for the practitioner to closely observe the patient's gait and/or posture on presentation for signs of lameness, reluctance to move, uncoordinated gait, sternal recumbency, painful mastication, and loose teeth. Pathological fractures can be present in any affected animal and are most frequently observed in the long bones (Towell 2010).

Radiographs may be helpful in diagnosing NSH and findings may include folding (greenstick) fractures, compression fractures of cancellous bone (vertebrae and epiphyses), wide medullary cavities, thin cortices, and normal height of growth plates with relatively white metaphyseal borders (Nap and Hazewinkel 1994; Aithal et al. 1999). Alternative differentials include inborn errors of metabolism such as mucopolysaccharidosis and osteogenesis imperfecta, neither of which have been reported in bears.

Clinical pathology values have not yet been established for bears affected with NSH. In domestic dogs with NSH, the total calcium (Ca) concentration is usually within normal limits (but the ionized calcium is low) and increases in serum calcitriol and parathyroid hormone may be detected (Nap and Hazewinkel 1994).

There is no standard treatment for NSH in bear cubs and therapeutic options should be extrapolated from small animal medicine and/or select zoo medicine cases. Following supportive care, the bear should be offered a complete and balanced diet, especially with regard to Ca and phosphorus (P). As in growing puppies, the absolute amount of calcium is likely more important than the Ca:P ratio. The diet should provide 0.8–1.2% dry matter Ca and the Ca:P should be kept within physiological

limits (1.1:1 to 2:1). In 3–4 weeks, improved mineralization of the skeleton should be apparent on radiographs. During this time, the patient should have its activity strictly restricted in order to prevent pathological fractures. Calcium may be supplemented as calcium carbonate or calcium lactate (but not Ca phosphate or bone meal) at 50 mg Ca/kg body weight which may help to accelerate osteoid mineralization. Euthanasia should be considered when multiple fractures are present, joints in the limbs show signs of permanent conformational changes, or if vertebral fractures are present.

Chemical Immobilization

Chemical immobilization is typically required before handling bears in order to reduce the risk of human injury. Ultra-potent opioids (e.g., carfentanil) are commonly used on bear species in zoos and in field research but they are beyond the scope of this chapter as most private practitioners have neither access nor training to use these drugs.

A thorough history should be taken prior to any anesthetic event. Bears are often brought to veterinarians by wildlife biologists and may already have been chemically immobilized. It is important to ask which immobilization drugs were used in order to best interpret physiological responses (e.g., temperature, heart rate, involuntary reactions) and plan for continued anesthesia.

Prior to any immobilization event, it is essential for the practitioner to be prepared for all aspects of the procedure and anesthetic emergencies. This includes having a well-stocked immobilization kit with emergency, supplemental, and reversal drugs calculated, if not already drawn up. Try to limit the number of people associated with the procedure and make sure everyone knows their roles in advance in order to expedite the process.

It is important to try to isolate bears from their conspecifics prior to chemical immobilization. Bears are monogastrics and therefore prone to vomiting during induction and regurgitating during anesthesia. Recommended food and water fasting time for healthy bears is approximately 12 hours (Collins 2015). Ideally, a bear is immobilized in an enclosure with no access to climbing structures and is clinically stable prior to immobilization. Estimating the weight may be necessary if the bear has never been handled or it has not been immobilized recently. If the bear was presented by a biologist, ask if they obtained a recent weight. With experience, practitioners will be become better at estimating weights (Lecount 1986; Beausoleil and Lackey 2015).

Methods of administering immobilization drugs include hand injection, pole syringing, blow darting, and darting pistols/rifles. Hand injection and pole syringing have the advantage of being low cost but only small drug volumes can be used and the bear must be within close proximity, usually through an opening in the enclosure. Blow pipes and pistols/rifles require specific darts but have the advantage of remote delivery. However, they are more expensive and care must be taken not to project the dart with too much power which can cause severe injuries. Blow darting and darting rifles require training and technical expertise. Regardless of method, the injection should be delivered in the neck or shoulder region for reasons discussed earlier.

Once the bear has been anesthetized, vital signs should be carefully monitored for depth of anesthesia and patient health. The body temperature, heart rate, and respiratory rate differ throughout the year based on activity and environmental stressors. Normal heart rate may be as low as 20 beats per minute (bpm) during hibernation and as high as 90 bpm during peak summer activity. When stressed by the presence of humans, the adult heart rate may rise to as high as 250 bpm (Laske et al. 2011). Temperature, heart rate, and respiratory rate are also influenced by the type of drugs used for chemical immobilization. Bears administered tiletamine-zolazepam (Telazol®, Zoetis, Parsippany, NJ, USA; Zoletil®, Virbac, Fort Worth, TX, USA) will normally maintain the heart rate between 70 and 90 bpm and the body temperature will drop over time. The heart rate of bears given a combination of either xylazine-zolazepam-tiletamine or medetomindine-zolazepam-tiletamine ranges between 50 and 70 bpm and the body temperature tends to increase. Bradycardia (30–40 bpm) is often observed in medetomindine-ketamine immobilizations. Bears do not usually exhibit hypoxemia while sedated. A pulse oximeter can be placed on the tongue and if the hemoglobin saturation drops below 85%, a nasal catheter can be inserted and oxygen flow delivered to achieve 95–98% saturation. Recommended flow rates depend on body size: 0.5 L/min to bears up to 25 kg, 1 L/min to bears 25–100 kg, 2 L/min to bears 100–200 kg, and 3 L/min to bears 200–250 kg (Caulkett 2014). Rectal temperatures should be monitored throughout anesthesia. If body temperatures reach more than 41 °C, alpha-agonists should be reversed.

A variety of drugs, dosages, and combinations have been successfully used to immobilize black bears. Most drug combinations consist of a combination of a dissociative agent and an alpha-2 agonist or benzodiazepine (Collins 2015).

The combination of tiletamine and zolazepam is commonly used for bear anesthesia. This combination has the advantage of being more potent, on a milligram-per-kilogram basis, than ketamine and is available in powder form. This combination can provide effective doses in small volumes since it may be reconstituted with variable quantities of diluents or another immobilization agent. Flumazenil used to reverse the effects of zolazepam may aid in reducing the recovery time from anesthesia.

Xylazine and medetomidine are commonly used as alpha-2 agonists in combination with a dissociative agent (usually ketamine) for immobilizing bears to achieve a reliable state of analgesia. Advantages of using these two alpha-2 agonists include that they are nonnarcotic drugs that are commercially available in concentrated forms, they are reversible with yohimbine, tolazoline, or atipamezole, and medetomidine is 10% more potent than xylazine and has a higher alpha-2 agonist receptor affinity that produces sedation and analgesia. Spontaneous muscle contractions and partial arousal may be seen in some bears sedated with medetomidine.

Ketamine (at a dosage of 2.2 mg/kg, intramuscularly [IM]) may be used to supplement any immobilization combination if anesthesia time needs to be prolonged (Collins 2015). Alternatively, inhalant gas anesthesia can be used via intubation or mask to supplement chemical immobilization. A portable inhalant anesthetic machine is convenient for work outside the clinic.

Common Surgical Conditions

Trauma is a frequent finding on physical exam and surgical intervention is often required. Skin abrasions and lacerations, fractured bones, broken teeth, and damage to internal organs are common injuries in bears.

Before initiating treatment, the practitioner should first determine whether the injury or the treatment may result in the patient being nonreleasable and thus euthanasia should be considered if no permanent placement is possible. It is also important to consider postoperative management when deciding the best surgical method. Surgical techniques that require daily management are not usually practical as frequent sedation or chemical immobilization is not in the patient's best interest.

Skin lacerations requiring closure should be repaired using subcutaneous and subcuticular patterns with absorbable suture to limit postoperative management. Try to minimize shaving around the wound, especially in the late fall and winter, to reduce the loss of body heat. Drains may be required, but are generally only tolerated by young cubs and an Elizabethan collar may be necessary.

Fractures require a full orthopedic examination followed by radiographs to determine the most effective means of stabilization and repair. Like most procedures in bears, sedation is required for the evaluation. While the same surgical techniques used in domestic small animal medicine can be used, the practitioner should note that stabilization and fixation devices may not be tolerated depending on age. Soft bandages and splints may be quickly destroyed once the bear regains strength. Fiberglass casts work well in nondisplaced fractures of the long bones in cubs <6 months of age. External skeletal fixators should be avoided in bears >6 months old as they will quickly be removed by the patient. Internal fixation is the preferred choice for orthopedic injuries and intramedullary pins (single or stacked), Kirschner wires, interlocking nails, orthopedic wire, and bone plates may be used as they are in small animal medicine. If the hardware cannot be removed once healed, permission from the state or provincial bear biologist may be needed prior to release since bears may be hunted and consumed. This conversation is best carried out prior to surgery.

Dental pathology is common in bears and may include fractured teeth, darkly discolored teeth secondary to dental trauma, excessively worn teeth, and periodontal disease (Collins 2015). While in captivity, bears can develop dental pathology secondary to fighting with conspecifics and/or compulsively chewing on enclosure bars. An exposed pulp cavity must be promptly repaired to prevent ascending infection to the tooth apex which may result in tooth root abscesses and alveolar osteomyelitis. When possible, the tooth structure should be maintained through endodontic treatments rather than tooth extraction. Bear canines, premolars, and molars are large and difficult to extract and a veterinary dentist should be consulted (Figure 25.8).

Rectal prolapse is usually associated with trauma or secondary to enteritis or endoparasitism, although it may result from any condition that causes tenesmus (Hedlund and Fossum 2007). In black bear patients, it is most commonly seen after vehicular collision. It is important to differentiate between a rectal prolapse and ileocolic intussusception. An intussusception is diagnosed if a finger can be inserted alongside the prolapsed mass. This is not possible with a rectal prolapse where a fornix can be identified along the outer surface. Rectal prolapses can be incomplete or complete. An incomplete prolapse involves only the mucosa. A complete prolapse involves the entire circumference and all layers of the

rectal wall. The amount of rectal eversion can vary from a few millimeters to several centimeters depending on the presence of continued straining. Continued exposure of the prolapse can lead to excoriation, bleeding, desiccation, and, eventually, necrosis.

Rectal prolapses should be treated promptly to prevent the everted tissue from becoming more edematous and more difficult to reduce. This also prevents any further trauma being inflicted to the area. The prognosis and treatment depend on the cause, chronicity, and degree of prolapse. Acute rectal prolapses can be easily treated but chronic prolapses may require resection.

If the prolapse is determined to be acute (minimal tissue trauma), the clinician should promptly digitally reduce the prolapse and place a purse-string suture around the anus. This procedure should be performed under heavy sedation or general anesthesia depending on the attitude of the bear. Before reduction is attempted, the area should be copiously lavaged with warm saline and lubricated with a water-soluble gel. The purse-string suture should be tight enough to keep the area reduced but still allow passage of soft stool. An appropriately sized syringe (according to the size of the patient) can be inserted into the rectum prior to tying off the purse-string suture. This technique may prevent the clinician from tying off too tightly.

Postoperative care includes close monitoring for recurrence and self-trauma (consider placing an Elizabethan collar on younger cubs), correcting the cause of the prolapse (essential in order to prevent reoccurrence), feeding a low-fiber diet while the purse-string suture is in place, and limiting stressful situations for the patient. The purse-string suture is generally removed 3–5 days after reduction. Complications of manual reduction include hematochezia, dyschezia, tenesmus, and recurrence. If a prolapse is determined to be chronic (severely traumatized) or nonreducible, a resection is warranted. This procedure is outside the scope of this chapter. Please refer to a small animal surgery book and consider contacting a small animal surgeon.

When selecting any medication for a bear, the practitioner should consider the route of delivery and duration of effect. Unlike domestic animal medicine where you can restrain the patient for injections or pill delivery, medium to large sized bears cannot be handled without sedation or excessive stress or contact. Depot injections and medications that can reliably administered in the food or in a treat should be utilized wherever possible.

Release

As for any wild animal undergoing medical care or rehabilitation, established criteria should be met before contemplating release (Miller 2012). Specific considerations

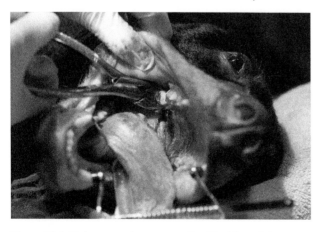

Figure 25.8 Molar extraction on a yearling black bear. Pain associated with this dead tooth resulted in severe emaciation which resolved shortly after surgery.

for bears include age, weight, time of year, and local hunting seasons (drug withdrawal times).

Black bears are a game species and drug withdrawal time needs to be considered if the intended release date falls within the legal hunting season. In order to protect humans from adverse reactions, the practitioner may extrapolate drug withdrawal times as they do not exist for bears (Cattet 2003; WAFWA 2010). The bear should be held until either the withdrawal period has expired or the hunting season has ended. If this is not possible, the bear should be clearly tagged/marked with a unique identification number and an appropriate notification warning. State/provincial wildlife officials should be involved in release decisions.

In the wild, bear cubs stay with the sow for 1.5–2 years before dispersing and living a largely solitary life. This duration may not be possible or practical in captive situations due to cost, available space, or increased human interaction. Bears are generally "hard released," meaning they are brought to a remote area with suitable habitat and released without ongoing support (Figure 25.9). Adult and juvenile bears may be released throughout the year as soon as their injuries heal. Bear cubs may be released in the spring/summer of their first year, the fall/winter of the first year, or in the spring following birth and each has its advantages and disadvantages.

Early releases have the advantage of decreased human contact time and fewer resources allocated to rehabilitation but are likely associated with a lower survival rate as the cubs may or may not be able to fend for themselves. Fall/winter releases are done by placing cubs into artificial dens and allowing them to hibernate for the rest of the winter to emerge naturally in the spring when there is often little human presence in the forest. These releases can be difficult logistically and often involve repeat sedation, once for initial transport and another to be placed in the artificial den. Spring releases after a year in captivity are most common as the cubs are large enough to naturally fend for themselves and survival is thought to be highest. The disadvantage includes increased human

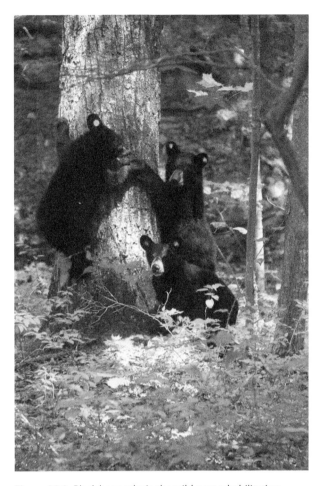

Figure 25.9 Black bear cubs in the wild post rehabilitation.

contact, especially after they awaken from captivity in the spring, and increased monetary and space resources throughout rehabilitation (Beecham 2006). Cubs found in the first 2–3 months following birth may be successfully placed in an active den with a surrogate sow. This is the best of all possible options for young cubs and emphasizes the importance of establishing a relationship with local bear biologists who may know of active dens.

References

Aithal, H., Singh, G., Kinjavdekar, P., and Setia, H. (1999). Fractures secondary to nutritional bone disease in dogs: a review of 38 cases. *Journal of Veterinary Medicine Series A* 46: 483–487.

Beausoleil, R. A. & Lackey, C. (2015). Responding to Human-Bear Conflict and Capture-Handling of Black Bears: A Field Techniques Guide for Agency Bear Biologists and Officers. www.bearbiology.org/wp-content/uploads/2018/09/agency_bear_manual_version-3.0_final-print-copy.pdf

Beecham, P. J. (2006). Orphan Bear Cubs: Rehabilitation and Release Guidelines. www.bearrehab.org/WSPA.pdf

Bronson, E., Spiker, H., and Driscoll, C.P. (2014). Serosurvey for selected pathogens in free-ranging American black bears (*Ursus americanus*) in Maryland, USA. *Journal of Wildlife Diseases* 50: 829–836.

Cattet, M. R. L. (2003). A CCWHC Technical Bulletin: Drug Residues in Wild Meat – Addressing A Public Health Concern. Canadian Cooperative Wildlife Health Centre: Newsletters & Publications. https://

digitalcommons.unl.edu/cgi/viewcontent.cgi?article=1045&context=icwdmccwhcnews

Caulkett, N.A. (2014). Ursids (bears). In: *Zoo Animal and Wildlife Immobilization and Anesthesia*, 2e (ed. G. West, D. Heard and N.A. Caulkett). Ames, IA: Wiley.

Chambers, D.L., Ulrey, W.A., Guthrie, J.M. et al. (2012). Seroprevalence of toxoplasma gondii from free-ranging black bears (*Ursus americanus*) from Florida. *Journal of Parasitology* 98: 674–675.

Collins, D.M. (2015). Ursidae. In: *Zoo and Wild Animal Medicine*, 8e (ed. R.E. Miller and M.E. Fowler). St Louis, MO: Elsevier Saunders.

Convy, J. (2002). Rehabilitation of black bear cubs. *Wildlife Rehabilitation Bulletin* 20: 16–43.

Cottrell, W.O., Keel, M.K., Brooks, J.W. et al. (2013). First report of clinical disease associated with canine distemper virus infection in a wild black bear (*Ursus americana*). *Journal of Wildlife Diseases* 49 (4): 1024–1027.

Deem, S.L., Spelman, L.H., Yates, R.A., and Montali, R.J. (2000). Canine distemper in terrestrial carnivores: a review. *Journal of Zoo and Wildlife Medicine* 31 (4): 441–451.

Dunbar, M.R., Cunningham, M.W., and Roof, J.C. (1998). Seroprevalence of selected disease agents from free-ranging black bears in Florida. *Journal of Wildlife Diseases* 34: 612–619.

Eager, J.T. and Pelton, M.R. (1979). *Panhandler Black Bears in the Great Smoky Mountains National Park*. Graduate Program in Ecology, University of Tennessee.

Fowler, M.E. (1995). *Restraint and Handling of Wild and Domestic Animals*. Ames, IA: Iowa State University Press.

Fox Valley 2016. www.mcssl.com/store/17128612/milk-replacers

Hedlund, C.S. and Fossum, T.W. (2007). Surgery of the perineum, rectum, and anus. In: *Small Animal Surgery*, 3e (ed. T.W. Fossum), 498–507. St Louis, MO: Mosby Elsevier.

Herrero, S. (1983). Social behaviour of black bears at a garbage dump in Jasper National Park. *Bears: Their Biology and Management* 54–70.

Herrero, S., Smith, T., Debruyn, T.D. et al. (2005). From the field: brown bear habituation to people – safety, risks, and benefits. *Wildlife Society Bulletin* 33: 362–373.

Herrero, S., Higgins, A., Cardoza, J.E. et al. (2011). Fatal attacks by American black bear on people: 1900–2009. *Journal of Wildlife Management* 75: 596–603.

Jenness, R., Erickson, A.W., and Craighead, J.J. (1972). Some comparative aspects of milk from four species of bears. *Journal of Mammalogy* 34–47.

Jordan, R. (1976). Threat behavior of the black bear (*Ursus americanus*). In: *Third International Conference on Bear Research and Management* (ed. M.R. Pelton, J.W. Lentfer

and G.E. Folk). Morges, Switzerland: International Union for the Conservation of Nature.

Lane, S.L., Koenig, A., and Brainard, B.M. (2015). Formulation and validation of a predictive model to correct blood glucose concentrations obtained with a veterinary point-of-care glucometer in hemodiluted and hemoconcentrated canine blood samples. *Journal of the American Veterinary Medical Association* 246: 307–312.

Laske, T.G., Garshelis, D.L., and Iaizzo, P.A. (2011). Monitoring the wild black bear's reaction to human and environmental stressors. *BMC Physiology* 11: 13.

Lecount, A. (1986). *Black Bear Field Guide: A Manager's Manual*. Phoenix, AZ: Research Branch, Arizona Game and Fish Department.

Lippo, N. and Byers, C.G. (2008). Hypophosphatemia and refeeding syndrome. *Standards of Care* 10: 6–10.

Matoff, K. and Komandarev, S. (1965). Comparative studies on the migration of the larvae of Toxascaris leonina and Toxascaris transfuga. *Parasitology Research* 25: 538–555.

Maughan, S. (2014). *Black Bear Rehabilitation Handbook*. Garden City, ID: Idaho Black Bear Rehabilitation, Inc.

Miller, E.A. (ed.) (2012). *Minimum Standards for Wildlife Rehabilitation*. St Cloud, MN: National Wildlife Rehabilitators Association.

Nap, R. and Hazewinkel, H. (1994). Growth and skeletal development in the dog in relation to nutrition; a review. *Veterinary Quarterly* 16: 50–59.

Nowak, R.M. (1999). *Walker's Mammals of the World*. Baltimore, MD: Johns Hopkins University Press.

Papageorgiou, S., Deghetto, D., and Convy, J. (2002). Black bear cubs. In: *Hand-Rearing Wild and Domestic Mammals* (ed. L.J. Gage). Ames, IA: Iowa State University Press.

Papini, R., Renzoni, G., Piccolo, S.L., and Casarosa, L. (1996). Ocular larva migrans and histopathological lesions in mice experimentally infected with Baylisascaris transfuga embryonated eggs. *Veterinary Parasitology* 61: 315–320.

Pelton, M.R. (1982). Black bear. In: *Wild Mammals of North America: Biology Management and Economics* (ed. J.A. Chapman and G.A. Feldhammer), 504–514. Baltimore, MD: Johns Hopkins University Press.

Pence, D.B., Crum, J.M., and Conti, J.A. (1983). Ecological analyses of helminth populations in the black bear, *Ursus americanus*, from North America. *Journal of Parasitology* 69: 933–950.

Ramsay, E.C. (2003). Ursidae and Hyaenidae. In: *Zoo and Wild Animal Medicine*, 5e (ed. M.E. Fowler and R.E. Miller). St Louis, MO: Saunders.

Ryan, C.W., Vaughan, M.R., Meldrum, J.B. et al. (2009). Retention time of telazol in black bears. *Journal of Wildlife Management* 73: 210–213.

Sajecki, J. (2016). Bear biologist, Virginia Department of Game and Inland Fisheries.

Sato, H., Matsuo, K., Osanai, A. et al. (2004). Larva migrans by *Baylisascaris transfuga*: fatal neurological diseases in Mongolian jirds, but not in mice. *Journal of Parasitology* 90: 774–781.

Sato, H., Une, Y., Kawakami, S. et al. (2005). Fatal Baylisascaris larva migrans in a colony of Japanese macaques kept by a safari-style zoo in Japan. *Journal of Parasitology* 91: 716–719.

Towell, T.L. (2010). Nutrition-related skeletal disorders. In: *Textbook of Veterinary Internal Medicine: Diseases of the Dog and Cat*, 7e (ed. S.J. Ettinger and E.C. Feldman). St Louis, MO: Saunders Elsevier.

WAFWA. (2010). A Model Protocol of Purchase, Distribution, and Use of Pharmaceuticals in Wildlife. Western Association of Fish and Wildlife Agencies, Wildlife Health Committee. www.wafwa.org/Documents% 20and%20Settings/37/Site%20Documents/Committees/ Wildlife%20Health/docs/WWHCDrugPrtc2010.pdf

White, T.H. Jr., Oli, M.K., Leopold, B.D. et al. (1996). Field evaluation of Telazol® and ketamine-xylazine for immobilizing black bears. *Wildlife Society Bulletin* 24: 521–527.

Wilson, D.E. and Reeder, D.M. (2005). *Mammal Species of the World: A Taxonomic and Geographic Reference*. Baltimore, MD: Johns Hopkins University Press.

Wolfe, L.L., Goshorn, C.T., and Baruch-Mordo, S. (2008). Immobilization of black bears (*Ursus americanus*) with a combination of butorphanol, azaperone, and medetomidine. *Journal of Wildlife Diseases* 44: 748–752.

Yunker, C., Binninger, C., Keirans, J. et al. (1980). Clinical mange of the black bear, *Ursus americanus*, associated with *Ursicoptes americanus* (Acari: Audycoptidae). *Journal of Wildlife Diseases* 16: 347–356.

Zimmerman, D. and Mitchell, M.A. (2006). Infectious diseases of north American black bears (*Ursus americanus*): parasites (part 2). *Wildlife Rehabilitation Bulletin* 24: 10.

26

Natural History and Medical Management of Felids

Emphasis on Bobcats

Bethany Groves and John R. Huckabee

PAWS Wildlife Center, Lynnwood, WA, USA

Natural History

Population Range

North America is home to seven native species of the family Felidae, three of which regularly inhabit the United States and Canada in significant numbers: bobcat (*Lynx rufus*), Canada lynx (*Lynx canadensis*), and cougar (*Puma concolor*). Cougars are also referred to as mountain lions or pumas, and include the endangered subspecies Florida panther (*Puma concolor coryi*). The other four species of North American felid are rarely, if ever, seen north of the US–Mexico border. The ocelot (*Leopardus pardalis*) maintains a small population in south Texas limited to roughly 80–120 individuals, with occasional sightings in Arizona (Sunquist and Sunquist 2002); their range stretches through eastern Mexico and lies primarily in Central and South America. Historically, the northern ranges of the jaguarundi (*Puma yagouaroundi*), jaguar (*Panthera onca*), and margay (*Leopardus wiedii*) also extended from Mexico into the southern US. This chapter will focus primarily on the bobcat with some information on the Canada lynx and cougar.

There are an estimated one million bobcats in North America, making them the most common and widely distributed species of native felid on the continent. Thirteen subspecies range from southern Canada through Mexico. Bobcats are found throughout the contiguous United States, although they maintain a very limited range in the midwestern states (Tesky 1995a). Habitat varies widely from forests and swamps to deserts and scrublands. Named for its short "bobbed" tail, the bobcat is easily distinguished from its northern relative, the Canada lynx, by its smaller size, shorter ear tufts (tufts typically exceed 5 cm in length on lynx), more prominent coat markings, and a black ring around the tail.

The Canada lynx remains more geographically restricted to northern Canada and Alaska, where it is specially adapted for the deep snow. Lynx typically have larger, more heavily furred paws than bobcats to provide better footing in deep snow. Their tail tip appears "dipped" in black as opposed to ringed.

While once as widespread as the bobcat, the cougar has been eliminated from over two-thirds of its original North American range and is now primarily limited to west of the Rocky Mountains and southward into Mexico. More recent reports of populations rebounding in the western US have been debated due to questions regarding methods of population and viability assessment. The Florida panther subspecies, once distributed throughout the southeastern US, is now estimated to be between 120 and 230 individuals isolated to southwestern Florida (https://myfwc.com/wildlifehabitats/wildlife/panther/).

Size and Lifespan

Body weight of the bobcat can be variable, ranging from 5 to 14 kg (9–40 lbs) (Banfield 1987); size tends to increase with latitude and elevation (Sikes and Kennedy 1992). The Canada lynx weighs in similarly at 6–14 kg (14–31 lbs) (Quinn and Parker 1987). Cougars are the largest of North American felids, with males (toms) weighing an average of 63–82 kg (140–180 lbs) and females weighing roughly 25% less (https://myfwc.com/wildlifehabitats/wildlife/panther/). In all species, males tend to be larger than females (queens) and gender confirmation is easily performed on physical exam based on appearance of external genitalia.

An average lifespan of bobcats in the wild is 2–5 years (Tesky 1995a), with a maximum reported of 12 years. A record of 32 years has been reported in captivity. Aging of bobcats and lynx under 1 year of age is possible based

Medical Management of Wildlife Species: A Guide for Practitioners, First Edition. Edited by Sonia M. Hernandez, Heather W. Barron, Erica A. Miller, Roberto F. Aguilar and Michael J. Yabsley.
© 2020 John Wiley & Sons, Inc. Published 2020 by John Wiley & Sons, Inc.

on tooth eruption patterns and is very similar to that for the domestic cat (*Felis catus*). Deciduous incisors begin erupting at 11–14 days of age, and all deciduous teeth are in by 40–60 days. Permanent teeth erupt between 120 and 240 days, with canine teeth erupting between 160 and 190 days. Crowe (1975) describes methods of aging by dentition and cementum annulum data.

The bobcat is an obligate carnivore. The diet may vary geographically and seasonally, but primarily consists of lagomorphs and rodents or other small mammals, birds, and even deer. The crepuscular lifestyle of the bobcat may also vary depending on factors including availability of prey, favoring a more nocturnal lifestyle in some areas during the spring. This adaptability in diet is believed to contribute to the bobcat's success in maintaining an expansive geographic range. Areas of intensive agriculture tend to deter the bobcat; predation of livestock is uncommon (McCord and Cardoza 1982). The Canada lynx, in comparison, is a "specialist predator" highly dependent on the snowshoe hare as its prey source. This specific predator–prey relationship results in a well-documented 9–11-year cycle of the lynx population directly following that of the hare (O'Donoghue et al. 1997). The cougar, like the bobcat, shows adaptability in diet dependent on geographic location and seasonality but tends to rely on ungulates as its primary prey source. Deer, elk, moose, and bighorn sheep are common targets although porcupine, beaver, hares, and rodents, as well as livestock, may also be consumed (Tesky 1995b).

Reproduction

The bobcat is a polygamous species with females reaching sexual maturity at 1 year of age and males at 2 years; both remain sexually reproductive throughout life. Females are seasonally polyestrous. Mating is variable based upon geographic location and possibly prey availability but typically occurs January through March. Kittens are typically born in late spring but reports exist of births in every month of the year, and in rare cases a queen may give birth to a second litter in September (Anderson 1987; Rolley 1987). Average litter size is 2–3 kittens but may be as large as five.

Compared to other felids, large gaps exist in the knowledge of estrous cycles and age of sexual maturity in the Canada lynx. Sexual maturity in females is reported as early as 9 months of age although more typically occurs in the second year of life (Ulev 2007). Breeding appears to be highly seasonal, taking place in late February to early April with a litter size of 1–6 kittens born between May and July (Poole 2003). Also unique to the lynx, a positive correlation has been demonstrated between snowshoe hare abundance and conception and birth rates, as well as average litter size and kitten survival

(Ruggiero et al. 2000; Poole 2003). It has been hypothesized that female lynx convert between spontaneous and induced ovulation dependent upon snowshoe hare density at the time of breeding season (Ruggiero et al. 2000).

Cougars, similar to bobcats, are polygamous and seasonally polyestrous, capable of breeding and producing successful litters in every month of the year (Chapman and Feldhamer 1982); peak numbers occur in summer. If a female loses her kittens, she may breed again shortly after (Hansen 1992). Sexual maturity is attained at 2–3 years of age. Females born during summer may enter their first breeding season in the winter following their second birthday. Females often do not breed until they have established a territory (Hansen 1992). Litter size may range from one to six with a first litter often limited to just one kitten (Tesky 1995b).

In all three felid species, kittens typically open their eyes at 2 weeks of age and wean at around 8 weeks. Female cougars may begin taking their kittens to kills at around this age (Hansen 1992), while bobcats begin to travel with the mother starting at around 3–5 months of age. In the case of bobcats and lynx, kittens stay with the mother until late fall or winter and must learn to hunt before dispersal. In northern latitudes, kittens may stay with the mother until the following spring (Tesky 1995a). While cougars can reportedly survive on their own as young as 6 months of age, they typically remain with the mother for the first 1–2 years. Siblings may stay together for several months following dispersal from the mother (Tesky 1995b).

Husbandry

Behavior assessment should be done continuously, and steps taken to keep felids wild and afraid of humans, including minimizing human contact to prevent habituation or inappropriate socialization. Kittens' eyes open at 10–14 days of age. By 4–6 weeks, they have developed a sense of fear and display defensive posturing, appropriate hissing, and vocalizing. This behavior is important for normal development and should not be discouraged; if it does not fully develop, ultimate survival may be compromised (Figure 26.1).

Providing an external heat source may be necessary until the kittens' eyes are open and they are old enough to thermoregulate. Using small blankets, fleece, or towels in their hide box or den will help to keep them warm. Towels or textiles that will unravel or have holes should not be used as entanglement and linear foreign body ingestion are common.

Healthy infant and juvenile bobcats should be housed with siblings or peer conspecifics when possible, and have access to both indoor and outdoor enclosures once

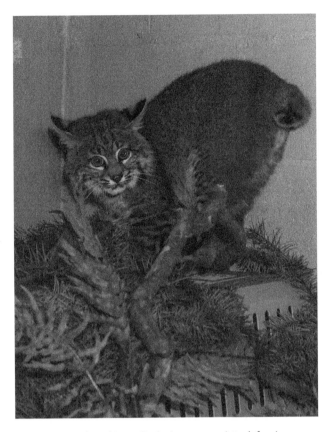

Figure 26.1 Bobcat kitten displaying appropriate defensive behavior toward humans. Note characteristic ear and tail markings. *Source:* Courtesy of PAWS Wildlife Center.

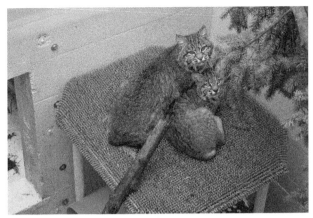

Figure 26.2 Two unrelated orphans housed together during rehabilitation, following appropriate quarantine, health screening, and vaccination. This pair was eventually released together. *Source:* Courtesy of PAWS Wildlife Center.

able to thermoregulate and ambulate (Figure 26.2). All domestic species, especially dogs, should not be housed with or allowed to socialize with bobcats of any age, as habituation will likely adversely affect survival. Subadult and adult bobcats are naturally solitary and fiercely territorial (Wack 2003); they should be housed individually and isolated from conspecifics and other species.

At least two shallow, freshwater sources should be provided as bobcats will often use one for defecation and urination. All logs and other cage furniture should be secured to prevent injury, and climbing logs, other substrates, and shallow water sources gradually added until the kittens are well coordinated and unlikely to drown or fall. Due to the extended periods of captive care, providing appropriate enrichment in addition to basic cage furniture can help prevent boredom and develop necessary survival skills.

Handling, Restraint, and Clinical Techniques

General principles regarding monitoring and management of anesthesia in domestic cats may be applied across species. During the anesthesia or immobilization

period, administration of fluids and maintaining normal blood pressure will reduce recovery time (Wack 2003).

Appropriate personal protective equipment (PPE) and safety procedures should always be employed and each facility should develop specific protocols for restraint and handling (Huckabee 2009). In addition to recognizing the inherent capabilities for bobcats to cause serious injury when defending themselves, their status as rabies vector species (RVS) throughout North America should be considered and appropriate precautions taken to prevent inadvertent scratch and bite exposure, including when they are fully immobilized or being necropsied.

Manual Handling and Restraint Techniques

Avoid handling whenever possible. When kittens must be physically handled, minimize the procedure time and avoid petting or any positive reinforcement associated with humans. Minimize or eliminate talking and other abnormal auditory stimuli, utilize solid/opaque visual barriers, and provide hide boxes or dens. Any bobcat that does not display fear and avoidance of humans should not be released.

When bobcats must be physically handled, the means of restraint largely depends on the age, size, condition, and presenting problems. Wild felid kittens develop the sharp teeth and claws, strong jaws, and rapid reflexes characteristic of their respective species very early.

General principles of handling and restraint are similar for all species of felid. All but the very youngest kittens (<2 weeks old) must be handled with an abundance of caution given the capability of a dangerous bite and retractable claws. Adult cougars, in particular, are capable of causing human fatality.

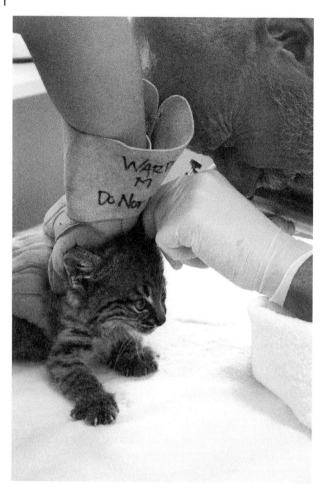

Figure 26.3 Manual restraint of bobcat kitten for physical exam. *Source:* Courtesy of PAWS Wildlife Center.

Bobcat kittens weighing under 1 kg can generally be restrained by scruffing and securing the hindlimbs, analogous to the restraint of a domestic cat (Figure 26.3). The eyes should be covered and noise should be eliminated to reduce stress from external stimuli. Kittens approaching 1 kg may require a blanket and Kevlar/leather gloves for capture and restraint. Special attention must be paid to preventing hyperthermia. A thorough physical exam and other veterinary procedures in kittens weighing over 1–2 kg are often more safely performed under chemical immobilization.

Operant conditioning is used in many zoos and sanctuaries to enable less stressful handling of their captive felines; however, in a rehabilitation setting this type of conditioning and behavioral modification may negatively affect ultimate release and survival success.

Ideally, facilities used for raising and rehabilitating bobcats for release are designed with effective visual and auditory barriers to prevent habituation and inappropriate socialization of the kittens through shifting between cages and enclosures without physical restraint or handling. Design can facilitate animal shifting via a series of guillotine/sliding doors or gates that can be activated remotely to prevent direct visual association with handlers. Though squeeze cages can also be effectively employed, they must be used cautiously to prevent panic and injury (Wack 2003).

Chemical Restraint

Juvenile bobcat and lynx may be captured with a net and briefly pinned down with a blanket for hand-injection of an appropriate anesthetic. If available, a squeeze cage is preferred for drug delivery in larger cats but must be used with appropriate caution. Use of pole syringes has been associated with fractured teeth. Remote drug delivery via blowgun is an excellent option but depends on the experience level of the operator. Use of other darting equipment (e.g., CO_2 pistol, rifle) is generally reserved for larger felids, such as cougar, as the delivery impact may cause significant soft tissue trauma in animals less than 10 kg.

Current drug protocols used to safely achieve chemical immobilization in wild felid species tend to include ketamine combined with an alpha-2 agonist. One study evaluated efficacy and physiological impact of ketamine and xylazine compared to ketamine, medetomidine, and butorphanol in field immobilization of bobcats for brief nonsurgical procedures (Rockhill et al. 2011). Both were found to be safe and reliable although the latter combination achieved a shorter recovery and drug processing time. Combinations of ketamine and xylazine or ketamine and medetomidine have also been routinely used in both captive and free-ranging lynx (Squires et al. 2004) and cougar (Elbroch et al. 2015). Emesis is a known potential side effect of alpha-2 agonists, particularly xylazine, though is not generally a concern in immobilization of nondomestic felids. Successful use of tiletamine/zolazepam has also been documented in these species for immobilization. Severe adverse reactions including fatality have been unofficially reported in several nondomestic felid species; however, a recent study called this risk into question (Kreeger and Armstrong 2010).

When prolonged immobilization or a surgical plane of anesthesia is required, intubation and maintenance on isoflurane gas are advised. Full reversal of any alpha-2 agonist should be administered at the end of a procedure; ensure any ketamine has had sufficient time to be metabolized (i.e., 30–40 minutes post injection) before reversal of the alpha-2 to avoid "stormy" recoveries.

Analgesics and Antiinflammatories

Analgesics commonly used in domestic cats can generally be used in nondomestic felids. The authors have used buprenorphine in bobcats both parenterally and transmucosally at the standard dose of 0.01–0.02 mg/kg BID. The sustained-release formulation of buprenorphine is widely used in domestic cats, providing analgesia for up to 72 hours. This formulation at the standard cat dose of 0.12 mg/kg SQ has been used in snow leopards following ovariohysterectomy with good clinical efficacy and no reported adverse effects (Helmick 2015, personal communication).

Fentanyl patches are also frequently used in domestic cats and have been anecdotally reported to be effective in snow leopards (Herrin et al. 2012) and African lions (Galloway et al. 2002) but safety and efficacy in individual nondomestic felid species need study. These patches generally require removal after 72 hours, which usually necessitates reimmobilization and should be considered prior to use. No anecdotal reports of ingestion of the patches are known, though this may be another consideration prior to use.

Tramadol has also been anecdotally used in a variety of nondomestic felids at doses ranging from 0.5 to 2 mg/kg orally every 12 hours. It should be considered that opioids may occasionally cause idiosyncratic excitatory effects. Although not formally documented in nondomestic felids, opioid-associated hyperthermia is occasionally reported in the literature for domestic cats and should be considered a possible adverse effect in any nondomestic felid.

Use of nonsteroidal antiinflammatory drugs (NSAIDs) in nondomestic cats should be undertaken with caution. Benefits should be weighed against risks and use avoided in those individuals that are dehydrated, hypovolemic, or suspected of hepatic or renal insufficiency. In a retrospective study evaluating renal lesions in 70 captive nondomestic felids of a wide range of species, 13 cases (including one cougar) were diagnosed as renal papillary necrosis and demonstrated a significant association with previous NSAID use (Newkirk et al. 2011).

Clinically Relevant Anatomy and Physiology

There are few clinically relevant anatomical and physiological features unique to individual felid species; the physiology of the domestic cat can be used as a model for all felids. All are obligate carnivores with a shorter digestive tract with smaller cecum and shorter colon than omnivores (Lamberski 2015).

The dental formula of felids is I 3/3, C 1/1, P 2–3/2, M 1/1. Due to the mechanical advantage of a shortened skull and mandibles, felids have a more powerful bite relative to muscle mass than other carnivores, except mustelids (Lamberski 2015).

Blood collection sites for bobcats are the same as for domestic cats; cephalic, medial saphenous, and jugular veins are most commonly used, with access dependent on means of restraint and individual preference. Similar to domestic cats, nondomestic felids have AB group blood types, underscoring the importance of cross-matching donors and recipients before blood transfusions or administering blood products (Wack 2003).

Laryngospasms are common in felids and may require topical anesthetic during endotracheal intubation.

Infectious and Parasitic Diseases of Concern

Biosecurity and disease control measures are essential in any facility in which felids are undergoing medical care and rehabilitation. As hosts for several zoonotic pathogens, management of wild felids in captivity carries a risk of disease transmission within the facility. It is important that each facility develops a customized disease control plan, including prevention of site and groundwater contamination, disinfection, vaccination, deworming, and parasite control (Huckabee 2009).

The following is intended to highlight those infectious diseases in wild North American felids of importance for clinical relevance, impact on release, biosecurity, and personnel exposure. Published data on pathogens of free-ranging species are often limited to seroprevalence studies which indicate exposure. Clinical case reports in captive individuals of the same species are relevant in documenting disease susceptibility and consequent rehabilitation considerations.

Viral Diseases

Feline Leukemia Virus
Infection with feline leukemia virus (FeLV) appears to be rare in most free-ranging nondomestic felids throughout North and South America. Only one published case of clinical disease and fatality in a bobcat exists (Sleeman et al. 2001). This animal was captive-bred and demonstrated anemia, immunosuppression, and lymphoproliferative disease similar to FeLV in domestic cats. A serological survey of free-ranging bobcats in California from 1992 to 1995 failed to identify seropositive individuals (Riley et al. 2004) but seropositive cougars have been documented in California and Washington (Rickard and Foreyt 1992; Foley et al. 2013). The first case report of clinical disease in a free-ranging North American felid was documented in a cougar near Sacramento (Jessup et al. 1993).

Despite the low risk of exposure and clinical disease in free-ranging felids, the potential impact in wild populations was realized when the virus appeared in the highly endangered Florida panther population in 2002 (Cunningham et al. 2008). Five viremic individuals were confirmed from 2002 to 2007; all died prematurely. Seropositive Florida panthers appeared to respond to FeLV similarly to domestic cats, proceeding toward regression, latency, or persistent infection. Experimental vaccination was initiated in 2006 in 52 Florida panthers; no viremic cases have been found since.

Feline leukemia virus screening may be prudent in nondomestic felids undergoing rehabilitation. Standard commercial ELISA kits used to screen domestic cats have been successfully used in other felid species (Franklin et al. 2007).

Feline Immunodeficiency Virus (FIV)

Historically, FIV was considered highly host specific. Eight related, but unique, lentiviral genetic variants have been documented in nondomestic felids. Puma lentivirus clade B (FIVpcoB) infects cougars throughout their geographic range while a second lineage (FIVpcoA) infects free-ranging bobcats and small numbers of cougars in southern California and Florida, with geographic distribution of viral subtypes reflecting evolution of host range (Franklin et al. 2007). This is the first documentation of cross-species transmission with perpetuation in the recipient species. Similar cross-species transmission and perpetuation of FIV variants outside of bobcats and cougar have not yet been demonstrated; however, further genomic studies on these two lineages have suggested that host–virus evolution of FIV in nondomestic cats is ongoing (Lee et al. 2014).

Despite high seroprevalence of FIV among many free-ranging felid populations, some as high as 100% (Franklin et al. 2007), FIV does not appear to be pathogenic. No correlation has been found between viral infection and clinical disease in free-ranging nondomestic felids, with the possible exception of the African lion (Franklin et al. 2007). However, FIV-like disease has occasionally been described in captive nondomestic cats in zoo settings (Barr et al. 1989). Although identification of FIV in an asymptomatic felid undergoing rehabilitation is unlikely to preclude release, documentation of the virus is encouraged.

Feline Panleukopenia Virus/Feline Parvovirus (FPV)

This virus is likely endemic in all populations of North American felids. Seroprevalence varies with geographic range and possibly correlates with proximity to feral cats and other potential host species. Despite serological evidence of exposure to this virus and detection of FPV and canine parvovirus DNA in feces or tissues of bobcats and cougars, clinical disease in free-ranging species is rarely reported (Allison et al. 2013). Five confirmed cases of fatality have been described in bobcats (Gaydos and Fischer 1999). This same study provided evidence that not all cases of infection are fatal in this species. Clinical signs, histopathological changes, and potential outcomes are believed to be similar as for domestic cats. It is standard protocol in the authors' facility to vaccinate juvenile bobcats against FPV within a multivalent vaccine (i.e., FVRCP vaccine).

Canine Distemper Virus (CDV)

Canine distemper virus can infect nondomestic felids. Historically, reports in North America were limited to captive felids (e.g., fatal infections in captive lions, tigers, leopards, and a jaguar at several institutions in California which correlated with a spike of CDV in the raccoon population that year) (Appel et al. 1994). CDV-induced encephalitis has been confirmed in free-ranging lynx and bobcat in eastern Canada (Daoust et al. 2009). No clinical disease in pumas has been reported and seroprevalence was low in one study (Foley et al. 2013). Decisions to vaccinate bobcat and lynx housed in rehabilitation facilities should be based on risk assessment, taking into consideration geographic location and housing of other CDV-susceptible species. Vaccination should never supplant proper biosecurity measures.

Rabies Virus

Rabies is endemic throughout much of North America and bobcats are considered a RVS. Between 1960 and 2000, 446 cases of rabies were confirmed in bobcats in the US, with a fivefold increase in the number of rabid bobcats between 1990 and 2000 compared to the previous decade (Krebs et al. 2003). In the United States in 2014, rabies was documented in a total of 18 bobcats (Monroe et al. 2016). Rabid cougars are much less frequently reported, with roughly one case every decade since 1960 (Krebs et al. 2003). Rabies should always be a differential for neurological signs in felids and appropriate precautions must be taken at all times. When considered geographically relevant, vaccination should be considered (see Chapter 7).

Other Pathogens

Feline coronavirus (FCoV), feline herpesvirus (FHV or rhinotracheitis), and feline calicivirus have all been detected by antibody testing of free-ranging North American felids. While seropositive bobcats, lynx, and cougar have been detected, prevalence is relatively low. Clinical disease or histological lesions have not been identified. At the authors' facility, juvenile bobcats are vaccinated against herpesvirus and calicivirus using the FVRCP vaccine.

Bacterial Diseases

Yersinia pestis, the causative agent of bubonic plague, is a risk in any felid species in endemic areas, especially the southwestern US. Humans have become infected following direct contact with bobcats and cougars that died from infection. Following a species reintroduction program in Colorado in 1999–2003, six out of 52 released Canada lynx died from pneumonic plague, providing the first documented cases of disease in this species (Wild et al. 2006).

Among other zoonotic concerns, causative agents of both tularemia and leptospirosis have been found capable of causing serological conversion without evidence of clinical disease in bobcats.

Parasitic Diseases

A high seroprevalence for *Toxoplasma gondii* and *Bartonella henselae* has been demonstrated in bobcats, lynx, and cougar. Serological screening for exposure to these pathogens may not be very useful in the rehabilitation setting. Although cases of clinical toxoplasmosis have been reported in juvenile free-ranging and captive bobcats (Dubey et al. 1987; Smith et al. 1995), clinical disease is generally considered rare. Bobcats also serve as the natural reservoir species for the tick-borne protozoal parasite *Cytauxzoon felis* (Shock et al. 2011); reports of clinical disease are rare (Nietfeld and Pollock 2002).

Notoedric mange, an often debilitating disease caused by the mite *Notoedres cati*, is known to affect free-ranging North American felids (Serieys et al. 2013). An epizootic occurring in the early 2000s in bobcats of southern California caused a significant impact on annual survival rate. In one study, 19 of 19 bobcats that died with severe notoedric mange showed elevated levels of anticoagulant residues, suggesting a possible link between rodenticide exposure and susceptibility to clinical mange. A similar correlation has been noted in cougars in the same geographic location (Riley et al. 2010). The potential for rodenticide exposure based on proximity to urbanized areas and clinical signs should be considered in cases of severe mange.

A wide variety of intestinal parasites, many shared with the domestic cat and dog population, have also been documented. Given the relatively high prevalence of endoparasitism and/or ectoparasites, empiric treatment of all bobcats admitted for rehabilitation with ivermectin and praziquantel may be considered, particularly for kittens. Standard deworming protocols used in domestic kittens are generally appropriate for nondomestic felids.

Common Reasons for Presentation

Traumatic injuries are common causes for presentation of juvenile and older bobcats. Collision with vehicles, gunshot wounds, and trap-related injuries are seen with some frequency in wildlife rehabilitation facilities. Parasitism and infectious disease problems are not frequent as a cause of presentation, though are frequently found on examination and diagnostic testing.

Neonates and orphans are generally not "found" unless a nursing queen has been shot, trapped, killed or excluded from returning to her den site. Further questioning of the finders may be necessary to determine if the kittens are truly orphaned, or if it may be possible to reunite with the queen. If the kittens have received care by the finders for more than a few days before presentation, a variety of iatrogenic issues may be present, such as hypothermia, dehydration, diarrhea, and nutritional deficiencies. Habituation and inappropriate socialization, sometimes irreversible, are also unfortunate results when untrained individuals try to keep a bobcat kitten as a pet.

All neonatal and infant kittens will need to be stimulated to defecate and urinate until soon after their eyes open, and may need to be stimulated immediately on presentation. Diagnostic and therapeutic approaches will be analogous to the domestic cat. Hydration and nutritional needs are essentially the same for all felids, regardless of size and age, and need to be assessed on presentation. A full physical examination and evaluation should be performed as soon as the patient is stable.

If the patient is in shock, starving/emaciated or severely injured, basic life-saving measures may be employed for patient stabilization. However, if it is clear that the patient will not have a chance of survival following recovery, the patient should be euthanized as part of a triage protocol.

Pre-release Conditioning and Postrelease Monitoring

Release juveniles with siblings or conspecifics when possible, in the fall of their first year if born early in the year and food availability is good. In northern areas, overwintering and release the following spring will help to ensure good food availability when the cats will be 10–12 months of age.

Bobcats must exhibit the following attributes for best chance of survival after their release: robust body and physical condition; disease free; fear and defense responses typical for the species, with appropriate posturing and vocalizations; strong aversion to humans and dogs with the response to run from a human presence rather than advance toward it; two functional eyes with no impairment in vision, hearing, smell, or touch; full use of all four limbs and able to run, jump, and climb well, demonstrating impeccable balance; thick pelage appropriate to the season of release; and fully intact and functional teeth capable of gripping and killing prey.

Live prey testing and practice is imperative for juvenile animals, and equally important in subadults and adults if recovery from an injury or condition leaves any doubt about the animal's full capabilities. By 5–6 months of age, they can begin live prey testing, and should be successful for at least three weeks prior to evaluation for release. Using video monitoring to observe live prey testing will provide valuable assessment regarding proficiency of prey prehension.

It is essential to plan ahead to ensure that bobcats are released as soon as possible after they are deemed ready; the longer a healthy wild animal is held, the greater the chance that problems associated with captivity will develop. They generally need to spend a few weeks in an outdoor enclosure for physical conditioning and weathering prior to release.

When performing the capture for release, the goal is to secure the bobcat as quickly and safely as possible to reduce exhaustion or injury. Often, capture may be simplified by utilizing a transport carrier for a den box in the enclosure days or weeks prior to the release. If the bobcat sees the carrier as a safe retreat, it may voluntarily enter it when intimidated on release day.

Agency Assistance with Release

Working closely with state or provincial wildlife agencies to determine best release sites and times is an important step in aiding the bobcat's survival after release. As cougars have significant potential for public health and safety, the agencies must be involved with planning and release of this species. Many states will not allow release of rehabilitated cougars, and young that have not been with their dam to learn survival skills may put human safety at risk if released. State or provincial wildlife agencies and universities are sometimes able to incorporate rehabilitated wildlife into existing studies and may be able to track the animal post release to provide invaluable information for the success of rehabilitation techniques.

Postrelease Monitoring

There are few published postrelease studies on rehabilitated bobcats. In the first report (Odell 1985), despite minimal handling when hand-rearing, five rescued bobcat kittens were habituated to humans to some degree. The Nebraska Game and Parks Commission directed that all be ear tagged and released; none were radio collared. Initially following release, there was contact with humans or human dwellings by four of the released bobcats; one was not seen following release. The only tag return was from the male that appeared to be most habituated of the five; he was released at 11 months old and was shot by a man hunting coyotes at 16 months old. He was in good body condition, and behavior reported as normal for age and species.

The second study (Convy and Zaremba 1998) described two bobcats that were raised with minimal human contact and showed no evidence of habituation. They were released together in western Washington State and dispersed from the release site at five and 10 days. Both wore radio collars and were tracked for 96 days (male) and 507 days (female). No human contact was reported, multiple sightings were reported for the female, and no mortality signals were received.

Clinical Pathology

In numerous studies of nondomestic felids, hematological and serum chemistry data are consistently within reference ranges for the domestic cat. However, some example data are provided in Appendix I.

References

Allison, A.B., Kohler, D.J., Fox, K.A. et al. (2013). Frequent cross-species transmission of parvoviruses among diverse carnivore hosts. *Journal of Virology* 87 (4): 2342–2347.

Anderson, E.M. (1987). Bobcat behavioral ecology in relation to resource use in southeastern Colorado. Doctoral dissertation. Colorado State University.

Appel, M.J., Yates, R.A., Foley, G.L. et al. (1994). Canine distemper epizootic in lions, tigers, and leopards in North America. *Journal of Veterinary Diagnostic Investigation* 6 (3): 277–288.

Banfield, A.W.F. (1987). *The Mammals of Canada*, 2e. Toronto, ON: University of Toronto Press.

Barr, M.C., Calle, P.P., Roelke, M.E. et al. (1989). Feline immunodeficiency virus infection in nondomestic felids. *Journal of Zoo and Wildlife Medicine* 20 (3): 265–272.

Chapman, J.A. and Feldhamer, G.A. (1982). *Wild Mammals of North America*. Baltimore, MD: Johns Hopkins University Press.

Convy, J.A. and Zaremba, M. (1998). Post-release survival and movements of captive-reared bobcats (*Felis rufus*).

In: *Wildlife Rehabilitation*, vol. 16 (ed. D.R. Ludwig), 115–122. St Cloud, MN: National Wildlife Rehabilitators Association.

Crowe, D.M. (1975). Aspects of ageing, growth, and reproduction of bobcats from Wyoming. *Journal of Mammalogy* 56 (1): 177–198.

Cunningham, M.W., Brown, M.A., Shindle, D.B. et al. (2008). Epizootiology of feline leukemia virus in the Florida puma. *Journal of Wildlife Diseases* 44 (3): 537–552.

Daoust, P.Y., McBurney, S.R., Godson, D.L. et al. (2009). Canine distemper virus-associated encephalitis in free-living lynx (*Lynx canadensis*) and bobcats (*Lynx rufus*) of eastern Canada. *Journal of Wildlife Diseases* 45 (3): 611–624.

Dubey, J.P., Quinn, W.J., and Weinandy, D. (1987). Fatal neonatal toxoplasmosis in a bobcat (*Lynx rufus*). *Journal of Wildlife Diseases* 23 (2): 324–327.

Elbroch, L.M., Lendrum, P.E., Alexander, P. et al. (2015). Cougar den site selection in the Southern Yellowstone Ecosystem. *Mammal Research* 60 (2): 89–96.

Foley, J.E., Swift, P., Fleer, K.A. et al. (2013). Risk factors for exposure to feline pathogens in California mountain lions (*Puma concolor*). *Journal of Wildlife Diseases* 49 (2): 279–293.

Franklin, S.P., Troyer, J.L., TerWee, J.A. et al. (2007). Variability in assays used for detection of lentiviral infection in bobcats (*Lynx rufus*), pumas (*Puma concolor*), and ocelots (*Leopardus pardalis*). *Journal of Wildlife Diseases* 43 (4): 700–710.

Galloway, D.S., Coke, R.L., Rochat, M.C. et al. (2002). Spinal compression due to atlantal vertebral malformation in two African lions (*Panthera leo*). *Journal of Zoo and Wildlife Medicine* 33 (3): 249–255.

Gaydos, J.K. & Fischer, J.R. (1999). Feline Panleukopenia in Free-Ranging Bobcats (Lynx rufus) from 3 States. International Virtual Conference on Veterinary Medicine – Diseases of Exotic Animals and Wildlife, November 15–30.

Hansen, K. (1992). *Cougar: The American Lion*. Flagstaff, AZ: Northland Publishing.

Herrin, K.V., Allan, G., Black, A. et al. (2012). Stifle osteochondritis dissecans in snow leopards (*Uncia uncia*). *Journal of Zoo and Wildlife Medicine* 43 (2): 347–354.

Huckabee, J.R. (2009). Biosecurity and disease control for wildlife rehabilitation facilities. In: *Topics in Wildlife Medicine: Infectious Diseases*, vol. 3 (ed. K. Shenoy), 1–19. St Cloud, MN: National Wildlife Rehabilitators Association.

Jessup, D.A., Pettan, K.C., Lowenstine, L.J. et al. (1993). Feline leukemia virus infection and renal spirochetosis in a free-ranging cougar (*Felis concolor*). *Journal of Zoo and Wildlife Medicine* 24 (1): 73–79.

Krebs, J.W., Williams, S.M., Smith, J.S. et al. (2003). Rabies among infrequently reported mammalian carnivores in the United States, 1960–2000. *Journal of Wildlife Diseases* 39 (2): 253–261.

Kreeger, T.J. and Armstrong, D.L. (2010). Tigers and Telazol: the unintended evolution of caution to contradiction. *Journal of Wildlife Management* 74 (6): 1183–1185.

Lamberski, N. (2015). Felidae. In: *Fowler's Zoo and Wild Animal Medicine*, vol. 8 (ed. R.E. Miller and M.E. Fowler), 467–476. St Louis, MO: Elsevier.

Lee, J.S., Bevins, S.N., Serieys, L.E.K. et al. (2014). Evolution of puma lentivirus in bobcats (*Lynx rufus*) and mountain lions (*Puma concolor*) in North America. *Journal of Virology* 88 (14): 7727–7737.

McCord, C.M. and Cardoza, J.E. (1982). Bobcat and lynx. In: *Wild Mammals of North America: Biology, Management, and Economics* (ed. J.A. Chapman and G.A. Felhamer), 728–766. Baltimore, MD: Johns Hopkins University Press.

Monroe, B.P., Yager, P., Blanton, J. et al. (2016). Rabies surveillance in the United States in 2014. *Journal of the American Veterinary Medical Association* 248 (7): 777–788.

Newkirk, K.M., Newman, S.J., White, L.A. et al. (2011). Renal lesions of nondomestic felids. *Veterinary Pathology Online* 48 (3): 698–705.

Nietfeld, J.C. and Pollock, C. (2002). Fatal cytauxzoonosis in a free-ranging bobcat (*Lynx rufus*). *Journal of Wildlife Diseases* 38 (3): 607–610.

Odell, C.H. (1985). Selection of release sites and post-release findings on five hand-reared bobcats. In: *Wildlife Rehabilitation*, vol. 3 (ed. P. Beaver), 155–162. St Cloud, MN: National Wildlife Rehabilitators Association.

O'Donoghue, M., Boutin, S., Krebs, C.J. et al. (1997). Numerical responses of coyotes and lynx to the snowshoe hare cycle. *Oikos* 80: 150–162.

Poole, K.G. (2003). A review of the Canada lynx, *Lynx canadensis*, in Canada. *Canadian Field-Naturalist* 117: 360–376.

Quinn, N.W.S. and Parker, G. (1987). Lynx. In: *Wild Furbearer Management and Conservation in North America* (ed. M. Novak, J.A. Barber, M.E. Obbard and B. Malloch), 683–694. Toronto, ON: Ontario Ministry of Natural Resources.

Rickard, L.G. and Foreyt, W.J. (1992). Gastrointestinal parasites of cougars (*Felis concolor*) in Washington and the first report of *Ollulanus tricuspis* in a sylvatic felid from North America. *Journal of Wildlife Diseases* 28 (1): 130–133.

Riley, S.P.D., Bromley, C., Poppenga, R.H. et al. (2010). Anticoagulant exposure and notoedric mange in bobcats and mountain lions in urban southern California. *Journal of Wildlife Management* 71 (6): 1874–1884.

Riley, S.P.D., Foley, J., and Chomel, B. (2004). Exposure to feline and canine pathogens in bobcats and gray foxes in urban and rural zones of a national park in California. *Journal of Wildlife Diseases* 40 (1): 11–22.

Rockhill, A.P., Chinnadurai, S.K., Powell, R.A. et al. (2011). A comparison of two field chemical immobilization techniques for Bobcats (*Lynx rufus*). *Journal of Zoo and Wildlife Medicine* 42 (4): 580–585.

Rolley, R.E. (1987). Bobcat. In: *Wild Furbearer Management and Conservation in North America*, 671–681. Toronto, ON: Ontario Ministry of Natural Resources.

Ruggiero, L.F., Aubry, K.B., Buskirk, S.W. et al. (2000). *Ecology and Conservation of Lynx in the United States*. Boulder, CO.: University Press of Colorado.

Serieys, L.E.K., Foley, J., Owens, S. et al. (2013). Serum chemistry, hematologic, and post-mortem findings in free-ranging bobcats (*Lynx rufus*) with notoedric mange. *Journal of Parasitology* 99 (6): 989–996.

Shock, B.C., Murphy, S.M., Patton, L.L. et al. (2011). Distribution and prevalence of *Cytauxzoon felis* in bobcats (*Lynx rufus*), the natural reservoir, and other wild felids in thirteen states. *Veterinary Parasitology* 175 (3): 325–330.

Sikes, R.S. and Kennedy, M.L. (1992). Morphologic variation of the bobcat (*Felis rufus*) in the eastern United States and its association with selected environmental variables. *American Midland Naturalist* 128 (2): 313–324.

Sleeman, J.M., Keane, J.M., Johnson, J.S. et al. (2001). Feline leukemia virus in a captive bobcat. *Journal of Wildlife Diseases* 37 (1): 194–200.

Smith, K.E., Fischer, J.R., and Dubey, J.P. (1995). Toxoplasmosis in a bobcat (*Felis rufus*). *Journal of Wildlife Diseases* 31 (4): 555–557.

Squires, J.R., McKelvey, K.S., and Ruggiero, L.F. (2004). A snow-tracking protocol used to delineate local lynx, *Lynx canadensis*, distributions. *Canadian Field-Naturalist* 118 (4): 583–589.

Sunquist, M. and Sunquist, F. (2002). Ocelots. In: *Wild Cats of the World*. Chicago, IL: University of Chicago Press.

Tesky, J.L. (1995a). Puma concolor. Fire Effects Information System. www.feis-crs.org/feis

Tesky, J.L. (1995b). Lynx rufus. Fire Effects Information System. www.feis-crs.org/feis

Ulev, E. (2007). *Lynx canadensis*. Fire Effects Information System. www.feis-crs.org/feis

Wack, R.F. (2003). Felidae. In: *Zoo and Wild Animal Medicine*, 5e (ed. M.E. Fowler and R.E. Miller), 491–501. St Louis, MO: Saunders Elsevier.

Wild, M.A., Shenk, T.M., and Spraker, T.R. (2006). Plague as a mortality factor in Canada lynx (*Lynx canadensis*) reintroduced to Colorado. *Journal of Wildlife Diseases* 42 (3): 646–650.

27

Natural History and Medical Management of Chiroptera

Linda E. Bowen

Bats101.info, Falls Village, CT, USA

Natural History

Bats are found on every continent with the exception of Antarctica. Over 1300 species occur worldwide, 46 in the United States. Most bats are nocturnal and many provide free, nontoxic insect control; bats save the agricultural industry in North America an estimated \$3.7 billion per year (Boyles et al. 2011). Scientists theorize that the evolution of bats from terrestrial beings was driven by heavy competition for food on the ground. Adjusting to boreal life created the need to leap from tree to tree to catch flying insects, eventually leading to a system of large, multiuse membranes that evolved into wings (Allen 1939; Burt and Grossenheider 1964).

Worldwide, bats fill many different niches. They catch and eat vertebrates such as fish and frogs; some drink nectar and eat fruit – behaviors that are essential for pollination of plants and seed dispersal – while a few species feed on blood from vertebrates. All bats have excellent hearing and most have very good vision, contrary to popular belief. When roosting, they hang upside down by their feet. With rare exceptions, rescued bats in the US are insectivorous (Kays and Wilson 2002).

It is important to identify bats, at least to the family level, to know about their care and dietary needs. Forearm length, weight, tragus characteristics, pinnae size, nose ornaments, and pelage may all be helpful in identification. The largest group and most likely to be encountered in the US are insectivorous bats from the family Vespertilionidae, and the information in this chapter is focused on that group unless otherwise stated. This family of bats ranges from very small to medium-sized bats (22–75 mm forearm) with mostly plain muzzles and small eyes. Many have tail membranes approximately the same length as the tail itself.

Bats from the family Molossidae are also frequently encountered in the US. They are small to medium insectivorous bats (27–85 mm forearm) with small projections on the nose tip. They have broad muzzles with thick, sometimes wrinkled lips and small eyes. Their tails extend beyond the edge of the tail membrane, hence the common name "free-tailed bats" (Nowak 1994).

A few species of bats from the family Phyllostomidae may rarely be presented for care in the southwestern US. These bats may eat fruit and flower parts or drink nectar, but they also eat insects (Kwiecinski and Dierenfeld 2011). Medium-sized (41–60 mm forearm) bats with long muzzles, they may have a leaf-like appendage at the nose tip (Nowak 1994). Medical concerns for these bats are the same as for other insectivorous bats.

Determining Age

Pups

Bat pups are born during the summer and are quite large in relation to the adult (as much as 30–40% of the mother's body weight). Most species are born naked with closed eyes. Eyes generally open within days after birth. The umbilical cord remains attached for a few days after birth then falls off naturally. Pups are reliant on the mother's milk for approximately 4–6 weeks and may begin short flights at 3–4 weeks. Hypothermia and dehydration are quite common in orphaned pups and should be addressed immediately. See Section 27.2.2.

Juveniles

This age group can be distinguished from adults by phalangeal joints that appear elongated due to uncalcified cartilage (Figure 27.1). Juveniles may be fully furred with adult teeth and behavior, but may not be capable of flight. If found inside a building and fully flighted, they should be immediately released outdoors as long as no human exposure has occurred.

Medical Management of Wildlife Species: A Guide for Practitioners, First Edition. Edited by Sonia M. Hernandez, Heather W. Barron, Erica A. Miller, Roberto F. Aguilar and Michael J. Yabsley.
© 2020 John Wiley & Sons, Inc. Published 2020 by John Wiley & Sons, Inc.

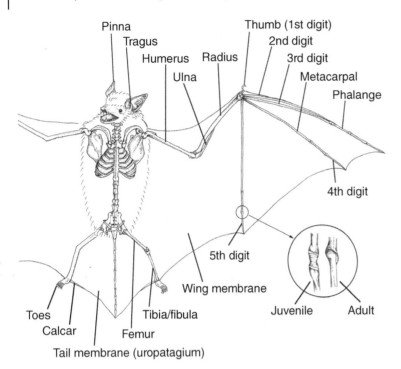

Figure 27.1 Anatomy of a bat. *Source:* Illustration by Victoria M. Campbell, based on Hill and Smith (1984). Reproduced with permission.

Adults

Phalangeal joints will be rounded and the bats will bite when handled.

Captive Management

Rabies is a concern when rehabilitating bats so the reader should refer to Chapters 2 and 4 for a detailed discussion of rabies and appropriate personal protective equipment (PPE) that should be used. White nose syndrome (WNS) is an emerging disease of bats in many parts of North America so proper quarantine and testing must be a consideration for anybody interested in rehabilitating bats. A full physical exam may reveal current or past wing lesions caused by WNS (Figure 27.2). Rehabilitators should contact the relevant state and federal agencies that have the most up-to-date recommendations for managing bats with WNS.

Housing of Adults

Bats may be kept in hard-sided plastic reptile containers (e.g., hermit crab enclosures) or zip-closed mesh carriers (e.g., Reptarium®, Apogee, Sabetha, KS, USA). The bats should have enough room to open and stretch both wings simultaneously. Bats should be housed only with conspecifics and only after a quarantine period, which can vary depending on the presentation. Aggressive bats or those displaying clinical signs of rabies (see Section 27.4) should always be housed alone. Specific

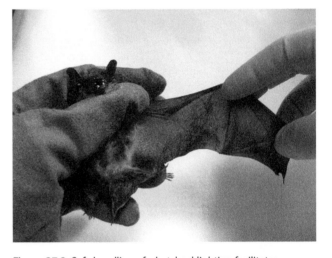

Figure 27.2 Safe handling of a bat; backlighting facilitates examination of the wings and may help to highlight lesions caused by diseases such as white nose syndrome. Big brown bat (*Eptesicus fuscus*) with normal wings shown. *Source:* Photo by the author.

guidelines regarding quarantine periods for wildlife have not been established; relying on best medical practice is recommended. Housing males and females separately is recommended and is often required by state law to prevent breeding (Rasweiler and Badwaik 2011).

Loosely woven cotton fabrics (not terry cloth because the loops tend to catch digits), folded in half, may be draped on the inside of the container to provide places to hang between the folds. Migratory and nectar-feeding bats (Phyllostomidae) may also use cloths to hang but often prefer hanging from the top of the carrier, away from the edges. Artificial foliage and thin branches provide good roosting areas.

Supplemental heat should be offered, depending on the season and patient's medical status. Heat for adult bats, if indicated, should be provided on a vertical surface to encourage hanging in a natural position. Electric heating pads, without an automatic shut-off, work well on the lowest setting. A bat disturbed from hibernation in colder months should be provided with heat until they are in suitable condition to return to torpor. Injured bats may be offered an area of heat to conserve energy and to promote healing, regardless of the time of year. Injured bats should not be allowed to enter torpor since lowering the metabolic rate reduces healing. Use the temperature, humidity, time of year, and region where the bat was found as a guideline to maintaining the bat while in captivity.

Caging should include two shallow dishes for water and mealworms (*Tenebrio molitor* larvae). Water dishes no deeper than one half inch are recommended to prevent drowning. Glass or ceramic mealworm dishes provide a slippery surface to slow mealworm escapes and should be one half inch deep.

Housing Infant Bats

Orphaned pups cannot thermoregulate so cold pups must be wrapped in a soft cloth (cotton T-shirt fabric is preferred, no synthetic material) and held in a warm hand until an enclosure is warmed and maintained between 80 and 90 °F (26–32 °C) with 50–85% humidity. Folded cotton cloths draped from the side of the enclosure to the bottom, along with a pile of cotton cloth placed directly on the bottom, provide places to hang, crawl under and hide. Fleece is not recommended as pups may ingest fibers, leading to an intestinal blockage. No dishes for food or water should be left in a pup's enclosure. At 3–4 weeks of age, once they have fur and can thermoregulate, they should have access to unheated areas in their enclosure. By weaning, they should no longer need supplemental heat.

Feeding Adults

Once the bat is hydrated, food should be offered. Fortified mealworms are recommended as a captive diet for insectivorous bats. As aerial predators, bats will not recognize mealworms as food or understand that food is in a dish. Bats must often be trained to eat in captivity. Offering mealworm viscera to an adult bat using hemostats or forceps can help encourage the bat to eat whole mealworms. Once the bat has eaten several whole live mealworms, move the bat's head close to the mealworms in the dish while offering them with hemostats. The bat will usually begin biting at the mealworms in the dish. Many learn this at the first feeding. Overfeeding bats in captivity is a common problem. Obese bats exhibiting bulging areas, particularly on their abdomen and rump, may develop health problems as seen in other overweight captive mammals, and may have difficulty flying.

To fortify mealworms, larvae should be maintained in a substrate of wheat bran, dark leafy greens, and sliced sweet potato. Use organic food to avoid pesticide exposure. Wash produce and place on top of the dry substrate. While still wet, sprinkle produce with pure calcium carbonate and powdered avian vitamins (adapted from Barnard 2011). In warm weather, refrigerate mealworms to slow morphing. Bring the worms to room temperature and allow them to feed on fresh substrate for 24 hours before feeding to bats. Remove beetles as soon as possible since they contain quinones shown to be harmful to bats (Ladisch et al. 1967; Thompson 1971).

Nectivorous bats may be temporarily fed a prepared sugar glider diet such as Instant HPW™ (Exotic Nutrition, Newport News, VA, USA) in addition to mealworm viscera. Since many nectivorous bats have no lower incisors, chitin or the mealworm exoskeleton may be chewed and spat out by the bat. Food may be presented in a small hummingbird feeder along with water in a shallow dish. Soft fruit, such as cantaloupe, banana, or strawberries, may also be offered with cut side presented for easier biting. Few nectivorous bats have been presented for rehabilitation, so few injuries have been reported. Many are simply found roosting in areas unacceptable to humans such as above doorways, in porches or car ports. For long-term care of these bats, see Delorme et al. (2011).

Hydration and Feeding of Pups

Once the pup is warm to the touch, it may be hydrated with electrolytes using subcutaneous (SQ) or oral routes, depending on the degree of dehydration. A small tipped cannula or plastic catheter tip on a 1 mL feeding syringe can facilitate oral feedings for mildly dehydrated neonates. A 25–28 gauge (ga) needle is recommended for SQ injections on pups exhibiting severe dehydration. The interscapular area or rump are appropriate injection sites.

After hydrating, food may be introduced via a commercial milk replacer such as Esbilac®, KMR®, Fox Valley 32/40®, powdered goat's milk, and fresh organic goat's milk.

Milk replacement formulas should be prepared according to package directions, using potable water. The portion to be fed initially should be diluted by 50%, maintaining the original 100% prepared formula in a separate container so that appropriate dilutions may be mixed when necessary. Probiotics should be added to aid digestion: either a small dab of plain yogurt containing active live cultures or powdered probiotics approved for use in humans. Feedings should be q2–3h around the clock. If fresh goat's milk is used, it may be diluted for one or two feedings as indicated above and then given at full strength.

Pups should be held in a horizontal position with their heads slightly lower to prevent aspiration – never on their backs. Feed until their stomachs are full, but not bulging. Dropping formula onto foam sponges or other porous material is not recommended since milk solids may be filtered through the sponge, depriving the pup of valuable nutrients. A milk line on the stomach will be visible after feeding. After feeding, clean pup of any residual formula with a warm, moist cloth to prevent bacterial skin infections. Stimulate the genitals gently with a soft cloth to promote elimination, and wipe clean (either prior to or after each feeding). Weigh pups daily at the same time and record to chart progress and development. If the stomach contents have not emptied completely by the next feeding, time between feedings may be extended, but should not exceed three hours.

A small amount of water should be offered after each feeding. Fortified mealworm viscera can be offered after each feeding to familiarize the pups with this taste. Eventually, whole, live mealworms will become 100% of their diet.

At 3–4 weeks old, pups should be offered formula in a dish. This helps to reduce handling and human interaction and starts the weaning process by teaching the pup to associate a dish with food. A dish containing the amount of formula the pup had previously taken via syringe should be held under its mouth while it hangs in the enclosure. The pup will usually lap the formula readily. After pinching the head off a mealworm, the viscera should be squeezed into the mouth and the pup allowed to suck on the remaining mealworm body to encourage eating the chitin. Very small pieces of chitin should be placed in the mouth with the viscera. Initially, the pup will spit out the chitin but it will eventually learn to eat the chitin and whole killed mealworms. Live mealworms should not be fed to pups less than 3 weeks of age since they may cause internal damage. At 4–6 weeks of age, pups should be fully weaned and eating whole live mealworms from a dish.

Handling and Examination

Adult Bats

Bats may bite when handled; heavy gloves are advised until control of the animal is obtained, at which point exam gloves may be used to facilitate the examination. Gloves are important because a rabies exposure occurs not just from bites but also from saliva. Remove a bat from its container while in a small, closed room, and close all openings such as heating vents, closets, etc. Grasping the bat firmly but gently with a thumb under the chin and the back of the animal toward the palm should position the animal to make biting difficult. Only slight pressure is needed to control the bat: pressing too hard on the chin and throat area could restrict breathing and cause harm (Figure 27.2).

During handling, even disabled bats become defensive and are likely to bite, urinate, extend wings, buzz, or hiss. These animals should not be considered overly aggressive as they are engaging in normal defensive responses to being captured and touched. Bat species encountered in the US are heterothermic so may be either cool or warm to the touch. Bats can go into daily torpor to conserve energy by lowering their body temperature and metabolic rate even in warm climates. Once disturbed, they usually warm up rapidly by vibrating or producing a steady rhythmic, pulsing motion of the body, and become more active as they warm.

The fur should be shiny and clean. Areas of alopecia may indicate a predator attack, contact with tacky material or excessive grooming incited by ectoparasites. Matted areas should be cleaned and the skin examined since matted hair may hide an underlying injury. Note any foreign material adhering to the fur. Examine the inside of the mouth for injuries, dirt or debris. If needed, an item can be gently tapped on their nose to encourage them to open the mouth. The gums, tongue, and mucous membranes should appear moist and pink. Eyes should be dark, clear, and moist. Note any discolored, broken or missing teeth. The number and type of teeth, and dental configuration vary between species (Koopman 1994). All observations should be recorded for future reference.

Gently extend each wing by holding the carpal then elbow joint for stability and note any external injuries (Figure 27.2). Check for fractures, bruising, wounds, ectoparasites (mites and lice are common) or membrane tears. Observing the wing with backlighting can help in detecting injuries or lesions related to WNS (discussed below). Extend each leg to examine for injuries, noting the grasping ability of each toe. The head of the femur can rotate 180° from the plantar surface facing posteriorly to facing anteriorly to accomplish both crawling and hanging, so the legs may appear "backward."

During the handling and examination process, strong odors may emanate from the bat. This is a normal occurrence and comes from gland secretions that are used as communication signals in mating, defensive warnings, and other behaviors (Bloss et al. 2002). The placement of the glands and the variety of odors vary greatly among species. Urine should be clear and straw colored; normal feces are black and coarse.

Several resources on the medical management of bats detail blood collection from large bats. Small volumes of blood can be collected from insectivorous, small bats by utilizing a small gauge needle and capillary tube (Figure 27.3).

General Presentation and Initial Exam

Bats presented for care are often disturbed from their daytime roosts by weather, construction, accidental entrapment or discovery in an indoor structure. Also, they may be roused from their hibernation sites by unexpected visitors. These bats may or may not exhibit signs of trauma. A thorough exam and history may indicate that rehydration is the only necessary treatment, and if no human or domestic animal exposure has taken place, the bat may then be released. Bats presented uninjured during the winter months may be allowed to return to torpor if their body condition is good. Such bats should be rehydrated and self-feeding prior to entering into torpor.

Recording an appropriate history of who has handled the bat and its condition is important, and may be mandated by local or state law. Noting names and contact information is critical in tracking possible exposure when rabies is of concern. Brochures and waivers explaining the risks of contracting rabies and what constitutes an exposure should always be provided to those presenting bats.

Fluid Therapy

Once a bat has been fully warmed, rehydration may begin. Assume that all animals coming into care will exhibit some degree of dehydration due to the circumstances and stress of capture. The high surface area of membranes results in evaporative water loss and is often the primary cause of dehydration in bats, especially in cold months when humidity levels can be low, both indoors and out. Mildly dehydrated bats may not exhibit clinical signs and may be rehydrated orally. Any bat over 5% dehydrated should be rehydrated subcutaneously with sterile electrolytes. Symptoms of moderate to severe dehydration include dry mucous membranes, decreased skin turgor, decreased urinary output, brittle patagia, or dry, sunken eyes. Mentation may be impaired in bats exhibiting severe dehydration.

A warmed, sterile electrolyte solution should be administered using an intraosseous (radius or femur) or intravenous (cephalic) catheter at a rate of 50–150 mL/kg/day either administered with a syringe pump or if not available, divided into 2–3 boluses given over 15–20 minutes per 24 hours period. Unless severely dehydrated, most bats rehydrate within 24 hours. Preferred injection sites are the interscapular region or along the hairline of the rump where the wing membrane meets the body. Brushing the hair toward the spine allows easy access to the latter site (Figure 27.4).

Prior to rehydration, ad lib water should be withheld as water intoxication has been observed in bats (Olsson 2009). Vitamins should not be added to water as the taste may cause the bat to avoid drinking. Feeding should not occur until rehydration has been provided.

Interfemoral membrane

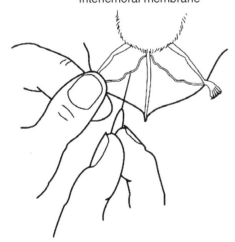

Figure 27.3 Blood collection of small bats can be achieved by puncturing a superficial vessel of the interfemoral membrane and collecting the blood that flows with a heparinized microcapillary tube. *Source:* Photo credit Amanda Lollar. Reproduced with permission from *The Rehabilitation and Captive Care of Insectivorous Bats* by Amanda Lollar, 2018.

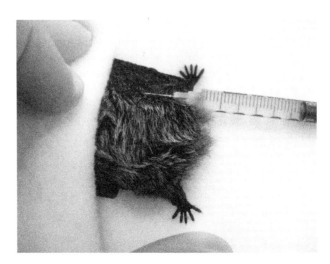

Figure 27.4 SQ injection site on the rump, near the hairline, of a silver haired bat (*Lasionycteris noctivagans*). *Source:* Photo by the author.

Medications

Analgesics, such as meloxicam, may be provided for slight to moderate pain. Meloxicam for oral administration can be diluted with distilled water and is generally stable for at least 28 days, although the solution should be shaken prior to use each time (Hawkins et al. 2006). Palatability is generally high. For more severe pain, opioid or partial opioid agonists such as buprenorphine may be given (see Appendix II: Formulary). As research on novel analgesics continues, the reader is encouraged to explore alternatives for analgesia in bats, for which safety and efficacy have not been tested.

Broad-spectrum antibiotics such as trimethoprim-sulfamethoxazole, enrofloxacin, amoxicillin-clavulanic acid or other antibiotics appropriate for mammals may be administered via injection or orally and must be dosed accordingly. Topical treatments such as povidone-iodine, chlorhexidine, silver sulfadiazine, honey, triple antibiotic ointment, and gentamicin ophthalmic drops may be applied sparingly to wounds.

Anesthetic and Surgical Considerations

When using an inhalant drug for induction, such as isoflurane, it may be administered at 4–5% via facemask with oxygen at a rate of 1–2 L/min. It can then be maintained at a level of 2–2.5% (Barrett and Olsson 2009). If sevoflurane is used, induction at 5–7%, with a maintenance level of 2–3.5%, is recommended (Muir et al. 2000). A dose of meloxicam prior to anesthesia allows the bat some pain relief upon awakening. Buprenorphine may be indicated in more invasive surgical procedures and may be given preoperatively (Heard 2007).

To begin induction, position the bat under a small cone. Once the bat becomes unconscious, it may be moved to a small mask for the remainder of the procedure. Using a hard plastic syringe container, tape a section of latex glove over the large end and make a small slit in the glove. Cut off the small end of the container to connect it to the anesthesia tubing and tape together to seal. Insert the entire head of the bat through the slit and tape the mask to the surgical drape. The drape should be placed on top of a heating pad set on low with the bat taped to the drape using either paper tape or autoclave tape. In dorsal recumbency, the wings may be opened and taped into position (Figure 27.5). Ophthalmic ointment may be sparingly applied to the bat's eyes. Administering warm SQ fluids during the anesthetic period maintains homeostasis (Molnár et al. 2004).

Infectious Diseases

Viral

Rabies cannot be diagnosed through observation alone. Aggressiveness (more than defensive biting), biting and holding on, chew marks on bedding, dirt or debris in the

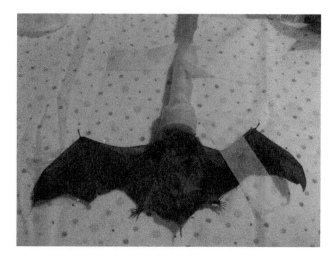

Figure 27.5 A big brown bat (*Eptesicus fuscus*) stabilized in dorsal recumbency using paper tape with head inserted into syringe holder connected to anesthesia tubing. *Source:* Photo by the author.

mouth, difficulty in swallowing, inappetance, paresis, paralysis, and seizures are signs that should be closely monitored and considered suspect for rabies. However, not all rabies cases present aggressively; some may act depressed or be moribund. Additional information is available in Chapter 2 and recommendations for PPE use in Chapter 4.

Fungal

Pseudogymnoascus destructans, the causative agent of WNS, has killed millions of bats in the US and Canada. Hairless portions of the bat's body (muzzle, ears, and wings) are most often affected. The fungus is rarely grossly visible on rescued bats, but certain clinical signs are a strong indication that the infection is present (Verant et al. 2014). Wings may have areas of depigmentation and scarring, tears or necrosis. Examining the wing with a backlit light source can be helpful in assessing wing damage (Reichard and Kunz 2009). Since the fungus does not survive above 15 °C (60 °F), transmission likely only occurs in caves where bats are hibernating; but the infected bat may be harboring microscopic spores which could spread to other bats prior to release so bats suspected of having WNS should be isolated. Once the fungus has infected a bat, it causes frequent episodes of arousal as a result of increased irritation. Energy stores can be quickly depleted during these arousal periods, leading to dehydration and/or starvation.

Affected, debilitated bats may be found outside the cave during cold temperatures. Isolating infected or potentially infected bats is essential. Emaciation protocols should be followed to avoid refeeding syndrome

(Winn 2006). A high-protein recovery diet such as Carnivore Care® (Oxbow Animal Health, Omaha, NE, USA) should be fed rather than a high-carbohydrate food once the animal has been properly hydrated. Because *P. destructans* grows best at low temperatures, maintain bats at 18.3–23.9 °C (65–75 °F). The application of topical treatments is not recommended since additional handling can cause stress and weaken the immune system. These treatments do not remediate the infection any more than properly provided supportive care, and in many cases actually produce an increased inflammatory response (Meteyer et al. 2011). If an infected bat survives without physical limitations, it may be considered for release if local and state laws allow it. Additional information is available from the manual *Rehabilitating Bats with White-Nose Syndrome* available for download at www.bats101.info.

Parasitic

Most lice or mites, which may be very small, can be removed with a cotton swab and alcohol. Larger, blood-sucking parasites in the family Cimicidae and Polyctenidae may also be present and are usually large enough to be removed with swabs or hemostats. No additional treatment is required. Changing roosting drapes daily can help to eliminate parasites from the environment. A small number of ectoparasites is common and these are generally removed during grooming. In large numbers, ectoparasites may indicate an underlying health condition. Insecticides should not be used on bats, but instead good husbandry practices and proper nutrition will usually control ectoparasite burdens.

Bats may also harbor endoparasites, most of which are innocuous in small numbers. Large infestations found on a fecal smear may be treated with antiparasitic agents used in other mammals and dosed accordingly.

Traumatic Injuries

Wing-related trauma is the most common type of injury encountered, from small tears to missing wing sections and fractured bones.

Membrane Lacerations

Minor wounds should be cleaned with a dilute povidone iodine or chlorhexidine solution. Small wing tears or punctures smaller than 2 cm should heal without intervention unless they occur on the trailing edge of the wing. Large wing tears or those along the trailing edge can be successfully treated with Tegaderm® transparent film. Tegaderm can be removed and reapplied if positioned

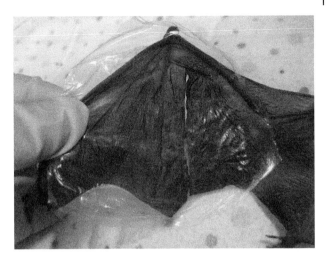

Figure 27.6 Application of Tegaderm on both dorsal and ventral surfaces of an extensive wing membrane tear of a big brown bat (*Eptesicus fuscus*). *Source:* Photo by the author.

incorrectly (Figure 27.6). Upon removal of Tegaderm, no adhesive remains on the bat.

Wing membrane repairs should always be done under anesthesia, regardless of the repair method. It may be necessary to freshen wound edges by scraping with a scalpel 1–1.5 mm to promote new tissue growth. Small pieces of jagged tissue may be trimmed off along with any necrotic tissue. Clean the edges with dilute povidone iodine and blot dry. Align the freshened edges within 1 mm of each other. Sandwich the wing membrane between two pieces of Tegaderm film with a border extending 2 cm or more beyond the edge of the tear to ensure adhesion to the wing.

Although glue has been used extensively on bat wing tears, it can be difficult to apply, may not hold, can cause irritation, and may be difficult to remove. If necessary, large tears may be spot glued at 1–1.5 cm intervals to enable apposition; however, where glue is applied, tissue may not grow.

A common injury is a wing membrane tear from ankle to axilla with only a narrow margin of membrane attached to the body. Using a depilatory, such as Nair™ (Church & Dwight Co. Inc., Ewing Township, NJ, USA) or Veet® (Reckitt Benckiser Group, Parsippany, NJ, USA), to remove a strip of body hair 1–2 mm from the ventral surface of the body near the wing membrane tear allows for adhesion of the ventral piece of Tegaderm. Anesthesia is not usually required for this step and it may be done 1–2 days prior to the repair. Apply the depilatory lotion with a cotton-tipped applicator and remove it with a clean cloth, rinse with warm water, and wipe dry with gauze. Allow the Tegaderm to extend beyond the trailing edge of the wing membrane on both dorsal and ventral surfaces to stabilize the tear.

Do not allow bats with wing trauma to roost in a hanging position, as this may exacerbate wounds by allowing edema to accumulate at or near the site of injury. Instead, use a small pile of cotton cloth in the bottom of a hard-sided enclosure to allow the bat to rest and hide.

Fractures

Closed humerus and radius/ulna fractures may be stabilized using a variety of techniques. Gluing lightweight (no more than 5% body weight) stiff material to span the fracture site may keep the bones stable while healing if the joints can be immobilized. Materials used are only limited by imagination and availability; toothpicks, wooden applicators, rolled tape, foam make-up sponges, straws split lengthwise, and thermoplastic splint materials have all been used.

Intermedullary pins have been used on both open and closed fractures; 22–25 ga hypodermic needles or catheters are the most readily available pins that will fit appropriately in the medulla of a bat bone. Determine the length and gauge based on the radiograph and insert the pin through the epiphysis and fracture site (Figure 27.7). Stabilize and protect the exposed pin using dental cement, glue, epoxy, or air-dried clay or retain the plastic hub of the needle and tape it to the membrane to prevent premature withdrawal. Fold the wing to its natural closed position and immobilize the joints above and below the fracture site using paper tape or Tegaderm. Radiographs should be taken after pin insertion to confirm placement and prior to removing the pin to determine the extent of healing.

If a bat begins to chew at splints, bandages or other stabilizers (a sign of pain or discomfort), acepromazine or butorphanol may be administered (Cottrell 2009). After three days, meloxicam should suffice for managing discomfort and preventing chewing.

Callous formation takes 4–6 weeks, but healing may take up to 100 days (Wellehan et al. 2001; Cottrell, personall communication). The above procedures may also be used on leg fractures.

Burns

Bats may present with burns from electrical sources, chimneys or fireplaces. Frequently, these injuries are fatal. If burns are extensive and severe, euthanasia should be considered.

The patagium is very sensitive to both heat and cold trauma, including the use of heat lamps or electrical blankets under anesthesia. Usually, the initial vesicle/bulla formation is followed by the membrane drying and falling off. Debridement should be delayed until this occurs. Minor burns may be treated topically with silver sulfadiazine or honey, along with rehydration therapy. Small areas of severe burns may also require systemic antibiotic treatment such as enrofloxacin. If a bat has been electrocuted, seizures or spasms may occur. Diazepam or midazolam may help control seizures, and may be repeated every 4–8 hours (Olsson 2009).

(a)

(b)

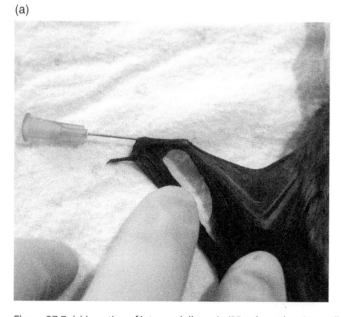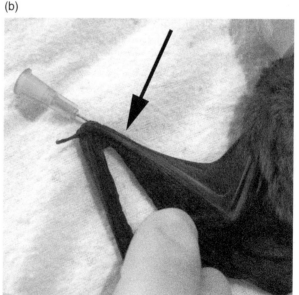

Figure 27.7 (a) Insertion of intermedullary pin (25 ga hypodermic needle) into the radius of a big brown bat (*Eptesicus fuscus*). (b) The needle placement after advancement through the fracture site (*arrow*) into the proximal fragment. *Source:* Photos by the author.

Contaminants

Bats may be exposed to contaminants such as paint, glue traps, tar, silicon, or other sticky, noxious materials. If the animal is attached to a larger piece of material, prior to attempting to free the bat, sprinkle the sticky areas with cornstarch, flour or cornmeal to prevent additional adherence and, if necessary, cut the larger piece of material to a more manageable size. It is not advisable to use talc due to potential inhalation. Mineral oil, vegetable oil or polysorbate 80 (available from most compounding pharmacies) may be gently rubbed on the contaminant to dissolve it; solvents such as turpentine, lighter fluid or acetone are potentially harmful and should be avoided. The mouth, nose and genital areas should be attended to immediately as contamination or blockage may be life threatening. Once these areas have been cleaned, other areas may be addressed in short intervals, allowing the bat to rest between cleaning sessions. Bats may lick or chew contaminants, so observe frequency and content of droppings for signs of blockage and other effects of ingestion. Attention to hydration status is critical due to stress and the possibility the bat was denied access to water prior to rescue.

Because of their roosting habits, bats are often sprayed with pesticides, such as wasp or ant spray. Exposed bats should be bathed gently in warm water with dilute original Dawn® liquid detergent (Proctor and Gamble, Cincinnati, OH, USA). Particular attention should be paid to the nose, mouth, and genitals. Rinse well, blot dry, and place the bat in a warm enclosure. Do not use a hair dryer or put in the sun to dry.

Health Issues in Pups

If, prior to feeding, the stomach is full or mostly full (an indication of bloat), discontinue feeding formula (Figure 27.8). Simethicone drops can be used to dissipate bloat. At the next feeding, if the stomach has emptied, return to the dilution of formula that was last tolerated.

Bat pups generally have good appetites and are eager to nurse; however, this can easily lead to overeating and bloat if they are not closely monitored.

Neonates can succumb quickly to aspiration pneumonia. Care must be taken to prevent aspiration of formula or water by following the previously recommended feeding position to monitor the flow of fluid into the pup's mouth. Stop feeding immediately if any fluid is seen exiting the pup's nostrils. In this author's experience, the pup can be turned upside down to allow gravity to remove the fluid in the nasal passages. Do not shake the pup, but wipe the nose continuously until no more fluid is seen. Listen for any crackling, ticking or abnormal breathing. Administering antibiotics or oxygen to neonatal bats for aspiration pneumonia may have some success.

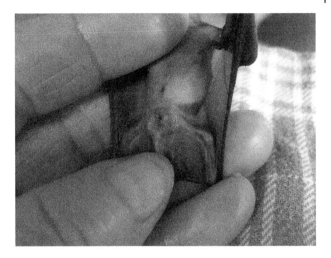

Figure 27.8 Milk line, after feeding, of an orphaned neonate big brown bat (*Eptesicus fuscus*) indicates that the stomach is full. *Source:* Photo by the author.

Release

Whatever the age, bats may have difficulty in achieving flight from the ground. When releasing them, place the bat on a platform, ledge or tree, or hold in the air 5–6 feet above the ground to provide altitude.

Adult Bats

Adult bats may be released if they meet the following criteria: (i) have recovered from presenting problem; (ii) can fly for five minutes nonstop; (iii) are capable of vocalization and echolocation; (iv) retain hearing; (v) are physically capable of capturing flying insects; and (vi) are capable of landing and climbing.

Hand-Raised Pups

All hand-raised pups will need extensive time in a large flight cage prior to release, until they can fly continuously for at least five minutes and are observed echolocating and catching flying insects (Kelly et al. 2008). If possible, at least one experienced conspecific adult should be placed in the flight cage with whom the pups can communicate, observe, and imitate (Scott and Dicks 1998, Kelly et al. 2012).

Euthanasia

If euthanasia is required, it should be performed using an acceptable method according to American Veterinary Medical Association guidelines (see Chapter 4). One of the simplest methods in a clinical setting is inhalant anesthesia by chamber induction followed by intracardiac or intraperitoneal injection of euthanasia solution.

Acknowledgments

The author would like to thank R. Averell Manes for her helpful comments on this manuscript; Victoria M. Campbell for her bat illustration and support; and Dick Wilkins and Susan Barnard for their advice on this chapter.

References

Allen, G.M. (1939). *Bats*, 174–176. Toronto, ON, Canada: General Publishing Company Ltd.

Barnard, S. (2011). Rearing insects for bat food. In: *Bats in Captivity*, vol. 3, 192. Washington, DC: Logos Press.

Barrett, J. and Olsson, A. (2009). Chemical restraint and anesthesia. In: *Bats in Captivity*, vol. 1 (ed. S. Barnard), 301. Washington, DC: Logos Press.

Bloss, J., Acree, T., Bloss, J.M. et al. (2002). Potential use of chemical clues for colony-mate recognition in the big Brown bat, *Eptesicus fuscus*. *Journal of Chemical Ecology* 28 (4): 819–834.

Boyles, J.G., Cryan, P.M., McCracken, G.F. et al. (2011). Conservation. Economic importance of bats in agriculture. *Science* 332 (6025): 41–42.

Burt, W.H. and Grossenheider, R.P. (1964). *The Field Guide to the Mammals*, 21–45. New York: Houghton Mifflin.

Cottrell, D. (2009). Chemical restraint and anesthesia. In: *Bats in Captivity*, vol. 1 (ed. S. Barnard), 303. Washington, DC: Logos Press.

Delorme, M., Williams, K.J., Halopulos, A.M. et al. (2011). Diet and feeding. In: *Bats in Captivity*, vol. 3 (ed. S. Barnard), 89–94. Washington, DC: Logos Press.

Hawkins, M.G., Karriker, M.J., Wiebe, V. et al. (2006). Drug distribution and stability in extemporaneous preparations of meloxicam and carprofen after dilution and suspension at two storage temperatures. *Journal of the American Veterinary Medical Association* 229 (6): 968–974.

Heard, D.J. (2007). Chiropterans. In: *Zoo Animal & Wildlife Immobilization and Anesthesia* (ed. G. West, D. Heard and N. Caulkett), 376. Ames, IA: Wiley.

Hill, J.E. and Smith, J.D. (1984). *Bats: A Natural History*. London: British Museum.

Kays, R.W. and Wilson, D.E. (2002). *Mammals of North America*, 140–159. Princeton, NJ: Princeton University Press.

Kelly, A., Goodwin, S., Grogan, A. et al. (2008). Post-release survival of hand-reared pipistrelle bats (*Pipistrellus* spp). *Animal Welfare* 17: 375–382.

Kelly, A., Goodwin, S., Grogan, A. et al. (2012). Further evidence for the post-release survival of hand-reared, orphaned bats based on radio-tracking and ring-return data. *Animal Welfare* 21: 27–31.

Koopman, K.F. (1994). Chiroptera: systematics. In: *Handbook of Zoology. A Natural History of the Phyla of the Animal Kingdom, vol. 8, Mammalia* (ed. J. Niethammer, H. Schliemann and D. Starck), 1–217. Berlin: Walter de Gruyter.

Kwiecinski, G.G. and Dierenfeld, E.S. (2011). Introduction and feeding ecology. In: *Bats in Captivity*, vol. 3 (ed. S. Barnard), 71. Washington, DC: Logos Press.

Ladisch, P.K., Ladisch, S.K., and Howe, P.M. (1967). Quinoid secretions in grain and flour beetles. *Nature* 215: 939–940.

Meteyer, C.U., Valent, M., Kashmer, J. et al. (2011). Recovery of little brown bats (*Myotis lucifugus*) from natural infection with *Geomyces destructans*, white-nose syndrome. *Journal of Wildlife Diseases* 47 (3): 618–626.

Molnár, V., Sós, E., & Beregi, A. (2004). Anaesthesia of Homeotherm and Heterotherm Bat Species. *5th Scientific Meeting of the European Association of Zoo and Wildlife Veterinarians (EAZWV) Proceedings*, Erken, A.H.M. & Dorrestein, G.M., eds (May 19–23). Denmark: Ebeltoft.

Muir, W.W., Hubbell, J.A.E., Skarda, R.T.K. et al. (2000). *Handbook of Veterinary Anesthesia*, 3e. St Louis, MO: Mosby.

Nowak, R.M. (1994). *Walker's Bats of the World*. Baltimore, MD: Johns Hopkins University Press.

Olsson, A. (2009). Common health disorders. In: *Bats in Captivity*, vol. 1 (ed. S. Barnard), 151–163. Washington, DC: Logos Press.

Rasweiler, J.J. and Badwaik, N.K. (2011). Environment and housing. In: *Bats in Captivity*, vol. 3 (ed. S. Barnard), 111–118. Washington, DC: Logos Press.

Reichard, J.D. and Kunz, T.H. (2009). White-nose syndrome inflicts lasting injuries to the wings of little brown myotis (*Myotis lucifugus*). *Acta Chiropterologica* 1b1 (2): 459.

Scott, C. and Dicks, C. (1998). Returning bats to the wild… an experiment in release. *Journal of Wildlife Rehabilitation* 21 (1): 22–25.

Thompson, R.H. (1971). *Naturally Occurring Quinones*. New York: Academic Press.

Verant, M.L., Meteyer, C.U., Speakman, J.R. et al. (2014). White-nose syndrome initiates a cascade of physiologic disturbances in the hibernating bat host. *BMC Physiology* 14: 10.

Wellehan, J.F.X., Zens, M.S., Bright, A.A. et al. (2001). Type 1 external fixation of radial fractures in microchiropterans. *Journal of Zoo and Wildlife Medicine* 32: 487–493.

Winn, D. (2006). When food can be fatal: recovery from emaciation. *Wildlife Rehabilitation Bulletin* 24 (1): 26–29.

28

Natural History and Medical Management of Terrestrial and Aquatic Chelonians

Terry M. Norton[1] and Matthew C. Allender[2]

[1] *Georgia Sea Turtle Center/Jekyll Island Authority, Jekyll Island, GA, USA*
[2] *Department of Veterinary Clinical Medicine, University of Illinois, Urbana, IL, USA*

Introduction

Several terrestrial and aquatic turtles and tortoises (chelonians) are experiencing population declines across the world. Currently, of the 328 total species of chelonians in the world, 178 (53%) are listed as near-threatened or worse with many species already extinct (Rhodin et al. 2010; van Dijk 2011). In the US, freshwater turtles have been exploited by the Southeast Asian turtle trade where tons of turtles, especially snapping turtles, softshells, and terrapins, have been captured and shipped abroad (IUCN 2015). Drowning in crab traps is a significant cause of mortality in the diamondback terrapin, particularly males due to their smaller size.

Natural History

Nearly 60 species of native turtles and tortoises exist in the United States, many of which are freshwater turtles. However, rehabilitation centers are commonly presented with terrestrial species such as box turtles (Brown and Sleeman 2002; Schrader et al. 2010), gopher tortoises (*Gopherus polyphemus*), desert tortoises (*Gopherus agassizii*) (Edwards and Berry 2013) and several aquatic species.

The eastern box turtle (*Terrapene carolina carolina*) has experienced significant population declines in numerous areas throughout its range (IUCN 2011). They are long-lived individuals, with some living over 100 years (Ernst and Lovich 2009). Sexual maturity occurs at 5–10 years of age for both sexes (Ernst and Lovich 2009).

There are five living species of North American tortoises: the gopher tortoise (*G. polyphemus*) from the southeastern US, desert tortoise (*G. agassizii*) from the

southwestern US, Texas tortoise (*G. berlandieri*) from south of Del Rio and San Antonio through eastern Coahuila, Nuevo Leon, and Tamaulipas to northeastern San Luis Potosi, Mexico, and Bolson's tortoise (*G. flavomarginatus*) from north central Mexico (Ernst et al. 1994c). Recently, desert tortoises occurring east and south of the Colorado River were described as a new species, *Gopherus morafkai* (Berry and Aresco 2014). Longevity is estimated at between 50 and 70 years, but annuli are only good indicators up to 13 years (Ernst and Lovich 2009). Sexual maturity is reached between nine and 21 years and is similar between both species (Ernst and Lovich 2009). All are adapted for burrowing, with shovel-like flattened forelimbs adapted for digging burrows. The gopher tortoise is considered to be the keystone species of the longleaf pine ecosystem. Its burrow provides shelter for 360 other animal species (Ernst et al. 1994c; Ashton and Ashton 2004).

North American genera of freshwater chelonians that are commonly presented for rehabilitation include *Trachchemys* (sliders), *Chrysemys* (painted turtles), *Kinosternon* (mud turtles), *Apalone* (softshelled turtles), *Pseudemys* (river cooters), and *Chelydra* (common snapping turtles). Longevity is variable among these genera and difficult to determine in wild populations, but when known can range from 20 to 50 years (Ernst and Lovich 2009). Similarly, sexual maturity is variable across geographic locations and is more defined based on size in most species (Ernst and Lovich 2009).

The diamondback terrapin (*Malaclemys terrapin*) is the only turtle species that resides predominantly in brackish coastal marshes of the eastern and southern United States. It has one of the largest ranges of all turtles in North America, stretching as far south as Florida Keys and as far north as Cape Cod with seven subspecies

Medical Management of Wildlife Species: A Guide for Practitioners, First Edition. Edited by Sonia M. Hernandez, Heather W. Barron, Erica A. Miller, Roberto F. Aguilar and Michael J. Yabsley.

within this range. It can survive in fresh water as well as full-strength ocean water but adults prefer intermediate salinities. Terrapins have high site fidelity and tend to live in the same areas for most or all of their lives, and do not make long-distance migrations (Ernst et al. 1994c). Sexual maturity occurs at 4–7 years in males and 8–10 years in females (Ernst and Lovich 2009). Longevity is reported from 20 to 40+ years (Ernst and Lovich 2009). Extreme sexual dimorphism exists in diamondback terrapins and map turtles, with females being much larger than males (Ernst et al. 1994a).

Common Diseases, Disorders, and Injuries of Chelonians

Chelonian species are at risk for a range of infectious and noninfectious diseases. In rehabilitation centers, the primary presentation and final diagnosis are most commonly associated with trauma (Brown and Sleeman 2002; Schrader et al. 2010; Rivas et al. 2014; Steen et al. 2014), but infectious diseases (e.g., upper respiratory infection, aural abscesses, etc.) are identified as the final diagnosis in ~10–18% of cases although cause of disease was not always investigated (Schrader et al. 2010).

Lethal disease outbreaks have emerged across the eastern US in chelonians (Harper et al. 1982; Brown and Sleeman 2002; Allender 2012; Allender et al. 2013a). Specifically, ranavirus and *Mycoplasma* have accounted for mortality events in box turtles and gopher tortoises in the eastern US (Feldman et al. 2006; Allender 2012). Moreover, herpesvirus infections have been demonstrated to be highly fatal in several captive US, European, and South African tortoise species, but its impact on free-ranging North American chelonians is unknown (Origgi et al. 2004; Marschang et al. 2006; Jacobson et al. 2012; Sim et al. 2015).

The family Iridoviridae consists of five genera of pathogens in invertebrates and ectothermic vertebrates including fish, amphibians, and reptiles (ICTV 2011), subsequently leading to the potential for pathogen transmission in rehabilitation facilities that house these vertebrate classes. Diseases caused by viruses in the genera *Ranavirus* are specifically a growing concern in free-ranging amphibian and reptile populations (Miller et al. 2011; Allender et al. 2013a). In box turtles, prevalence outside of an outbreak is often <1%, but may be as high as 3% in a rehabilitation center in the same geographic area (Allender et al. 2011).

Mycoplasmosis (caused by *Mycoplasma agassizii and M. testudineum*) is a bacterial disease characterized by rhinitis and conjunctivitis in wild tortoises and has been associated with population declines in free-ranging tortoises

within the US (Jacobson et al. 1991; Brown et al. 1999; Wendland et al. 2006). Mortality is rare, but morbidity can affect all animals in a population, and can lead to carrier states (Wendland et al. 2006). Most tortoises develop chronic disease and may serve as a reservoir for transmission. Similar disease has been noted in *Mycoplasma*-infected box turtles, but the prevalence in and impact on free-ranging turtles are poorly understood (Feldman et al. 2006). However, prevalence in free-ranging bog turtles (70%), box turtles (100%), and spotted turtles (18%) demonstrated widespread occurrence of this pathogen (Ossiboff et al. 2015). Herpesviruses are double-stranded DNA viruses that affect numerous species of animals (Origgi et al. 2004). They have been recognized in all orders of reptiles, with mortality rates up to 100% in experimental studies (Origgi et al. 2004). Clinical signs most commonly associated with herpesvirus infections in tortoises are rhinitis, stomatitis, and conjunctivitis (Origgi et al. 2004). Oral plaques can develop and may be mild or large enough to impair eating (Figure 28.1).

Few studies have determined the prevalence, pathogenesis, or phylogenetic relatedness of herpesviruses in wild chelonians, but a new herpesvirus was recently characterized in captive and free-ranging eastern box turtles (Jacobson et al. 2012; Sim et al. 2015). A variety of adenovirus species appear to be emerging in both captive and wild populations (Rivera et al. 2009; Doszpoly et al. 2013). Testudine intranuclear coccidiosis (TINC) is a serious parasite in captive tortoises and turtles (Innis et al. 2007) and has the potential to be a problem in wild populations.

Aural abscesses are often seen in box turtles presented to rehabilitation centers (Brown and Sleeman 2002; Schrader et al. 2010), but they also occur in other free-ranging chelonian species (Figure 28.2).

The etiological agents are variable and are believed to be secondary to an altered aural microbial environment (Joyner et al. 2006). Other studies have resulted in mixed findings for the correlation of aural abscesses and organochlorine exposure leading to hypovitaminosis A (Sleeman et al. 2008). Despite the common occurrence, its presence likely has minimal contagious capabilities.

The most common medical issues seen in freshwater turtles presented for rehabilitation are injuries sustained from automobile strikes and fishhook and line ingestion. Both of these issues are depleting populations drastically (Steen et al. 2014; Crawford et al. 2014a).

Husbandry: Enclosures

Chelonians may be housed in a wide range of environments, such as tanks, cages, or runs. The size will vary with the species, but should be large enough for them to

(a)

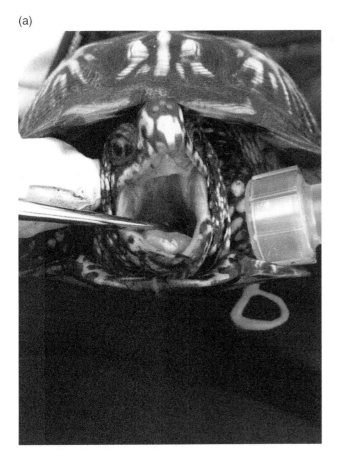

(b)

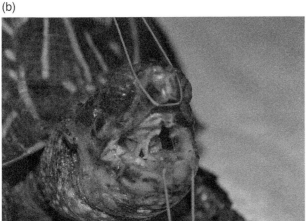

Figure 28.1 Presence of minimal (a) and severe (b) oral plaques observed in a free-ranging eastern box turtle (*Terrapene carolina carolina*) during an oral examination. *Source:* Courtesy of Matt Allender (a) and CROW (b).

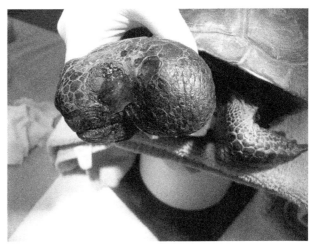

Figure 28.2 Aural abscess in a free-ranging gopher tortoise (*Gopherus polyphemus*). *Source:* Courtesy of Terry Norton.

waterproofed. Access to natural sunlight is preferred, especially in young animals, even if only a few times per week. If not possible, vitamin D3 should be supplemented in the diet. In the absence of natural sunlight, artificial ultraviolet (UV) light sources have been evaluated and should be referenced to acquire full-spectrum UVA and UVB (Adkins et al. 2003; Burger et al. 2007).

For *Gopherus*, in a rehabilitation setting, outdoor enclosures work best but indoor housing may be necessary for critically ill patients or when it is too cold. Tortoises are much more likely to eat if housed outdoors where there is access to grass for grazing. They are much more comfortable in larger outdoor areas with grass to graze upon and dirt to dig. The perimeter should have sides extending well below the surface. Solid walls are preferred over fencing. The outdoor enclosure should drain properly and not become overly wet. The tortoise burrow is a very stable environment, an important consideration when attempting to care for them.

Large stock tanks, for horses, work very well for indoor housing. A sand/dirt mix is best as a substrate unless open wounds are present. Wearing down the claws is a real problem if improper substrate is used. An overhead heat source should be positioned at one end of the enclosure to provide a basking spot of approximately 32 °C (90 °F) with cooler areas available 21–24 °C (70–75 °F) for thermoregulation. A full-spectrum fluorescent light should be provided for UVB.

Freshwater turtles and diamondback terrapins in critical condition may need to be dry docked, especially if the shell integrity is compromised or the turtle is in shock or weak. Small tubs with a thermogradient and a towel as a bottom substrate work well. Once the turtle can be placed in water, a small plastic container tilted with water at one end and a towel on the other works well for short periods.

demonstrate normal temperature-seeking behavior and include a hide box (terrestrial species) or basking site (aquatic species). The enclosure should also provide an environment that prevents injury or damage during recovery, such that turtles with fractures should not be allowed to submerge in water unless the injury has been

For the stable aquatic patient, housing requirements vary according to size and species. In a rehabilitation setting, we recommend housing freshwater turtles individually. For example, diamondback terrapin are not aggressive but if they are overcrowded, especially juveniles, they will bite each other. Adult terrapins seem to benefit from group housing if a large enough enclosure and basking spot are provided. If the terrapins are from the same location, they can be housed together. Male aquatic turtles may need to be kept separated from females in a rehabilitation setting due to constant attempts to mount.

A rule of thumb for minimum enclosure size in a relatively active and recovering aquatic turtle patient is that the combined surface area of the carapace should not exceed 25% of the floor space surface area. Floor surface area does not include inaccessible areas that the turtle cannot rest on. Water depths of 2 ft and lots of surface area to swim around are important. The simpler the set-up, the easier it will be to keep clean. Avoid gravel or sand substrates because they will make cleaning much more difficult and the turtle may ingest them (Boyer and Boyer 1992).

Clean water is crucial to good health and best achieved through frequent full water changes and enclosure cleaning. The water can be kept cleaner if the turtle is fed in a separate container. If the turtles are fed in their enclosure, the water should be changed within 12 hours of feeding. Portable electric submersible pumps can drain large volumes of water very quickly, making cleaning much easier. Drains can be installed in the bottom of the tank to empty into a floor drain, which also saves time and staff resources. The enclosure should be thoroughly disinfected and rinsed after the water has been drained and prior to refilling. Waterland Tubs (www.waterlandtubs.com) have designed a variety of tanks for aquatic turtles that work well for rehabilitation of freshwater turtles and diamondback terrapins. Abrupt changes in water temperature can cause mortality, so make sure water temperature after cleaning is similar to what it was prior to cleaning. Water should be at least as deep as the width of the widest turtle's shell so that if overturned, the turtle will be able to right itself and avoid drowning. Filtration can decrease the frequency of complete water changes but not eliminate them. The best filters are external canister filters with refillable charcoal cartridges that are changed every 1–2 weeks. Water quality should be monitored regularly for pH, ammonia, nitrites, and nitrates.

Water temperature for most species should be 24–28 °C (75–80 °F). Some species, such as mud and musk turtles and common snapping turtles, prefer it a bit cooler. A submersible aquarium heater is typically needed. A basking area is needed and should be around 32 °C (90 °F) for most species and provide a full-spectrum light source during the day. The basking area should be large enough for the turtle to completely emerge from the water and dry off and secure enough so that it will not fall over and trap the turtle. A cinderblock with rubber matting that allows the turtle to climb up onto the basking area works well (Figure 28.3).

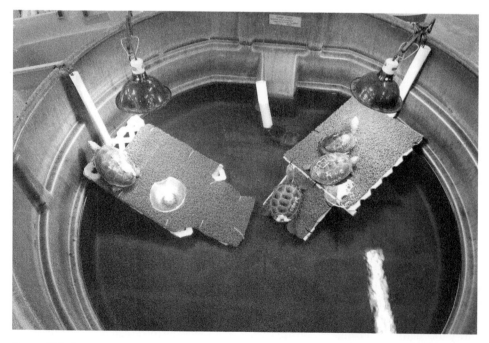

Figure 28.3 An appropriate aquatic turtle rehabilitation setting with a basking site covered in 3M matting, UV light source, and clean water. *Source:* Courtesy of Terry Norton.

Avoid rough surfaces that cause skin and shell abrasions. Snapping turtles do not need basking areas. Full-spectrum UV and basking lights that provide heat are necessary (Adkins et al. 2003).

The stable adult diamondback terrapin undergoing rehabilitation is best maintained in brackish water (15 parts per thousand [ppt]). The terrapin can be fed in a separate container with fresh water which will aid in hydration and maintaining water quality.

In general, to avoid pathogen transmission, turtles of different species or different populations of the same species should not be housed in contact with each other. Shared equipment should not be used in these cases and strict biosecurity should be followed.

Diet

Diets of species commonly found in a rehabilitation setting range widely from piscivorous to herbivorous. All attempts must be made to provide a high-quality, balanced diet consistent with natural diets. Omnivorous species, such as the box turtle, should be offered a range of vegetables (including dark leafy greens and orange and red vegetables) and insect protein sources. Fruit may be offered food 3–4 times weekly. Caloric content may be calculated, but offering *ad libitum* is usually acceptable for the brief time they are in rehabilitation.

Gopherus are all strict herbivores and typically eat a mixed diet of grasses, leaves, and wild fruits (Ashton and Ashton 2004). Grasses and grass-like plants are the principal foods of adults and broad-leaved weeds are preferred by juvenile tortoises, with dependence upon them increasing as the growing season progresses and grass becomes dryer and less nutritious. In captivity, a high-fiber, low-protein, and calcium-rich diet will ensure good digestive tract function and smooth growth. *Opuntia* cactus, grass hay, assorted weeds, leafy greens, and dandelions are all good additions to the diet. Providing the opportunity to graze on grass is nutritious and behaviorally stimulating. Nutritionally complete pellets formulated for tortoises can be provided as part of the diet, especially if the tortoise is under weight. Calcium supplementation is particularly important in juvenile tortoises. Cuttlebones are a good source of calcium and will help with beak maintenance.

A balanced diet for freshwater turtles is very important for good health. A wide variety of foods should be fed. A variety of whole chopped fish, chopped mice, earthworms, and commercial pellets work well for most species. Many sliders and cooters become more herbivorous as they mature, thus dark leafy greens can be added to their diet.

For diamondback terrapins, various types of fish, shrimp, crab, and squid can be fed. Live prey such as fiddler crabs and periwinkle snails should be fed regularly. Hatchling and juvenile diamondback terrapins should be fed a mixture of commercial foods and small live prey once they are large enough to handle without injury (Helms 2006).

Diagnostic Evaluation

Physical Examination

There are several limitations in performing a physical examination of a chelonian but it often directs the prognosis and management. There is no prescribed method for performing the examination, but each examination should follow a similar pattern.

Evaluation of the eyes and nares should confirm symmetry and describe the presence and nature of any discharge. Conjunctivitis and rhinitis are common signs of diseases and careful attention should be paid to these structures. Symmetry and presence or absence of swelling of the tympanic membranes should be recorded. An oral examination should be performed in each animal; it is often the most revealing component of the examination as it may demonstrate the clinical signs of dehydration, anemia, septicemia, infectious disease, and vitamin deficiency. Access to the oral cavity is difficult in most chelonians and may require sedation in some species (e.g., softshells and snapping turtles). In most species, careful elevation with a probe can be successful without sedation (Figure 28.1).

The physical examination should continue with evaluation of the axial and appendicular musculoskeletal structures. Presence of swelling, flaking, pitting, ulcerations, erosions, discharge, and fractures of the limbs or shell should be recorded. Appearance of the skin and nails should then be recorded. A neurological examination that includes the ability to use the fore- and hindlegs is critical in trauma cases.

Sample Collection

Venipuncture is most often performed through collection of venous blood from the jugular vein, subcarapacial sinus, brachial vein, femoral vein, or tail veins (Lloyd and Morris 1999). The jugular vein can be accessed with the neck in full extension, but may require sedation. Samples from this site are least likely to result in lymph contamination (Gottdenker and Jacobson 1995) (Figure 28.4c). The subcarapacial sinus is often used in box turtles and freshwater turtles smaller than 1 kg (Hernandez-Divers et al. 2002) (Figure 28.4a). This site can be accessed with

(a)

(b)

(c)

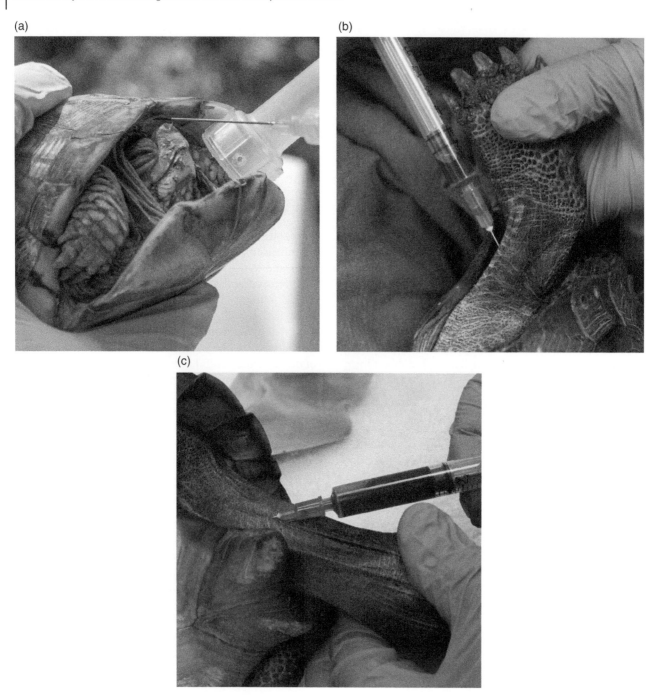

Figure 28.4 Sites for venipuncture include the subcarapacial sinus (a; eastern box turtle), brachial vein (b; gopher tortoise), and jugular vein (c; gopher tortoise). *Source:* Courtesy of Terry Norton and Matt Allender.

the turtle still contained within the shell, providing an easy site for free-ranging box turtles. However, blood from this site is often mixed with lymphatic fluid and thus can alter results by lowering packed cell volume (PCV) and total solids (TS) (or TP), increasing sodium, and decreasing potassium and many enzymes on a biochemistry panel. The brachial vein is most useful for *Gopherus* spp. and is accessed with the forelimb in extension

near the caudal aspect of the leg; however, there is also a high risk of lymphatic contamination (Figure 28.4b).

The femoral vein is accessed with the animal in dorsal recumbency and leg in extension. The landmarks are similar to other animals. The dorsal and ventral tail veins are attractive options for large animals or those that are aggressive (e.g., snapping turtles). An approach to the occipital sinus has been reported for aquatic turtles by extending the head and accessing the vessel with a 25 gauge needle on the dorsal midline (Martinez-Silvestre et al. 2002).

Maximum blood volume that can be collected in a chelonian is recommended to be 5–8% of the blood volume (~0.5–0.8% of the body weight) (Smits and Kozubowski 1985; Sykes and Klaphake 2015). Samples collected from the subcarapacial sinus can be accomplished with the use of a 1.5 in. needle or butterfly set attached to an appropriately sized syringe. Samples from the brachial, femoral, and tail veins can be collected with a 22–25 gauge 0.75 in. needle on 1–6 mL syringes. Most samples should be placed in lithium heparin (Muro et al. 1998) after fresh whole blood smears are made (Sykes and Klaphake 2015), but the authors have utilized heparinized syringes and made blood smears within five minutes of collection. Some freshwater turtle blood has been successfully stored in dipotassium EDTA (Martinez-Jimenez et al. 2007), but many other reports indicate lysis of blood cells in chelonians (Anderson et al. 1997; Budischak et al. 2006; Campbell 2006; Chansue et al. 2011; Christopher et al. 1999; Chung et al. 2009; Sykes and Klaphake 2015).

Oral and cloacal swabs often lead to the most rewarding diagnostic results for common upper respiratory and gastrointestinal pathogens of chelonians. Oral swabbing needs to include both the respiratory epithelium accessed from the choanae on the roof of the oral cavity as well as the oral epithelium itself. Sampling can occur using many types of swabs, but sterile cotton-tipped applicators are the most common. Synthetic swabs, such as nylon flocked swabs, produce superior samples for culture, virus isolation, and molecular diagnostics and may improve the ability to detect a pathogen.

Radiography is helpful in diagnosing lower respiratory diseases, gastrointestinal (GI) foreign bodies (fish hook and line), fractures, ileus, and many other conditions. Proper positioning is integral to accurate interpretation in chelonians, similar to mammal and bird patients. Unlike mammals and birds, chelonian radiographs require three views. The patient should be maintained in a horizontal plane: dorsal-ventral, right or left lateral, and cranial-caudal. Failure to acquire the horizontal beam of the cranial-caudal projection prevents accurate diagnoses of pulmonary disease as this is the only view that separates the lung fields and does not have superimposing GI or reproductive structures.

Clinical Pathology

A single complete blood count result in a chelonian is rarely helpful in identifying disease, but serial samples or comparisons among similarly grouped animals may detect significant changes. A single sample in certain cases can help direct therapy in cases of nonregenerative anemia, hypoglycemia, hypoproteinemia, or increased PCV/TS. Several studies have reported reference ranges for free-ranging chelonians (see Appendix I) but these studies have also demonstrated the effect that season, age class, sex, venipuncture site, and disease status can have on the hemogram (Stacy et al. 2011; Sykes and Klaphake 2015). Thus, with all of the demographic and physiological differences between individuals, interpretation of the hemogram should be undertaken with caution (Chung et al. 2009). Wild chelonians may present with chronic debilitation and common abnormalities to clinical pathology parameters may include low PCV, hypoproteinemia, and hypoalbuminemia, low BUN in carnivorous turtles, low cholesterol and triglycerides, low calcium and high phosphorus. Follow-up sampling after rehydration therapy is recommended.

Infectious Diseases

There are several infectious diseases that have been described in free-ranging chelonians, including ranaviral disease, herpes, and mycoplasmosis.

Ranaviral disease in chelonians is caused by Frog 3-virus. Affected wild turtles commonly present with upper respiratory signs, oral plaques, stomatitis, facial edema, severe chemosis, lethargy, and dehydration but may also include red skin lesions and conjunctivitis (Hausmann et al. 2013). Diagnosis includes histopathology, molecular diagnostics, virus isolation, ELISA, electron microscopy, and cytology (Hyatt et al. 2000; Gray et al. 2009; Miller et al. 2011; Allender and Mitchell 2013; Allender et al. 2006, 2013b, 2013c). Immunohistochemistry is useful in quickly confirming the presence of a pathogen in formalin-fixed tissue (Cunningham et al. 2008; Balseiro et al. 2009; Cinkova et al. 2010). In chelonians, tissues are most commonly tested, while antemortem sampling has only been evaluated in red-eared sliders that demonstrated whole blood was the most sensitive and specific, while oral and cloacal swabs showed the same specificity but lower sensitivity (Allender et al. 2011). Quantitative polymerase chain reaction (qPCR) has been developed to detect lower amounts of genetic material than conventional PCR and is the preferred method (Daszak et al. 2000, De Voe et al. 2004, Allender et al. 2011). Serological assays have been developed to detect antibodies against FV3 antigen, but are not currently commercially available (Johnson et al. 2010).

Herpesvirus (caused by herpesviruses 1–4) causes upper respiratory tract disease (URTD) and necrotizing stomatitis with high mortality rates. Diagnosis is accomplished through histopathology, PCR/qPCR, and ELISA. Characteristic intranuclear inclusions may be observed in affected cells of the respiratory or GI cells/tissues of infected patients. The most widely used molecular test is a herpesvirus-wide conventional PCR (van Devanter et al. 1996; Sim et al. 2015). This method requires sequencing of products but some may or may not be associated with clinical disease. Herpesvirus diagnosis in many species of tortoises has been reported based on results of an ELISA (Origgi et al. 2004). However, this requires the use of species-specific antibodies or interpretation of the results based on the assay being validated in other species.

Infection with *Mycoplasma* spp. in turtles and tortoises causes URTD which can present with various signs such as oculonasal discharge, "bubbling" from the nare, and open-mouth breathing. Disease due to *Mycoplasma* is often associated with cyclical recurrent disease that makes traditional methods of pathogen detection difficult. Diagnosis includes pathogen detection (culture and qPCR) and demonstrating previous infections (serology). Culture is ideal but mycoplasmas are difficult to grow and may produce false negatives (Brown et al. 2001). Quantitative PCR assays are highly sensitive for testing *Mycoplasma* in desert tortoise nasal lavage samples (duPre et al. 2011). Conventional PCR has been used in swabs of the choanae of other species, including box turtles (Feldman et al. 2006). Importantly, a PCR-positive sample does not confirm that *Mycoplasma* is causing the disease, and more importantly, it does not indicate it is acting alone. Coinfections with *Mycoplasma* and herpesvirus and even ranavirus are reported in box turtles (Sim et al. 2012; Hausmann et al. 2013) and should be considered likely.

Many times in rehabilitation settings, clinical signs are nonspecific and therefore diagnosis may require a broad approach (Hanley and Hernandez-Divers 2003). Histopathology of specific lesions obtained through biopsies and endoscopy are often the most efficient at obtaining a diagnosis of unknown diseases. Additionally, consensus PCRs are available for many bacterial, fungal, and viral pathogens, but are specific to classes of pathogens and thus require some knowledge of pathogens involved.

Emergency Care and Medical Management

Most chelonians presented for emergency care are dehydrated and hypovolemic, thus rehydration is often the first step in treatment. Debilitated chelonians may be anemic and hypoproteinemic, which may mask the extent of dehydration (Norton 2005). Depending on the species and the severity of the problem, drawing blood may be too stressful for the patient upon presentation and may have to wait until it is more stable. Serial PCV, total solids and other bloodwork will help assess the status of the patient, target the most appropriate therapeutic regimen, and aid in prognostication and response to therapy.

Selecting the route, rate, and type of fluids to administer depends on the species of chelonian and condition of the patient. Fluid choice is frequently dictated by clinician preference, the patient's presenting problem, clinical pathology, and acid–base abnormalities, if available. Mammalian crystalloid fluid preparations are suitable for chelonians. It is critical to correct hydration status of the ill chelonian before starting oral nutritional support. Whole-blood transfusions, ideally using homologous donors, may be indicated in cases of acute hemorrhage and life-threatening anemia and other sources should be referenced (Norton 2005). Alternatively, fluid therapy, careful iron supplementation, and nutritional support may be successful.

Soaking mildly dehydrated patients in shallow lukewarm water 23.8–26.6 °C (75–80 °F), which reaches to just below the chin when the head is retracted, will assist in rehydration and maintaining hydration status (Boyer 1998). This is a preferred method for mildly dehydrated turtles and is recommended for 15–30 minutes per soak once to twice daily initially, with eventual decrease in frequency as the turtle improves. The turtle has the ability to absorb water in the colon actively through negative pressure induced by cloacal contractions.

Intravenous (IV) or intraosseous (IO) routes of fluid administration allow for rapid rehydration and emergency therapy; however, placement, and maintenance of catheters can be technically challenging and should be reserved for patients that are unconscious or minimally responsive. The jugular vein is the preferred site for IV catheter placement in most chelonians. A small skin incision allows direct visualization of the vessel. After catheter placement, secure the catheter to the skin with tape and/or suture (Boyer 1998; Bonner 2000; Norton 2005). Maintaining patency of the jugular catheter may be difficult, especially in active turtles (Whitaker and Krum 1999). IV or IO routes are necessary for administration of whole blood, colloidal fluids, and fluids containing greater than 5% dextrose (McCracken et al. 1994; Divers 1997; Bonner 2000; Rosskopf 2000; Wilkinson 2004). IO catheters may be placed in the distal humerus, distal femur or plastron-carapacial bridge (Mader 1997; Whitaker and Krum 1999).

The primary disadvantages associated with IO catheters are that the fluid flow rate is limited due to the small bone marrow space, fluid and drug administration may be painful, and the metal of the spinal needle may fatigue and break (Wellehan et al. 2004).

Bolus IV fluid therapy via the subcarapacial vein is the authors' choice for initial stabilization. Advantages of the bolus IV method include easy vessel accessibility and minimal stress to the patient due to rapid access.

The epicoelomic fluid administration site is useful in chelonians that are completely retracted into their shell and difficult to coerce out (McArthur 2004). The intracoelomic (IC) route is not recommended by the authors because of the potential of compromising the lung space, perforating the lungs or GI tract, urinary bladder, or an ovarian follicle in mature females. Hypoproteinemic patients may have fluid in the coelomic cavity, which will further complicate absorption.

Subcutaneous fluids can be given into any accessible fold of skin, but are typically placed into the inguinal fossa, front limb fossa, or ventral neck fold. Administering the fluids in multiple sites may improve absorption. Disadvantages to this route include poor absorption in severely debilitated chelonians (Norton 2005).

The oral route of fluid administration should be reserved for use in patients with functional GI tracts that are mildly to moderately dehydrated and for maintenance fluid therapy. Severely dehydrated and weak turtles tend to regurgitate orally administered fluids (Norton 2005). Fluids can be administered directly into the stomach using an appropriately sized, well-lubricated red rubber or metal feeding tube. For long-term oral medication, fluid therapy and nutritional support, an esophagostomy tube should be considered (see Section 28.9). The stomach volume in most chelonian patients is about 2% of the body weight or 20 mL/kg (Bonner 2000; Wilkinson 2004). Procedures for placement are described elsewhere (Norton 2005).

Maintenance fluid rates range from 15 to 40 mL/kg/day depending on the degree of dehydration and size of the patient. Smaller patients should be given more fluids per kg than larger patients. Infusion or syringe pumps can be used to accurately control the flow rate. Care should be taken not to overhydrate anemic and hypoproteinemic patients (Norton 2005).

Nutritional Support

Nutritional support is an important component of chelonian critical care. Patients respond more quickly to therapy if their nutritional status is positive. The critically ill chelonian is often immunosuppressed secondary to starvation. Regurgitation and aspiration may occur in dehydrated and debilitated chelonians. These turtles may not be able to digest solid food and the material may remain in the stomach as a result of decreased GI motility. Thus, GI nutritional support should not be instituted until the patient has been rehydrated and attains normal blood glucose and GI motility. The volume of formula fed by stomach tube is approximately 0.5–2% or 20 mL/kg of the turtle's body weight. Begin with smaller volumes and more dilute solutions and steadily increase the volume

and concentration to meet the turtle's nutritional requirements. The turtle should be weighed daily during the convalescent period, and the measurement of weight gain or loss can be used as a guide for dietary management (Norton 2005).

Cardiopulmonary Resuscitation Principles in Chelonians

For chelonians presented in respiratory or cardiovascular arrest, determine if the animal has a heartbeat with a Doppler probe, electrocardiogram, and/or ultrasound. Proceed only if cardiac electrical activity is present. Keep in mind that the heart will continue to beat for hours to even a day after the chelonian is dead. Second, extend the head and neck, swab the mouth to remove any materials blocking the glottis, and intubate the patient with an uncuffed endotracheal (ET) tube. Use suction and/or gravity to remove any material from the ET tube. Ventilate the patient with oxygen. A self-inflating bag or manual resuscitator (Ambu bag) can be used for field emergencies. Lubricate the eyes if they are open. Administer fluids IV or IO as described earlier, obtain blood for a minimum database if possible, and then bolus fluids and emergency medications. If the heart rate remains low (variable for each species) with ventilation and bolus fluids, glycopyrrolate IV or atropine IV should be administered. Epinephrine can be given IV, IO, IP, intratracheally, or intracardiac (Norton 2005).

Therapeutic Agents Used in Chelonians

Although several pharmacokinetic studies have been conducted on chelonians (Lawrence et al. 1984; Caligiuri et al. 1990; Prezant et al. 1994; Raphael et al. 1994; Holz et al. 1997; Stamper et al. 1999; Wimsatt et al. 1999; Kolmstetter et al. 2001; Mallo et al. 2002; Jacobson et al. 2003; James et al. 2003; Manire et al. 2003), limited information is available on accurate dosing for the numerous species presented to rehabilitation centers (see Appendix II: Formulary). Because sick chelonians do not necessarily absorb drugs well, it is important to correct hypothermia, dehydration, hypoglycemia, acid–base, and electrolyte imbalances before or in conjunction with starting other therapeutic agents. Drug absorption is temperature dependent in reptiles so the patient's core body temperature should be within its preferred optimal temperature zone (POTZ).

Antimicrobial Therapy in Critically Ill Chelonians

Sick and injured turtles are usually given broad-spectrum antibiotics as a treatment for established bacterial infections or as a preventive measure (see Appendix II: Formulary). Diagnostic samples should be obtained for culture and antimicrobial sensitivity testing before starting antibiotic therapy whenever possible. Although controversial, the front half of the body, including the soft tissues of the forelimbs and neck, should be used for injections (Beck et al. 1995; Holtz et al. 1997; Bonner 2000), especially when using nephrotoxic drugs. Enrofloxacin is a commonly used antibiotic in chelonians and has good efficacy against aerobic gram-negative bacteria. Unfortunately, it can cause tissue necrosis when injected multiple times IM or SQ and is painful on administration, which can be minimized by diluting it in saline and only using the SQ route for injection. Anaerobic bacteria can also cause significant morbidity in chelonians and should be considered when deciding on a therapeutic plan.

Many critically ill chelonians are painful and benefit from analgesics (see Appendix II: Formulary). Chelonians are relatively stoic and challenging to assess for pain. Pain may be exhibited in chelonians by decreased appetite, depression, or alteration in normal behavior such as lameness or not using a limb. Butorphanol and buprenorphine have been demonstrated to be ineffective as opioid analgesics in reptiles (Sladky 2014). Tramadol (5 mg/kg PO) administered to red-eared sliders significantly increased withdrawal latencies for 12–24 hours post drug administration, and 6–96 hours after administration of the higher tramadol dosages (10 or 25 mg/kg PO) (Baker et al. 2011). Plasma concentrations of tramadol and O-desmethyltramadol remained ≥100 ng/mL for 48 hours when administered at a dose of 5 mg/kg orally and for 72 hours at a dose of 10 mg/kg orally in loggerhead sea turtles (Norton et al. 2015). Respiratory depression associated with tramadol administration in red-eared sliders was approximately 50% less than that measured after morphine administration (Baker et al. 2011).

For heavy debridement, low-dose dexmedetomidine (5–10 μg/kg) intranasally, IM, or IV has been beneficial in selected sea turtle patients, while some sea turtles require much higher doses. Dexmedetomidine is also useful for short painful procedures in other chelonians. The dose is extremely variable among species and individuals within a species. The reversibility of this drug is attractive. It should not be used in critical unstable chelonian patients due to the cardiovascular side effects.

Lidocaine at a maximum dose of 5 mg/kg may be helpful alone or in combination with other drugs in chelonians for selected procedures. Topical 4% lidocaine placed directly on a wound after initial cleaning may provide pain relief in some situations.

Nonsteroidal antiinflammatory drugs (NSAIDs) are frequently used in chelonians for both analgesic and antiinflammatory properties. Ball pythons administered meloxicam (0.3 mg/kg IM) prior to surgical placement of an arterial catheter showed no physiological changes indicative of analgesia (Olesen and Perry 2009). Plasma concentrations of meloxicam (0.2 mg/kg PO) administered as a single dose to green iguanas were at levels considered analgesic in mammals, and these levels were measureable out to 24 hours post administration (Divers et al. 2010). In loggerhead sea turtles, meloxicam (0.1 mg/kg) administered both IM and IV did not reach plasma concentrations consistent with analgesia in humans, horses, or dogs (Lai et al. 2015). Ketoprofen (2 mg/kg IV) administered to green iguanas had a long half-life (31 hours) compared to ketoprofen pharmacokinetics in mammals, but the bioavailability after IM administration was only 78% with a relatively short half-life (8.3 hours) (Tuttle et al. 2006). Since there are no efficacy data and few pharmacokinetics studies on NSAID administration in reptiles, appropriate dosages and frequency of administration can only be extrapolated. There are several potential deleterious side effects documented in other species (e.g., renal impairment, GI ulceration/inflammation, hematological abnormalities), so these drugs should be used with caution. Chelonian pain management may be best approached using a multimodal analgesia drug paradigm (Sladky 2014).

Wound Management Techniques

Wound management techniques used for the various chelonian species are similar to those for humans and domestic animals. Initially, the wound is cleaned and larger debris is removed from the wound. Copious lavage with saline or lactated Ringer's, dilute chlorhexidine, or povidone-iodine is critical. Regular debridement of necrotic and infected tissue is critical, especially in the early stages of wound management.

A variety of topical products for open wound management have been successfully used by the authors. The choice of a particular product depends on the wound, stage of healing, and frequency of treatment. Silver-containing products have been shown to be antimicrobial and speed wound healing. For example, SilvaKlenz® and Silvion® (Molecular Therapeutics, Athens, GA, USA) are pH-balanced potentiated ionic silver solutions that are showing promising results for wound cleansing and flushing. The turtle should be positioned so the flushed solution drains ventrally, especially if the coelomic cavity integrity is compromised. For relatively minor wounds on the shell, silver collasate postoperative dressing® (PRN Pharmacal, Pensacola, FL, USA) and silver sulfadiazine cream (SSD, Kings Pharmaceutical, Bristol, TX, USA) mixed with ilex paste (Medcon Biolab Technologies,

Grafton, MA, USA) for waterproofing in aquatic species can be applied after cleaning and debridement.

Honey is another topical antimicrobial that may be used. Frequent wound management is usually necessary and a waterproof bandage is often needed for aquatic species to keep the honey in place. Honey will attract ants so if the patient is being managed outdoors, an alternative will be needed.

A waterproof bandage consists of petroleum-impregnated gauze over the topical product, Tegaderm® or similar sticky bandaging material with superglue placed around the edges, and finally waterproof tape placed over the entire area with another application of superglue.

Rediheal® (Avalon Medical, Stillwater, MN, USA), a borate-based biological glass containing factors that promote angiogenesis, can be applied to deep wounds with exposed bone, and has been effective in the authors' experience. For deep shell wounds, it can be placed within the wound and then covered with bone cement impregnated or not with an antibiotic. Doxirobe® gel (doxycycline, Zoetis, Parsippany, NJ, USA) has been useful for treating exposed bone and stays on well in aquatic environments. Superglue can be used to lightly cover the Doxirobe or bone cement once it is dry to provide further waterproofing. Weekly wound management is usually adequate when using these products in aquatic species.

Large skin defects are often difficult to bandage. The wound is packed with the preferred topical product and petroleum-impregnated gauze and then suture loops or staples are placed around the wound and umbilical tape or suture material is placed through the loops or staples to hold the dressing in place. Vacuum-assisted wound care has been very effective in treating a variety of wounds in chelonians (Lafortune et al. 2014) (Figure 28.5a,b).

Surgical Management

Anesthesia

Anesthetic and analgesic protocols should provide muscle relaxation and analgesia when performing surgery on chelonian patients. Supplemental heat, consistent with the patient's POTZ, is necessary during an anesthetic procedure to allow normal metabolism of the anesthetics for both induction and recovery.

Dissociative anesthetic agents (e.g., ketamine), alpha-2 agonists (e.g., dexmedetomidine), propofol, inhalants (e.g., isoflurane), local anesthetics (e.g., lidocaine, bupivicaine), and more recently neuroactive steroid (alfaxalone) have been found to provide the most reliable results in reptiles and have been summarized well in other texts (Read 2004; Ziolo and Bertelsen 2009; Schroeder and Johnson 2013; Knotek 2014; Vigani 2014) (Box 28.1).

Fracture Repair

Shell repair is the most common indication for surgery in rehabilitated chelonian species. The procedures and approaches for repair in turtles and tortoises are similar to other species: provide stability in normal anatomical position for a sufficient time to allow bone healing (Fleming 2008). Bone healing in reptiles, in general, may take between six and 30 months (Mitchell 2002), necessitating the need for long-term housing. Specific approaches to repair involve either external coaption or internal fixation (Mitchell 2002; Fleming 2008; Vella 2009).

If the fracture is nondisplaced and stable or if it involves the appendicular skeleton, then external coaption with bandaging and protection may be used. Additionally, this

(a)

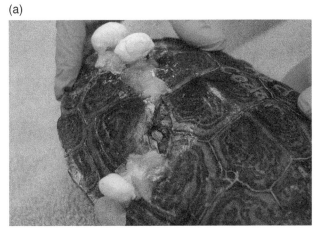

(b)

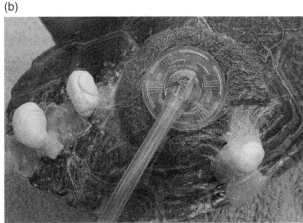

Figure 28.5 Carapace fracture repair utilizing screws and wires covered with marine epoxy, and bone cement within the fracture site before (a) and after (b) application of the vacuum-assisted closure. *Source:* Courtesy of Terry Norton.

Box 28.1 Meshing Rehabilitation, Education, and Research: the GSTC Diamondback Terrapin Model

The Georgia Sea Turtle Center (GSTC) is a conservation organization that focuses its efforts on native chelonians and integrates rehabilitation, education, and research. A Diamondback Terrapin (*Malaclemys terrapin*) Conservation Initiative started with rescuing them off the road after being hit, rehabilitating them, recovering their eggs for incubation and eventual release of any that were successfully rehabilitated or hatched. Over the last ten years, this has evolved into a multifaceted conservation program which is serving as a model for other similar initiatives around the world (Crawford et al. 2014a, b, 2015; Grosse et al. 2015). Thousands of reproductively mature female diamondback terrapins are injured and killed by motor vehicles on causeways going to developed barrier islands throughout their range during the nesting season. On the Jekyll Island Causeway (JIC) alone, an average of 163 and a range of 91–223 terrapins have been hit annually and a total of 980 have been hit over a six-year period.

Initial research focused on investigating the extent of the problem on the JIC and demonstrated that per capita terrapin mortality from vehicle strikes and nest predation rates is sufficient to cause population decline along the JIC. Additionally, we demonstrated where the hot and warm spots for terrapin nesting and crossing occur and that there is a three-hour window surrounding high tide when a large percentage of the terrapins come up to nest. Annual sampling of the terrapin population in two creeks next to the JIC over several years demonstrated a male-biased (4:1 male:female) population which is suspected to be due to a combination of adult female mortality from being struck on the road while nesting and the extensive shrub vegetation that shades nesting habitats resulting in the production of male hatchlings. These results were critical to designing our management strategies, which included nest mounds to attract the terrapins to nest and avoid crossing the road and electrified nest boxes that allow the terrapins through but not raccoons and other predators. Nest mounds and boxes were strategically placed in the hot and warm spots along the JIC. The most successful barrier was modified over several years and consisted of six nest boxes which were designed to block terrapins from getting to the road and provide attractive nesting habitat. We have observed subsequent reductions in the number of turtles on the road and the number of nests being depredated at this location which is no longer a hot spot.

Early on, eight static signs were dispersed along the JIC to alert drivers that terrapins were nesting but over the last two seasons, two flashing warning signs similar to a school crossing sign were used in addition to the other signs. We estimate that the rate of mortality due to vehicles has decreased 30–50% from the rates observed prior to sign installation, which suggests the flashing signs are reducing road mortality. Little is known about the movements of females during the nesting season, thus spatial ecology of the nesting females is being investigated by initially using radiotransmitters and now GPS telemetry.

Education programs have been developed for the general public, school children, scientists, veterinary students, and veterinarians. The GSTC is open to the public and has an interactive diamondback terrapin exhibit, a treatment room window where various rehabilitation activities can be observed up close, and displays of hatchling and adult terrapins. Several interactive education programs have been developed for kids to adults. An AmeriCorps training program and a veterinary student externship program train young professionals on a variety of terrapin-related conservation activities.

Despite our research successes, substantial numbers of terrapins are still struck by vehicles, and there is work to be done to translate our research into fewer terrapin deaths on the JIC. A structured decision-making approach is currently being implemented to ensure the most effective mitigation strategies and research are being used and implemented as the program moves forward (Crawford, personal communication).

---

may be a temporary method prior to surgery. Bandaging should be nonadherent and securely affixed to the shell so as to prevent movement of bone fragments. In our experience, bioglass and bone cement alone may be used, but the wound needs to be monitored weekly by removing the cement, flushing, and reapplying cement. If the limb is fractured, then the bandage can splint the limb to the shell or within the shell to prevent natural movement (Mitchell 2002).

Complete shell fractures in rehabilitated turtles should be considered open and contaminated. Generally, the duration of the injury is unknown (Mitchell 2002). When reducing shell fractures, maintain strict asepsis. Shell fractures can be reduced using different types of surgical hardware, including metal sutures, cerclage wire, or plates (Rosskopf and Woerpel 1981). It is the authors' preference in a variety of wild chelonian species to utilize screws and cerclage wires for fracture repairs with bioglass and bone cement along fracture lines. Routine principles of repair should be followed. A marine putty like epoxy can be used to cover the wires and top portion of the screws to waterproof and provide further stabilization

(Figure 28.5). Other noninvasive methods to oppose shell fragments include the use of zip-ties, hook-eye, or boot-lace fasteners as they do not require drilling into the shell (Figure 28.6). For aquatic chelonians, waterproof bandaging over the repair can be monitored by the use of fluorescein strips (Figure 28.7).

Esophagostomy tubes (E-tubes) are useful for nutritional management in some critically ill chelonians, depending on the species and size of the patient. If nutritional support is deemed necessary, the authors try to tube feed the patient initially. The decision to place an E-tube is usually based on how difficult it is to get their head out and mouth open for tube feeding and that the patient is of appropriate size to tolerate an E-tube. Many patients will start to eat on their own if provided with an appropriate environment and can be supplemented with tube feeding nutritional support until they start maintaining or gaining weight, if appropriate. In some patients, the E-tube may be left in place for months and is usually well tolerated by the turtle. The tube should be left in until the animal is eating normally. An E-tube may be stressful to patients where the tube prevents them from withdrawing into the shell, and therefore may be contraindicated in such patients.

Possible complications of E-tube placement include cellulitis or abscess information at the stoma site and ulceration or erosion with or without perforation of the gastric wall at the point where the tube contacts the stomach. Smaller patients are at greater risk of developing problems from the E-tube. Smaller tube size and the propensity to clog with thick solutions may limit the ability to meet the patient's nutritional needs.

The technique for placing an E-tube has been described by Norton (2005). Briefly, test the formula to be used before tube placement to ensure it will pass through the tube without clogging. The tube should enter at the mid to lower esophagus rather than the upper esophagus or pharyngeal region. Premeasure the tube and obtain radiographs after E-tube placement to confirm tube positioning. A purse-string suture and Chinese finger lock suture pattern will secure the tube. Flexible tubing should be used that allows for flexion and extension of the neck. After feeding, the tube should be flushed with a small amount of water or saline to remove any gruel. Enteral tube feeding formulas have been used in various species of chelonians (Norton 2005).

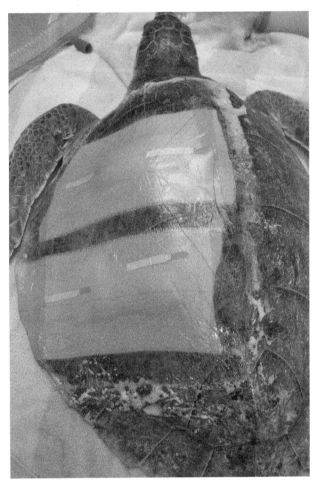

Figure 28.7 A green sea turtle with a waterproof bandage in place. Traditional bandages are used for the first layer and then covered with an iodine-impregnated self-adhesive bandage. A fluorescein strip provides a visual cue in case of leakage. A second layer of clear plastic cling wrap is placed over the first layer with an adhesive spray and then sealed around the edges with a waterproof silicon sealant. *Source:* Courtesy of CROW.

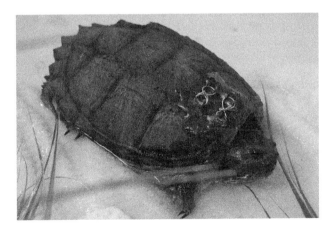

Figure 28.6 There are many ways to close shell fractures. Zip-ties or bootlace fasteners secured with epoxy have the advantage of being less invasive than screws and work well with minimally displaced, low-tension fixation.

Rigid endoscopy has been used for gender determination, evaluation of reproductive activity, exploring the coelomic cavity, and organ biopsy for histopathology. A 2.7 mm endoscope with a 30° lens is the most versatile. A trochar/cannula with multiple ports for various types of instruments and saline and CO_2 administration is recommended. Both rigid and flexible systems can be used to visualize the location of fish hooks in the esophagus in aquatic species. In larger turtle patients, flexible endoscopes/bronchoscopes may be used to evaluate the upper and lower gastrointestinal tract (GIT). Saline can be instilled through the scope to distend the cloaca, giving a better view of the bladder, rectum, distal ureteral openings, and reproductive tract. A more detailed radiographic evaluation of the lower GIT can be performed by instilling contrast media directly into the lower colon through the endoscope. Similar techniques can be used to perform an enema with saline or other solutions.

Release Criteria

It is the goal of every rehabilitation setting to provide care to injured or ill wildlife that results in release of the patient to conserve populations. This requires careful consideration of rehabilitated patients to avoid releasing individuals that may transmit pathogens jeopardizing conservation efforts. Health assessments should be performed on each animal even if the presenting complaint is most likely trauma. A study in rehabilitated box turtles found that several turtles that presented for trauma by automobiles had underlying infectious diseases (Schrader et al. 2010). Health assessments should be directed toward both the individual and the recipient population (Esque et al. 2009). In desert tortoise populations, specific criteria for movement of desert tortoises have been established and include physical examination, as well as *Mycoplasma* and herpesvirus testing (Esque et al. 2009).

In releasing turtles, the health of the individual has to be similar to the health of population to which it is being returned. Box turtles, specifically, have shown a strong desire to return to their natural home range when displaced, and the home range of displaced/translocated turtles may be up to 7.5 times larger (Hester et al. 2008). Thus, release of a turtle outside its range with a history of an infectious disease or unknown disease status may increase intraspecific transmission of pathogens. Health assessments and disease surveillance have rarely been performed in most populations, thereby making it even more important to determine that the released individual poses no infectious disease risk. The health assessment protocols are likely to be species specific, but need to be based on the "Do No Harm" principle.

In box turtles, ranavirus, *Mycoplasma*, terrapene herpesvirus 1, and box turtle adenovirus have all been observed in free-ranging individuals and the animal's status needs to be confirmed. No chelonian should be released if it has a history of a positive ranavirus test. The disease risk to the population is too great, as ranavirus has been documented to cause significant (>80%) mortality in several species. Captive box turtles that were successfully treated for ranaviral infection were then observed to continue to shed virus into the environment when reexposed to the virus (Hausmann et al. 2013). The release criteria for turtles with *Mycoplasma*, herpesvirus, and adenovirus are less well understood. These pathogens are contagious and mortality may be great in some instances, but recent surveys in emydid turtles indicate a high prevalence of these pathogens in free-ranging populations (Ossiboff et al. 2015). If pathogen prevalence is high in natural settings, then release of positive turtles at the site of capture may pose no greater risk to the population and appears a reasonable course of action.

Conclusions and Approach to Population Impacts

The uncertainty of diseases leading to presentation at rehabilitation centers hinders the ability to effectively conserve these species. Here we present criteria for establishing a health assessment protocol that can be applied to rehabilitated chelonians. It is imperative that health monitoring and disease surveillance of both individual turtles in rehabilitation facilities and the free-ranging populations occur. This would allow reasonable, practical decisions to be made about the fate of individual turtles so as to maximize conservation efforts. In the absence of these data, every effort should be made to not reintroduce animals with pathogens known to cause mortality, such as ranavirus, *Mycoplasma*, and herpesvirus. However, as has been observed from studies in desert tortoises (Sandmeier et al. 2009) and bog turtles (Ossiboff et al. 2015), updated recommendations may weaken these restrictions, specifically as they relate to *Mycoplasma*.

Wildlife in rehabilitation facilities have been proposed as sentinels of wildlife health (Sleeman 2008) and continued disease surveillance of rehabilitated turtles is integral to conservation efforts. Future studies should continue to fill gaps in our knowledge, such as the fate of reintroduced turtles.

References

Adkins, E., Driggers, T., Ferguson, G. et al. (2003). Roundtable: ultraviolet light and reptiles, amphibians. *Journal of Herpetological Medicine and Surgery* 13: 27–37.

Allender, M.C. (2012). Characterizing the epidemiology of ranavirus in North American chelonians: diagnosis, surveillance, pathogenesis, and therapy. PhD dissertation. University of Illinois.

Allender, M.C. and Mitchell, M.A. (2013). Hematologic response to experimental infections of frog virus 3-like virus in red-eared sliders (*Trachemys scripta elegans*). *Journal of Herpetological Medicine Surgery* 23: 25–31.

Allender, M.C., Fry, M.M., Irizarry, A.R. et al. (2006). Intracytoplasmic inclusions in circulating leukocytes from an eastern box turtle (*Terrapene carolina carolina*) with Iridoviral infection. *Journal of Wildlife Diseases* 42: 677–684.

Allender, M.C., Abd-Eldaim, M., Schumacher, J. et al. (2011). PCR prevalence of Ranavirus in free-ranging eastern box turtles (*Terrapene carolina carolina*) at rehabilitation centers in three southeastern US states. *Journal of Wildlife Diseases* 47: 759–764.

Allender, M.C., Mitchell, M.A., McRuer, D. et al. (2013a). Prevalence, clinical signs, and natural history characteristics of frog virus 3-like infections in eastern box turtles (*Terrapene carolina carolina*). *Herpetological Conservation and Biology* 8: 308–320.

Allender, M.C., Mitchell, M.A., Torres, T. et al. (2013b). Pathogenicity of frog virus 3-like virus in red-eared slider turtles (*Trachemys scripta elegans*) at two environmental temperatures. *Journal of Comparative Pathology* 149: 356–367.

Allender, M.C., Bunick, D., and Mitchell, M.A. (2013c). Development and validation of TaqMan quantitative PCR for detection of frog virus 3 in eastern box turtles (*Terrapene carolina carolina*). *Journal of Virological Methods* 188: 121–125.

Anderson, N.L., Wack, R.F., and Hatcher, R. (1997). Hematology and clinical chemistry reference ranges for clinically normal, captive New Guinea snapping turtle (*Elseya novaguineae*) and the effects of temperature, sex and sample type. *Journal of Zoo and Wildlife Medicine* 28: 394–403.

Ashton, P.S. and Ashton, R.E. (2004). Daily life. In: *The Gopher Tortoise: A Life History*, 29–43. Sarasota, FL: Pineapple Press.

Baker, B.B., Sladky, K.K., and Johnson, S.M. (2011). Evaluation of the analgesic effects of oral and subcutaneous tramadol administration in red-eared slider turtles. *Journal of the American Veterinary Medical Association* 238: 220–227.

Balseiro, A., Dalton, K.P., del Cerro, A. et al. (2009). Pathology, isolation and molecular characterisation of a ranavirus from the common midwife toad *Alytes obstetricans* on the Iberian Peninsula. *Diseases of Aquatic Organisms* 84: 95–104.

Beck, K., Loomis, M., Lewbart, G. et al. (1995). Preliminary comparisons of plasma concentrations of gentamicin injected into the cranial and caudal limb musculature of the eastern box turtle, (*Terrapene carolina carolina*). *Journal of Zoo and Wildlife Medicine* 26: 265–268.

Berry, K.H. and Aresco, M.J. (2014). Threats and conservation for north American tortoises. In: *Biology & Conservation of North American Tortoises* (ed. D.C. Rostal, E.D. McCoy and H.R. Mushinsky), 149–158. Baltimore, MD: Johns Hopkins University Press.

Bonner, B.B. (2000). Chelonian therapeutics. *Veterinary Clinics of North America: Exotic Animal Practice* 3: 257–332.

Boyer, T.H. (1998). Emergency care of reptiles. *Veterinary Clinics of North America: Exotic Animal Practice* 1: 191–206.

Boyer, T.H. and Boyer, D.M. (1992). Care in captivity: aquatic turtle care. *Bulletin of the Association of Reptilian and Amphibian Veterinarians* 2: 13–17.

Brown, J.D. and Sleeman, J.M. (2002). Morbidity and mortality of reptiles admitted to the Wildlife Center of Virginia, 1991 to 2000. *Journal of Wildlife Diseases* 38 (4): 699–705.

Brown, M.B., McLaughlin, G.S., Klein, P.A. et al. (1999). Upper respiratory tract disease in the gopher tortoise is caused by *Mycoplasma agassizii*. *Journal of Clinical Microbiology* 37: 2262–2269.

Brown, M.B., Brown, D.R., Klein, P.A. et al. (2001). Mycoplasma agassizii sp. nov., isolated from the upper respiratory tract of the desert tortoise (*Gopherus agassizii*) and the gopher tortoise (*Gopherus polyphemus*). *International Journal of Systemic Evolutionary Microbiology* 51 (Pt 2): 413–418.

Budischak, S.A., Hester, J.M., Price, S.J. et al. (2006). Natural history of *Terrapene carolina* (box turtles) in an urbanized landscape. *Southeastern Naturalist* 5: 191–204.

Burger, R.M., Gehrmann, W.H., and Ferguson, G.W. (2007). Evaluation of UVB reduction by materials commonly used in reptile husbandry. *Zoo Biology* 26: 417–423.

Caligiuri, R., Kollias, G.V., Jacobson, E. et al. (1990). The effects of ambient temperature on amikacin pharmacokinetics in gopher tortoises. *Journal of Veterinary Pharmacology and Therapeutics* 13: 287–291.

Campbell, T.W. (2006). Clinical pathology of reptiles. In: *Reptile Medicine and Surgery*, 2e (ed. D.R. Mader), 453–470. Philadelphia, PA: Saunders, Elsevier.

Chansue, N., Sailasuta, A., Tangtrongpiros, J. et al. (2011). Hematology and clinical chemistry of adult yellow-headed temple turtles (*Hieremys annandalii*) in Thailand. *Veterinary Clinical Pathology* 40: 174–184.

Christopher, M.M., Berry, K.H., Wallis, I.R. et al. (1999). Reference intervals and physiologic alterations in hematologic and biochemical values of free-ranging desert tortoises in the Mojave desert. *Journal of Wildlife Diseases* 35: 212–238.

Chung, C.S., Cheng, C.H., Chin, S.C. et al. (2009). Morphologic and cytochemical characteristics of Asian yellow pond turtle (*Ocadia sinensis*) blood cells and their hematologic and plasma biochemical reference values. *Journal of Zoo and Wildlife Medicine* 40: 76–85.

Cinkova, K., Reschova, S., Kulich, P. et al. (2010). Evaluation of a polyclonal antibody for the detection and identification of ranaviruses from freshwater fish and amphibians. *Diseases of Aquatic Organisms* 89: 191–198.

Crawford, B.A., Maerz, J.C., Nibbelink, N.P. et al. (2014a). Estimating the impacts of multiple threats and management strategies for diamondback terrapins (*Malaclemys terrapin*). *Journal of Applied Ecology* 51: 359–366.

Crawford, B.A., Maerz, J.C., Nibbelink, N.P. et al. (2014b). Hot spots and hot moments of diamondback terrapin road-crossing activity. *Journal of Applied Ecology* 51: 367–375.

Crawford, B.A., Poudyal, N.C., and Maerz, J.C. (2015). When drivers and terrapins collide: assessing stakeholder attitudes toward wildlife management on the Jekyll Island causeway. *Human Dimensions of Wildlife* 20: 1–14.

Cunningham, A.A., Tems, C.A., and Russell, P.H. (2008). Immunohistochemical demonstration of Ranavirus antigen in the tissues of infected frogs (*Rana temporaria*) with systemic haemorrhagic or cutaneous ulcerative disease. *Journal of Comparative Pathology* 138: 3–11.

Daszak, P., Cunningham, A.A., and Hyatt, A.D. (2000). Emerging infectious diseases of wildlife – threats to biodiversity and human health. *Science* 287: 443–449.

De Voe, R.K., Geissler, K., Elmore, S. et al. (2004). Ranavirus-associated morbidity and mortality in a group of captive eastern box turtles (*Terrapene carolina carolina*). *Journal of Zoo and Wildlife Medicine* 35: 534–543.

Divers, S.J. (1997). Emergency Care of the Critically Ill Reptiles. Annual Conference of the Association of Reptilian and Amphibian Veterinarians, Houston, TX, pp. 153–162.

Divers, S.J., Papich, M., McBride, M. et al. (2010). Pharmacokinetics of meloxicam following intravenous and oral administration in green iguanas (*Iguana iguana*). *American Journal Veterinary Research* 71: 1277–1283.

Doszpoly, A., Wellehan, J.F.X., Childress, A.L. et al. (2013). Partial characterization of a new adenovirus lineage discovered in testudinoid turtles. *Infection, Genetics, and Evolution* 17: 106–112.

duPre, S.A., Tracy, C.R., and Hunter, K.W. (2011). Quantitative PCR method for detection of mycoplasma spp. DNA in nasal lavage samples from the desert tortoise (*Gopherus agassizzi*). *Journal of Microbiological Methods* 86: 160–165.

Edwards, T. and Berry, K.H. (2013). Are captive tortoises a reservoir for conservation? An assessment of genealogical affiliation of captive *Gopherus agassizii* to local, wild popualtions. *Conservation Genetics* 14: 649–659.

Ernst, C.H. and Lovich, J.E. (2009). *Turtles of the United States and Canada*, 2e. Baltimore, MD: Johns Hopkins University Press.

Ernst, C.H., Lovich, J.E., and Barbour, R.W. (1994a). Malaclemys terrapin, diamondback terrapin. In: *Turtles of the United States and Canada*, 429–442. Washington, DC: Smithsonian Institution Press.

Ernst, C.H., Lovich, J.E., and Barbour, R.W. (1994b). Eastern box turtle. In: *Turtles of the United States and Canada*, 250–265. Washington, DC: Smithsonian Institution Press.

Ernst, C.H., Lovich, J.E., and Barbour, R.W. (1994c). Testudinidae: Tortoises. In: *Turtles of the United States and Canada*, 443–466. Washington, DC: Smithsonian Institution Press.

Esque, T.C., Nussear, K.E., Drake, K.K., et al. (2009). Amendment to Desert Tortoise Translocation Plan for Fort Irwin's Land Expansion Program at the US Army National Training Center (NTC) and Fort Irwin. https://www.energy.ca.gov/sitingcases/genesis_solar/documents/others/testimony_centr_biological_diversity/exhibits/Exh.%20813.%20Esque%20et%20al.%202009.%20%20Amendment%20to%20DT%20trans.%20Plan..pdf

Feldman, S.H., Wimsatt, J., Marschang, R.E. et al. (2006). A novel mycoplasma in association with upper respiratory disease syndrome in free-ranging eastern box turtles (*Terrapene carolina carolina*) in Virginia. *Journal of Wildlife Diseases* 42: 279–289.

Fleming, G.J. (2008). Clinical technique: chelonian shell repair. *Journal of Exotic Pet Medicine* 17: 246–258.

Gottdenker, N.L. and Jacobson, E.R. (1995). Effect of venipuncture sites on hematologic and clinical biochemical values in desert tortoises (*Gopherus agassizzi*). *American Journal of Veterinary Research* 56: 19–21.

Gray, M.J., Miller, D.L., and Hoverman, J.T. (2009). Ecology and pathology of amphibian ranaviruses. *Diseases of Aquatic Organisms* 87: 243–266.

Grosse, A.M., Crawford, B.M., Maerz, J.C. et al. (2015). Effects of vegetation structure and artificial nesting habitats on hatchling sex determination and nest survival of diamondback terrapins. *Journal of Fish and Wildlife Management* 6: 19–28.

Hanley, C.S. and Hernandez-Divers, S. (2003). Practical gross pathology of reptiles. *Seminars in Avian and Exotic Pet Medicine* 12: 71–80.

Harper, P.A., Hammond, D.C., and Heuschele, W.P. (1982). A herpesvirus-like agent associated with a pharyngeal abscess in a desert tortoise. *Journal of Wildlife Diseases* 18: 491–494.

Hausmann, J.C., Wack, A.N., Allender, M.C., et al. (2013). Experimental Challenge Study of Ranavirus Infection in Previously Infected Eastern Box Turtles (*Terrapene carolina carolina*) to Assess Immunity. 2013 International Symposium on Ranaviruses, Knoxville, TN.

Helms, J. (2006). Diamondback Terrapins (*Malaclemys terrapin*) Care. World Chelonian Trust. www.chelonia.org.

Hernandez-Divers, S.M., Hernandaz-Divers, S.J., and Wyneken, J. (2002). Angiographic, anatomic and clinical technique descriptions of a subcarapacial venipuncture site for chelonians. *Journal of Herpetological Medicine and Surgery* 21: 32–37.

Hester, J.M., Price, S.J., and Dorcas, M.E. (2008). Effects of relocation on movements and home ranges of eastern box turtles. *Journal of Wildlife Management* 72: 772–777.

Holz, P., Barker, I.K., Crawshaw, G.J. et al. (1997). The anatomy and perfusion of the renal portal system in the red-eared slider (*Trachemys scripta elegans*). *Journal of Zoo and Wildlife Medicine* 28: 386–393.

Hyatt, A.D., Gould, A.R., Zupanovic, Z. et al. (2000). Comparative studies of piscine and amphibian iridoviruses. *Archives of Virology* 145: 301–331.

ICTV. (2011). Iridovirus: Virus Taxonomy 2011 Release. https://talk.ictvonline.org/ictv-reports/ictv_9th_report/dsdna-viruses-2011/w/dsdna_viruses/113/iridoviridae

Innis, C.J., Garner, M.M., Johnson, A.J. et al. (2007). Antemortem diagnosis and characterization of nasal intranuclear coccidiosis in Sulawesi tortoises (*Indotestudo forsteni*). *Journal of Veterinary Diagnostic Investigation* 19: 660–667.

International Union for Conservation of Nature (IUCN). (2011). Tortoise & Freshwater Turtle Specialist Group 1996. Terrapene carolina. IUCN Red List of Threatened Species. www.iucnredlist.org.

International Union for Conservation of Nature (IUCN) 2015). IUCN Red List of Threatened Species. Version 2015.1. www.iucnredlist.org

Jacobson, E.R., Gaskin, J.M., Brown, M.B. et al. (1991). Chronic upper respiratory tract disease of free-ranging desert tortoises (*Xerobates agassizii*). *Journal of Wildlife Diseases* 27: 296–316.

Jacobson, E.R., Harman, G., Laille, E. et al. (2003). Plasma concentrations of praziquantel in loggerhead sea turtles *Caretta caretta* following oral administration of single & multiple doses. *American Journal of Veterinary Research* 64: 304–309.

Jacobson, E.R., Berry, K.H., Wellehan, J.F.X. Jr. et al. (2012). Serologic and molecular evidence for Testudinid herpesvirus 2 infection in wild Agassiz's desert tortoises, *Gopherus agassizii*. *Journal of Wildlife Diseases* 48: 747–757.

James, S.B., Calle, P.P., Raphael, B.L. et al. (2003). Comparison of injection versus oral enrofloxacin pharmacokinetics in red-eared slider turtles, *Trachemys scripta elegans*. *Journal of Herpetological Medicine and Surgery* 13: 5–10.

Johnson, A.J., Wendland, L., Norton, T.M. et al. (2010). Development and use of an indirect enzyme-linked immunosorbent assay for detection of iridovirus exposure in gopher tortoises (*Gopherus polyphemus*) and eastern box turtles (*Terrapene carolina carolina*). *Veterinary Microbiology* 142: 160–167.

Joyner, P.H., Brown, J.D., Holladay, S. et al. (2006). Characterization of the bacterial microflora of the tympanic cavity of eastern box turtles with and without aural abscesses. *Journal of Wildlife Diseases* 42: 859–864.

Knotek, Z. (2014). Alfaxalone as an induction agent for anesthesia in terrapins and tortoises. *Veterinary Record* 175: 327–329.

Kolmstetter, C.M., Frazier, D., Cox, S. et al. (2001). Pharmacokinetics of metronidazole in yellow rat snakes, *Elaphe obsolete quadrivittata*. *Journal of Herpetological Medicine and Surgery* 11: 4–8.

Lafortune, M., Norton, T., and Mettee, N. (2014). Vacuum assisted wound closure in chelonians. In: *Current Therapy in Reptile Medicine and Surgery* (ed. D.R. Mader and S.J. Divers). St Louis, MO: Elsevier.

Lai, O.R., di Bello, A.V.F., Soloperto, S. et al. (2015). Pharmacokinetic behavior of meloxicam in loggerhead sea turtles (*Caretta caretta*) after intramuscular and intravenous administration. *Journal of Wildlife Diseases* 51: 509–512.

Lawrence, K., Muggleton, P.W., and Needham, J.R. (1984). Preliminary study on the use of ceftazidime, a broad spectrum cephalosporin antibiotic, in snakes. *Research in Veterinary Science* 36: 16–20.

Lloyd, M. and Morris, P. (1999). Chelonian venipuncture techniques. *Bulletin of the Association of Reptilian and Amphibian Veterinarians* 9: 26–28.

Mader, D.R. (1997). Trauma management in reptiles and amphibians. *Proceedings of the North American Veterinary Conference* 10: 742–743.

Mallo, K., Harms, C.A., Lewbart, G.A. et al. (2002). Pharmacokinetics of fluconazole in loggerhead sea turtles (*Caretta caretta*) after single intravenous and subcutaneous injections, and multiple subcutaneous injections. *Journal of Zoo and Wildlife Medicine* 33: 29–35.

Manire, C.A., Rhinehart, H.L., Pennick, G.J. et al. (2003). Plasma concentrations of itraconazole after oral administration in Kemp's Ridley Sea turtles, *Lepidochelys kempi. Journal of Zoo and Wildlife Medicine* 34: 171–178.

Marschang, R.E., Gleiser, C.B., Papp, T. et al. (2006). Comparison of 11 herpesvirus isolates from tortoises using partial sequences from three conserved genes. *Veterinary Microbiology* 117: 258–266.

Martinez-Jimenez, D., Hernandez-Divers, S.J., Floyd, T.M. et al. (2007). Comparison of the effects of dipotassium ethylenediaminetetraacetic acid and lithium heparin on hematologic values in yellow-blotched map turtles, *Braptemys flavimaculata. Journal of Herpetological Medicine and Surgery* 17: 36–41.

Martinez-Silvestre, A., Perpinan, D., Marco, I. et al. (2002). Venipuncture technique of the occipital venous sinus in freshwater aquatic turtles. *Journal of Herpetological Medicine and Surgery* 12: 31–32.

McArthur, S. (2004). Feeding techniques and fluids. In: *Medicine and Surgery of Tortoises and Turtles* (ed. S. McArthur, R. Wilkinson and J. Meyer), 257–272. Ames, IA: Blackwell Publishing.

McCracken, H., Hyatt, A.D., Slocombe, R.F. (1994). Two Cases of Anemia in Reptiles Treated with Blood Transfusion: (1) Hemolytic Anemia in a Diamond Python Caused by an Erythrocytic Virus, (2) Nutritional Anemia in a Bearded Dragon. Proceedings of the Annual Conference of the American Association of Zoo Veterinarians, Pittsburgh, PA, pp. 47–51.

Miller, D., Gray, M., and Storfer, A. (2011). Ecopathology of Ranaviruses infecting amphibians. *Viruses-Basel* 3: 2351–2373.

Mitchell, M.A. (2002). Diagnosis and management of reptile orthopedic injuries. *Veterinary Clinics of North America* 5: 97–114.

Muro, J., Cuenca, R., Pastor, J. et al. (1998). Effects of lithium heparin and tripotassium EDTA on hematologic values of Hermann's tortoises (*Testudo hermannii*). *Journal of Zoo and Wildlife Medicine* 29: 40–44.

Norton, T.M. (2005). Chelonian emergency and critical care. *Seminars in Avian and Exotic Pet Medicine* 14: 106–130.

Norton, T.M., Sladky, K., Cox, S. et al. (2015). Pharmacokinetics of tramadol and o-desmethyltramadol in Loggerhead Sea turtles (*Caretta caretta*). *Journal of Zoo and Wildlife Medicine* 46: 262–265.

Olesen, M.G. and Perry, S.F. (2009). Effects of preoperative administration of butorphanol or meloxicam on physiologic responses to surgery in ball pythons. *Journal of the American Veterinary Medical Association* 233: 1883–1888.

Origgi, F.C., Romero, C.H., Bloom, D.C. et al. (2004). Experimental transmission of a herpesvirus in Greek tortoises (*Testudo graeca*). *Veterinary Pathology* 41: 50–61.

Ossiboff, R.J., Raphael, B.L., Ammazzalorso, A.D. et al. (2015). A *Mycoplasma* species of emydidae turtles in the northeastern USA. *Journal of Wildlife Diseases* 51: 466–470.

Prezant, R.M., Isaza, R., and Jacobson, E.R. (1994). Plasma concentrations with disposition kinetics of enrofloxacin in gopher tortoises (*Gopherus polyphemus*). *Journal of Zoo and Wildlife Medicine* 25: 82–87.

Raphael, B.L., Papich, M., and Cook, R.A. (1994). Pharmacokinetics of enrofloxacin after a single intramuscular injection in Indian star tortoises (*Geochelone elegans*). *Journal of Zoo and Wildlife Medicine* 25: 88–94.

Read, M.R. (2004). Evaluation of the use of anesthesia and analgesia in reptiles. *Journal of the American Veterinary Medical Association* 224: 547–552.

Rhodin, A.G.J., van Dijk, P. P., Iverson, J.B., et al. (2010). Turtles of the World, 2010 Update: Annotated Checklist of Taxonomy, Synonymy, Distribution, and Conservation Status. www.iucn-tftsg.org/wp-content/uploads/file/Accounts/crm_5_000_checklist_v3_2010.pdf

Rivas, A.E., Allender, M.C., Mitchell, M. et al. (2014). Morbidity and mortality in reptiles presented to a wildlife care facility in Central Illinois. *Human-Wildlife Interactions* 8: 78–87.

Rivera, S., Wellehan, J.F.X., McManamon, R. et al. (2009). Systemic adenovirus infection in Sulawesi tortoises (*Indotestudo forsteni*) caused by a novel siadenovirus. *Journal of Veterinary Diagnostic Investigation* 21: 415–426.

Rosskopf, W.J. (2000). Disorders of reptilian leukocytes and erythrocytes. In: *Laboratory Medicine: Avian and Exotic Pets* (ed. A.M. Fudge), 198–204. Philadelphia, PA: WB Saunders.

Rosskopf, W.J. and Woerpel, R.W. (1981). Repair of shell damage in tortoises. *Modern Veterinary Practice* 62: 938–939.

Sandmeier, F.C., Tracy, C.R., duPre, S. et al. (2009). Upper respiratory tract disease (URTD) as a threat to desert tortoise populations: a reevaluation. *Biological Conservation* 142: 1255–1268.

Schrader, G.M., Allender, M.C., and Odoi, A. (2010). Diagnosis, treatment, and outcome of eastern box turtles (*Terrapene carolina carolina*) presented to a wildlife clinic in Tennessee, USA, 1995–2007. *Journal of Wildlife Disease* 45: 1079–1055.

Schroeder, C.A. and Johnson, R.A. (2013). The efficacy of intracoelomic fospropofol in red-eared sliders (*Trachemys scripta*). *Journal of Zoo and Wildlife Medicine* 44: 941–950.

Sim, R.R., Wack, A.N., Allender, M.C., et al. (2012). Management of a Concurrent Ranavirus and

Herpesvirus Epizootic Event in Captive Eastern Box Turtles (*Terrapene carolina carolina*). Annual Conference of the American Association of Zoo Veterinarians, Oakland, CA.

Sim, R.R., Norton, T.M., Bronson, E. et al. (2015). Identification of a novel herpesvirus in captive eastern box turtles (*Terrapene carolina carolina*). *Veterinary Microbiology* 175: 218–223.

Sladky, K.K. (2014). Analgesia. In: *Current Therapy in Reptile Medicine and Surgery*, 3e (ed. D.R. Mader and S. Divers), 217–228. St Louis, MO: Elsevier-Saunders.

Sleeman, J.M. (2008). Use of wildlife rehabilitation centers as monitors of ecosystem health. In: *Zoo and Wild Animal Medicine: Current Therapy*, 6e (ed. M.E. Fowler and R.E. Miller), 97–104. St Louis, MO: Elsevier Health Sciences.

Sleeman, J.M., Brown, J., Steffen, D. et al. (2008). Relationships among aural abscesses, organochlorine compounds, and vitamin a in free-ranging eastern box turtles (*Terrapene carolina carolina*). *Journal of Wildlife Diseases* 44: 922–929.

Smits, A.W. and Kozubowski, M.M. (1985). Partitioning of body fluids and cardiovascular responses to circulatory hypovolemia in the turtle *Pseudemys scripta elegans*. *Journal of Experimental Biology* 116: 237–250.

Stacy, N.I., Alleman, A.R., and Sayler, K.A. (2011). Diagnostic hematology of reptiles. *Clinical Laboratory Medicine* 31: 87–108.

Stamper, M.A., Papich, M.G., Lewbart, G.A. et al. (1999). Pharmacokinetics of ceftazidime in loggerhead sea turtles (*Caretta caretta*) after single intravenous and intramuscular injections. *Journal of Zoo and Wildlife Medicine* 30: 32–35.

Steen, D.A., Hopkins, B.C., van Dyke, J.U. et al. (2014). Prevalence of ingested fish hooks in freshwater turtles from five rivers in southeastern United States. *PLOS One* 9: 1–6.

Sykes, J.M. and Klaphake, E. (2015). Reptile hematology. *Veterinary Clinics of North America: Exotic Animal Practice* 18: 63–82.

Tuttle, A.D., Papich, M., Lewbart, G.A. et al. (2006). Pharmacokinetics of ketoprofen in the green iguana (*Iguana iguana*) following single intravenous and intramuscular injections. *Journal of Zoo and Wildlife Medicine* 37: 567–570.

Van Devanter, D.R., Warrener, P., Bennett, L. et al. (1996). Detection and analysis of diverse herpesviral species by consensus primer PCR. *Journal of Clinical Microbiology* 34: 1666–1671.

van Dijk, P.P. (2011). *Terrapene carolina*. IUCN Red List of Threatened Species. www.iucnredlist.org/species/21641/97428179

Vella, D. (2009). Management of aquatic turtle shell fractures. *Lab Animal* 38: 52–53.

Vigani, A. (2014). Chelonia (tortoises, turtles, and terrapins). In: *Zoo Animal and Wildlife Immobilization and Anesthesia*, 2e (ed. G. West, D. Heard and N. Caulkett), 365–387. Ames, IA: John Wiley & Sons.

Wellehan, J.F.X., Lafortune, M., Gunkel, C. et al. (2004). Coccygealvascular catheterization in lizards and crocodilians. *Journal of Herpetological Medicine and Surgery* 14: 26–28.

Wendland, L.D., Brown, D.R., Klein, P.A. et al. (2006). Upper respiratory tract disease (Mycoplasmosis) in tortoises. In: *Reptile Medicine and Surgery*, 2e (ed. D.R. Mader), 931–938. Philadelphia, PA: Saunders Elsevier.

Whitaker, B.R. and Krum, H. (1999). Medical management of sea turtles in aquaria. In: *Zoo & Wild Animal Medicine*, 4e (ed. M.E. Fowler and R.E. Miller), 217–231. Philadelphia, PA: WB Saunders.

Wilkinson, R. (2004). Therapeutics. In: *Medicine and Surgery of Tortoises and Turtles* (ed. S. McArthur, R. Wilkinson and J. Meyer), 465–503. Ames, IA: Blackwell Publishing.

Wimsatt, J., Johnson, J., Mangone, B.A. et al. (1999). Clarithromycin pharmacokinetics in the desert tortoise. *Journal of Zoo and Wildlife Medicine* 30: 36–43.

Ziolo, M.S. and Bertelsen, M.F. (2009). Effects of propofol administered via the supravertebral sinus in red-eared sliders. *Journal of the American Veterinary Medical Association* 234: 390–393.

29

Natural History and Medical Management of Amphibians

Leigh Ann Clayton

Animal Care and Welfare, National Aquarium, Baltimore, MD, USA

Natural History

The Amphibia class is diverse and contains three orders: Anura (frogs and toads), Caudata (salamanders, newts, and sirens), and Gymnophiona (caecilians). The order Anura has the greatest diversity, with over 6500 species, while Caudata and Gymnophiona contain approximately 650 and 250 species respectively.

Amphibians occupy a wide range of environments on every continent except Antarctica (Wright 2001a; Amphibiaweb 2015). Habitat needs vary widely; amphibians may be aquatic, semiaquatic, terrestrial, fossorial, or arboreal. Amphibians are not found in salt water and only a few species of anurans are documented in brackish water. Anurans occupy all habitat niches, while caudatans and gymnophionans are typically aquatic, terrestrial, or fossorial.

Adult amphibians are insectivorous or carnivorous and may be active or sit-and-wait predators. Anurans and caudatans rely primarily on sight for hunting so ensuring adequate vision prior to release is critical. Caecilians use a chemosensory-tactile organ for hunting and are generally blind, though some species may sense general light levels (Wright 2001a–c; Helmer and Whiteside 2005; Baitchman and Herman 2014; Chai 2014; Clayton and Mylniczenko 2014).

Anatomy and Physiology

Highlights of major clinical anatomy and physiology are presented here; more detailed clinical reviews are available (Wright 2001a–c; Pessier and Pinkerton 2003; Helmer and Whiteside 2005; Pessier 2009; Poole and Grow 2012; Baitchman and Herman 2014; Chai 2014; Clayton and Mylniczenko 2014).

Amphibians are ectotherms and depend on environmental temperature to maintain appropriate internal temperature. Nonaquatic amphibians require microclimates of high humidity. During periods of environmental extremes, some species will hibernate or estivate.

Pulmonary, buccopharyngeal, cutaneous, and branchial modes of respiration have been described in amphibians and it is typical for amphibians to rely on multiple modes to varying degrees. Most amphibians have well-developed, sac-like lungs and the respiratory cycle demonstrates a gular and abdominal phase. Amphibians have a three-chambered heart (two atria, one ventricle).

The main nitrogen excretory product depends on the natural habitat. Aquatic amphibians primarily excrete ammonia while more terrestrial amphibians excrete urea. Uric acid production has been described in a few species of tree frogs. Nitrogenous waste is primarily removed via the renal system, though the skin and gills may play a role in aquatic species.

The integumentary, lymphatic, and renal systems have a significant role in osmoregulation. An excellent clinical review is available (Pessier 2009). Passive diffusion across the integument is the major mechanism of water intake, while electrolytes are actively transported. Many semiaquatic and terrestrial species of anurans have a specialized "drink patch" on the caudoventral body, which has increased surface area and vascularity to promote water uptake.

Amphibians have an extensive lymphatic system and in anurans the subcutaneous space around the body is composed of lymph sacs. The vascular system is "leaky" with an estimated 50× plasma volume turnover via the lymphatic system in 24 hours; the composition of blood plasma and lymphatic fluid is similar (Wright 2001c; Pessier 2009; Reynolds et al. 2009). Plasma osmolality is >200 mOsmol, but significant fluctuations regularly occur

Medical Management of Wildlife Species: A Guide for Practitioners, First Edition. Edited by Sonia M. Hernandez, Heather W. Barron, Erica A. Miller, Roberto F. Aguilar and Michael J. Yabsley.

(Wright 2001c; Pessier 2009). For example, in dehydrated terrestrial amphibians, blood osmotic concentration increases significantly to facilitate water absorption.

Amphibian kidneys have no loop of Henle, so they cannot concentrate urine. The glomerular filtration rate is relatively high (25–100 mL/kg/h) (Wright 2001c; Pessier 2009). The bladder serves as a storage location for water, urea, and electrolytes and plays an active role in normal osmoregulation.

Aquatic amphibians are continually "water loaded" as water from the environment diffuses into the body, and normal physiological mechanisms retain electrolytes and reduce water accumulation via production of large urine volumes. Terrestrial amphibians are generally at risk of dehydration, and normal physiological mechanisms are directed toward water retention.

Husbandry While in Captivity

The basic principles and standards of care applied to rehabilitation of other classes can be translated to use with amphibians (Miller 2012). Appropriate management of humidity levels and water quality is more important with amphibians than other classes. Online and textbook reviews of captive husbandry are available and should be consulted (Barnett et al. 2001; Whitaker 2001; Wright 2001d; Pessier and Mendelson 2010; Poole and Grow 2012; Baitchman and Herman 2014; Chai 2014; Clayton and Mylniczenko 2014; Latney and Clayton 2014). A suggested list of questions to guide appropriate husbandry decisions is provided in Box 29.1.

Box 29.1 Amphibian Husbandry Checklist

The following list can be used to guide preparation for an amphibian patient.

1) Enclosure review
   a) What is normal habitat of the amphibian and how does it use it (e.g., fossorial, aquatic, semiaquatic, arboreal)?
   b) What enclosure will best mimic this habitat?
   c) Where can the enclosure be placed to reduce stressful stimuli?
   d) What hides and other visual barriers will be used?
   e) What substrate will be provided?
   f) How much aquatic and terrestrial habitat is needed?
   g) How will humidity be maintained?
   h) Will modifications be needed as the animal heals?
2) Water quality
   a) What is the source water and does it need to be conditioned or reconstituted?
   b) How will water quality be evaluated and on what schedule?
   c) For aquatic animals, can a recirculating system be established or will dump and fill be used?
   d) How and when will water changes be conducted?
   e) How will appropriate water be provided for procedures (e.g., misting for humidity, cleaning/moistening gloves prior to handling)?
3) Temperature
   a) What is the appropriate temperature?
   b) How will it be maintained without reducing humidity levels?
4) Food and feeding
   a) What does the animal naturally eat?
   b) What can be fed that mimics the natural diet?
   c) How will prey items be kept and fed to ensure they are nutritious for the amphibian?
   d) What type of supplements will be used and at what frequency?
5) Cleaning, disinfection, and quarantine
   a) What cleaning protocol will be used while the animal is in the enclosure?
   b) What cleaning and disinfection protocol will be used on the enclosure and cage furniture after the case is finished?
   c) What materials will be disposed of and how?
   d) What biosecurity protocols will be used to limit the risk of disease transmission?

Enclosures

Enclosure design should account for species' natural habitat and provide opportunities for normal behaviors (e.g., burrowing, hiding, climbing, soaking), as medically indicated. Hospital enclosures provide these opportunities using minimal organic material and limited space. As the animal heals, more organic material and additional space may be offered.

While amphibian-specific enclosures are available, repurposed glass aquaria or plastic containers (e.g., animal carriers, sweater boxes, food storage containers, livestock water troughs) are more commonly used. If lids are needed to prevent escape, they should be tight fitting but facilitate airflow (e.g., mesh covers, perforations in tops of plastic food containers). Surfaces should be smooth to reduce injury. There are no standards for enclosure size but guidelines for reptile rehabilitation may be used (e.g., width and length 3–5× the amphibian's length) (Miller 2012).

Visual barriers within the enclosure, hiding space, and opaque enclosure walls limit potentially stressful visual stimuli. Items used in the tank should be easily cleaned and disinfected or discarded after use to reduce disease transmission. A wide variety of items may be appropriate and some examples are given. Plastic aquarium plants and live *Pothos* spp. leaves make good visual barriers. Hide structures can be made from modified plastic plant pots (Figure 29.1).

Transparent enclosures should have opaque material applied to the outside. Noise and vibration should also be reduced, and enclosures should be placed in quiet areas with minimal foot traffic.

Amphibians require cooler, moister environments than reptiles. Ideal ambient temperatures vary by species, but a range of 23.8–26.7°C (75–80°F) is an appropriate starting point. Many North American amphibians can be kept at the lower end of the range. Appropriate temperature should be achieved by adjusting the ambient temperature around the enclosure. Heating elements (e.g., radiant heat panels, under-tank heaters) placed on the outside of the tank can provide supplemental heat support. Temperature should be monitored in multiple areas of the tank (horizontally and vertically). Based on current knowledge, provision of ultraviolet (UV) light is not critical for short-term rehabilitation (Poole and Grow 2012).

High ambient humidity is needed to maintain hydration in terrestrial amphibians and should be above 50% (70–90% is preferred). In top-opening enclosures, an impervious barrier (e.g., plastic wrap, plastic sheeting) over part of the top can improve humidity while allowing air circulation. Cage substrate should be kept moist at all times; frequent misting of the tank is typically needed. Areas of water (e.g., standing pools, shallow

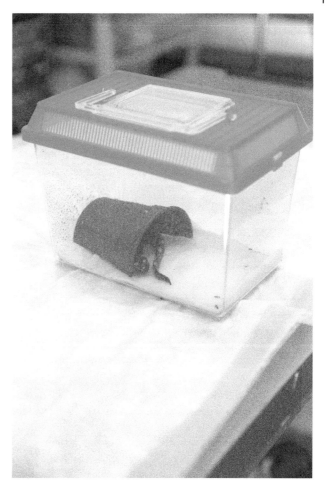

Figure 29.1 Transportation carrier with a hide (modified plastic flowerpot) for short-term terrestrial amphibian holding.

water bowls, soaked sponges) also increase humidity and allow soaking.

Substrate needs will vary with species and health status. Sick amphibians should be managed in simple enclosures with minimal organic material. Hospital enclosures for terrestrial amphibians should have wet paper towels (nonbleached and fragrance free) or other moisture-retaining, disposable materials (e.g., absorbent "pee pads") on the bottom.

Hospital enclosures for aquatic and semiaquatic amphibians require larger amounts of water. Semiaquatic amphibians should be provided with larger pools that cover 40–60% of the tank bottom. Any pool areas should have gently sloped edges to allow easy egress. Fully aquatic amphibians should be held in aquarium systems similar to those used for freshwater fish. If used, water heaters should be in a sleeve to prevent direct contact with the amphibian and reduce the risk of burns. If fully aquatic animals are severely debilitated, they may need to be housed in limited water, with the head supported above the water line.

Water Quality and Life Support Systems

Ensuring appropriate water quality is essential for amphibian health; this applies to all water used in the enclosure (e.g., misting, spot cleaning, pools, bowls). Detailed reviews are available (Barnett et al. 2001; Whitaker 2001; Poole and Grow 2012).

Water Quality Basics

Simple colorimetric water quality test kits are available from pet shops or fish hobbyist websites. Ammonia, pH, and chlorine levels are commonly tested, but additional parameters to consider monitoring include nitrite, nitrate, hardness (mineral content), and alkalinity (buffering capacity). Guidelines for freshwater fish systems are an appropriate starting point for amphibians (Table 29.1).

Many amphibians can tolerate values outside these limits, but healing and long-term health may be impacted. Some species may be adapted to parameters outside these ranges, although this would be unlikely for most species presented for rehabilitation.

Water pH should be near neutral. High or low pH can cause irritation and negatively impact basic physiological functions, such as electrolyte transport. Chlorine and ammonia are known toxins and should be below detection limits of colorimetric tests. Clinical signs of toxicity include agitation, increased respirations, equilibrium loss, increased mucus production, and death. Common sources of chlorine include tap water (see Section

Conditioning Water) and exposure to bleach cleaning products. Common sources of ammonia include normal protein breakdown products.

Water Quality Testing

Testing frequency should be established with the goal of ensuring that animals are not exposed to known and easily controlled environmental changes or toxins. Water temperature should be checked daily. If present, the life support system should be evaluated for normal function at this time. In an established system with appropriate life support for the nitrogen load, water quality will be stable and water chemistry testing and water changes can be done relatively infrequently (typically every two weeks). In contrast, systems that are newly established, have newly added animals (increased bioload), or have had an acute change in environmental parameters (e.g., temperature or pH change) should have water quality tested daily until the system is stable.

Conditioning Water

Water from municipal sources typically needs to be "conditioned" to remove residual chlorine or chloramine used in disinfection prior to use with amphibians. Chlorine is reactive and readily removed by simple off-gassing. The necessary volume of tap water is "aged" for about 24 hours in an open-topped container. Aeration will increase the speed of off-gassing. Sodium thiosulfate binds chlorine and is readily available from pet shops or

Table 29.1 Water quality parameter ranges for amphibians, acute toxicity signs, and review of management responses.

Parameter	Recommended range	Acute toxicity	Notes
Temperature	23.9–26.7 °C (75–80 °F)	Slower or increased metabolism. Clinical signs vary with magnitude and speed of change	Review life support system. Adjust heating or cooling system in room and enclosure
pH	6.5–8; usually close to 7	Increases mucus, hemorrhage of skin and gills	Prevent with appropriate system management. Water change, buffer addition if ammonia normal
Chlorine	Undetectable	Increases mucus, gill necrosis, restlessness, death	Water change, sodium thiosulfate
Ammonia	Undetectable	Restless, agitation; irregular or increased respiration, loss of equilibrium, muscle spasms, death	Prevent with appropriate system management. Water change, reduce bioload, zeolite, or sodium hydroxymethanesulfonate (SH). Zeolite or SH may be needed to condition tap water if chloramine used by municipal water company
Nitrite	<1 mg/L	Methemoglobinemia, torpor, loss of orientation, nonreactive	Water change, reduce bioload, sodium chloride addition (competes with nitrite uptake)
Nitrate	<50 mg/L	—	
Hardness (mineral ions)	<150 mg/L	—	Primarily calcium and magnesium ions
Alkalinity (buffering capacity)	15–50 mg/L	—	

fish hobbyist websites. While carbon will adsorb chlorine, carbon filters on an animal system will not remove it quickly enough to eliminate the risk of toxicity.

Chloramine has ammonia bound to the chlorine and is more stable than chlorine. It does not off-gas quickly, but chemical treatment products are available from pet stores or fish hobbyist websites. The ammonia–chlorine bond is broken and chlorine can then off-gas or be removed with sodium thiosulfate. Ammonia is removed with sodium hydroxymethanesulfonate or zeolite.

If concerns exist regarding other contaminates in the water (e.g., nitrates, heavy metals), reconstituted "purified" water (e.g., deionized, reverse osmosis) can be used. The processed water lacks necessary solutes and these must be re-added (Poole and Grow 2012). Commercial salt mixtures designed for saltwater fish aquaria can be used to create an approximately 100 mg/L solution. Bottled and mineral water can be used, but water chemistry varies significantly between brands; at a minimum, pH should be checked prior to use.

Life Support Basics

Water quality is particularly important for fully aquatic and semiaquatic amphibians and the aquarium life support system is critical to maintaining acceptable water quality. Major components of simple freshwater life support systems include mechanisms for filtration (mechanical, biological, chemical) and gas exchange.

Mechanical filtration removes suspended material from the water by using physical filters and screens to filter out particles. Biological filtration is the process where bacteria oxidize toxic ammonia and nitrite to less toxic nitrate. Water changes are then used to remove nitrates. "Cycling a tank" refers to allowing nitrifying bacteria to colonize the tank to a level that will oxidize the anticipated nitrogen burden from the animal(s). These bacteria are normal components of an aquatic biofilm and will grow on any surface in the system; they do best in dark conditions with high oxygen levels. In small aquarium systems, the mechanical filter mesh usually provides the surface area for the biological filter. Chemical filtration removes dissolved organic material and is accomplished using activated carbon filters. Large areas of air–water interface support gas exchange and appropriate dissolved gas levels, but it is advisable to use waterfalls or air diffusers to further increase surface area and prevent stratification of water.

Animals can be held in systems without life support components (commonly called "dump-and-fill" systems). Despite being simple, these systems are prone to developing high ammonia, low pH, and low oxygen levels due to the limited mechanical and biological filtration and lack of water movement.

Cleaning, Disinfection, and Quarantine

Enclosures should be evaluated daily. While daily physical cleaning (e.g., removing feces/uneaten food, flushing with water) is appropriate in both terrestrial and aquatic enclosures, chemical cleaning and disinfection is usually unnecessary and inappropriate. Amphibians are sensitive to these products and exposure can cause toxicity.

Water in soaking bowls for terrestrial amphibians should be changed at least once daily. Water changes and filter maintenance in aquatic systems are also important. A two-week frequency is acceptable for most small aquaria that have life support, while more frequent changes are needed in dump-and-fill systems.

Appropriate biosecurity protocols (e.g., quarantine, eliminating cross-contamination) are critical in order to reduce the risk of introducing potentially fatal infectious diseases to wild populations (Poole and Grow 2012). While basic standards for wildlife rehabilitation are a starting point for amphibians, more rigorous standards specific for amphibians need to be implemented (Mendelson et al. 2009; Miller 2012; Pessier and Mendelson 2010; Pessier 2011; Poole and Grow 2012).

Enclosures and cage furniture, like hides, should be cleaned and disinfected after use. Protocols that are sufficient to kill chytrid fungus and ranavirus should be utilized (Table 29.2) (Pessier and Mendelson 2010; Pessier 2011, 2014b; Poole and Grow 2012; Scheele et al. 2014; Miller et al. 2015). Care must be taken to remove any residual soaps or disinfectants prior to the next use. Organic material and anything that cannot be disinfected should be discarded.

Food and Feeding

Most amphibians will need to be fed live insects or other invertebrate prey. Prey animals need to be managed to optimize nutritional value by providing moisture and high-quality food. Prior to being fed to amphibians, most insects need additional mineral and vitamin supplementation to enhance their nutritional value, such as by "gut loading" with high-calcium food and/or applying calcium dusts. More detailed reviews are available and should be consulted for specific details (Wright 2001d; Latney and Clayton 2014).

Handling, Restraint, and Clinical Techniques

Amphibians can tolerate handling for physical exams, diagnostics, and treatments, but well-planned procedures will reduce time and stress. Reviews of clinical management techniques are available (Stetter 2001;

Table 29.2 A partial list of disinfectants for inactivating *Batrachochytrium dendrobatidis* and ranavirus on surfaces.

Method/chemical	Concentration	Comments
Batrachochytrium dendrobatidis[a]		
Sodium hypochlorite (NaH)	1–4%	30 seconds Household bleach is 5–6% NaH
Ethanol (95%)	70%	1 minute
Virkon	1 mg/mL	20 seconds
Heat	47 °C (116.6 °F) 37 °C (98.6 °F) 32 °C (89.6 °F)	30 minutes 4 hours 96 hours
Desiccation	Complete drying	3 hours
Ranavirus[b]		
Sodium hypochlorite (NaH)	3% or greater	1 minute minimum Household bleach is 5–6% NaH
Virkon	1%	1 minute minimum
Nolvasan	0.75%	1 minute minimum

[a] Pessier (2014a).
[b] Miller (2014).

Whitaker and Wright 2001; Wright 2001e; Wright and Whitaker 2001; Clayton and Gore 2007; Poole and Grow 2012; Wright and DeVoe 2012; Baitchman and Herman 2014; Chai 2014).

Manual Restraint and Physical Exam

There is limited risk to humans from amphibian patients. Dermal toxins present in some species can cause topical irritation or, rarely, systemic effects (Wright 2001b,e; Helmer and Whiteside 2005). Some toads (especially the cane toad, *Rhinella marina*) can produce toxic secretions from the parotid gland. Amphibians can carry zoonotic diseases (e.g., nontuberculous mycobacteria, enteric pathogens, *Chlamydia pneumoniae*) (Latney and Klaphake 2013). Basic personal protective equipment and hygiene standards (e.g., gloves, hand washing, protective glasses) are typically sufficient.

Moistened powder-free gloves are recommended for handling amphibians. They should be changed between animals to reduce the risk of disease transmission. Latex and vinyl gloves are toxic to some larval forms; nitrile gloves appear safest (Poole and Grow 2012).

Amphibians will be stressed by observation and handling. Procedures should be well planned so that restraint times are minimized. Most amphibians will initially freeze when threatened, and then attempt to escape. Animals can be injured during escape events.

The physical exam starts with a visual evaluation of the respiratory rate/effort (gular and abdominal), skin quality,

coloration, body condition, posture, ambulatory ability, and responsiveness. Once restrained, these parameters may change (e.g., anurans may inflate the lungs and appear edematous). Animals can be moved into small, clear containers (e.g., petri dishes, plastic bags) that facilitate evaluation of the ventral body without manual restraint. Heart rates via visual exam or Doppler can be obtained through the container, as can diagnostic procedures such as radiographs and ultrasounds (Figure 29.2).

Appropriate manual restraint technique varies according to the animal species and size. Larger amphibians, particularly those with powerful back legs (e.g., bullfrogs and leopard frogs, *Lithobates* spp.), are classically restrained with one hand encircling the body cranial to the hips, extending the hind legs backward, while the other hand supports the body (Figure 29.3).

Small anurans and caudatans are restrained between the thumb and forefinger. Caecilians, particularly aquatic species, are most safely restrained in a moistened plastic bag. When capturing aquatic amphibians, plastic bags or bag nets are less traumatic than standard nets.

Magnification aids in performing a detailed examination of the eyes, nares, and skin in small amphibians. Transillumination (using a cold light) may be helpful in small species to evaluate the coelom for organ size and masses. When dehydrated, animals may feel tacky and have obvious skin tenting or sunken eyes. Limbs should be palpated for fractures or bony abnormalities.

Oral speculums are typically needed to open the mouth. Guitar picks come in a variety of sizes and thickness and work well (Figure 29.4). Small squares of waterproof paper can be used in animals <30 g and various sized rubber spatulas may be useful in larger animals. The flat, narrow edge of the object is inserted upward, between the lip edges at the tip of the mouth or along the lateral edges.

Sedation, Anesthesia, and Analgesia

Sedation and general anesthesia can be used to obtain biological samples or perform treatments. Depth of anesthesia is evaluated via loss of the righting and withdrawal reflexes, decreased gular and abdominal respiration, and a delayed corneal reflex. Surgical depth is generally achieved at the point that respiration ceases. Heart rate monitoring is critical for evaluating anesthesia depth. Amphibians have significantly lower heart rates than similarly sized mammals; rates of 20–60 are common. The heart rate should remain fairly stable throughout the procedure. The amphibian should be kept moist using conditioned fresh water, tank water, anesthetic water, or physiological fluid. Adding supplemental oxygen to the water limits hypoxia and acidosis. Detailed reviews of anesthesia and analgesia are available and there is increasing literature on the subject (Wright 2001e; Koeller 2009; Coble et al. 2011; McMillan and Leece 2011; Minter et al. 2011; Stevens 2011; Poole and Grow 2012; Wright and DeVoe 2012; Posner et al. 2013; Baitchman and Stetter 2014; Sladakovic et al. 2014; Whiteside 2014).

Tricaine methanesulfonate (MS-222) as a topical bath consistently induces sedation and anesthesia safely in adult amphibians and is readily available as a fish anesthetic. For anesthesia, terrestrial or semiaquatic species are typically induced at 1–2 g (weight of powder)/

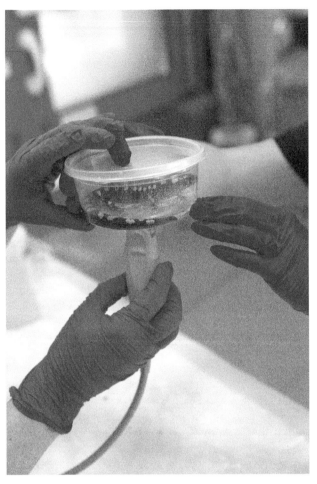

Figure 29.2 Ultrasound examination of a spotted salamander (*Ambystoma maculatum*) through a container.

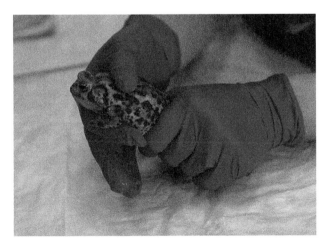

Figure 29.3 Manual restraint technique demonstrated on an American toad (*Anaxyrus americanus*); fingers of one hand encircling body just cranial to the hind legs with the other hand supporting the body.

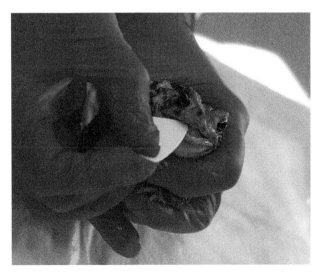

Figure 29.4 Guitar pick used to assist in opening the mouth of an American toad (*Anaxyrus americanus*).

L. Aquatic species and larval forms require lower doses: 0.1–0.2 g (weight of powder)/L. The MS-222 solution is acidic and buffer (e.g., calcium carbonate, baking soda) is needed to achieve neutral pH. Buffer is added at equal weight to the MS-222, but pH should be evaluated prior to use. Appropriate nonanesthetic water is needed for maintenance of and recovery from anesthesia.

Isoflurane applied topically (e.g., gel matrix, bubbled into water, applied directly) or via inhalation has also been used. To produce an isoflurane gel, 3 mL isoflurane can be mixed with 1.5 mL water and 2.5 mL water-based gel, which is then administered at 0.025–0.035 mL/g body weight. The inhalant agent must be scavenged appropriately to ensure staff safety. Large amphibians can be intubated and manually ventilated for longer procedures; the trachea is extremely short and bronchial intubation should be avoided.

Intramuscular alfaxalone (10–30 mg/kg) appears to be a safe sedative, based on limited studies, but does not reliably produce general anesthesia (Posner et al. 2013; Sladakovic et al. 2014). Alfaxalone topically (bath) maintained surgical anesthesia in an aquatic axolotl, *Ambystoma mexicanum*, but only produced light sedation in other species studied (McMillan and Leece 2011; Posner et al. 2013).

Signs of pain in amphibians include abnormal postures, reduced movement and reaction to stimuli, resting in atypical locations, anorexia, and color changes (generally darkening). Pain response is most typical in the first 72 hours after a trauma (Koeller 2009). While amphibians benefit from analgesia, the stress of handling during administration should be balanced against the benefits of use, particularly after the first three days (Stevens 2011; Baitchman and Stetter 2014; Whiteside 2014).

Local analgesia (e.g., lidocaine, bupivacaine) and systemic medications at the time of surgery can be beneficial in amphibians, as in other species.

Nonsteroidal antiinflammatories are commonly used in clinical work. In one study on African clawed frogs, *Xenopus laevis*, flunixin meglumine at 25 mg/kg SQ produced analgesia but meloxicam at 0.2 mg/kg did not (Coble et al. 2011). That study utilized a flunixin meglumine dosage much higher than the meloxicam dosage, when compared to those commonly used in mammals. Higher meloxicam dosages may show greater efficacy. In the author's experience, meloxicam at 0.1–1 mg/kg PO, IM, or SQ SID to q48h in dendrobatid frogs has been safe.

Experiments have demonstrated efficacy of injectable and topical (bath) opioid analgesics at dosages much higher than those used in mammals (Koeller 2009; Coble et al. 2011; Stevens 2011). In eastern red spotted newts (*Notophthalmus viridescens*), buprenorphine 50 mg/kg intracoelomic and butorphanol 0.5 mg/L tank water were effective at reducing postoperative pain in an experimental setting (Koeller 2009). Tramadol is commonly used at 5–10 mg/kg PO SID to q24–48h, although no formal studies have been conducted. One author reports using tramadol 25 mg/kg PO q48h to manage arthropathies in geriatric cane toads (Whiteside 2014).

Clinical Techniques

Amphibian medicine follows the same basic principles of diagnostics and treatment as for other classes. Detailed reviews of clinical techniques are available (Stetter 2001; Whitaker 2001; Wright 2001c,e–g; Wright and Whitaker 2001; Pessier and Pinkerton 2003; Allender and Fry 2008; Wright and DeVoe 2012; Baitchman and Stetter 2014).

Cytology of lesions, aspirated fluid, or masses is an important diagnostic tool in amphibians. Skin preparation for such procedures is accomplished by flushing with sterile physiological fluid, such as 0.9% saline, or dilute chlorhexidine (0.05%). Importantly, soaps and other disinfectants commonly used in mammals, birds, and reptiles are generally toxic to amphibians.

Cytology should include direct microscopy, gram stain, Romanowsky-type stain (e.g., Diff-Quik), and modified Ziehl–Neelsen (acid-fast) stain. Chronic mycobacterial infection is common in amphibians and an acid-fast stain should routinely be included in any cytology (Chai 2011). Cytology can help guide treatment and culture decisions. While gram-negative aerobic bacterial infections are common, gram-positive and anaerobic infections can also occur (Taylor 2001; Taylor et al. 2001; Chai 2011). Whole blood or lymph fluid cultures are useful in cases where systemic bacterial infection is suspected.

Fecal exams (direct, float, and cytology) should be considered for ill amphibians. In anorexic animals, assisted feeding may be necessary to obtain a fecal. Eggs from nematode parasites (gastrointestinal and pulmonary) are passed in the feces. Intestinal protozoa are common and generally not associated with disease (Poynton and Whitaker 2001).

In anurans, blood can be obtained from the ventral vein, heart, lingual venous plexus, femoral plexus, axillary plexus, and facial vein (Allender and Fry 2008; Forzán et al. 2012). Due to the high plasma turnover, lymphatic fluid may be appropriate for evaluating biochemistry values. A technique utilizing a temporary ligature around the body cranial to the hind legs is described for anurans (Reynolds et al. 2009). In caudatans, blood is most commonly obtained from the ventral tail vein using the same techniques as for lizards. In caecilians, blood is obtained from the heart. Sedation may be needed if animals are struggling. Lithium heparin, which does not lyse amphibian erythrocytes, is the preferred anticoagulant for blood samples.

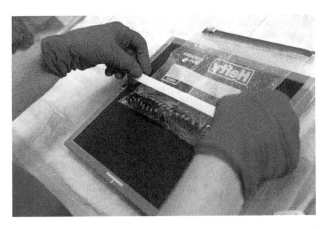

Figure 29.5 Plastic bag and tape being used to position a spotted salamander (*Ambystoma maculatum*) for radiographs.

Radiographs are useful, although there is limited radiographic contrast in the normal amphibian coelom. Amphibians should not be taped to the plate and are typically restrained in plastic bags or containers, depending on the imaging needed (Figure 29.5). For lateral views, animals tolerate a horizontal lateral beam better than being placed in lateral recumbency. Ultrasound can be easily accomplished in amphibians by placing the animal and a small amount of water in a container and scanning through the container or immersing the probe in the water (Figure 29.2).

Endoscopy can be used to obtain diagnostic samples in amphibians. Rigid endoscopes commonly used in other small exotics and thin fiberscopes (e.g., feline bronchoscope) are most appropriate. Amphibians also tolerate surgery, including coelomic exploratory exams and fracture fixation.

Many wildlife rehabilitation clinics will have equipment appropriate for amphibians (e.g., gram scales and 25–30 gauge needles). Medication can be administered using topical (cutaneous), oral, or injectable (IM or SQ) routes. For amphibians with a waxy coating or thick skin, topical medication should be delivered onto the thinner skin of the lateral body wall or lateral/ventral thigh to improve absorption. Micropipettes are ideal for appropriate oral or topical medication administration in small patients. Dilutions of medications are often necessary. Ocular medications are convenient to use topically and are nonirritating, but actual doses should be computed to avoid toxicity. Exotic animal formularies and publications should be consulted for up-to-date recommendations (Wright and DeVoe 2012).

Fluid support can be readily accomplished through soaking in electrolyte solutions used for IV fluid administration and is a viable means of rehydration. Intraosseous or intralymphatic routes may be needed in cases of severe skin disease and electrolyte abnormalities, such as with severe chytridiomycosis (Young et al. 2012).

Debilitated amphibians should be provided with nutritional support. Feeding frequency varies with species' needs. Small, active foragers may need daily food support while sit-and-wait predators can be fed less frequently. Enteral formulas made for carnivores or insectivores are appropriate and volumes of 1–3% body weight are well tolerated and appropriate for maintaining or improving condition.

Infectious and Parasitic Diseases

Systemic bacterial infection is common in amphibians and clinical signs include lethargy, collapse, edema, and erythema. Erythema is particularly noticeable on the ventrum and hindlimbs and historically cases were called "red leg disease" due to *Aeromonas* spp. However, in reality, a diversity of bacteria can cause septicemia. Additionally, bacterial septicemia is frequently secondary to immunosuppression from other infectious diseases or husbandry factors. *Batrachochytrium dendrobatidis* (Bd) (chytrid fungus) and ranavirus infections can cause the same clinical signs and/or lead to secondary bacterial infections.

Batrachochytrium dendrobatidis and ranaviruses are important primary pathogens of wild amphibians and cause mortality events in wild and captive populations. Rehabilitators should work with state wildlife biologists to understand the regional occurrence of infectious diseases to reduce the risk of introducing diseases through the rehabilitation process. Clinically relevant summaries are available (Pessier and Mendelson 2010; Crawshaw 2011; Pessier 2011, 2014a; Baitchman and Pessier 2013; Latney and Klaphake 2013; Miller 2014; Miller et al. 2015).

Batrachochytrium dendrobatidis was initially reported in the 1990s, has been documented to infect over 500 species of amphibians from all three orders, and is responsible for the extinction of multiple species in the wild. A second amphibian chytrid, *B. salamandrivorans*, has been described in Europe and linked to population declines in free-ranging fire salamanders (*Salamandra salamandra*) (Martel et al. 2013). Transmission is via a motile zoospore that needs a moist environment. The amphibian stratum corneum thickens and life-threatening hypokalemia and hypernatremia develop. Clinical signs are most obvious in postmetamorphic animals and include increased skin shedding or thickening (dysecdysis), skin discoloration (e.g., erythema, darkening), postural changes, increased soaking in water, neurological abnormalities, and dehydration. Secondary bacterial infection may develop. Mortality rates as high as 100% are reported. A carrier state has been described. Recently, the US Fish and Wildlife Service has banned the importation and interstate movement of over 200 species of salamanders due to *B. salamandrivorans* concerns.

Multiple strains of ranavirus have been identified and some can be transmitted between classes (e.g., amphibian to reptiles or fish). Ranaviruses are transmitted via consumption of infected tissue, direct and indirect contact, water, and fomites. Animals often present acutely moribund and may develop systemic secondary bacterial infections. The classic presentation for ranavirus infection in tadpoles is edema, hemorrhage, and erythema of the body cavity and/or organs. Mortality events in anuran and caudate metamorphs and adults have also described. As with Bd, a carrier state exists.

Ranid herpesvirus 1 causes rapidly developing kidney adenocarcinomas in northern leopard frogs (*Lithobates pipiens*). Virus replication and transmission occur at cooler temperatures and tumor growth develops with warmer temperatures. Animals may present with edema in the body cavity or obviously enlarged kidneys.

Amphibians have a number of different parasites. Many healthy amphibians have low parasite burdens without clinical disease. Heavy parasite burdens cause disease and may develop in debilitated animals or captive settings. Many gastrointestinal and pulmonary nematodes have direct life cycles and transmission within captive settings can occur. Amphibians with heavy infections may be weak and thin. Protozoa are normal commensals in the gastrointestinal tract, but occasionally overgrowth may be associated with enteritis. Anurans are intermediate hosts for cestodes and trematodes and clinical disease is rare. In some populations, *Ribeiroia* spp. metacercariae have been associated with supernumerary limbs. Alveolate protozoan infections have been reported in tadpoles of numerous ranid species throughout the eastern United States and sporadically in other areas. Generally large acute die-offs are noted with tadpoles presenting with erratic swimming, coelomic effusion, and enlarged liver, spleen, and kidney.

Common Reasons for Presentation

Trauma and collection as pets are major reasons amphibians present for rehabilitation (Hartup 1996). Presentation due to infectious diseases is infrequent.

Traumatic lesions include bone fractures or other musculoskeletal injuries, internal bleeding, wounds, and desiccation, and animals can be responsive to care (Hartup 1996; Johnson 2003; Royal et al. 2007; van Bonn 2009). Supportive care should be instituted on a case-by-case basis. Closed fractures, particularly of limbs without significant muscle mass, may respond to conservative management by confining the animal to a small hospital tank and limiting mobility. Surgical fixation is more appropriate if the limb has significant muscle mass, such as the hindlimbs of bullfrogs. Successful surgical repair of a femoral fracture has been described (Royal et al. 2007). Internal fixation reduces secondary osteomyelitis compared to external fixation (Johnson 2003; Royal et al. 2007). Skin wounds may be closed primarily (e.g., suture, methyl-2-cyanoacrylate), although amphibians also readily heal via second intention (Wright 2001g; Rosa and Fernández-Loras 2012). Antibiotics and analgesics are indicated post fracture repair and with significant skin wounds.

Blunt trauma can cause internal bleeding. Supportive care with fluids, oxygen, and confinement to a hospital cage is indicated and animals can be successfully managed.

Amphibian healing rates have not been well studied in a clinical setting. In the author's experience, integument and musculoskeletal injuries heal readily in 1–4 weeks, depending on the extent of the injury. If healing is not clearly progressing, a secondary issue is usually present, such as low environmental temperature, infection, or continued trauma and if wounds are not healing, then the husbandry and diagnosis should be reevaluated.

Secondary bacteria infections, including mycobacteria, are common. Infections may be localized (e.g., in a wound, ulceration, abscess, osteomyelitis site) or systemic. Underlying etiologies may include inappropriate caging (i.e., skin trauma during feeding), cutaneous parasitic disease, bite wounds (from cagemates or prey items), or traumatic lacerations. Systemic antibiotics are frequently indicated. First-line antibiotics are typically those appropriate for gram-negative infections, such as fluoroquinolones. Healthy amphibians are capable of mounting an effective response to localized infection and treatment is often successful. In addition to antibiotic administration, topical wound care is often beneficial. Infected wounds should be left to heal by second intention. Wound cleaning with 0.9% saline or 0.05% chlorhexidine solution followed by application of 1% silver sulfadiazine every 24–48 hours is a good first-line therapeutic.

Aquatic amphibians may develop "water mold" infections on wounds (saprolegniasis), as described in fish. These appear as white, fluffy growths on the animal and are typically secondary to skin trauma. Increasing the salinity of the water to 1–2 ppt can reduce the fungal lesions and help with osmoregulation, though topical treatment may be necessary.

Clinical Pathology

As in reptiles and birds, amphibians have nucleated red cells. Plasma color can vary with species and may be clear to light yellow, orange, green, or blue depending on the species. Reviews of obtaining, preparing, and interpreting blood samples, as well as some expected values, are available (Wright 2001f; Allender and Fry 2008; Wright and DeVoe 2012).

Hemogram and biochemistry values vary based on age, sex, and season of the year, among other environmental factors, and this makes defining normal values challenging. While monitoring trends in individual cases may be helpful, management is rarely dependent on bloodwork. Anuran hematocrits tend to be <30% and amphibian blood glucose values <50 mg/dL (Wright 2001f). Blood biochemistry values are not maintained within a tight range; during periods of dehydration significant increases in certain analytes (e.g., blood urea nitrogen, sodium) are expected.

Pre-Release Condition and Postrelease Monitoring

Release standards for amphibians can be based on those developed for other classes (Miller 2012). It is imperative to evaluate the individual animal's ability to hunt, prehend and consume prey, and escape predators.

Population concerns are important due to chytridiomycosis and ranavirus infections. Ranavirus has the added potential for transmission to other classes (e.g., reptiles and fish); in North America, box turtles are particularly susceptible. Rehabilitators working with amphibians should ensure individual animals are released to the site of origin and not exposed to amphibians from other locations during their time at the facility (Mendelson et al. 2009; Scheele et al. 2014).

References

Allender, M.C. and Fry, M.M. (2008). Amphibian hematology. *Veterinary Clinics of North American: Exotic Animal Practice* 11 (3): 463–480.

AmphibiaWeb (2015) http://amphibiaweb.org/amphibian/speciesnums.html

Baitchman, E.J. and Herman, T.A. (2014). Caudata (Urodela): tailed amphibians. In: *Fowler's Zoo and Wild Animal Medicine*, vol. 8 (ed. R.E. Miller and M.E. Fowler), 13–20. St Louis, MO: Saunders.

Baitchman, E.J. and Pessier, A.P. (2013). Pathogenesis, diagnosis, and treatment of amphibian chytridiomycosis. *Veterinary Clinics of North America: Exotic Animal Practice* 16 (3): 669–685.

Baitchman, E. and Stetter, M. (2014). Amphibians. In: *Zoo Animal and Wildlife Immobilization and Anesthesia*, 2e (ed. G. West, D. Heard and N. Caulkett), 303–311. Ames, IA: Wiley-Blackwell.

Barnett, S.L., Cover, J.F., and Wright, K.M. (2001). Amphibian husbandry and housing. In: *Amphibian Medicine and Captive Husbandry* (ed. K.M. Wright and B.R. Whitaker), 35–61. Malabar, FL: Krieger.

Chai, N. (2011). Mycobacteriosis in amphibians. In: *Fowler's Zoo and Wild Animal Medicine Current Therapy*, vol. 7 (ed. R.E. Miller and M.E. Fowler), 224–230. St Louis, MO: Saunders.

Chai, N. (2014). Anurans. In: *Fowler's Zoo and Wild Animal Medicine*, vol. 8 (ed. R.E. Miller and M.E. Fowler), 1–13. St Louis, MO: Saunders.

Clayton, L.A. and Gore, S.R. (2007). Amphibian emergency medicine. *Veterinary Clinics of North America: Exotic Animal Practice* 10 (2): 587–620.

Clayton, L.A. and Mylniczenko, N.D. (2014). Caecilians. In: *Fowler's Zoo and Wild Animal Medicine*, vol. 8 (ed. R.E. Miller and M.E. Fowler), 20–26. St Louis, MO: Saunders.

Coble, D.J., Taylor, D.K., and Mook, D.M. (2011). Analgesic effects of meloxicam, morphine sulfate, flunixin meglumine, and xylazine hydrochloride in African-clawed frogs (*Xenopus laevis*). *Journal of the American Association of Laboratory Animal Science* 50 (3): 355–360.

Crawshaw, G. (2011). Amphibian viral diseases. In: *Fowler's Zoo and Wild Animal Medicine Current Therapy*, vol. 7 (ed. R.E. Miller and M.E. Fowler), 231–238. St Louis, MO: Saunders.

Forzán, M.J., Vanderstichel, R.V., Ogbuah, C.T. et al. (2012). Blood collection from the facial (maxillary)/musculo-cutaneous vein in true frogs (family Ranidae). *Journal of Wildlife Disease* 48 (1): 176–180.

Hartup, B.K. (1996). Rehabilitation of native reptiles and amphibians in DuPage County, Illinois. *Journal of Wildlife Diseases* 32 (1): 109–112.

Helmer, P.J. and Whiteside, D.P. (2005). Amphibian anatomy and physiology. In: *Clinical Anatomy and Physiology of Exotic Species: Structure and Function of Mammals, Birds, Reptiles, and Amphibians* (ed. B. O'Malley), 3–14. Philadelphia, PA: Elsevier Saunders.

Johnson, D. (2003). External fixation of bilateral tibial fractures in an American bullfrog. *Exotic DVM* 5 (2): 27–30.

Koeller, C.A. (2009). Comparison of buprenorphine and butorphanol analgesia in the eastern red-spotted newt (*Notophthalmus viridescens*). *Journal of the American*

Association of Laboratory Animal Science 48 (2): 171–175.

Latney, L. and Clayton, L.A. (2014). Updates on amphibian nutrition and nutritive value of common feeder insects. *Veterinary Clinics of North America: Exotic Animal Practice* 17 (3): 347–367.

Latney, L.V. and Klaphake, E. (2013). Selected emerging diseases of amphibia. *Veterinary Clinics of North America: Exotic Animal Practice* 16 (2): 283–301.

Martel, A., Spitzen-van der Sluijs, A., Blooi, M. et al. (2013). *Batrachochytrium salamandrivorans* sp. nov. causes lethal chytridiomycosis in amphibians. *Proceedings of the National Academy of Sciences USA*, 110 (38): 15325–15329.

McMillan, M.W. and Leece, E.A. (2011). Immersion and branchial/transcutaneous irrigation anaesthesia with alfaxalone in a Mexican axolotl. *Veterinary Anaesthesia and Analgesia* 38 (6): 619–623.

Mendelson, J.R., Pramuk, J.B., Gagliardo, R. et al. (2009). Considerations and recommendations for raising live amphibians in classrooms. Letter to the editors. *Herpetological Review* 40 (2): 142–144.

Miller, E.A. (2012). *Minimum Standards for Wildlife Rehabilitation*, 4e. St Cloud, MN: National Wildlife Rehabilitators Association.

Miller, D.L. (2014). Ranavirus. In: *Current Therapy in Reptile Medicine and Surgery* (ed. D.R. Mader and S.J. Divers), 277–280. St Louis, MO: Saunders Elsevier.

Miller, D.L., Pessier, A.P., Hicks, P. et al. (2015). Comparative pathology of ranaviruses and diagnostic techniques. In: *Ranaviruses* (ed. M.J. Gray and V.G. Chinchar), 171–208. SpringerOpen. https://link. springer.com/book/10.1007/978-3-319-13755-1.

Minter, L.J., Clarke, E.O., Gjeltema, J.L. et al. (2011). Effects of intramuscular meloxicam administration on prostaglandin E2 synthesis in the north American bullfrog (*Rana catesbeiana*). *Journal of Zoo and Wildlife Medicine* 42 (4): 680–685.

Pessier, A.P. (2009). Edematous frogs, urinary tract disease, and disorders of fluid balance in amphibians. *Journal of Exotic Pet Medicine* 18 (1): 4–13.

Pessier, A.P. (2011). Diagnosis and control of amphibian chytridiomycosis. In: *Fowler's Zoo and Wild Animal Medicine Current Therapy*, vol. 7 (ed. R.E. Miller and M.E. Fowler), 217–223. St Louis, MO: Saunders.

Pessier, A.P. (2014a). Infectious disease of amphibians: it isn't just redleg anymore. In: *Current Therapy in Reptile Medicine and Surgery* (ed. D.R. Mader and S.J. Divers), 247–254. St Louis, MO: Saunders Elsevier.

Pessier, A.P. (2014b). Chytridiomycosis. In: *Current Therapy in Reptile Medicine and Surgery* (ed. D.R. Mader and S.J. Divers), 255–270. St Louis, MO: Saunders Elsevier.

Pessier, A.P. & Mendelson, J.R. 2010. A Manual for Control of Infectious Diseases in Amphibian Survival Assurance Colonies and Reintroduction Programs. IUCN/SSC Conservation Breeding Specialist Group, Apple Valley. www.cpsg.org/sites/cbsg.org/files/documents/ AMPHIBIAN_DISEASE_MANUAL_2017.pdf

Pessier, A.P. and Pinkerton, M. (2003). Practical gross necropsy of amphibians. *Seminars in Avian and Exotic Pet Medicine* 12 (2): 81–88.

Poole, V.A. and Grow, S. (2012). *Amphibian Husbandry Resource Guide*, 2.0e. Silver Spring, MD: Association of Zoos and Aquariums www.speakcdn.com/assets/2332/ amphibianhusbandryresourceguide.pdf.

Posner, L.P., Bailey, K.M., Richardson, E.Y. et al. (2013). Alfaxalone anesthesia in bullfrogs (*Lithobates catesbeiana*) by injection or immersion. *Journal of Zoo and Wildlife Medicine* 44 (4): 965–971.

Poynton, S.L. and Whitaker, B.R. (2001). Protozoa and metazoan infecting amphibians. In: *Amphibian Medicine and Captive Husbandry* (ed. K.M. Wright and B.R. Whitaker), 193–221. Malabar, FL: Krieger.

Reynolds, S.J., Christian, K.A., and Tracy, C.R. (2009). Application of a method of obtaining lymph from anuran amphibians. *Journal of Herpetology* 43 (1): 148–153.

Rosa, G.M. and Fernández-Loras, A. (2012). Emergency procedures in the field: a report of wound treatment and fast healing in the giant ditch frog (*Leptodactylus fallax*). *Animal Welfare* 21 (4): 559–562.

Royal, L.W., Grafinger, M.S., Lascelles, B.D.X. et al. (2007). Internal fixation of a femur fracture in an American bullfrog. *Journal of the American Veterinary Medical Association* 230 (8): 1201–1204.

Scheele, B.C., Hunter, D.A., Grogan, L.F. et al. (2014). Interventions for reducing extinction risk in chytridiomycosis-threatened amphibians. *Conservation Biology* 28 (5): 1195–1205.

Sladakovic, I., Johnson, R.S., and Vogelnest, L. (2014). Evaluation of intramuscular alfaxalone in three Australian frog species (*Litoria caerulea, Litoria aurea, Litoria booroolongensis*). *Journal of Herpetological Medicine and Surgery* 24 (1–2): 36–42.

Stetter, M.D. (2001). Diagnostic imaging of amphibians. In: *Amphibian Medicine and Captive Husbandry* (ed. K.M. Wright and B.R. Whitaker), 253–272. Malabar, FL: Krieger.

Stevens, C.W. (2011). Analgesia in amphibians: preclinical studies and clinical applications. *Veterinary Clinics of North America: Exotic Animal Practice* 14 (1): 33–44.

Taylor, S.K. (2001). Mycoses. In: *Amphibian Medicine and Captive Husbandry* (ed. K.M. Wright and B.R. Whitaker), 181–191. Malabar, FL: Krieger.

Taylor, S.K., Green, K., Wright, K.M. et al. (2001). Bacterial diseases. In: *Amphibian Medicine and Captive*

Husbandry (ed. K.M. Wright and B.R. Whitaker), 159–179. Malabar, FL: Krieger.

Van Bonn, W. (2009). Clinical technique: extra-articular surgical stifle stabilization of an American bullfrog (*Rana catesbeiana*). *Journal of Exotic Pet Medicine* 18 (1): 36–39.

Whitaker, B.R. (2001). Water quality. In: *Amphibian Medicine and Captive Husbandry* (ed. K.M. Wright and B.R. Whitaker), 147–157. Malabar, FL: Krieger.

Whitaker, B.R. and Wright, K.M. (2001). Clinical techniques. In: *Amphibian Medicine and Captive Husbandry* (ed. K.M. Wright and B.R. Whitaker), 89–110. Malabar, FL: Krieger.

Whiteside, D.P. (2014). Analgesia. In: *Zoo Animal and Wildlife Immobilization and Anesthesia*, 2e (ed. G. West, D. Heard and N. Caulkett), 83–108. Ames, IA: Wiley-Blackwell.

Wright, K.M. (2001a). Taxonomy of amphibians kept in captivity. In: *Amphibian Medicine and Captive Husbandry* (ed. K.M. Wright and B.R. Whitaker), 3–14. Malabar, FL: Krieger.

Wright, K.M. (2001b). Anatomy for the clinician. In: *Amphibian Medicine and Captive Husbandry* (ed. K.M. Wright and B.R. Whitaker), 15–30. Malabar, FL: Krieger.

Wright, K.M. (2001c). Applied physiology. In: *Amphibian Medicine and Captive Husbandry* (ed. K.M. Wright and B.R. Whitaker), 31–34. Malabar, FL: Krieger.

Wright, K.M. (2001d). Diets for captive amphibians. In: *Amphibian Medicine and Captive Husbandry* (ed. K.M. Wright and B.R. Whitaker), 63–72. Malabar, FL: Krieger.

Wright, K.M. (2001e). Restraint techniques and euthanasia. In: *Amphibian Medicine and Captive Husbandry* (ed. K.M. Wright and B.R. Whitaker), 111–122. Malabar, FL: Krieger.

Wright, K.M. (2001f). Amphibian hematology. In: *Amphibian Medicine and Captive Husbandry* (ed. K.M. Wright and B.R. Whitaker), 129–146. Malabar, FL: Krieger.

Wright, K.M. (2001g). Surgical techniques. In: *Amphibian Medicine and Captive Husbandry* (ed. K.M. Wright and B.R. Whitaker), 273–283. Malabar, FL: Krieger.

Wright, K. and DeVoe, R.S. (2012). Amphibians. In: *Exotic Animal Formulary*, 4e (ed. J.W. Carpenter), 53–82. St Louis, MO: Elsevier Saunders.

Wright, K.M. and Whitaker, B.R. (2001). Pharmacotherapeutics. In: *Amphibian Medicine and Captive Husbandry* (ed. K.M. Wright and B.R. Whitaker), 309–330. Malabar, FL: Krieger.

Young, S., Speare, R., Berger, L. et al. (2012). Chloramphenicol with fluid and electrolyte therapy cures terminally ill green tree frogs (*Litoria caerulea*) with chytridiomycosis. *Journal of Zoo and Wildlife Medicine* 43 (2): 330–337.

Appendix I

Clinical Pathology of Common Wildlife Species

Erica A. Miller

Wildlife Medicine, Department of Clinic Studies, University of Pennsylvania School of Veterinary Medicine, Philadelphia, PA, USA

Medical Management of Wildlife Species: A Guide for Practitioners, First Edition. Edited by Sonia M. Hernandez,
Heather W. Barron, Erica A. Miller, Roberto F. Aguilar and Michael J. Yabsley.
© 2020 John Wiley & Sons, Inc. Published 2020 by John Wiley & Sons, Inc.

Hematology Values of Rodents

	Units	North American Porcupine *Erethizon dorsatum* Range (Median)	Beaver *Castor canadensis* Range (Median)	Gray Squirrel *Sciurus carolinensis* Male	Gray Squirrel *Sciurus carolinensis* Female	Gray Squirrel *S. carolinensis*	Fox Squirrel *Sciurus niger*
WBCs	(10³/µL)	2.78–16.64 (7.65)	5.35–23.84 (11.61)	1.113–3912			
RBCs	(10⁶/µL)	2.66–5.29 (3.86)	3.04–4.63 (3.83)			4.43	3.93
Hematocrit	(%)	24.4–46.1 (36.3)	28.2–46.9 (37.3)	32.5–48.0	28.5–36.0	37	41
Hemoglobin	(g/dL)	8.9–15.2 (12.2)	10.0–15.5 (12.7)	12.7–16.3	9.3–12.0		
MCV	(fL)	75.5–112.4 (90.5)	77.5–108.9 (93.2)				
MCH	(pg)	25.8–36.8 (30.8)	27.9–38.2 (33.1)				
MCHC	(g/dL)	27.5–40.3 (34.2)	29.7–40.6 (35.2)	28.8–40.0	29.7–37.9		
Neutrophils	(10³/µL)	0.01–0.19 (0.04)	0.02–0.12 (0.05)	0–6		0.08	0.07
Segmented neutrophils	(10³/µL)	0.50–9.53 (3.24)	1.09–15.76 (6.83)	1–14		2.55	2.28
Lymphocytes	(10³/µL)	1.05–9.29 (3.5)	0.92–8.96 (3.02)	75–91		1.14	1.14
Monocytes	(10³/µL)	55–1051 (255)	60–1076 (286)	0–1		6	5
Eosinophils	(10³/µL)	30–925 (218)	0–809 (315)	0–3		0	0
Basophils	(10³/µL)			0–1		0.7	0.2
Platelets	(10³/µL)	83–698 (390)	4–388 (196)			1.28	1.18
Neutrophils	(%)						
Band neutrophils	(%)						
Lymphocytes	(%)						
Monocytes	(%)						
Eosinophils	(%)						
Basophils	(%)						
References		Teare (2013)	Teare (2013)	Guthrie and Mosby (1966)		Murnane and Miller (1993)	Murnane and Miller (1993)

ALP, alkaline phosphatase; ALT, alanine aminotransferase; AST, aspartate aminotransferase; CPK, creatine phosphokinase; GGT, gamma-glutamyl transferase; LDH, lactate dehydrogenase; MCH, mean corpuscular hemoglobin; MCHC, mean corpuscular hemoglobin concentration; MCV, mean corpuscular volume; RBC, red blood cell; WBC, white blood cell.

Biochemical Values of Rodents

	Units	North American Porcupine *Erethizon dorsatum* Range (Median)	Beaver *Castor canadensis* Range (Median)	Gray Squirrel *Sciurus carolinensis* Range	Gray Squirrel *S. carolinensis* Range	Fox Squirrel *Sciurus niger* Range	Woodchuck *Marmota monax* Range
Total protein	(g/dL)	4.7–8.3 (6.7)	4.9–8.0 (6.6)	3.7–6.6	5.8–6.0	5.8–6.4	4–4.4
Glucose	(mg/dL)	54–266 (143)	24–127 (84)	25–255	130	120–180	180–250
Blood urea nitrogen (BUN)	(mg/dL)	9–39 (18)	9–38 (20)	4–70	26–40	15–40	26–80
Uric acid	(mg/dL)	1.4–1.5 (1.4)					
Creatinine	(mg/dL)	0.2–1.5 (0.7)	0.4–2.0 (1.2)		0.17–0.4	0.56–0.78	0.24–0.28
BUN/creatinine ratio		12.4–63.8 (26.3)	6.7–35.0 (15.6)		24.92–59.26	19.23–60.61	108.3–296.3
Total bilirubin	(mg/dL)	0.0–0.6 (0.1)	0.0–0.7 (0.2)				
Direct bilirubin	(mg/dL)						
Indirect billirubin	(mg/dL)						
Triglycerides	(mg/dL)	0–290 (120)		20–496			
Cholesterol	(mg/dL)	42–205 (112)	51–134 (79)	124–448	133.7–272.3	152.6–161.8	195.65–9.95
Amylase	(IU/L)	0–3393 (1316)	0–425 (171)				
ALP	(IU/L)	27–381 (96)	53–610 (178)		202.9–249.6	138.7–163.5	28–73
ALT	(IU/L)	2–26 (7)	8–47 (20)		0	2–8	18–42
AST	(IU/L)	43–349 (157)	37–190 (75)		34–56	59–76	30–47
CPK	(IU/L)						
LDH	(IU/L)				1098–1199	1487–1635	1510–1786
GGT	(IU/L)	0–13 (6)	0–11 (3)				
Albumin (A)	(g/dL)	2.3–5.7 (4.2)	2.1–4.4 (3.5)		1.8–2.98	3.11–3.51	1.88–2.12
Globulin (G)	(g/dL)	1.1–4.1 (2.3)	1.8–5.5 (3.1)		3.42–4.2	2.68–2.89	1.64–2.12
A/G ratio		0.9–4.1 (1.9)			0.43–0.87	1.08–1.21	0.89–1.44
Phosphorus (P)	(mg/dL)	2.0–9.6 (5.6)	2.9–10.0 (6.2)	3.1–21.8			
Calcium (C)	(mg/dL)	8.6–12.6 (10.6)	8.7–11.5 (10.1)	7.0–14.5	7.96–9.94	10.77–11.91	9.21–11.43
Ca/P ratio		0.9–4.1 (1.9)	1.0–3.7 (1.6)				
Sodium (Na)	(mEq/L)	128–145 (136)	121–143 (132)				
Potassium (K)	(mEq/L)	3.1–6.7 (4.6)	3.1–6.6 (4.2)				

(Continued)

(Continued)

	Units	North American Porcupine *Erethizon dorsatum* Range (Median)	Beaver *Castor canadensis* Range (Median)	Gray Squirrel *Sciurus carolinensis* Range	Gray Squirrel *S. carolinensis* Range	Fox Squirrel *Sciurus niger* Range	Woodchuck *Marmota monax* Range
Na/K ratio		18.0–44.1 (29.8)	19.8–42.5 (30.8)				
Chloride	(mEq/L)	93–111 (101)	81–104 (89)	80–155			
Creatinine kinase	(IU/L)	0–2852 (813)	0–1833 (743)				
Lipase	(IU/L)						
Bicarbonate	(mEq/L)	12.8–28.1 (20.5)	12.3–37.4 (24.8)				
Magnesium	(mg/dL)			1.3–5.3			
Iron	(µg/dL)						
Carbon dioxide	(mEq/L)	12.3–28.5 (20.4)	15–36 (25)				
TT4	(µg/dL)						
References		Teare (2013)	Teare (2013)	Hoff et al. (1976)	Murnane and Miller (1993)	Murnane and Miller (1993)	Murnane and Miller (1993)

References

Guthrie, D.R. and Mosby, H.S. (1966). Hematological values for the Eastern Gray Squirrel (*Sciurus carolinensis*). *Canadian Journal of Zoology* 44: 323–327.

Hoff, G.L., McEldowny, L.E., Bigler, W.J. et al. (1976). Blood and urinary values in the gray squirrel. *Journal of Widlife Diseases* 12 (3): 349–352.

Murnane, J. & Miller, E.A. (1993). Forming a Clinical Pathology Database for Wildlife. Poster Presentation, National Wildlife Rehabilitators Association

Symposium, Oakland, CA. Values are averages from 8–12 animals, determined using Unopettes and Neubauer hemocytometers and blood smear stained with Wright's Giemsa.

Teare, J.A. (ed.) (2013). *ISIS Physiological Reference Intervals for Captive Wildlife: A CD-ROM Resource.* Bloomington, MN: International Species Information System.

Hematology Values of Lagomorphs

| | | Eastern Cottontail Rabbit (*Sylvilagus floridanus*) | | | | | Black-tailed Jackrabbit (*Lepus californicus*) | |
| | | Adult | Adults (Sept–Oct) | Adults (Dec–Jan) | Adults (Mar–Apr) | Adults (Jul–Aug) | Adults | Juveniles |
	Units	Range	Range (Median)	Range (Median)	Range (Median)	Range (Median)	Range (Mean)	Range (Mean)
WBCs	(10³/µL)						2.20–14.70 (8.0)	2.0–16.0 (6.0)
RBCs	(10⁶/µL)						6.59–8.56 (7.7)	6.45–9.02 (7.6)
Hematocrit	(%)	43.1–46.2	11.0–45.0 (28)	24.0–50.0 (42)	26.0–49.0 (38)	21.0–46.0 (35)	42.00–53.00 (47.5)	42.00–55.00 (48.7)
Hemoglobin	(g/dL)						13.70–17.50 (15.9)	13.50–18.30 (15.8)
MCV	(fL)						57.60–65.60 (61.0)	58.80–68.90 (63.4)
MCH	(pg)							
MCHC	(g/dL)						31.50–34.70 (33.5)	31.10–34.50 (32.4)
Neutrophils	(10³/µL)						1.342–12.789 (33.6)	0.378–3.416 (1.73)
Segmented neutrophils	(10³/µL)							
Lymphocytes	(10³/µL)						0.682–8.549 (3.3)	1.540–11.431 (3.19)
Monocytes	(10³/µL)						0.198–0.820 (0.40)	
Eosinophils	(10³/µL)						0.0–0.864 (0.19)	0.0–0.840 (0.29)
Basophils	(10³/µL)						0.0–0.130 (0.05)	0.0–0.112 (0.02)
Platelets	(10³/µL)	41.2–57.9	0.5–44.5 (4.5)	1.5–21.5 (9)	3.0–60.0 (7)	5.0–61.5 (22)		
Neutrophils	(%)						13.00–81.50 (50.3)	14.0–57.5 (32.0)
Band neutrophils	(%)	31.3–48.6	48.0–96.5 (90.5)	71.5–96.0 (86.5)	31.5–93.0 (83)	22.0–91.5 (71)		
Lymphocytes	(%)	8.4–12.6	0.0–2.0 (1)	1.0–4.0 (2.2)	0.0–5.0 (1.5)	0.0–4.5 (2.5)	25.0–83.0 (42.6)	32.0–80.0 (57.2)
Monocytes	(%)		0.0–9.5 (1)	0.0–1.5 (0)	0.0–5.0 (2)	0.0–7.5 (0.5)	2.0–10.0 (4.0)	1.0–16.0 (6.1)
Eosinophils	(%)	1.7–3.4	0.0–1.5 (0)	0.0–1.3 (0.7)	0.0–3.5 (1)	0.0–6.5 (1)	0.0–8.0 (2.1)	0.0–11.0 (4.1)
Basophils	(%)						0.0–1.5 (0.41)	0.0–2.0 (0.35)
References		Jacobson and Kirkpatrick (1975)	Jacobson et al. (1978)	Jacobson et al. (1978)	Jacobson et al. (1978)	Jacobson et al. (1978)	Fetters (1971)	Fetters (1971)

Biochemical Values of Lagomorphs

	Units	Eastern Cottontail Rabbit (Sylvilagus floridanus)					Black-tailed Jackrabbit (Lepus californicus)
		Adult	Adults (Sept–Oct)	Adults (Dec–Jan)	Adults (Mar–Apr)	Adults (Jul–Aug)	Adults
		Range	Range (Median)	Range (Median)	Range (Median)	Range (Median)	Range (Mean)
Total protein	(g/dL)	5.4–8.3	3.6–12.0 (8.7)	3.0–8.7 (6.1)	3.7–11.3 (6)	6.6–11.6 (10)	3.8–8.3 (5.6)
Glucose	(mg/dL)						
Blood urea nitrogen (BUN)	(mg/dL)		7.0–61.0 (18)	18.0–37.0 (27)	18.0–132.0 (31)	4.0–27.0 (14)	7–47 (21.0)
Uric acid	(mg/dL)						0.4–4.8 (1.7)
Creatinine	(mg/dL)						0.1–2.0 (1.1)
BUN/creatinine ratio							
Total bilirubin	(mg/dL)						0–0.4 (0.18)
Direct bilirubin	(mg/dL)						
Indirect bilirubin	(mg/dL)						
Triglycerides	(mg/dL)						
Cholesterol	(mg/dL)						14–86 (35.3)
Amylase	(IU/L)						
ALP	(IU/L)						18–276 (94.6)
ALT	(IU/L)						19–296 (92.1)
AST	(IU/L)						20–293 (106.9)
CPK	(IU/L)						
LDH	(IU/L)						
GGT	(IU/L)						
Albumin (A)	(g/dL)	3.4–4.9	1.6–8.6 (4.5)	2.0–4.6 (3.8)	2.4–5.2 (3.5)	2.9–8.6 (4.7)	2.3–3.5 (2.9)
Globulin (G)	(g/dL)	2.0–3.8	0.6–5.7 (2.6)	0.3–4.9 (1.7)	1.1–6.1 (2.7)	2.3–7.1 (4.1)	
A/G ratio							0.5–1.7 (1.2)
Phosphorus (P)	(mg/dL)						
Calcium (Ca)	(mg/dL)						6.4–15 (10.9)
Ca/P ratio							
Sodium (Na)	(mEq/L)						123–149 (138.7)

(Continued)

(Continued)

| | | Eastern Cottontail Rabbit (*Sylvilagus floridanus*) | | | | | Black-tailed Jackrabbit (*Lepus californicus*) |
| | | Adult | Adults (Sept–Oct) | Adults (Dec–Jan) | Adults (Mar–Apr) | Adults (Jul–Aug) | Adults |
	Units	Range	Range (Median)	Range (Median)	Range (Median)	Range (Median)	Range (Mean)
Potassium (K)	(mEq/L)						2.8–9.5 (6.4)
Na/K ratio							
Chloride	(mEq/L)						84–115 (100.2)
Creatinine kinase	(IU/L)						
Lipase	(IU/L)						
Bicarbonate	(mEq/L)						
Magnesium	(mg/dL)						
Iron	(µg/dL)						
Carbon dioxide	(mEq/L)						7–16 (19.0)
TT4	(µg/dL)						
References		Jacobson and Kirkpatrick (1975)	Jacobson et al. (1978)	Jacobson et al. (1978)	Jacobson et al. (1978)	Jacobson et al. (1978)	Fetters (1971)

References

Fetters, M.D. (1971). Hematology of the black-tailed jackrabbit (*Lepus californicus californicus*). *Laboratory Animal Sciences* 22 (4): 546–548.

Jacobson, H.A. and Kirkpatrick, R.L. (1975). Effects of parasitism on selected physiological measurements of the cottontail rabbit. *Journal of Wildlife Diseases* 10 (4): 384–391.

Jacobson, H.A., Kirkpatrick, R.L., Burkhart, H.E., and Davis, W. (1978). Hematologic comparisons of shot and live trapped cottontail rabbits. *Journal of Wildlife Diseases* 14 (1): 82–88.

Hematology Values of Passerines

	Units	Blue Jay — *Cyanocitta cristata* Range (Median)	American Crow — *Corvus brachyrhynchos* Range (Median)	Nothern Flicker — *Colaptes auratus* Range (Median)	Common Grackle — *Quiscalus quiscula* Range (Median)	Mourning Dove — *Zenaida macroura* Range (Median)	American Robin — *Turdus migratorius* Range (Median)	Rock Pigeon — *Columba livia* Range
WBCs	$(10^3/\mu L)$	409–985 (790)	210–640 (395)	560–805 (672)	151–221 (184)	121–220 (179)	260–339 (297)	10–30
RBCs	$(10^6/\mu L)$	92–301 (115)	292–640 (414)	100–152 (125)	293–440 (348)	116–460 (231)	125–401 (349)	2.1–4.2
Hematocrit	(%)	40–49 (42)	31–55 (48)	20–48 (45)	32–46 (44)	30–50 (36)	30–50 (40)	39.3–59.4
Hemoglobin	(g/dL)							
MCV	(fL)							
MCH	(pg)							
MCHC	(g/dL)							
Heterophils	$(10^3/\mu L)$							
Segmented heterophils	$(10^3/\mu L)$							
Lymphocytes	$(10^3/\mu L)$							
Monocytes	$(10^3/\mu L)$							
Eosinophils	$(10^3/\mu L)$							
Basophils	$(10^3/\mu L)$							
Thrombocytes	$(10^3/\mu L)$							
Heterophils	(%)	32–66 (48)	33–50 (45)	29–42 (36)	28–46 (38)	33–66 (48)	28–48 (36)	15–50
Segmented heterophils	(%)							
Lymphocytes	(%)	24–47 (36)	30–44 (38)	38–45 (42)	36–52 (45)	20–46 (31)	29–45 (36)	25–70
Monocytes	(%)	2–10 (5)	4–10 (7)	4–8 (6)	2–8 (6)	2–10 (6)	2–11 (6)	1–3
Eosinophils	(%)	3–12 (8)	3–15 (8)	12–8 (14)	3–14 (8)	4–23 (11)	9–26 (19)	0–1.5
Basophils	(%)	0–5 (4)	0–6 (3)	0–4 (2)	3–9 (5)	0–6 (1)	0–6 (2)	0–1
Thrombocytes	$(10^3/\mu L)$	109–400 (202)	341–700 (501)	115–219 (163)	209–375 (303)	201–310 (264)	215–365 (265)	
#individuals sampled		22	23	16	21	16	21	
References		Murnane and Miller (1993)	Murnane and Miller (1993)	Murnane and Miller (1993)	Murnane and Miller (1993)	Murnane and Miller (1993)	Murnane and Miller (1993)	Carpenter (2013)

Biochemical Values of Passerines

	Units	Blue Jay *Cyanocitta cristata* Range (Median)	American Crow *Corvus brachyrhynchos* Range (Median)	Northern Flicker *Colaptes auratus* Range (Median)	Common Grackle *Quiscalus quiscula* Range (Median)	American Robin *Turdus migratorius* Range (Median)	Northern Cardinal *Cardinalis cardinalis* Range (Median)	Mourning Dove *Zenaida macroura* Range (Median)	Mourning Dove *Z. macroura*[1998] Male Range	Female Range	Mourning Dove *Z. macroura*[1996] Male Range	Female Range	Rock Pigeon *Columba livia* Range
Total protein	(g/dL)	3.8–4.2 (3.8)	4.1–4.7 (4.6)	3–4 (3.8)	4–4.2 (4.1)	3.4–4.6 (4.4)	2.5–5.05 (5.0)	5.6–5.7 (5.6)	1.80–3.90	1.70–3.90	2.1–5.1	2.0–3.5	2.1–3.3
Glucose	(mg/dL)	180–400 (180)	180–220 (180)	130–180 (130)	200–280 (250)	300–450 (400)	180–400 (250)	130–180 (150)	310.0–822.0	342.0–1116.0	351.0–663.0	340.0–718.0	232.0–269.0
Blood urea nitrogen (BUN)	(mg/dL)												
Uric acid	(mg/dL)	3.5–7.8 (6.5)	10.7–18.4 (12.8)	6–6.6 (6.2)	9.9–12.4 (12.1)	4.3–9.6 (7.2)	2.5–12.6 (8.8)	9.8–12.8 (10.9)	3.0–14.2	2.6–17.1	1.9–10.0	1.5–13.3	2.5–12.9
Creatinine	(mg/dL)	0.06–0.15 (0.11)	0.12–0.25 (0.22)	0.14–0.21 (0.18)	0–0.06 (0.02)	0.6–1.19 (1.01)	0.04–0.8 (0.06)						0.3–0.4
BUN/creatinine ratio													
Total bilirubin	(mg/dL)												
Direct bilirubin	(mg/dL)												
Indirect bilirubin	(mg/dL)												
Triglycerides	(mg/dL)												
Cholesterol	(mg/dL)	78.9–134.1 (128.7)	81–167.1 (97.3)	107.9–127.8 (123.4)	190–195.3 (192.2)	140.1–181.1 (159)	122.4–203.9 (189.9)	184.9–290.6 (189.5)	122.0–550.0	84.0–485.0	175.0–441.0	141.0–506.0	
Amylase	(IU/L)												
ALP	(IU/L)	410–730 (692)	481–778 (588)	317–434 (341)	283–311 (300)	59–314 (176)	187–318 (204)	1248–1339 (1301)					160.0–780.0
ALT	(IU/L)	22–58 (37)	41–72 (57)	8–11 (9)	91–122 (92)	14–76 (42)	89–220 (89)	0–2 (2)					19.0–48.0
AST	(IU/L)	110–244 (186)	132–245 (237)	151–179 (166)	182–336 (241)	116–142 (130)	200–215 (206)	91–98 (93)	94.0–709.0	143.0–659.0	81.0–663.0	93.0–757.0	45.0–123.0
CPK	(IU/L)												
LDH	(IU/L)	644–905 (886)	1457–1782 (1657)	866–979 (898)	345–455 (398)	1769–1899 (1887)	489–538 (499)	870–901 (870)	312–1822.0	320–8528.0	445.0–8117.0	425.0–9168.0	30.0–205.0
GGT	(IU/l)								9.0–37.0	9.0–27.0	5.0–48.0	5.0–29.0	0.0–2.9

(Continued)

(Continued)

	Units	Blue Jay *Cyanocitta cristata* Range (Median)	American Crow *Corvus brachyrhynchos* Range (Median)	Northern Flicker *Colaptes auratus* Range (Median)	Common Grackle *Quiscalus quiscula* Range (Median)	American Robin *Turdus migratorius* Range (Median)	Northern Cardinal *Cardinalis cardinalis* Range (Median)	Mourning Dove *Zenaida macroura* Range (Median)	Mourning Dove *Z. macroura*[1998] Male Range	Female Range	Mourning Dove *Z. macroura*[1996] Male Range	Female Range	Rock Pigeon *Columba livia* Range
Albumin (A)	(g/dL)	0.93–1.76 (1.72)	2.03–2.26 (2.03)	1.27–1.5 (1.34)	2.02–2.2 (2.17)	2.25–3.28 (3.08)	0.31–2.76 (2.69)	1.61–1.71 (1.65)	0.9–1.7	1.0–1.7	1.0–2.0	1.0–1.6	1.5–2.1
Globulin (G)	(g/dL)	2.08–2.87 (2.44)	2.07–2.67 (2.34)	1.66–2.73 (2.3)	1.83–2.08 (2.0)	1.15–1.32 (1.32)	2.19–2.36 (2.24)	3.89–4.05 (3.99)	0.9–2.6	0.7–2.6	1.1–3.4	1.0–2.0	0.6–1.2
A/G ratio		0.32–0.83 (0.72)	0.76–0.98 (0.97)	0.47–0.81 (0.65)	0.97–1.19 (1.10)	1.96–2.48 (2.33)	0.14–1.23 (1.14)	0.4–0.44 (0.41)					1.5–3.6
Phosphorus (P)	(mg/dL)								2.1–8.4	2.1–8.1	1.9–7.4	1.5–6.6	1.8–4.1
Calcium (Ca)	(mg/dL)	9.86–10.96 (10.7)	10.15–12.23 (10.17)	8.25–9.32 (8.52)	11.11–11.56 (11.16)	10.15–13.69 (10.17)	6.54–9.41 (8.39)	9.58–11.29 (11.06)	7.2–11.5	8.1–25.1	7.6–12.1	6.4–12.0	7.6–10.4
Ca/P ratio													
Sodium (Na)	(mEq/L)								137.0–154.0	125.0–156.0	137.0–160.0	138.0–153.0	141.0–149.0
Potassium (K)	(mEq/L)								4.0–14.9	4.5–12.0	3.6–12.5	3.9–13.0	3.9–4.7
Na/K ratio													
Chloride	(mEq/L)								107.0–121.0	96.0–123.0	104.0–137.0	101.0–119.0	101.0–113.0
Creatinine kinase	(IU/l)												
Lipase	(IU/L)												
Bicarbonate	(mEq/L)												
Magnesium	(mg/dL)								2.1–3.9	2.1–3.7	1.9–3.6	1.7–3.4	
Iron	(μg/dL)												
Carbon dioxide	(mEq/L)								24.0–40.0	22.0–40.0	17.0–36.0	21.0–37.0	
TT4	(μg/dL)												
References		Murnane and Miller (1993)	Murnane and Miller (1993)	Murnane and Miller (1993)	Murnane and Miller (1993)	Murnane and Miller (1993)	Murnane and Miller(1993)	Murnane and Miller (1993)	Schulz et al. (2000)		Schulz et al. (2000)		Carpenter (2013)

References

Carpenter, J.W. (2013). *Exotic Animal Formulary*, 4e. St Louis, MO: Saunders.

Murnane, J. & Miller, E.A. (1993). Forming a Clinical Pathology Database for Wildlife. Poster Presentation, National Wildlife Rehabilitators Association Symposium, Oakland, CA. Values are determined using Unopettes and Neubauer hemocytometers and blood smear stained with Wright's Giemsa.

Schulz, J.H., Bermudez, A.J., Tomlinson, J.L. et al. (2000). Blood plasma chemistries from wild mourning doves held in captivity. *Journal of Wildlife Diseases* 36 (3): 541–545.

Hematology Values of Galliforms

	Units	Turkey *Meleagris gallopavo* Range	Greater Sage Grouse *Centrocercus urophasianus* Mean (SD)
WBCs	$(10^3/\mu L)$	16–25.5	5.539 (1.918)
RBCs	$(10^6/\mu L)$	1.74–3.7	
Hematocrit	(%)	30.4–45.6	53 (8)
Hemoglobin	(g/dL)	8.8–13.4	
MCV	(fL)	112–168	
MCH	(pg)	32–49.3	
MCHC	(g/dL)	23.2–35.3	
Heterophils	$(10^3/\mu L)$		2.048 (1.250)
Segmented heterophils	$(10^3/\mu L)$		
Lymphocytes	$(10^3/\mu L)$		3.376 (1.370)
Monocytes	$(10^3/\mu L)$		50 (123)
Eosinophils	$(10^3/\mu L)$		11 (36)
Basophils	$(10^3/\mu L)$		44 (127)
Thrombocytes	$(10^3/\mu L)$		
Heterophils	(%)	29–52	36 (16)
Segmented heterophils	(%)		
Lymphocytes	(%)	35–48	62 (16)
Monocytes	(%)	3–10	1 (2)
Eosinophils	(%)	0–5	0.2–1
Basophils	(%)	1–9	1 (2)
References		Carpenter (2013)	Dunbar et al. (2005)

Biochemical Values of Galliforms

	Units	Turkey *Meleagris gallopavo* Range	Greater Sage Grouse *Centrocercus urophasianus* Mean (SD)
Total protein	(g/dL)	4.9–7.6	5.3 (1.2)
Glucose	(mg/dL)	275–425	320.2 (34.6)
Blood urea nitrogen (BUN)	(mg/dL)		
Uric acid	(mg/dL)	3.4–5.2	5.4 (2.2)
Creatinine	(mg/dL)	0.8–0.9	
BUN/creatinine ratio			
Total bilirubin	(mg/dL)		
Direct bilirubin	(mg/dL)		
Indirect bilirubin	(mg/dL)		
Triglycerides	(mg/dL)		
Cholesterol	(mg/dL)	81.0–129.0	
Amylase	(IU/L)		
ALP	(IU/L)		
ALT	(IU/L)		
AST	(IU/L)		430.3 (77.2)
CPK	(IU/L)		
LDH	(IU/L)		
GGT	(IU/L)		
Albumin (A)	(g/dL)	3.0–5.9	2.1 (0.2)
Globulin (G)	(g/dL)	1.7–1.9	
A/G ratio			
Phosphorus (P)	(mg/dL)	5.4–7.1	7.3 (2.4)
Calcium (Ca)	(mg/dL)		21.4 (7.4)
Ca/P ratio			
Sodium (Na)	(mEq/L)	149.0–155.0	
Potassium (K)	(mEq/L)	6.0–6.4	
Na/K ratio			
Chloride	(mEq/L)		
Creatinine kinase	(IU/L)		2395.9 (1017.1)
Lipase	(IU/L)		
Bicarbonate	(mEq/L)		
Magnesium	(mg/dL)		
Iron	(μg/dL)		
Carbon dioxide	(mEq/L)		
TT4	(μg/dL)		
References		Carpenter (2013)	Dunbar et al. (2005)

References

Carpenter, J.W. (2013). *Exotic Animal Formulary*, 4e. St Louis, MO: Saunders.

Dunbar, M.R., Gregg, M.A., Crawford, J.A. et al. (2005). Normal hematologic and biochemical values for prelaying greater sage grouse (*Centrocercus urophasianus*) and their influence on chick survival. *Journal of Zoo and Wildlife Medicine* 36 (3): 422–429.

Hematology Values of Raptors

Parameter	Units	Turkey Vulture	Red-Tailed Hawk	Golden Eagle	Bald Eagle	Red Shouldered Hawk	Harris' Hawk	Sharp Shinned Hawk	American Kestrel	Peregerine Falcon	Barn Owl	Great Horned Owl	Barred Owl	Screech Owl
		Cathartes aura	*Buteo jamaicensis*	*Aquila chrysaetos*	*Haliaeetus leucocephalus*	*Buteo lineatus*	*Parabuteo unicinctus*	*Accipiter striatus*	*Falco sparverius*	*Falco peregrinus*	*Tyto alba*	*Bubo virginianus*	*Strix varia*	*Megascops asio*
		Range (Median)	Range (Median)	Range (Median)	Range (Median)	Range (Median)	Range (Median)	Range (Median)	Range (Median)	Range (Median)	Range (Median)	Range (Median)	Range (Median)	Range (Median)
WBCs	($10^3/\mu L$)	3.78–33.94 (13.27)	3.3–28.4 (10.7)	5.9–24 (12.3)	3.61–26.73 (11.32)		3.12–23.69 (8.23)	7.7–16.8	1.87–21.12 (5.96)	3.77–22.73 (9.08)	3.17–28.85 (10.32)	3.18–26.63 (12.02)	3.89–27.44 (10.84)	2.98–37.49 (11.23)
RBCs	($10^6/\mu L$)	1.7–3.9 (2.49)	0.87–3.68 (2.38)	1.05–3.68 (2.37)	1.23–4.03 (2.63)	116–460 (231)	1.49–3.68 (2.59)	–	1.48–5.11 (3.29)	1.62–3.99 (2.81)	1.41–3.59 (2.5)	1.42–3.06 (2.24)		1.30–4.16 (2.73)
Hematocrit	(%)	34–54 (45)	26–54 (41)	29–55 (41)	32.3–58.4 (46)	32.1–53.4 (42.9)	30–50 (40)	44–52	34.8–58.1 (45.9)	33.1–55.1 (46.3)	31.8–55.2 (42.6)	31.7–48.5 (41.2)	29.0–50.1 (39.7)	30.6–54.8 (42.5)
Hemoglobin	(g/dL)	15.7–17.3 (16.3)	11.6–14.6 (12.9)	9.8–17.2 (13.5)	9.5–21.2 (15.3)	121	16–185 (121)		(135)		110–174 (142)	(125)		71–188 (130)
MCV	(fL)	19–282 (184)	75–253 (166.7)	76.8–277.7 (177.2)	65.4–273.4 (169.4)	108.6–236.8 (172.7)	120.1–260.3 (172.7)		83.2–188.5 (135.9)	(164.1)	109.4–257.9 (183.7)	(179.2)		86.7–221.9 (154.3)
MCH	(pg)		19.1–33.4	56.3–62.7 (53.3)	35.8–79.7 (57.8)					40–48.4	54.3	–		16.8–80.9 (48.8)
MCHC	(g/dL)	28.6–32.0 (30.2)	297–345	261–282 (322)	232–432 (332)	(258)	35–418 (258)		(311)	319–352	222–395 (309)	(318)		177–449 (313)
Heterophils	($10^3/\mu L$)	1.64–19.82 (7.16)	1.38–13.25 (4.44)	2.37–22.67 (7.67)	2.21–19.99 (7.34)		1.11–12.89 (4.21)		0.63–9.17 (2.77)	1.77–12.98 (5.05)	1.41–17.63 (5.67)	1.29–17.54 (6.50)	0.0–8.51 (3.71)	1.15–14.79 (4.26)
Segmented heterophils	($10^3/\mu L$)													
Lymphocytes	($10^3/\mu L$)	0.52–25.6 (3.68)	0.48–11.68 (3.29)	0.34–12.2 (2.71)	0.22–7.19 (2.13)		0.37–11.12 (2.74)		0.39–8.81 (2.31)	0.87–9.68 (2.81)	0.64–11.16 (3.20)	0.82–10.45 (3.47)	1.15–13.77 (4.74)	0.95–17.00 (4.16)
Monocytes	($10^3/\mu L$)	0.0–0.014	0.083–2.877 (5.23)	0.087–0.20 (3.73)	0.063–2.215 (4.61)		0.039–1.376 (3.0)		0.018–1.238 (1.94)	0.0–1.286 (3.98)	0.058–1.683 (2.7)	0.0–24.07 (4.69)	0.0–17.40 (5.77)	0.45–31.95 (4.9)
Eosinophils	($10^3/\mu L$)	0.15–0.75	0.086–4.337 (10.86)	0.047–0.25 (0.44)	0.085–3.102 (7.39)		0.051–3.164 (6.1)		0.0–0.357 (1.45)	1.23	0.064–2.820 (3.22)	0.0–30.54 (3.09)	0.0–21.80 (6.88)	0.51–88.1 (14.3)
Basophils	($10^3/\mu L$)	0.0–0.023	0.046–1.321 (3.79)	0.0–0.06 (0.292)	0.042–0.869 (1.72)		0.038–0.985 (1.79)		0.0–0.50 (1.86)	–	0.049–0.867 (2.36)	0.0–9.49 (4.1)	0.0–9.38 (3.04)	0.40–17.77 (3.17)
Thrombocytes	($10^3/\mu L$)	7–22 (14)								0–7.12 (2.03)				
Heterophils	(%)	32–66 (48)	35±11	49–86	19–61 (44)	33–66 (48)		16–24	47±3	65±12	15–50	47±11		

Segmented heterophils (%)	16–24						54–75			40–70	27±7		
Lymphocytes (%)	59–64	44±9	23–60 (38)	36–52 (45)	20–46 (31)			46±3	35±13	0–3	9±3.6		
Monocytes (%)	0–3	6±3	0–8 (4)	2–8 (6)	2–10 (6)		0–3	2±0.2	0	5.0–25	1±1.2		
Eosinophils (%)	0–5	13±4	4–26 (13)	3–14 (8)	4–23 (11)		5.0–11	1+=0.2	0	0.0–2.0	rare		
Basophils (%)	0–1	Rare	0.1	3–9 (5)	0–6 (1)		0–1	2±0.2	0				
#individuals sampled	82	97	74	120	16	91		71	57	143	53	48	147
References	Samour (2015) and Teare (2013)	Carpenter (2013) and Teare (2013)	Carpenter (2013) and Teare (2013)	Carpenter (2013) and Teare (2013)	Carpenter (2013)	Carpenter (2013) and Teare (2013)	Carpenter (2013)	Carpenter (2013) and Teare (2013)	Carpenter (2013) and Teare (2013)	Carpenter (2013) and Teare (2013)	Carpenter (2013) and Teare (2013)	Teare (2013)	Teare (2013)

Biochemical Values of Raptors

	Units	Turkey Vulture (*Cathartes aura*)	Red Tailed Hawk (*Buteo jamaicensis*)	Golden Eagle (*Aquila chrysaetos*)	Bald Eagle (*Haliaeetus leucocephalus*)	Red Shouldered Hawk (*Buteo lineatus*)	Harris' Hawk (*Parabuteo unicinctus*)	Sharp Shinned Hawk (*Accipiter striatus*)	American Kestrel (*Falco sparverius*)	Peregrine Falcon (*Falco peregrinus*)	Barn Owl (*Tyto alba*)	Great Horned Owl (*Bubo virginianus*)	Barred Owl (*Strix varia*)	Screech Owl (*Megascops asio*)
		Range	Range	Range	Range	Range	Range	Range	Range	Range	Range	Range	Range	Range
Total protein	(g/dL)	2.8–5.7	2.5–5.6	2.4–5.2	2.6–5.3	—	2.2–4.5	2.4–3.2	2.0–5.1	2.1–4.9	1.9–4.2	2.6–5.6	2.9–6.0	2.1–5.8
Glucose	(mg/dL)	170–334	248–432	208–462	218–403	—	247–400	—	213–483	259–411	149–345	235–423	234–406	204–462
Blood urea nitrogen (BUN)	(mg/dL)	—	—	—	9	—	7	—	—	4	—	6	11	8
Uric acid	(mg/dL)	41.7–13.8	1.9–21.4	1.9–14.0	2.4–24	—	2.7–20.4	—	2.3–33.9	2.4–29.3	2.1–27.9	2.9–20.0	2.5–19.5	2.1–17.2
Creatinine	(mg/dL)	0.2	—	—	0.0–0.8	—	—	—	—	—	—	—	—	—
Cholesterol	(mg/dL)	2123–273	119–306	66–251	134–299	—	125–337	—	129–410	100–351	120–312	88–262	110–314	107–300
ALP	(IU/L)	0–105	0–87	0–57	11–98	—	1.0–89	—	0–732	0–304	0–109	0–125	0–90	0–135
ALT	(IU/L)	—	0–47	0–49	3–56	—	0–58	—	—	14–93	0–59	0–59	0–141	87
AST	(IU/L)	10–71	114–480	9.0–16.2	102–415	—	127–645	—	25–196	22–200	71–261	89–375	104–459	77–579
LDH	(IU/L)	0–367	0–1754	0–992	0–1060	—	0–713	—	1065	781	0–938	0–941	0–1430	0–1098
GGT	(IU/L)	—	0–16	—	0–10	—	0–12	—	—	0–7	0–15	0–4	—	0–4
Albumin (A)	(g/dL)	0.8–2.5	0.6–2.4	0.6–2.3	0.7–2.7	—	0.7–3.0	—	0.0–2.4	0.0–2.1	0.6–2.5	0.7–2.8	0.6–2.4	0.5–2.2
Globulin (G)	(g/dL)	0.4–3.7	0.3–3.7	0.8–3.6	0.8–4.1	—	0.1–3.0	—	0.2–3.5	0.6–3.5	0.2–2.8	0.3–4.1	0.8–3.8	0.1–3.7
A/G ratio		—	—	—	—	—	0.45–0.55	—	—	0.4–0.6	—	—	—	—
Phosphorus (P)	(mg/dL)	0.7–5.9	1.0–7.2	0.8–6.5	1.0–7.1	—	1.0–5.9	—	0.6–9.4	0.4–6.1	0.6–7.8	1.8–10.9	0.7–7.8	1.2–9.4
Calcium (Ca)	(mg/dL)	7.1–11.8	7.5–11.5	7.8–11.8	8.1–12.4	—	7.4–1.5	—	6.2–11.1	7.2–10.9	6.9–11.2	7.5–11.6	7.9–12.0	6.1–11.4
Ca/P ratio		1.7–11.0	1.2–7.7	1.2–8.6	1.6–8.8	—	1.6–8.4	—	—	0.0–5.7	1.2–7.1	0.9–4.7	0.3–4.7	0.9–6.4
Sodium (Na)	(mEq/L)	141–164	144–170	142–167	139–167	—	138–171	—	141–176	148–168	142–167	146–175	143–168	141–171
Potassium (K)	(mEq/L)	1.4–2.6.2	0.9–5.1	0.4–4.7	1.0–4.8	—	0.7–4.3	—	0.0–5.0	0.0–5.3	0.8–4.2	1.2–5.2	0.6–4.4	0.5–5.1
Na/K ratio		21.0–107.0	29.8–152.6	7.7–109.4	30.1–133.1	—	38.3–197.9	—	0.1–121.4	1.0–131.9	11.9–109.3	29.2–114.9	12.6–110.7	4.6–103.8
Chloride	(mEq/L)	104–127	111–129	107–130	102–128	—	110–131	—	104–128	109–129	104–133	105–131	111–130	104–131
Creatinine kinase	(IU/L)	134–1030	276–2575	144–1209	138–915	—	176–1372	—	383–2377	75–957	391–3670	67–1626	0–1134	92–1169
Amylase	(IU/L)	0–321	0–471	0–1115	0–2363	—	32–448	—	0–560	0–518	0–672	0–878	0–372	0–534
Total bilirubin	(mg/dL)	0.2	—	0.0–0.4	0.0–0.4	—	0.2	—	0.5	0.5	—	0.2	—	—
Magnesium	(mg/dL)	—	—	1.8	—	—	—	—	—	—	—	—	—	—
Bicarbonate	(mEq/L)	—	—	—	18.0	—	—	—	—	—	—	—	—	—
Triglyceride	(mg/dL)	—	—	—	—	—	99	—	—	—	—	—	—	—
References		Samour (2015) and Teare (2013)	Carpenter (2013) and Teare (2013)	Carpenter (2013) and Teare (2013)	Carpenter (2013) and Teare (2013)	Carpenter (2013)	Carpenter (2013) and Teare (2013)	Carpenter (2013)	Carpenter (2013) and Teare (2013)	Carpenter (2013) and Teare (2013)	Carpenter (2013) and Teare (2013)	Carpenter (2013) and Teare (2013)	Teare (2013)	Teare (2013)

References

Carpenter, J.W. (2013). *Exotic Animal Formulary*, 4e. St Louis, MO: Saunders.

Samour, J. (2015). *Avian Medicine and Surgery*. St Louis, MO: Elsevier.

Teare, J.A. (ed.) (2013). *ISIS Physiological Reference Intervals for Captive Wildlife: A CD-ROM Resource*. Bloomington, MN: International Species Information System.

Hematology Values of Waterfowl

	Units	Canvasback *Aythya valisineria*	Tundra Swan *Cygnus columbianus*	Mallard *Anas platyrhynchos*	Nene Goose *Branta sandvicensis*	White-winged Scoter *Melanitta deglandi*	Canada Goose *Branta canadensis*	Greater Snow Goose *Chen caerulescens*
		Range	Range	Range	Range	Range	Range	Range
WBCs	$(10^3/\mu L)$		18.26–19.7	23.4–24.8		16.5	13.0–21.8	18.8–21
RBCs	$(10^6/\mu L)$	2.5–2.61		2.7–3.6	2.6	0.0899	1.6–12.2	2.1–2.7
Hematocrit	(%)	46.3–60	44.6–45	37–46	46	50	38–58	41–54
Hemoglobin	(g/dL)	13.8–18.1		13.9–16	15.25–15.72		12–19.1	13.8–14.7
MCV	(fL)	165–209		163.4–181			145–229.5	
MCH	(pg)	47–63		51.0–52.6	32.5–34.7		53.7–70	
MCHC	(g/dL)	28–31		29.1–31.2	5.6–6.3		27.6–34.7	
Heterophils	$(10^3/\mu L)$		67–67.4	24.3–51			17.1–50	7.0–53.0
Segmented heterophils	$(10^3/\mu L)$							
Lymphocytes	$(10^3/\mu L)$		27.8–28.4	32–61.7			39–58.4	12.3–73.0
Monocytes	$(10^3/\mu L)$		0.21–0.45	4–10.8			1.6–6	0.2–1.3
Eosinophils	$(10^3/\mu L)$		2.94–3.48	2.1–7			1.9–21.2	0.1–1.31
Basophils	$(10^3/\mu L)$		1.09–1.34	1.5–5			1.6–7	0.5–3.5
Thrombocytes	$(10^3/\mu L)$			207			179	
Heterophils	(%)							
Segmented heterophils	(%)							
Lymphocytes	(%)							
Monocytes	(%)							
Eosinophils	(%)							
Basophils	(%)							
References		Perry et al. (1986), Wallach and Boever (1983)	Milani et al. (2012)	Fairbrother et al. (1990), Humphreys (1978), Olsen (1994)	Olsen (1994)	Olsen and Perry (2008)	Charles-Smith et al. (2014), Murnane and Miller (1993), Olsen (1994), Williams and Trainer (1971)	Shave (1986)

Biochemical Values of Waterfowl

		Canvasback	Tundra Swan	Mallard	Nene Goose	White-winged Scoter	Canada Goose
		Aythya valisineria	*Cygnus columbianus*	*Anas platyrhynchos*	*Branta sandvicensis*	*Melanitta deglandi*	*Branta canadensis*
	Units	Range	Range	Range	Range	Range	Range
Total protein	(g/dL)	3.6–6.8	3.49–3.57	3.8–4.2	4.4	4.83	4.26–5.6
Glucose	(mg/dL)	180–549		180–215	185–192	188.31	120–320.3
Blood urea nitrogen (BUN)	(mg/dL)	2.4–3.5			2		
Uric acid	(mg/dL)	4.9–5.8	7.63–8.34	3.6–10.6	8	6.1	5.5–6.7
Creatinine	(mg/dL)	0.9–1.0		0.25–0.28	0.8	0.74	0–0.06
BUN/creatinine ratio		2.8–3.9					
Total bilirubin	(mg/dL)	0.20–0.25		0.16	0.12		
Direct bilirubin	(mg/dL)	0.05–0.06					
Indirect bilirubin	(mg/dL)						
Triglycerides	(mg/dL)	181–192			163		145.2–258
Cholesterol	(mg/dL)	237–293			230–233	279	156.3–307
Amylase	(IU/L)		3890–4258	2631–2766	824	549.13	
ALP	(IU/L)	56–75	706–729	26.3–44.2	33	137.69	323–450
ALT	(IU/L)	70–89		26.3–52		19.563	16–31
AST	(IU/L)	82–95	31–37.1	9.0–16.2		23.375	22–60
CPK	(IU/L)						
LDH	(IU/L)	308–332	636.6–688	147–199	256		1644–1689
GGT	(IU/L)	2.5–2.6		7.7–8.0	2	3	
Albumin (A)	(g/dL)	1.6–2.08	1.27–1.31	1.5–1.7	1.7–1.9	1.55	
Globulin (G)	(g/dL)	2.6–2.8	2.22–2.26		2.6	3.3	
A/G ratio							
Phosphorus (P)	(mg/dL)		2.34–2.45	2.9–3.0	2.4	2.56	
Calcium (Ca)	(mg/dL)	10–10.4	8.92–9.11	9.40–12.96	10–10.5	9.79	12.05–12.1
Ca/P ratio							
Sodium (Na)	(mEq/L)	149–152	148–149	138	146		
Potassium(P)	(mEq/L)	2.6–2.7	2.48–2.66	3.4	2.5		
Na/K ratio							
Chloride	(mEq/L)	111–113					
Creatinine kinase	(IU/L)		1191–1775			300.75	
Lipase	(IU/L)						
Bicarbonate	(mEq/L)						
Magnesium	(mg/dL)			1.8			
Iron	(μg/dL)	159–186					
References		Perry et al. (1986), Wallach and Boever (1983)	Milani et al. (2012)	Fairbrother et al. (1990), Humphreys (1978), Olsen (1994)	Olsen (1994)	Olsen and Perry (2008)	Charles-Smith et al. (2014), Murnane and Miller (1993), Olsen (1994), Williams and Trainer (1971)

References

Charles-Smith, L.E., Rutledge, E., Meek, C.J. et al. (2014). Hematologic parameters and hemoparasites of nonmigratory Canada geese (*Branta canadensis*) from Greensboro, North Carolina, USA. *Journal of Avian Medicine and Surgery* 28 (1): 16–23.

Fairbrother, A., Craig, M.A., Walker, K. et al. (1990). Changes in mallard (*Anas platyrhynchos*) serum chemistry due to age, sex, and reproductive condition. *Journal of Wildlife Diseases* 26 (1): 67–77.

Humphreys, P. (1978). Ducks, geese, swans (anseriformes). In: *Zoo and Wild Animal Medicine, Vol 1* (ed. M.E. Fowler), 181–210. Philadelphia, PA: W.B. Saunders.

Milani, J.F., Wilson, H., Ziccardi, M. et al. (eds.) (2012). Hematology, plasma chemistry, and bacteriology of wild tundra swans (*Cygnus columbianus)* in Alaska. *Journal of Wildlife Diseases* 48 (1): 212–215.

Murnane, J. & Miller, E.A. (1993). Forming a Clinical Pathology Database for Wildlife. Poster Presentation, National Wildlife Rehabilitators Association Symposium, Oakland, CA.

Olsen, G.H. & Perry, M.E. (2008) Behavioral and Physiological Observations of White-winged Scoters with Surgically Implanted Transmitters. In: Proceedings of the 3rd North American Sea Duck Conference. USGS Patuxent Wildlife Research Center, Laurel, MD.

Olsen, J. (1994). Anseriformes. In: *Avian Medicine: Principles and Application* (ed. B.W. Ritchie and G.J. Harrison), 1343–1344. Lake Worth, FL: Wingers Publishing.

Perry, M.C., Obrecht, H.H. III, Williams, B.K. et al. (1986). Blood chemistry and hematocrit of captive and wild canvasbacks. *Journal of Wildlife Management* 50 (3): 435–441.

Shave, H. (1986). Ducks, geese, swans and screamers (anseriformes). In: *Zoo and Wild Animal Medicine, Vol 2* (ed. M.E. Fowler), 333–364. Philadelphia, PA: W.B. Saunders.

Wallach, J.D. and Boever, W.J. (1983). Game birds, waterfowl and ratites. In: *Diseases of Exotic Animals: Medical and Surgical Management*, 831–889. Philadelphia, PA: Saunders.

Williams, J.L. and Trainer, D.O. (1971). A hematological study of snow, blue and Canada Geese. *Journal of Wildlife Diseases* 7: 258–265.

Hematology Values of Seabirds

	Units	Common Murre *Uria aalge* Range	Glaucous-winged Gull *Larus glaucescens* Range	Great Frigatebird *Fregata minor* Range	Sooty Tern *Onychoprion fuscatus* Range	Brown Pelican *Pelecanus occidentalis* Range	Imperial Cormorant *Phalacrocorax atriceps* Range
WBCs	$(10^3/\mu L)$	9350 ± 1348	5077 ± 4470	5.74–13.7	6.7–49.2	16.7+/−4.7	2.4–24.0
RBCs	$(10^6/\mu L)$					2.6 ± 0.4	0.4–6.3
Hematocrit	(%)	39 ± 4	38 ± 8	43–53	41–55	45+/f5	44–54
Hemoglobin	(g/dL)						
MCV	(fL)						
MCH	(pg)						
MCHC	(g/dL)						
Heterophils	$(10^3/\mu L)$			3.87–16.1		8.3 ± 2.1	1.2–7.1
Segmented heterophils	$(10^3/\mu L)$						
Lymphocytes	$(10^3/\mu L)$			0.4–11.8	4.3–41.4	7.3 ± 2.2	1.8–7.2
Monocytes	$(10^3/\mu L)$			0–0.6	0–0.7	0.2 ± 0.3	0.0–1.0
Eosinophils	$(10^3/\mu L)$			0.5–3.8	0.1–3.9	0.87 ± 1.0	0.0–4.3
Basophils	$(10^3/\mu L)$			0–0.3	0–0.8	0	0.0–0.1
Thrombocytes	$(10^3/\mu L)$						
Heterophils	(%)	31 ± 28	53 ± 20				
Segmented heterophils	(%)						
Lymphocytes	(%)	51 ± 21	43 ± 16				
Monocytes	(%)	2 ± 2	1 ± 1				
Eosinophils	(%)	16 ± 6	3 ± 4				
Basophils	(%)	0	0				
References		Newman et al. (1997), Work (1996)	Newman et al. (1997), Work (1996)	Newman et al. (1997), Work (1996)	Newman et al. (1997), Work (1996)	Zaias et al. (2000)	Gallo et al. (2013)

Biochemical Values of Seabirds

	Units	Common Murre *Uria aalge* Range	Glaucous-winged Gull *Larus glaucescens* Range	Great Frigatebird *Fregata minor* Range	Sooty Tern *Onychoprion fuscatus* Range	Brown Pelican *Pelecanus occidentalis* Range	Imperial Cormorant *Phalacrocorax atriceps* Range
Glucose	(mg/dL)	313+/-119	320+/-60	76–167	201–387	220 ± 28	110–300
Blood urea nitrogen (BUN)	(mg/dL)					4.3 ± 0.7	1.0–24.0
Uric acid	(mg/dL)	19 ± 16	28 ± 11	3.0–11.2	4.1–28	12.3 ± 7	2.4–10.1
Creatinine	(mg/dL)						
BUN/creatinine ratio							
Total bilirubin	(mg/dL)						
Direct bilirubin	(mg/dL)						
Indirect bilirubin	(mg/dL)						
Triglycerides	(mg/dL)	211 ± 211	163 ± 178			283 ± 383	37–207
Cholesterol	(mg/dL)	376 ± 244	268 ± 92			165 ± 45	155–591
Amylase	(IU/L)					993 ± 119	
ALP	(IU/L)	69 ± 21					130–4886
ALT	(IU/L)	85 ± 31				45 ± 18	26–151
AST	(IU/L)	164 ± 33		247–528	315–928	286 ± 100	108–530
CPK	(IU/L)	624 ± 379	1629 ± 1468		22–239	981 ± 545	276–1973
LDH	(IU/L)	1304 ± 345	1010 ± 877			2352 ± 701	306–1259
GGT	(IU/l)					12 ± 3	
Albumin (A)	(g/dL)			1.3–1.8			
Globulin (G)	(g/dL)			1.7–2.7			
A/G ratio							
Phosphorus (P)	(mg/dL)			6.1–13.5	1.6–6.5		2.4–6.1
Calcium (Ca)	(mg/dL)			8.1–11.3	7.7–11.1		6.5–14.1
Ca/P ratio							
Sodium (Na)	(mEq/L)					147 ± 3	
Potassium (K)	(mEq/L)					5.1 ± 0.8	
Na/K ratio							

				References
Chloride	(mEq/L)			
Creatinine kinase	(IU/L)			
Lipase	(IU/L)	10–1589		
Bicarbonate	(mEq/L)			
Magnesium	(mg/dL)			
Iron	(µg/dL)			
Carbon dioxide	(mEq/L)			
TT4	(µg/dL)			
References	Newman et al. (1997), Work (1996)	Newman et al. (1997), Work (1996)	Newman et al. (1997), Work (1996)	Newman et al. (1997), Work (1996)
				Zaias et al. (2000)
				Gallo et al. (2013)

References

Gallo, L., Quintana, F., Svagelj, W.S., and Uhart, M. (2013). Hematology and blood chemistry values in free-living imperial cormorants (*Phalacrocorax atriceps*). *Avian Diseases* 57 (4): 737–743.

Newman, S.H., Piatt, J.F., and White, J. (1997). Hematological and plasma biochemical reference ranges of Alaskan seabirds: their ecological significance and clinical importance. *Colonial Waterbirds* 20 (3): 492–504.

Work, T.M. (1996). Weights, hematology, and serum chemistry of seven species of free-ranging tropical pelagic seabirds. *Journal of Wildlife Diseases* 32 (4): 643–657.

Zaias, J., Fox, W.P., Cray, C., and Altman, N.H. (2000). Hematologic, plasma protein, and biochemical profiles of brown pelicans (*Pelecanus occidentalis*). *American Journal Veterinary Research* 61 (7): 771–774.

Hematology Values of Cervids

	Units	White-tailed Deer (Odocoileus virginianus) Range ≤7 days	White-tailed Deer Mean + SD 90–120 days	White-tailed Deer Mean + SD 154–175 days	White-tailed Deer Range (Median) Adult	Mule Deer (Odocoileus hemionus) Range (Median) Adult	Caribou (Rangifer tarandus) Range (Median) Adult	Moose (Alces alces americanus) Range (Median) Adult	Elk (Cervus canadensis) Range Adult
WBCs	$(10^3/\mu L)$	1.0–6.2	4.1 + 1.3	3.7 + 0.1	1.05–8.60 (3.16)	1.94–10.73 (4.54)	1.59–11.65 (4.91)	2.40–13.11 (6.53)	6.5–14.6
RBCs	$(10^6/\mu L)$	5.6–10.7	19.0 + 1.8	19.1 + 0.37	5.56–18.76 (11.78)	4.69–13.19 (8.94)	6.75–12.73 (9.6)	2.45–8.58 (5.51)	9.36–13.2
Hematocrit	(%)	19.0–42.0	52.5 + 3.1	48.3 + 0.8	20.9–56.7 (37.1)	19.7–47.8 (34.6)	31.7–58.9 (43.4)	21.0–52.6 (34.2)	58–76.5
Hemoglobin	(g/dL)	5.9–11.4	18.5 + 1.2	17.5 + 0.4	7.0–19.8 (13.2)	7.6–18.4 (13)	10.8–21.3 (15.8)	5.0–18.5 (11.7)	16.2–22.0
MCV	(fL)	29.0–43.0	27.6 + 2.6	30.2 + 0.5	21.3–46.3 (31.2)	29.5–49.4 (39.4)	38.5–53.7 (46)	47.7–82.1 (64.9)	57.5–65.0
MCH	(pg)	8.0–13.0	9.8 + 1.3	11.0 + 0.1	7.8–16.4 (11)	10.6–17.5 (14.1)	13.3–19.2 (16.8)	15.4–29.5 (22.5)	
MCHC	(g/dL)	24.0–33.0	35.2 + 2.8	35.8 + 0.3	28.7–41.5 (35.7)	30.2–40.9 (35.5)	27.5–40.6 (36.3)	26.0–41.3 (33.7)	
Neutrophils	$(10^3/\mu L)$								
Segmented neutrophils	$(10^3/\mu L)$				0.20–5.53 (1.67)	1.06–8.62 (2.85)	0.55–8.03 (2.73)	1.16–8.78 (4.09)	
Lymphocytes	$(10^3/\mu L)$				0.13–2.74 (0.91)	0.28–2.95 (1.08)	0.35–3.80 (1.47)	0.36–4.55 (1.68)	
Monocytes	$(10^3/\mu L)$				0.012–0.367 (0.088)	0–0.420 (0.125)	0.032–0.642 (0.164)	0.046–0.639 (0.191)	
Eosinophils	$(10^3/\mu L)$				0.023–0.732 (0.143)	0–0.747 (0.192)	0.028–1.330 (0.287)	0–0.503 (0.144)	
Basophils	$(10^3/\mu L)$				0–0.093 (0.034)	(0.050)	0.011–0.232 (0.073)	(75)	
Platelets	$(10^3/\mu L)$				0–1043 (404)		61–666 (319)	28–645 (336)	
Neutrophils	(%)								
Band Neutrophils	(%)								
Lymphocytes	(%)								
Monocytes	(%)								
Eosinophils	(%)								
Basophils	(%)								
References		Powell et al. (2005)	Kendall et al. (1998)	Tumbleson et al. (1970)	Taere (2013)	Taere (2013)	Taere (2013)	Taere (2013)	Pederson and Pedersen (1975)

Biochemical Values of Cervids

	Units	White-tailed Deer (Odocoileus virginianus) Range ≤7 days	White-tailed Deer Mean + SD 90–120 days	White-tailed Deer Mean + SD 154–175 days	White-tailed Deer Range (Median) Adult	Mule Deer (Odocoileus hemionus) Range (Median) Adult	Caribou (Rangifer tarandus) Range (Median) Adult	Moose (Alces alces americanus) Range (Median) Adult	Elk (Cervus canadensis) Range Adult
Total protein	(g/dL)	3.2–7.3	5.4 (0.4)	7.8 (0.4)	4.2–8.2 (6.2)	4.1–7.7 (6.1)	4.4–9.1 (7.2)	3.5–10.0 (6.7)	7.2 (0.76)
Glucose	(mg/dL)		114.0 (35.0)	133.0 (30.0)	42–325 (146)	59–341 (149)	68–270 (124)	47–218 (125)	135.97 (56.09)
Blood urea nitrogen (BUN)	(mg/dL)	9.0–41.0	13.0 (5.0)	30.0 (5.0)	7.0–46.0 (26)	6.0–47.0 (24)	14–53 (34)	5.0–64.0 (28)	26.34 (7.22)
Uric acid	(mg/dL)	0.0–1.7					0.0–3.9 (0.1)		0.31 (0.13)
Creatinine	(mg/dL)		1.2 (0.05)	2.5 (0.3)	0.6–2.3 (1.3)	0.5–2.3 (1.3)	0.7–2.3 (1.4)	0.4–3.6 (1.5)	
BUN/creatinine ratio					8.0–36.1 (19.1)	4.7–33.8 (19.3)	12.0–42.7 (24.3)	4.3–43.2 (16)	1.23 (0.48)
Total bilirubin	(mg/dL)			0.4 (0.1)	0.2–2.2 (0.6)	0.0–0.7 (0.3)	0.1–1.1 (0.2)	0.1–1.4 (0.5)	
Direct bilirubin	(mg/dL)						0.0–0.5 (0)		
Indirect bilirubin	(mg/dL)						0.0–0.7 (0.1)		
Triglycerides	(mg/dL)	5.0–186.0			0–26 (12)		5.0–98 (23)		
Cholesterol	(mg/dL)	16.0–80.0		118.0 (29.0)	23–102 (63)	(50)	40–128 (76)	33–113 (73)	85.72 (13.26)
Amylase	(IU/L)				0–167 (60)		1–168 (54)		
ALP	(IU/L)		551.0 (101.0)	42 (11)	14–455 (58)	0–717 (68)	32–633 (111)	0–406 (136)	187 (93.7)
ALT	(IU/L)				14–99 (38)	0–58 (27)	4–121 (42)	0–58 (27)	
AST	(IU/L)		115.0 (23.0)	115.0 (23.0)	45–285 (116)	43–179 (84)	42–139 (75)	28–144 (64)	
CPK	(IU/L)								
LDH	(IU/L)			551.0 (63.0)	(571)		188–1120 (448)		
GGT	(IU/L)		136.0 (15.0)		0–137 (60)	6–132 (69)	6.0–60.0 (23)	0–57 (25)	
Albumin (A)	(g/dL)		2.7 (0.2)	2.7 (0.3)	1.1–4.0 (2.8)	1.6–3.9 (2.8)	1.9–5.3 (3.7)	1.5–5.0 (3.2)	
Globulin (G)	(g/dL)		2.7 (0.5)		1.9–5.5 (3.3)	1.9–5.0 (3.4)	1.4–5.5 (3.4)	1.5–5.5 (3.2)	
A/G ratio									1.12 (0.29)
Phosphorus (P)	(mg/dL)	7.4–14.3	11.9 (1.6)	11.8 (0.9)	3.6–13.2 (7.3)	2.9–11.7 (7.3)	4.0–11.3 (7.5)	3.0–11.9 (7.4)	5.5 (1.67)
Calcium (Ca)	(mg/dL)	7.7–14.4	9.4 (0.3)	11.5 (0.5)	7.3–11.7 (9)	7.2–11.1 (9.1)	7.8–11.8 (9.6)	8.2–12.1 (10.1)	9.4 (0.9)

		Powell et al. (2005)	Kendall et al. (1998)	Tumbleson et al. (1970)	Teare (2013)	Teare (2013)	Teare (2013)	Teare (2013)	Pedersen and Pedersen (1975)
Ca/P ratio				1.0 (0.05)	0.7–2.4 (1.2)	0.5–2.0 (1.3)	0.9–2.1 (1.3)	0.9–2.1 (1.3)	0.9–2.6 (1.3)
Sodium (Na)	(mEq/L)	139.0–155.0	140.0 (0.6)	159.0 (4.0)	133–150 (155)	134–152 (143)	135–155 (143)	135–155 (143)	131–149 (139)
Potassium (K)	(mEq/L)	3.9–6.4	4.5 (0.2)	6.4 (0.7)	3.2–6.3 (4.2)	2.8–6.0 (4.4)	3.4–6.1 (4.4)	3.4–6.1 (4.4)	3.4–6.4 (4.8)
Na/K ratio					17.0–44.8 (34.3)	20.3–43.7 (32)	21.6–42.1 (32.4)	21.6–42.1 (32.4)	19.8–38.1 (28.8)
Chloride	(mEq/L)		102 (3.5)	111.0 (3.0)	97–114 (104)	94–112 (103)	92–110 (100)	92–110 (100)	91–108 (97)
Creatinine kinase	(IU/L)	64–2055	426 (213)		0–635 (238)	0–715 (180)	53–825 (185)	53–825 (185)	0–243 (105)
Lipase	(IU/L)						0–52 (12)	0–52 (12)	
Bicarbonate	(mEq/L)					12.6–35.8 (24.2)	11.8–30.5 (23.1)	11.8–30.5 (23.1)	(26)
Magnesium	(mg/dL)		2.2 (0.2)		0.95–2.73 (1.84)	1.03–2.72 (1.87)	1.24–2.77 (2.01)	1.24–2.77 (2.01)	1.21–2.81 (2.01)
Iron	(µg/dL)						15–406 (187)	15–406 (187)	
Carbon dioxide	(mEq/L)		22.0 (3.9)		12.9–33.9 (23.4)	(23.5)	12.1–31.3 (23.2)	12.1–31.3 (23.2)	18.1–32.0 (25.1)
TT4	(µg/dL)								
Fibrinogen					0–378 (141)	0–589 (218)	53–731 (200)	53–731 (200)	0–954 (438)
References		Powell et al. (2005)	Kendall et al. (1998)	Tumbleson et al. (1970)	Teare (2013)	Teare (2013)	Teare (2013)	Teare (2013)	Pedersen and Pedersen (1975)

References

Kendall, L.V., Kennett, M.J., and Rish, R.E. (1998). Short-term care of white-tailed deer fawns (*Odocoileus virginianus*) in a conventional laboratory animal facility. *Journal of the American Association for Laboratory Animal Science* 37 (5): 96–100.

Pedersen, R.J. and Pedersen, A.A. (1975). Blood chemistry and hematology of elk. *Journal of Wildlife Management* 39 (3): 617–620.

Powell, M.C. and DelGiudice, G. (2005). Birth, morphologic, and blood characteristics of free-ranging White-Tailed Deer neonates. *Journal of Wildlife Diseases* 41 (1): 171–183.

Teare, J.A. (ed.) (2013). *ISIS Physiological Reference Intervals for Captive Wildlife: A CD-ROM Resource.* Bloomington, MN: International Species Information System.

Tumbleson, M.E., Cuneio, J.D., and Murphy, D.A. (1970). Serum biochemical and hematological parameters of captive white-tailed deer fawns. *Canadian Journal of Comparative Medicine* 24: 66–71.

Hematology Values of Raccoons

		Raccoons (*Procyon lotor*)						
	Units	Mean (SD)	Range (Mean) Adults	Mean (SD) Adult Male	Mean (SD) Adult Female	Range (Mean) Adult Male	Range (Mean) Adult Female	Range (Mean) Juvenile Male	Range (Mean) Juvenile Female
RBCs	(10^6/µL)	8.74 (1.20)	5.29–8.78 (7.32)	7.77 (1.03)	6.42 (1.06)				
Hematocrit	(%)	36.8 (5.4)	27–51 (40)	42 (6.4)	36 (7.8)	25–52 (40)	29–48 (39)	27–48 (38)	26–47 (38)
Hemoglobin	(g/dL)	12.2 (1.5)	10.0–18.5 (13.1)	13.7 (2.2)	11.7 (1.5)	8.7–15.8 (12.2)	9.0–14.7 (11.8)	8.7–14.6 (11.5)	7.8–14.8 (11.6)
MCV	(fL)	42.8 (5.2)	48–62 (54.7)						
MCH	(pg)	14.2 (1.4)	15–21 (18.1)						
MCHC	(g/dL)	32.9 (2.2)	30–37 (32.9)						
Neutrophils	(10^3/µL)	4.844 (3.650)							
Segmented neutrophils	(10^3/µL)								
Lymphocytes	(10^3/µL)	3.942 (1.982)							
Monocytes	(10^3/µL)	0.333 (0.254)							
Eosinophils	(10^3/µL)	0.784 (0.656)							
Basophils	(10^3/µL)	0.058 (0.041)							
Platelets	(10^3/µL)	470 (160)							
Neutrophils	(%)		45–88 (66.4)	65 (15.8)	69 (22.1)	27–97 (72)	42–99 (72)	12–97 (73)	23–57 (66)
Band neutrophils	(%)								
Lymphocytes	(%)		10–51 (29.1)	30 (14.6)	28 (20.7)	0–66 (23)	0–45 (24)	2–88 (26)	2–72 (31)
Monocytes	(%)		1–8 (3.6)	4.2 (2.4)	2.3 (1.5)	0–11 (1)	0–10 (2)	0–5 (1)	0–4 (1)
Eosinophils	(%)		0–3 (0.9)	1.2 (1.3)	0.3	0–28 (2)	0–13 (2)	0–5 (1)	0–14 (2)
Basophils	(%)					0–2 (0)	0–0 (0)	0–0 (0)	0–3 (0)
References		Denver (2003)	Strolle et al. (1978)	Strolle et al. (1978)	Strolle et al. (1978)	Hoff et al. (1974)	Hoff et al. (1974)	Hoff et al. (1974)	Hoff et al. (1974)

Biochemical Values of Raccoons

	Units	Mean (SD)	Raccoons (Procyon lotor)					
			Range (Mean) Adult Male	Range (Mean) Adult Female	Range (Mean) Juvenile Male	Range (Mean) Juvenile Female	Mean (SE) Adults	Mean (SE) Juveniles
Glucose	(mg/dL)	65 (22)	53–154 (99)	75–150 (106)	51–158 (103)	65–160 (104)	82.3 (6.16)	96.0 (9.17)
Blood urea nitrogen (BUN)	(mg/dL)	20 (7)	8–36 (17)	5–38 (18)	10–35 (22)	9–41 (20)	19.0 (1.92)	38.8 (5.03)
Uric acid	(mg/dL)	1.2 (0.5)	1.0–2.9 (2.0)	1.0–2.5 (2.0)	1.3–4.2 (2.2)	1.2–7.3 (2.4)	2.40 (0.10)	2.21 (0.14)
Creatinine	(mg/dL)	0.9 (0.2)					0.41 (0.02)	0.39 (0.03)
BUN/creatinine ratio								
Total bilirubin	(mg/dL)	0.2 (0.1)						
Direct bilirubin	(mg/dL)	0.0 (0.1)						
Indirect bilirubin	(mg/dL)	0.1 (0.1)						
Triglycerides	(mg/dL)	33 (17)					54.1 (6.19)	73.1 (17.65)
Cholesterol	(mg/dL)	211 (63)	136–382 (245)	178–380 (277)	92–464 (275)	164–450 (273)	185.5 (14.65)	270.4 (11.86)
Amylase	(IU/L)	3119 (917)						
ALP	(IU/L)	60 (31)						
ALT	(IU/L)	121 (36)						
AST	(IU/L)	85 (26)						
CPK	(IU/L)	306 (198)						
LDH	(IU/L)	1299 (673)						
GGT	(IU/L)	4 (2)						
Albumin (A)	(g/dL)	3.4 (0.3)					1.96 (0.06)	1.94 (0.07)
Globulin (G)	(g/dL)	3.7 (0.7)					7.47 (0.17)	6.86 (0.29)
A/G ratio								
Phosphorus (P)	(mg/dL)	4.7 (1.2)						
Calcium (Ca)	(mg/dL)	9.0 (0.7)						
Ca/P ratio								
Sodium (Na)	(mEq/L)	146 (4)					145.7 (0.82)	146.0 (1.63)
Potassium (K)	(mEq/L)	4.3 (0.4)					4.41 (0.11)	4.53 (0.15)
Na/K ratio								

		Denver (2003)	Hoff et al. (1974)	Hoff et al. (1974)	Hoff et al. (1974)	Hoff et al. (1974)	Hoff et al. (1974)	Lotze and Fleischman (1978)	Lotze and Fleischman (1978)
Chloride	(mEq/L)	110 (3)							
Creatinine kinase	(IU/L)								
Lipase	(IU/L)	252 (0)							
Bicarbonate	(mEq/L)	21.0 (0.0)							
Magnesium	(mg/dL)	3.05 (0.07)							
Iron	(µg/dL)	146 (29)							
Carbon dioxide	(mEq/L)	20.8 (4.4)							
TT4	(µg/dL)								
References									

References

Denver, M. (2003). Procyonidae and Viverridae. In: *Zoo and Wild Animal Medicine*, 5e (ed. M.E. Fowler and R.E. Miller), 516–523. St Louis, MO: Saunders (Elsevier Science).

Hoff, G.L., Bigler, W.J., McEldowny, L.E. et al. (1974). Blood and urinary value of free-ranging raccoons (*Procyon lotor*) in Florida. *American Journal of Veterinary Research* 35 (6): 861–864.

Lotze, J.H. and Fleischman, A.I. (1978). *The Raccoon (Procyon Lotor) on St. Catherines Island, Georgia: 1. Biochemical Parameters of Urine and Blood Serum,* American Museum Novitates 2644. New York: American Museum of Natural History.

Strolle, L.A., Nielsen, S.W., and Diters, R.W. (1978). Bone marrow and hematological values of wild raccoons. *Journal of Wildlife Diseases* 14 (4): 409–415.

Hematology Values of Mustelids

	Units	Striped Skunk	Fisher	North American River Otter	Sea Otter
		Mephitis mephitis	*Martes pennanti*	*Lontra canadensis*	*Enhydra lutris*
		Range (Median)	Range (Median)	Range (Median)	Range (Median)
		Male and Female	Male and Female	Male and Female	Male and Female
WBCs	$(10^3/\mu L)$	1.68–11.96 (5.57)	0.02–10.14 (5.08)	4.7–33.2 (11.3)	3.00–15.42 (6.67)
RBCs	$(10^6/\mu L)$	5.28–11.13 (7.43)	(8.5)	6.10–14.50 (10.99)	3.60–6.63 (4.85)
Hematocrit	(%)	24.0–53.9 (36.5)	32.6–56.2 (44.4)	32.2–60.8 (47.6)	41.2–62.7 (54.3)
Hemoglobin	(g/dL)	7.5–17.1 (11.8)	11.3–18.3 (14.8)	10.4–19.0 (15.1)	13.0–22.7 (4.85)
MCV	(fL)	39.3–60.5 (48.6)	(56.6)	38.3–49.0 (43.3)	82.5–135.4 (114.1)
MCH	(pg)	13.5–18.7 (15.8)		11.3–15.8 (13.7)	28.5–46.7 (39.6)
MCHC	(g/dL)	27.3–38.1 (32.3)	24.5–38.5 (31.5)	27.8–39.2 (31.4)	28.8–40.9 (35.2)
Neutrophils	$(10^3/\mu L)$	0.51–7.05 (2.68)	0.0–5.21 (2.4)	3.0–28.22 (8.87)	1.45–9.45 (3.70)
Segmented neutrophils	$(10^3/\mu L)$	0.01–0.06 (0.02)	0.0–0.06 (0.02)	0–0.48 (0.09)	0.01–0.37 (0.03)
Lymphocytes	$(10^3/\mu L)$	0.62–5.55 (2.27)	0.0–4.08 (1.84)	0.123–4.95 (1.25)	0.51–5.15 (2.04)
Monocytes	$(10^3/\mu L)$	36–788 (207)	0.0–0.416 (0.147)	0.05–2.38 (0.45)	0.04–0.91 (0.25)
Eosinophils	$(10^3/\mu L)$	31–1238 (223)	0–0.99 (0.362)	0–1.83 (0.31)	0.0–1.14 (0.34)
Basophils	$(10^3/\mu L)$			0–0.22 (0.08)	
Platelets	$(10^3/\mu L)$	37–575 (281)		298–931 (565)	108–501 (305)
Neutrophils	(%)				
Band neutrophils	(%)				
Lymphocytes	(%)				
Monocytes	(%)				
Eosinophils	(%)				
Basophils	(%)				
References		Teare (2013)	Teare (2013)	Tocidlowski et al. (2000)	Teare (2013)

Biochemical Values of Mustelids

	Units	Striped Skunk	Fisher	North American River Otter	Sea Otter
		Mephitis mephitis	*Martes pennanti*	*Lontra canadensis*	*Enhydra lutris*
		Range (Median)	Range (Median)	Range (Median)	Range (Median)
		Male and Female	Male and Female	Male and Female	Male and Female
Total protein	(g/dL)	4.8–8.9 (6.7)	5.0–7.2 (6.1)	5.7–9.0 (7.3)	5.1–7.3 (6.4)
Glucose	(mg/dL)	55–149 (96)	44–172 (108)	56–225 (130)	66–182 (109)
Blood urea nitrogen (BUN)	(mg/dL)	10–42 (20)	0–38 (19)	17–56 (31)	25–102 (46)
Uric acid	(mg/dL)			0.6–3.6 (1.7)*	
Creatinine	(mg/dL)	0.2–1.0 (0.6)	0.2–1.1 (0.7)	0.4–0.8 (0.5)	0.2–1.0 (0.5)
BUN/creatinine ratio		16.4–95.7 (36.3)	0.0–68.2 (32.3)		38.2–264.9 (86.0)
Total bilirubin	(mg/dL)	0.1–0.5 (0.1)	0.0–1.0 (0.4)	0.1–0.6 (0.2)*	0.0–0.6 (0.2)
Direct bilirubin	(mg/dL)			0.0–0.3 (0.1)*	
Indirect bilirubin	(mg/dL)			0.0–0.3 (0.1)*	
Triglycerides	(mg/dL)	0–127 (59)	(59)	9–72 (31)	
Cholesterol	(mg/dL)	89–306 (158)	133–392 (262)	63–279 (152)	99–238 (168)
Amylase	(IU/L)	75–336 (205)		2–22 (12)	0–32 (2)
ALP	(IU/L)	5–147 (40)	0–137 (65)	29–282 (85)	46–280 (117)
ALT	(IU/L)	29–323 (77)	0–162 (76)	46–990 (194)	70–821 (175)
AST	(IU/L)	47–171 (85)	6–218 (112)	34–1260 (85)	0–571 (179)
CPK	(IU/L)			67–1300 (219)	
LDH	(IU/L)	0–1869 (508)		36–10 820 (149)	
GGT	(IU/L)	0–11 (3)		8–38 (19)	0–56 (23)
Albumin (A)	(g/dL)	2.1–4.3 (3.2)	2.6–4.2 (3.4)	2.4–4.1 (3.3)	2.5–3.6 (2.9)
Globulin (G)	(g/dL)	2.0–6.0 (3.3)	1.6–3.7 (2.6)	2.9–5.8 (4.0)	2.3–4.4 (3.4)
A/G ratio					
Phosphorus (P)	(mg/dL)	2.7–10.5 (4.7)	1.7–8.5 (5.1)	3.2–8.3 (5.8)	3.3–9.5 (5.5)
Calcium (Ca)	(mg/dL)	7.9–11.4 (9.7)	8.3–10.9 (9.4)	6.8–10.0 (8.4)	8.0–10.3 (8.9)
Ca/P ratio		1.0–3.5 (2.0)	0.7–3.0 (1.9)		0.8–2.4 (1.6)
Sodium (Na)	(mEq/L)	134–160 (149)	141–157 (149)	136–158 (152)	143–163 (152)
Potassium (K)	(mEq/L)	3.8–6.4 (4.9)	3.4–5.4 (4.4)	3.5–5.3 (4.4)	3.4–5.6 (4.2)
Na/K ratio		23.3–40.0 (30.3)	25.6–41.5 (33.6)		28.1–44.5 (36.0)
Chloride	(mEq/L)	104–122 (112)	107–124 (116)	94–121 (113)	108–125 (114)
Creatinine kinase	(IU/L)	0–1262 (421)	(401)	78–1528 (310)*	0–2196 (420)
Lipase	(IU/L)	0–1219 (581)		4–55 (22)*	12–36 (24)
Bicarbonate	(mEq/L)		(18.0)	13.3–31.3 (24)*	18.9–32.1 (25.5)
Magnesium	(mg/dL)	0.97–3.19 (2.08)		1.46–2.62 (1.90)*	
Iron	(µg/dL)		38–270 (154)	25–318 (172)*	
Carbon dioxide	(mEq/L)	16.1–35.1 (25.6)		15.1–33.1 (24.3)*	11.6–35.8 (23.7)
TT4	(µg/dL)				
References		Teare (2013)	Teare (2013)	Tocidlowski et al. (2000)	Teare (2013)

References

Teare, J.A. (ed.) (2013). *ISIS Physiological Reference Intervals for Captive Wildlife: A CD-ROM Resource.* Bloomington, MN: International Species Information System.

Tocidlowski, M.E., Spelman, L.H., Sumner, P., and Stoskopf, M.K. (2000). Hematology and serum biochemistry parameters of north american river otters (*Lontra canadensis*). *Journal of Zoo and Wildlife Medicine* 31 (4): 484–490.

Hematology Values of Virginia Opossums

	Units	*Didelphis virginiana* Range Male	Range Female	Range Unknown
WBCs	($10^3/\mu$L)	4.20–9.80	3.90–12.60	6.0–8.0
RBCs	($10^6/\mu$L)	4.92–6.50	3.78–6.02	3.3–5.9
Hematocrit	(%)	41.5–51.0	33.0–49.0	40–50
Hemoglobin	(g/dL)	13.8–17.9	12.4–17.0	13.3–16.2
MCV	(fL)	79–90	73–103	64–80
MCH	(pg)	26.8–31.0	24.4–34.6	22.5–35.9
MCHC	(g/dL)	32.7–35.2	33.5–40.0	30–40
Neutrophils	($10^3/\mu$L)			1800–4000
Segmented neutrophils	($10^3/\mu$L)			0
Lymphocytes	($10^3/\mu$L)			2400–4800
Monocytes	($10^3/\mu$L)			0–160
Eosinophils	($10^3/\mu$L)			0–160
Basophils	($10^3/\mu$L)			0–160
Platelets	($10^3/\mu$L)			>200
Neutrophils	(%)	14–48	11–42	30–50
Band neutrophils	(%)	one seen	one seen	0
Lymphocytes	(%)	42–76	26–73	40–60
Monocytes	(%)	0–6	1–7	0–2
Eosinophils	(%)	6–17	11–38	0–2
Basophils	(%)	one seen	0–3	0–2
References		Giacometti et al. (1972), Lewis (1974)		Henness (2006)

Biochemical Values of Virginia Opossums

	Units	Virginia Opossum (Didelphis virginiana)			
		Range	Range	Range	Range
		Male	Female	Unknown	Unknown
Total protein	(g/dL)	5.1–6.0	3.8–7.1		5.0–7.5
Glucose	(mg/dL)	97–127	64–130		80–100
Blood urea nitrogen (BUN)	(mg/dL)	23–38	16–38		20–40
Uric acid	(mg/dL)	0.5–2.0	0.4–2.3		0.9–2.2
Creatinine	(mg/dL)	0.4–3.3	0.4–14.0		0.5–1.2
BUN/creatinine ratio					10–40
Total bilirubin	(mg/dL)	0.2–0.8	0.1–0.6		0.3–0.8
Direct bilirubin	(mg/dL)			0–0.1	
Indirect bilirubin	(mg/dL)				
Triglycerides	(mg/dL)				
Cholesterol	(mg/dL)	95–195	85–203		80–151
Amylase	(IU/L)				
ALP	(IU/L)			85–196	13–135
ALT	(IU/L)			35–144	<80
AST	(IU/L)			171–575	<150
CPK	(IU/L)			891–7400	
LDH	(IU/L)			128–7400	
GGT	(IU/L)				
Albumin (A)	(g/dL)	1.3–2.3	0.3–4.9		2.0–3.0
Globulin (G)	(g/dL)				3.0–4.0
A/G ratio					0.5–1.0
Phosphorus (P)	(mg/dL)	1.8–5.7	3.0–8.4		4.6–8.2
Calcium (Ca)	(mg/dL)			8.9–10.5	8.0–11.0
Ca/P ratio					4.6–8.2
Sodium (Na)	(mEq/L)	135–145	131–145		143–155
Potassium (K)	(mEq/L)	3.45–5.1	3.10–4.8		4.1–6.2
Na/K ratio					
Chloride	(mEq/L)	102–115	101–129		100–108
Creatinine kinase	(IU/L)				<1000
Lipase	(IU/L)				
Bicarbonate	(mEq/L)	21.2–25.8	17.3–28.0		
Magnesium	(mg/dL)	1.56–1.77	1.15–1.71		
Iron	(µg/dL)	43–55	52–58		
Carbon dioxide	(mEq/L)				
TT4	(µg/dL)				
References		Giacometti et al. (1972), Lewis (1974)			Henness (2006)

References

Giacometti, L., Berntzen, A.K., and Bliss, M.L. (1972). Hematologic parameters of the opossum (*Didelphis virginiana*). *Comparative Biochemistry and Physiology Part A* 43 (2): 287–292.

Henness, A.M. (2006). *Opossum Blood and Urine Normals*. Catonsville, MD: National Opossum Society, Inc.

Lewis, J.H. (1974). Comparative hematology: studies on opossums Didelphis marsupialis (*virginianus*). *Comparative Biochemistry and Physiology Part A* 51: 275–280.

Hematology Values of Canids

	Units	Red Fox *Vulpes vulpes* Range (Median)	Cascade Red Fox *Vulpes vulpes cascadensis* Range	Gray Fox *Urocyon cinereoargenteus* Range (Median)	Island Fox *Urocyon littoralis* Mean (SD)	Coyote *Canis latrans* Range (Median)	Coyote *C. latrans* Mean (SD) Adult Male	Coyote *C. latrans* Mean (SD) Adult Female	Gray Wolf *Canis lupus* Range (Median)	Gray Wolf *C. lupus* Mean (SD) Adult
		Adults	Adults		Adults	Adults				Adult
WBCs	(10³/μL)	0.59–9.64 (5.11)	5.5–19.8 (12.9)	0.64–12.11 (6.37)	15.84 (3.86)	4.30–16.75 (8.33)	20.3 (8.5)	15.5 (5.8)	4.53–18.53 (9.24)	
RBCs	(10⁶/μL)	4.37–11.4 (9.2)	6.7–10.9 (9.15)	2.87–8.19 (5.53)	6.34 (0.82)	4.48–8.42 (6.45)			4.35–9.21 (7.01)	
Hematocrit	(%)	26.8–61.0 (44.1)	32.4–55.7 (45.85)	22.2–56.7 (39.4)	40.48 (4.51)	31.6–59.4 (47.4)	47.7 (8.7)	49.0 (0.8)	30.6–61.6 (48.4)	63.6 (2.0)
Hemoglobin	(g/dL)	9.2–19.1 (15.3)	11.4–17.5 (15.95)	7.8–17.4 (12.6)	12.76 (1.51)	10.4–19.2 (15.8)	14.2 (2.5)	15.0 (0.8)	10.1–21.5 (16.8)	19.9 (0.07)
MCV	(fL)	40.6–56.3 (48.4)	48–58 (50.5)	56.9–86.3 (71.6)	64.11 (2.36)	62.7–81.7 (72.2)			58.1–78.3 (69.5)	
MCH	(pg)	14.4–18.3 (16.4)	16.1–17.7 (16.85)	17.1–29.2 (23.2)	20.17 (0.82)	20.4–27.7 (24)			20.6–26.5 (23.9)	
MCHC	(g/dL)	27.8–41.7 (33.6)	29.1–35.4 (34.45)	26.0–38.3 (32.2)	31.53 (0.87)	26.9–38.4 (33.2)	29.8	30.6	29.3–38.5 (34.3)	
Band neutrophils	(10³/μL)	0.00–0.05 (0.02)		0.00–0.06 (0.03)		0.02–0.11 (0.04)			0.02–0.16 (0.04)	
Segmented neutrophils	(10³/μL)	0.00–5.89 (2.6)		0.00–8.92 (3.96)	12.292 (3.75)	2.37–11.70 (5.26)			2.71–13.69 (6.17)	
Lymphocytes	(10³/μL)	0.00–3.63 (1.34)		0.00–3.24 (1.58)	1.623 (0.832)	0.43–4.01 (1.48)			0.41–4.61 (1.65)	
Monocytes	(10³/μL)	0–0.503 (0.181)		0–0.538 (0.193)	0.720 (0.391)	0.051–1.032 (0.339)			0.074–1.363 (0.384)	
Eosinophils	(10³/μL)	0–1.284 (0.414)		0.0–1.121 (0.350)	1.065 (0.623)	0.083–2.607 (0.646)			0.077–1.821 (0.443)	
Basophils	(10³/μL)				0.314 (0.209)				0.007–0.271 (0.085)	
Platelets	(10³/μL)	120–596 (358)				91–516 (304)			108–454 (246)	
Neutrophils	(%)				76.95 (8.46)		80	89		
Band neutrophils	(%)									
Lymphocytes	(%)				10.53 (5.25)		12	5		
Monocytes	(%)				4.58 (2.23)		4	5		
Eosinophils	(%)				7.14 (4.50)		4	–		
Basophils	(%)				1.95 (1.17)					
References		Teare (2013)	Aubry (1983)	Teare (2013)	Crooks et al. (2000)	Teare (2013)	Smith and Rongstad (1980)		Teare (2013)	Butler et al. (2006)

Biochemical Values of Canids

	Units	Red Fox *Vulpes vulpes* Range (Median)	Cascade Red Fox *Vulpes vulpes cascadensis* Range (Median) Adults	Gray Fox *Urocyon cinereoargenteus* Range (Median)	Island Fox *Urocyon littoralis* Mean (SD)	Coyote *Canis latrans* Range (Median)	Coyote *C. latrans* Mean (SD) Adult Male	Coyote Adult Female	Gray Wolf *Canis lupus* Range (Median)	Gray Wolf *C. lupus* Range (Median) Adults – Spring
Total protein	(g/dL)	4.3–7.6 (5.8)	5.3–6.3 (5.9)	4.7–7.7 (6.2)	7.8 (0.62)	4.8–7.4 (6.2)	6.4 (0.5)	6.4 (0.6)	4.6–7.6 (6.1)	
Glucose	(mg/dL)	80–218 (126)	98–277 (120)	55–162 (108)	111.42 (49.28)	60–185 (110)	161 (44)	181 (47)	64–176 (111)	118.7 (7.4)
Blood urea nitrogen (BUN)	(mg/dL)	10–40 (21)	13–48 (34.5)	7–27 (17)	17.58 (9.23)	9–45 (21)	28.2 (13.2)	21.2 (8.3)	9–40 (19)	52.9 (3.4)
Uric acid	(mg/dL)								0.0–1.3 (0.3)	1.3 (0.09)
Creatinine	(mg/dL)	0.4–1.5 (0.9)	0.6–1.3 (0.8)	0.5–1.5 (1)	0.65 (0.06)	0.6–2.0 (1.1)			0.4–1.7 (1.1)	1.1 (0.1)
BUN/creatinine ratio		11.1–57.2		4.2–32.7 (18.4)	26.87 (13.15)	10.3–39.2 (20.2)			9.8–40.0 (19.1)	
Total bilirubin	(mg/dL)	0.2–1.9 (0.8)	0.5–2.1 (0.85)	0.0–0.5 (0.2)	0.1 (0.02)	0.0–0.5 (0.1)	0.1 (0.1)	0.2 (0.1)	0.0–0.6 (0.2)	
Direct bilirubin	(mg/dL)	0.0–1.0 (0.3)	0.1–0.4 (0.2)		0.04 (0.05)	mean = 0.1			0.0–0.1 (0.0)	
Indirect bilirubin	(mg/dL)	0.1–1.1 (0.6)			0.06 (0.05)	mean = 0.1			0.0–0.5 (0.1)	
Triglycerides	(mg/dL)	0–88 (44)				2–76 (39)				51.8 (5.8)
Cholesterol	(mg/dL)	92–323 (175)	100–235 (156)	107–318 (212)	146.21 (34.35)	92–351 (182)	153 (35)	157 (40)	100–349 (186)	
Amylase	(IU/L)	0–1160 (517)				68–491 (280)			129–988 (333)	
ALP	(IU/L)	3–73 (24)	55–695 (69.5)	0–25 (12)	14.29 (4.89)	7–75 (26)			8–112 (31)	49.8 (6.7)
ALT	(IU/L)	29–166 (68)	78–684 (134.5)	17–106 (61)	101.39 (59.55)	17–93 (42)			19–110 (45)	
AST	(IU/L)	10–98 (50)	55–695 (280.5)	23–101 (62)	91.76 (37.55)	0–103 (46)			18–83 (38)	
CPK	(IU/L)									
LDH	(IU/L)	0–509 (147)		mean = 92					24–482 (101)	306.7 (22.7)
GGT	(IU/L)	0–10 (4)			2.00 (0.99)	0–11 (4)			0–15 (5)	226.5 (23.8)
Albumin (A)	(g/dL)	2.2–4.1 (3.1)	2.1–3.5 (3.05)	2.5–4.2 (3.3)	2.71 (0.19)	2.3–4.1 (3.1)	2.9 (0.2)	3.1 (0.4)	2.3–4.3 (3.2)	
Globulin (G)	(g/dL)	1.2–4.5 (2.7)	0.9–3.5 (2.7)	1.5–4.3 (2.9)	5.09 (0.64)	1.9–4.2 (3)	3.5 (0.4)	3.3 (0.5)	1.5–4.2 (2.8)	1.0 (0.06)
A/G ratio		0.6–1.5 (1.0)	0.6–1.5 (1.0)		0.54 (0.09)		0.9 (0.1)	1.0 (0.2)		
Phosphorus (P)	(mg/dL)	2.1–8.1 (3.8)	1.9–13.2 (5.0)	2.3–5.9 (4.1)	3.67 (0.51)	1.7–7.9 (3.6)	3.4 (0.5)	3.5 (0.7)	1.7–8.5 (3.7)	4.4 (0.4)

		Teare (2013)	Aubry (1983)	Teare (2013)	Crooks et al. (2000)	Teare (2013)	Smith and Rongstad (1980)		Teare (2013)	Butler et al. (2006)
Calcium (Ca)	(mg/dL)	8.1–11.4 (9.4)	8.6–10.8 (9.3)	8.3–10.6 (9.4)	8.53 (0.34)	7.5–11.3 (9.6)	8.6 (0.6)	8.8 (0.7)	8.5–11.5 (9.9)	8.9 (0.3)
Ca/P ratio		1.1–4.4 (2.4)		1.4–3.2 (2.3)		1.3–5.4 (2.6)			1.2–5.1 (2.6)	
Sodium (Na)	(mEq/L)	138–156 (148)	145–159 (152.5)	138–157 (148)	145.87 (2.74)	139–153 (147)			139–156 (147)	
Potassium (K)	(mEq/L)	3.5–5.5 (4.3)	3.0–5.4 (4.0)	3.1–5.5 (4.3)	4.15 (0.26)	3.5–5.8 (4.5)			3.8–5.5 (4.5)	
Na/K ratio		25.8–41.2 (34.3)	25.6–42.9 (34.3)		35.21 (2.34)	24.2–40.2 (32.2)			26.0–39.3 (32.4)	
Chloride	(mEq/L)	108–121	109–124 (120)	106–123 (114)	7.8 (0.62)	105–121 (113)			107–124 (115)	161.1 (4.0)
Creatinine kinase	(IU/L)	0–514 (140)			948.11 (1049.28)	0–631 (196)			47–455 (138)	
Lipase	(IU/L)				7.8 (0.62)	mean = 330			29–1000 (221)	
Bicarbonate	(mEq/L)				7.8 (0.62)	12.5–22.5 (17.5)			12.3–25.7 (19.5)	
Magnesium	(mg/dL)	mean = 1.7							1.26–2.40 (1.71)	
Iron	(µg/dL)								36–280 (137)	47.4 (4.5)
Carbon dioxide	(mEq/L)	12.7–29.8 (21.3)	11–25 (16)	mean = 23.2					12.1–29.8 (20.2)	
TT4	(µg/dL)								0.0–3.2 (1.4)	

References

Aubry, K.Bl (1983). The Cascade red fox: distribution, morphology, zoogeography and ecology. PhD dissertation. University of Washington.

Butler, M.J., Ballard, W.B., and Whitlaw, H.A. (2006). Physical characteristics, Hematology, and Serum Chemistry of freeranging Gray Wolves, *Canis lupus*, in Southcentral Alaska. *Canadian Field-Naturalist* 120 (2): 205–212.

Crooks, K.R., Scott, C.A., Bowen, L., and Van Vuren, D. (2000). Hematology and serum chemistry of the island Fox on Santa Cruz Island. *Journal of Wildlife Diseases* 36 (2): 397–404.

Smith, G.J. and Rongstad, O.J. (1980). Serologic and hematologic values of wild coyotes in Wisconsin. *Journal of Wildlife Diseases* 16 (4): 491–497.

Teare, J.A. (ed.) (2013). *ISIS Physiological Reference Intervals for Captive Wildlife: A CD-ROM Resource.* Bloomington, MN.: International Species Information System.

Hematology Values of Ursids

| | Units | Black Bear *Ursus americanus* | |
		Range (Mean)	N
WBCs	$(10^3/\mu L)$	0.6–9.65 (5.87)	#
RBCs	$(10^6/\mu L)$		
Hematocrit	(%)	17–40 (29.38)	#
Hemoglobin	(g/dL)		
MCV	(fL)		
MCH	(pg)		
MCHC	(g/dL)		
Neutrophils	$(10^3/\mu L)$	0.24–6.369 (3.49)	#
Segmented neutrophils	$(10^3/\mu L)$	0–0.202 (0.01)	#
Lymphocytes	$(10^3/\mu L)$	0.065–3.65 (2.04)	#
Monocytes	$(10^3/\mu L)$	0–0.77 (0.18)	#
Eosinophils	$(10^3/\mu L)$	0–0.58 (0.08)	#
Basophils	$(10^3/\mu L)$	<0.01–<0.01 (<0.01)	#
Platelets	$(10^3/\mu L)$	0–60 (33.57)	#
Neutrophils	(%)		
Band neutrophils	(%)		
Lymphocytes	(%)		
Monocytes	(%)		
Eosinophils	(%)		
Basophils	(%)		

Values taken from American black bear cubs admitted to the Wildlife Center of Virginia between January 1st and July 31st, 2013–2015, and determined to be "clinically healthy" (no abnormalities on physical examination, normal body condition score, and no more than mild dehydration).

Biochemical Values of Ursids

	Units	Black Bear *Ursus americanus* Range (Mean)	N
Total protein	(g/dL)	3.7–5.6 (4.81)	#
Glucose	(mg/dL)	48–128 (95.59)	#
Blood urea nitrogen (BUN)	(mg/dL)	1–26 (9)	#
Uric acid	(mg/dL)		
Creatinine	(mg/dL)	0.19–0.73 (0.47)	#
BUN/creatinine ratio		5.3–35.6 (19.1)	#
Total bilirubin	(mg/dL)	0.1–0.7 (0.31)	#
Direct bilirubin	(mg/dL)		
Indirect bilirubin	(mg/dL)		
Triglycerides	(mg/dL)		
Cholesterol	(mg/dL)	105–408 (235)	#
Amylase	(IU/L)	9–19 (13.67)	3
ALP	(IU/L)	45–266 (145.82)	#
ALT	(IU/L)	31–49 (38.67)	3
AST	(IU/L)	24–114 (53.38)	#
CPK	(IU/L)		
LDH	(IU/L)		
GGT	(IU/L)		
Albumin (A)	(g/dL)	1.2–3.8 (2.42)	5
Globulin (G)	(g/dL)	1.2–2.3 (1.73)	3
A/G ratio			
Phosphorus (P)	(mg/dL)	3.1–11.3 (8.37)	#
Calcium (Ca)	(mg/dL)	7.2–10.8 (9.28)	#
Ca/P ratio		1.1–2.3 (1.1)	#
Sodium (Na)	(mEq/L)	134–163 (142.65)	#
Potassium (K)	(mEq/L)	2.8–5.7 (4.22)	#
Na/K ratio		28.6–47.9 (33.8)	#
Chloride	(mEq/L)	101–128 (110.57)	#
Creatinine kinase	(IU/L)	69–1024 (329.5)	#
Lipase	(IU/L)		
Bicarbonate	(mEq/L)		
Magnesium	(mg/dL)		
Iron	(µg/dL)		
Carbon dioxide	(mEq/L)		
TT4	(µg/dL)		

Hematology Values of Felids

	Units	Bobcat	Lynx	Cougar
		Lynx rufus	*Lynx canadensis*	*Puma concolor*
		Range (Median)	Range (Median)	Range (Median)
WBCs	$(10^3/\mu L)$	2.61–13.16 (5.97)	4.50–19.31 (9.03)	3.43–12.15 (6.43)
RBCs	$(10^6/\mu L)$	5.07–10.41 (7.73)	4.70–9.54 (7.12)	5.17–10.52 (8.04)
Hematocrit	(%)	24.8–49.4 (36.4)	24.7–49.4 (35.9)	25.7–50.0 (37.4)
Hemoglobin	(g/dL)	8.3–15.7 (11.9)	8.2–15.6 (12.2)	8.7–16.4 (12.5)
MCV	(fL)	37.5–54.9 (47.1)	44.0–59.3 (51.7)	38.5–55.9 (46.4)
MCH	(pg)	13.3–17.6 (15.4)	15.0–20.6 (17.8)	12.9–18.6 (15.8)
MCHC	(g/dL)	28.3–36.9 (32.7)	26.6–37.8 (34.2)	29.6–38.4 (33.5)
Neutrophilic band cells	$(10^3/\mu L)$	0.01–0.06 (0.03)	0.02–0.46 (0.05)	0.01–0.07 (0.03)
Segmented neutrophils	$(10^3/\mu L)$	0.10–8.44 (3.47)	2.22–13.63 (5.92)	1.57–8.87 (4.18)
Lymphocytes	$(10^3/\mu L)$	0.50–4.26 (1.72)	0.69–5.09 (2.33)	0.54–4.18 (1.66)
Monocytes	$(10^3/\mu L)$	0.034–0.536 (0.153)	0.072–0.703 (0.281)	0.044–0.719 (0.216)
Eosinophils	$(10^3/\mu L)$	0.040–1.261 (0.318)	0.0–0.464 (0.186)	0.031–0.659 (0.149)
Basophils	$(10^3/\mu L)$	0.0–0.120 (0.042)		0.0–0.154 (0.069)
Platelets	$(10^3/\mu L)$	100–723 (399)	(406)	76–587 (282)
Neutrophils	(%)			
Band beutrophils	(%)			
Lymphocytes	(%)			
Monocytes	(%)			
Eosinophils	(%)			
Basophils	(%)			
References		Teare (2013)	Teare (2013)	Teare (2013)

Biochemical Values of Felids

	Units	Bobcat *Lynx rufus* Range (Median)	Lynx *Lynx canadensis* Range (Median)	Cougar *Puma concolor* Range (Median)
Total protein	(g/dL)	5.5–8.4 (5.1)	5.1–8.7 (7)	5.8–8.5 (7.3)
Glucose	(mg/dL)	89–323 (156)	73–306 (139)	82–250 (132)
Blood urea nitrogen	(mg/dL)	18–48 (29)	19–59 (32)	17–54 (29)
Uric acid	(mg/dL)	0–1.0 (0.3)	(0.1)	0.0–1.2 (0.1)
Creatinine	(mg/dL)	0.9–3.7 (2)	0.5–4.2 (2)	0.6–3.6 (2.2)
BUN/creatinine ratio		8.5–29.0 (14.4)	9.7–42.3 (16.1)	7.1–34.1 (12.9)
Total bilirubin	(mg/dL)	0.1–0.8 (0.3)	0.1–0.5 (0.2)	0.0–0.6 (0.2)
Direct bilirubin	(mg/dL)	0.0–0.3 (0.1)	(0.1)	0.0–0.1 (0.1)
Indirect bilirubin	(mg/dL)	0.0–0.4 (0.2)	(0.1)	0.0–0.4 (0.1)
Triglycerides	(mg/dL)	10–59 (23)	0–65 (27)	8–69 (25)
Cholesterol	(mg/dL)	67–231 (134)	79–224 (142)	114–286 (186)
Amylase	(IU/l)	345–1390 (728)	44–2342 (1193)	187–738 (360)
ALP	(IU/l)	3–45 (12)	10–64 (26)	3–60 (12)
ALT	(IU/l)	17–83 (34)	13–126 (41)	20–100 (41)
AST	(IU/l)	17–76 (32)	12–71 (30)	14–72 (32)
CPK	(IU/l)			
LDH	(IU/l)	0–322 (99)	0–597 (108)	29–330 (87)
GGT	(IU/l)	0–9 (1)	0–6 (1)	0–9 (1)
Albumin	(g/dL)	2.3–4.4 (3.5)	2.6–4.6 (3.8)	2.7–4.5 (3.7)
Globulin	(g/dL)	2.4–5.4 (3.6)	1.8–5.3 (3.1)	2.4–5.4 (3.6)
Phosphorus	(mg/dL)	2.8–8.4 (7.1)	3.7–10.7 (5.6)	2.9–9.1 (4.9)
Calcium	(mg/dL)	8.4–11.0 (9.7)	8.1–11.9 (9.8)	9.0–11.9 (10.3)
Ca/P ratio		1.2–2.9 (1.9)	1.0–2.6 (1.7)	1.2–3.4 (2.1)
Sodium	(mEq/L)	145–162 (153)	142–167 (153)	145–165 (154)
Potassium	(mEq/L)	3.5–5.3 (4.4)	3.4–5.6 (4.3)	3.5–5.2 (4.2)
Na/K ratio		28.7–43.8 (35.1)	26.6–45.1 (35.6)	29.2–44.0 (36.9)
Chloride	(mEq/L)	111–129 (120)	110–128 (118)	110–129 (120)
Creatine kinase	(IU/l)	96–1119 (333)	0–1042 (393)	68–877 (259)
Lipase	(IU/l)	0–41 (11)	0–116 (13)	0–46 (4)
Bicarbonate	(mEq/L)	7.3–23.3 (15.3)		10.9–22.6 (16.8)
Magnesium	(mg/dL)	1.12–2.68 (1.9)		1.36–2.62 (1.99)
Iron	(µg/dL)			27–145 (86)
Carbon dioxide	(mEq/L)	9.7–22.6 (15.7)	8.2–24.5 (16.4)	10.9–22.8 (16.9)
TT4	(µg/dL)	0.0–2.7 (1.4)		0.0–3.6 (1.8)

Reference

Teare, J.A. (ed.) (2013). *ISIS Physiological Reference Intervals for Captive Wildlife: A CD-ROM Resource.* Bloomington, MN: International Species Information System.

Hematology Values of Chelonians

	Units	Gopher tortoise	Common Box turtles	Desert tortoises
		Gopherus polyphemus	*Terrapene carolina*	*Gopherus agassizii*
		Median (Range)	Median ± SD	Median ± SD
WBCs	$(10^3/\mu L)$	15.7 (10–22)	7.0 ± 4.6	6.6–8.9
RBCs	$(10^6/\mu L)$	0.54 (0.24–0.91)	0.5 ± 0.3	1.2–3.0
Hematocrit	(%)	23 (15–30)	22 ± 7	23–27
Hemoglobin	(g/dL)	6.4 (4.2–8.6)	5.1 ± 0.1	6.9–7.7
MCV	(fL)	—	421 ± 257	377–607
MCH	(pg)	—	102	113–126
MCHC	(g/dL)	—	28 ± 3	19–34
Heterophils	(%)	30 (10–57)	—	35–60
Lymphocytes	(%)	57 (32–79)	—	25–50
Monocytes	(%)	7 (3–13)	—	0–4
Eosinophils	(%)	—	—	0–4
Basophils	(%)	6 (2–11)	—	15 Feb

Biochemical Values of Chelonians

	Units	Common Box Turtle	Desert Tortoise	Gopher Tortoise
		Terrapene carolina	*Gopherus agassizii*	*Gopherus polyphemus*
		Median ± SD	Median (Range)	Median (Range)
Total protein	(g/dL)	5.6 ± 1.4	3.6 (3.4–3.8)	3.1 (1.3–4.6)
Glucose	(mg/dL)	84 ± 35	75 (69–82)	75 (55–128)
Blood urea nitrogen (BUN)	(mg/dL)	49 ± 29	46 (30–62)	30 (1–130)
Uric acid	(mg/dL)	1.6 ± 1.0	2.2–9.2	3.5 (0.9–8.5)
Creatinine	(mg/dL)	0.4	0.13 (0.12–0.14)	0.3 (0.1–0.4)
BUN/creatinine ratio		—	—	—
Total bilirubin	(mg/dL)	0.5 ± 0.3	0.1 ± 0.1	0.02 (0–0.1)
Direct bilirubin	(mg/dL)	—	—	—
Indirect bilirubin	(mg/dL)	—	—	—
Triglycerides	(mg/dL)	—	—	—
Cholesterol	(mg/dL)	240 ± 157	74 (60–89)	76 (19–150)
Amylase	(IU/L)	—	—	—
ALP	(IU/L)	62 ± 27	32 (29–35)	39 (11–71)
ALT	(IU/L)	7 ± 6	6.1 (3.8–8.3)	15 (2–57)
AST	(IU/L)	124 ± 148	59 (47–70)	136 (57–392)
CPK	(IU/L)	—	—	—
LDH	(IU/L)	206 ± 82	25–250	273 (18–909)
GGT	(IU/L)	—	—	—
Albumin (A)	(g/dL)	2.2 ± 0.6	1.1 (1.0–1.2)	1.5 (0.5–2.6)
Globulin (B)	(g/dL)	3.4 ± 0.9	2.5 (2.3–2.6)	—
A/G ratio		—	—	—
Phosphorus (P)	(mg/dL)	4.0 ± 1.5	2.2–4.5	2.1 (1.0–3.1)
Calcium (Ca)	(mg/dL)	13.6 ± 5.1	10 (9.6–10.3)	12 (10–14)
Ca/P ratio		—	—	—
Sodium (Na)	(mEq/L)	144 ± 5	130–157	138 (127–148)
Potassium (K)	(mEq/L)	5.6 ± 2.4	3.7 (3.5–3.9)	5.0 (2.9–7.0)
Na/K ratio		—	—	—
Chloride	(mEq/L)	106 ± 5	110 (109–112)	102 (35–128)
Creatinine kinase	(IU/L)	463 ± 337	2079 ± 1783	160 (32–628)
Lipase	(IU/L)	—	—	—
Bicarbonate	(mEq/L)	—	—	—
Magnesium	(mg/dL)	4.2	2.52 (2.16–2.88)	4.92 (3.96–5.76)
Iron	(µg/dL)	—	—	—
Carbon dioxide	(mEq/L)	—	—	—
TT4	(µg/dL)	—	—	—

Hematology Values of Amphibians

	Units	American Bullfrog *Lithobates catesbeiana* Range	Leopard Frog *Lithobates pipiens* Range	Tiger Salamander *Ambystoma spp* Range
WBCs	$(10^3/\mu L)$	11.3–29.7	3.1–22.2	0.05–1.67
RBCs	$(10^6/\mu L)$	0.80–1.82	0.223–0.77	0.08–9.5
Hematocrit	(%)	19.3–40.9	19–52	26–64
Hemoglobin	(g/dL)	—	—	3.3–14.3
MCV	(fL)	—	722–916	60–7200
MCH	(pg)	—	182–221	8.95–1760
MCHC	(g/dL)	—	22.70–26.8	7.5–271.9
Heterophils	(%)	—	—	—
Lymphocytes	(%)	17–36.6	—	16–70
Monocytes	(%)	0.7–5.1	—	0–10
Eosinophils	(%)	2.6–9	—	4–63
Basophils	(%)	1.1–5.9	—	0–15
		Gibbons et al. (2019)	Gibbons et al. (2019)	Brady et al. (2016)

Biochemical Values of Amphibians

	Units	American Bullfrog *Lithobates catesbeiana* Range	Leopard Frog *Lithobates pipiens* Range	Tiger Salamander *Ambystoma californiense* Range
Total protein	(g/dL)	3.02–5.66	—	3–4
Glucose	(mg/dL)	25.8–74.0	—	17–40
Blood urea nitrogen (BUN)	(mg/dL)	—	—	—
Uric acid	(mg/dL)	0–7.1	—	—
Creatinine	(mg/dL)	0.24–0.73	—	—
BUN/creatinine ratio	—	—	—	—
Total bilirubin	(mg/dL)	—	—	—
Direct bilirubin	(mg/dL)	—	—	—
Indirect bilirubin	(mg/dL)	—	—	—
Triglycerides	(mg/dL)	22–67.9	—	—
Cholesterol	(mg/dL)	34–89.6	—	—
Amylase	(IU/L)	—	—	—
ALP	(IU/L)	155.1–158.9	—	—
ALT	(IU/L)	10.52–14.28	—	—
AST	(IU/L)	—	—	261–1759
CPK	(IU/L)	—	—	—
LDH	(IU/L)	72–161	—	—
GGT	(IU/L)	—	—	—
Albumin (A)	(g/dL)	0.92–2.24	—	1–1.5
Globulin (G)	(g/dL)	—	—	0–2.3
A/G ratio		–	–	–
Phosphorus (P)	(mg/dL)	5.23–12.41	–	3.5–10.2
Calcium (Ca)	(mg/dL)	6.89–9.73	–	5.8–15.4
Ca/P ratio		–	–	–
Sodium (Na)	(mEq/L)	108.7–111.4	–	114–135
Potassium (K)	(mEq/L)	2.5–2.9	–	3.5–7.5
Na/K ratio		–	–	–
Chloride	(mEq/L)	96–121.2	–	–
Creatinine kinase	(IU/L)	262–602	–	–
Lipase	(IU/L)	–	–	–
Bicarbonate	(mEq/L)	–	–	–
Magnesium	(mg/dL)	–	–	–
Iron	(µg/dL)	–	–	–
Carbon dioxide	(mEq/L)	–	–	–
TT4	(µg/dL)	–	–	–

References

Brady, S., Burgdorf-Moisuke, A., Kass, P.H., and Brady, J. (2016). Hematology and plasma biochemistry intervals for captive-born California Tiger salamanders (*Ambystoma californiense*). *Journal of Zoo and Wildlife Medicine* 47 (3): 731–735.

Gibbons, P.J., Whitaker, B.R., Carpenter, J.W. et al. (2019). Hematology and biochemistry tables. In: *Mader's Reptile and Amphibian Medicine and Surgery* (ed. S.J. Divers and S.J. Stahl). St Louis, MO: Elsevier.

Appendix II

Formulary for Common Wildlife Species

Heather W. Barron

Clinic for the Rehabilitation of Wildlife, Sanibel, FL, USA

Medical Management of Wildlife Species: A Guide for Practitioners, First Edition. Edited by Sonia M. Hernandez,
Heather W. Barron, Erica A. Miller, Roberto F. Aguilar and Michael J. Yabsley.

Analgesics and Nonsteroidal Antiinflammatory Drugs

	Birds	Mammals	Reptiles and Amphibians
Buprenorphine can be used at this dose q24h in the concentrated 1.8 mg/ml formulation (Simbadol®)	0.1–0.6 mg/kg SQ q12h (Adamcak and Otten 2000)	Most species: 0.01–0.05 mg/kg SQ, IM, IV, IP, OTM q6–12h (Adkesson et al. 2011; Baker et al. 2011) Felids: 0.01–0.02 mg/kg SQ, IM q12h; may be administered via transmucosal route at higher dosage of 0.02–0.03 mg/kg q12h (Barnard 2009) Bats: 0.1 mg/kg SQ q24h (Bechert et al. 2010)	Currently not recommended for reptiles (Beynon et al. 1996; Black et al. 2010) Amphibians: 75 mg/kg into dorsal lymph sac q4–6h (Blankespoor et al. 2001)
Bupivacaine	2 mg/kg Toxic effects seen at 3 mg/kg in some species	Carnivores: 2 mg/kg Rabbits: 1 mg/kg Rodents: 1–2 mg/kg (Caligiuri et al. 1990) Cervids: up to 5 mg/kg Toxic dose varies with species; use lowest dose possible	1–2 mg/kg Toxic dose 4 mg/kg
Buprenorphine-SR (compounding pharmacy; sustained release; shelf-life 1 year, refrigerate)	1.8 mg/kg IM, SQ q12–24h	Carnivores: 0.06–0.12 mg/kg SQ q72h (Bloomfield et al. 1997) Rodents: 1–2 mg/kg SQ q 48–72h (Bodri et al. 2001; Bonar et al. 2003)	Currently not recommended
Butorphanol (can be compounded at 30–50 mg/mL by compounding pharmacy)	Most species: 1–4 mg/kg SQ, IM, IV q2–3h (Bowles 2006; Bowerman et al. 2010) Not recommended for use in American kestrels (Brown and Donnelly 2012) Very low oral bioavailability and short plasma half-life	Carnivores: 0.1–0.5 mg/kg SQ, IV, IM q2–4h Rabbits, small rodents: 0.1–0.5 mg/kg SQ, IM, IV q4–6h (Bush et al. 1981) Prairie dog: 2 mg/kg IM, SQ q4h (Caligiuri et al. 1990) Ruminants: 0.2–0.25 mg/kg IV, SQ q4h; do not recommend using alone (Barnard 2009)	Currently not recommended (Carpenter et al. 2005)
Carprofen	Use with caution (Catbagan et al. 2011) 3 mg/kg IM q 6–12h (Ceulemans et al. 2014)	Canids: 2.2mg/kg PO q12h Not recommended for felids Rabbits: 1–2 mg/kg PO q12h; 4 mg/kg SQ q24h Rodents: 2–5 mg/kg PO, SQ, IM q12–24h (Chitty 2003)	Use with caution (Coke et al. 2003) 2 mg/kg IM q 24h (Cole et al. 2009)
Fentanyl	Loading dose 2–5µg/kg SQ, IM + CRI 0.15–0.50 µg/kg/min IV (Cooper and Penaliggon 1997)	Most species: transdermal patch 1–5 µg/kg/h; dysphoria more prevalent at higher end of dose range (Barnard 2009)	Transdermal patch 12.5–25 µg/h may have some application in reptiles (Cybulski et al. 1996)
Gabapentin (compounded suspension has a shelf-life of ~90 days at 5°C/41°F)	10–80 mg/kg PO q8–12h (Dahlhausen 2006; Diaz-Figueroa and Mitchell 2006)	100 mg/kg (de la Navarre 2003)	Not commonly used

Drug	Birds	Mammals	Reptiles/Amphibians
Ketoprofen	Currently not recommended (Deeb and Carpenter 2004)	Rodents: 5 mg/kg SQ (Delk et al. 2014) Bats: 2–5 mg/kg SQ q24h Cervids: 3 mg/kg IV, IM q24h	2 mg/kg IM q 24h (DeMarco et al. 2002)
Lidocaine	2–3 mg/kg Potentially toxic dose (varies with species): 4–6 + mg/kg	Canids: <4 mg/kg Felids: <3 mg/kg Rabbits, rodents: 1–2 mg/kg (Caligiuri et al. 1990) Toxic dose varies with species; use lowest dose possible	Reptiles: 2–5 mg/kg Toxic dose varies with species; use lowest dose possible Amphibians: 1.0 mg/kg of 2% lidocaine topically
Meloxicam	0.5–2 mg/kg PO, IM, SQ q12–24h (Divers 1996; Desmarchelier et al. 2012) (use with caution in xerophilic species or hospitalized wild birds not able to have access to free- choice drinking water; discontinue if decrease in appetite seen) Compounded sustained-release meloxicam in kestrels 1.8 mg/kg q 24–48h (Blankespoor et al. 2001)	Canids: 0.2 mg/kg PO, IV, SQ, then 0.1 mg/kg PO q24h (Barnard 2009) Felids: Label dosage: 0.3 mg/kg SQ once for 3–4 day effect (Barnard 2009) Extralabel dosage: 0.2 mg/kg PO once, then 0.1 mg/kg PO q24h in food for 3–4 days Bats: 0.1 mg/kg PO q24h (Bechert et al. 2010) Rabbits: 1 mg/kg PO SID (di Somma et al. 2007) Rodents: 1–2 mg/kg PO, SQ q24 (a compounded sustained-release meloxicam reportedly used in rodents at 4 mg/kg q72h and rabbits 0.6 mg/kg q72h) (Donnelly 2004)	Reptiles: 0.2–0.4 mg/kg PO, SQ, IM q24h (Fernández-Varón et al. 2006) Amphibians: 0.1–0.4 mg/kg PO, SQ, ICe, IM q24h (Flammer 2002)
Morphine	Not commonly used in avian species	Canids: 0.5–2 mg/kg IM, SQ q4–6h Felids: 0.1–0.5 mg/kg IM, SQ q4–6h; do not recommend using alone (Barnard 2009) Rabbits, rodents: 2–5 mg/kg IM, SQ q2–4h (Caligiuri et al. 1990)	Most reptile species: 1–5 mg/kg IM q24h; monitor for respiratory depression (Flammer 1993) May be ineffective in snakes (Flammer et al. 2011) Amphibians: 30–100 mg/kg IM, SQ, topical; peak analgesia 60–90 m (Flammer 2002)
Tapentadol	No data at this time	Studies in domestic species only	Chelonians: 5 mg/kg IM q10h (Flecknell et al. 1999; Flecknell 2001)
Tramadol (compounded suspension has a shelf-life of 90 days at 5°C/41°F) (Fleming and Robertson 2012)	Most species: 5–30 mg/kg PO q6–12h (Gauvin 1993; Gentz et al. 1995; Gades et al. 2000; Funk and Diethelm 2006; Gamble 2008; Foley et al. 2011) (dosage inversely proportional to size; smaller birds may need higher doses given more frequently)	Canids: 3–5 mg/kg PO q8–12h (Barnard 2009) Felids: 0.5–2 mg/kg PO q12h (Barnard 2009) Rodents: 10–40 mg/kg PO q12–24h (weak analgesic; combine with NSAIDs) (Georoff et al. 2013) Not currently recommended for rabbits or deer	Chelonians: 5–10 mg/kg PO, SQ q24–72h (Gibbons 2014; Giorgi et al. 2014, 2015) No data in snakes

Anesthetic/Sedative Agents

	Birds	Mammals	Reptiles and Amphibians
Acepromazine	Currently not recommended	Prairie dog: 0.5–2.5 mg/kg IM (Graham et al. 2014) Beaver, porcupine: 0.1 mg/kg IM (Graham et al. 2014)	Currently not recommended
Alfaxalone	2 mg/kg IV (Griggs et al. 2015)	Most species: 5–10 mg/kg IM or 1.5 mg/kg IV (Guinotte et al. 1993)	Most reptile species: 6–30 mg/kg IM, IV (Guzman et al. 2011) Amphibians: 20–30 mg/kg IM (Guinotte et al. 1993)
Atipamezol	Give same volume as medetomidine or dexmedetomidine SQ, IV, IM	Give same volume as medetomidine or dexmedetomidine SQ, IV, IM	Give same volume as medetomidine or dexmedetomidine SQ, IM (IV use may cause severe hypotension)
Atropine sulfate (preanesthetic dose)	Most species: 0.01–0.02 mg/kg SQ, IM (not routinely used in smaller birds due to risk of increased viscosity of secretions plugging endotracheal tube)	Most species: 0.03–0.05 mg/kg SQ (Bechert et al. 2010) (may not be effective in lagomorphs and some rodents)	Most species but rarely indicated; 0.01–0.04 mg/kg SQ, IM
Dexmedetomidine	80 mg/kg IN with midazolam (Greenacre et al. 2006) 25–75 mg/kg IM (Guinotte et al. 1993) (given alone at this dose, adequate sedation for handling, but not intubation)	Generally insufficient alone to produce sedation in most wild mammals. Carnivores: 20–30 mg/kg + ketamine 3 mg/kg IM	30 mg/kg + ketamine 6 mg/kg IV in hatchling sea turtles (Guzman et al. 2011) Dexmedetomidine 70–100 mg/kg + midazolam 1–2 mg/kg + ketamine 1–5 mg/kg SQ/IM
Diazepam (available as a 1 mg/mL oral solution)	Most species: daily anxiolytic dose: 1–4 mg/kg PO q12h Most species: 0.05–1 mg/kg IV or IM	Prairie dog: 1–2.5 mg/kg IM, IP, PO Beaver, porcupine: 0.1–1.0 mg/kg IM, PO Bats: 0.5–2 mg/kg IM, SQ, PO (Bechert et al. 2010)	0.2–1 mg/kg IM, IV (generally used in combination with other chemical restraint agents like ketamine)
Flumazenil	0.05–0.1 mg/kg IM, IV (Greenacre et al. 2005) 0.05–0.3 mg/kg IN (Harris 2003)	0.01–0.05 mg/kg IM, IV, IO; repeat q1h PRN If using 5 mg/mL midazolam and 0.1 mg/mL flumazenil, use 2× the volume of midazolam given	0.008–0.01 mg/kg IM, IV, IO
Glycopyrrolate	0.02 mg/kg IM, IV (slower onset than atropine)	Prairie dog: 0.05 mg/kg SQ, IM (Giorgi et al. 2014) Beaver, porcupine: 0.01 mg/kg SQ, IM (Giorgi et al. 2014)	0.01 mg/kg IM, IV; rarely indicated
Ketamine combined with benzodiazepines or alpha-2 agonists	Rarely used; 5–30 mg/kg IM, IV, IO (Harrison et al. 2006)	Bats: 30–100 mg/kg SQ (Bechert et al. 2010) Rodents: 0.1–0.4 mg/kg/h CRI for postoperative analgesia (Hawkins and Pascoe 2007)	Most species: 5–50 mg/kg IM, IV (Hawkins and Pascoe 2012)
Midazolam	Raptors: 0.5–1 mg/kg IM, IV q8h (sedative, anticonvulsant) 2–5 mg/kg IN Waterfowl: 2–6 mg/kg IM	Carnivores: 0.2–0.4 mg/kg IV, IM 0.05–0.5 mg/kg/h IV CRI for recurrent seizures Rabbits, rodents: 1–2 mg/kg IV, IM Prairie dog: 1–2 mg/kg IM, IP (Giorgi et al. 2014) Beaver, porcupine: 0.1–0.5 mg/kg IM (Giorgi et al. 2014)	Most species: 1–2 mg/kg IM, IV

Propofol:
reduce dose with hypoproteinemia; supplemental oxygen recommended; induces profound respiratory depression; be prepared to ventilate

Most species:
1–15 mg/kg IV, IO slow bolus to effect (Hernandez-Divers 2001, 2003; Hawkins et al. 2003; Heard 2007)
0.5–1 mg/kg/min CRI (Hess 2004)
May experience rough recovery from CRI

Carnivores:
3–7 mg/kg IV slowly to effect
0.1–0.6 mg/kg/min CRI (sedation at lower doses; light anesthesia at higher doses)
Rabbits: 3–6 mg/kg IV slowly to effect; 1.2–1.3 mg/kg/min IV CRI
Rodents: 6–10 mg/kg IV slowly to effect (Giorgi et al. 2014)

Snakes:
5–10 mg/kg IV slow bolus
Chelonians:
7–10 mg/kg IV slow bolus (Hilf et al. 1991)

Amphibians: 10–30 mg/kg ICe; 75 ml/L immersion bath (lower dose for sedation or light anesthesia, induction within 30 min, recovery in 24h; bath provides sedation but duration/depth highly variable (Hillyer 1997)

Chemical immobilization: example combinations frequently used by the authors. Most can be followed by intubation and inhalant anesthetic drugs if general anesthesia is required

Ketamine 10–40 mg/kg + 0.2–2.0 mg/kg midazolam (Harrison et al. 2006)
OR
Butorphanol 1–2 mg/kg + 1 mg/kg midazolam (adequate sedation for physical therapy or lateral recumbancy or premedication prior to induction with inhalant anesthetic); reverse with flumazenil at 2× the volume of midazolam

Bear:
tiletamine-zolazepam 3–7 mg/kg (can concentrate up to 250 mg/mL; reconstitute with concentrated ketamine 2–5 mg/kg); prolonged recoveries
OR
medetomidine (20 mg/mL) 0.05 mg/kg + ketamine (200 mg/mL) 5 mg/kg for escapes/free-ranging wildlife; lower doses for routine immobilizations
medetomidine 0.02–0.025 mg/kg + ketamine 2–3 mg/kg
Reverse with atipamezole at 0.2 mg/kg IM
AND
To any of the above can add buprenorphine SR 0.06–0.12 mg/kg SQ q3d +/– meloxicam SR 0.6 mg/kg SQ q3d for analgesia

Snakes:
propofol 5–10 mg/kg IV slow bolus
OR
midazolam 1–2 mg/kg + dexmedetomidine 0.05 mg/kg and ketamine 10–40 mg/kg IM; reverse dexmedetomidine with equal volume of atipamezole IM

Chelonians:
propofol 7–10 mg/kg IV slow bolus
OR
Mild–moderate sedation – ketamine 5–10 mg/kg + dexmedetomidine 0.03–0.05 mg/kg IM +/– hydromorphone 0.3–0.5 mg/kg IM; reverse dexmedetomidine with equal volume of atipamezole IM

Concentrated formulations of ketamine (200 mg/mL), butorphanol (30–50 mg/mL) and medetomidine (20 mg/mL) are available from compounding pharmacies and are advised for larger mammals

Deer:
butorphanol 0.2–0.4 mg/kg + azaperone 0.15–0.30 mg/kg + medetomidine 0.05–0.1 mg/kg
OR
xylazine 2–3 mg/kg IM + ketamine 1 mg/kg IV once head down to prevent sudden arousal.
Reverse with yohimbine 0.2 mg/kg half IM and half IV

Bobcat:
0.01 mL per pound IM each of ketamine (100 mg/mL), dexmedetomidine (0.5 mg/mL), and butorphanol (10 mg/mL).
Deepen anesthesia with isoflurane for invasive procedures.
Reverse dexmedetomidine with equal volume of atipamezole IM (wait at least 30 min after ketamine is administered)

SR = sustained-release products available from compounding pharmacies

Coyote/fox:
dexmedetomidine 0.02 mg/kg with butorphanol 0.04 mg/kg IM; +/– ketamine 4 mg/kg IM or inhalant anesthetic for invasive procedures. Reverse with 0.2 mg/kg atipamezole IM (wait at least 30 min after ketamine is administered)

Raccoon/skunk:
ketamine 5 + 0.06 mg/kg medetomidine IM

Antibiotics

	Birds	Mammals	Reptiles and Amphibians
Amikacin	7–10 mg/kg SQ, IV, IM q12h (may cause myositis with IM injection; monitor renal function; maintain hydration) (Bloomfield et al. 1997) 3 g/40 g packet bone cement for PMMA bead formation; apply at site of infection, remove in 30 days	Rodents: 10–15 mg/kg SQ, IM, IV q12h (Yarto-Jaramillo 2015) Bats: 20 mg/kg SQ; q24h (Barnard 2009) *To make AIPMMA beads:* 1.25 g/20 g methylmethacrylate (Vennen and Mitchell 2009)	Reptiles: 2.5–5 mg/kg IM q48–72h (Caligiuri et al. 1990) Amphibians: 5 mg/kg IM, SQ, ICe q24–48h (Letcher and Papich 1994; Wright and Whitaker 2001)
Amoxicillin/ clavulanic acid (Clavamox®, Pfizer) or amoxicillin	Clavamox: 125–150 mg/kg PO q12h (Samour 2000) Amoxicillin: 100–150 mg/kg PO q12h (Mitchell and Tully 2009)	DO NOT USE in rabbits and certain species of rodents. OK in rats, mice, squirrels, bats, raccoons, opossums, wild felids and canids. Clavamox: 13–22 mg/kg PO q8–12h (Barnard 2009; Plumb 2015; pers. comm. Schott 2015) Amoxicillin: 10–20 mg/kg PO q8h (Plumb 2015)	Reptiles: amoxicillin (use with an aminoglycoside): 10–22 mg/kg PO, IM q12–24h (Mitchell and Tully 2009)
Ampicillin sodium + subbactam (Unasyn®, Pfizer) stable for 3 days refrigerated and 3 months frozen	200–300 mg/kg IM, IV slow q8h (Fernández-Varón et al. 2004, 2006)	For infections susceptible to amoxicillin–clavulanate in patients unable to receive oral doses (extra-label): 10–20 mg/kg IV or IM q8h (Plumb 2015)	No information available
Ampicillin trihydrate	100 mg/kg IM q4–8h (Harrison et al. 2006)	DO NOT USE in rats, mice, squirrels, raccoons, opossums: 20–30 mg/kg SQ, IM, IV q8h (Plumb 2015; pers. comm. Schott 2015) Canids and felids: 6.6 mg/kg SQ, IM q12h (Plumb 2015) Cervids: for respiratory infections, 11–22 mg/kg SQ q12–24h (Plumb 2015)	May use with an aminoglycoside 20–50 mg/kg IM q12–24h (Mitchell and Tully 2009; Schumacher 2011)
Azithromycin (Zithromax®)	40–45 mg/kg PO q24h for infection with intracellular organisms (*Chlamydophila, Mycobacteria, Plasmodium, Cryptosporidium*) (Carpenter et al. 2005) 10–20 mg/kg PO q48h for nonintracellular infections (Carpenter et al. 2005)	Carnivores: 5–10 mg/kg PO q24h × 3–5 days (Plumb 2015) Rabbits, rodents: 15–30 mg/kg PO q24h (Yarto-Jaramillo 2015) Bats: 20 mg/kg PO q24h (Barnard 2009)	10 mg/kg PO q2–7d (Coke et al. 2003)
Cefazolin sodium	Raptors: 50–100 mg/kg PO, IM q12h (Scott 2010) Other species: 25–75 mg/kg IM, IV q12h (Ritchie and Harrison 1997)	DO NOT USE in rabbits and rodents. Carnivores: 10–30 mg/kg SQ, IM, IV q8h (Plumb 2015) For making AIPMMA beads: 2 g per 20 g methylmethacrylate (Vennen and Mitchell 2009)	Chelonians: 22 mg/kg IM q24h (Johnson 2002)

Cefovecin (Convenia®)	Not currently recommended for use in birds due to short half-life (Thuesen et al. 2009; Wernick and Muntener 2010)	Carnivores: 8 mg/kg SQ once, repeat in 10 days if indicated (author experience in raccoons)	Not currently recommended for use in reptiles due to short half-life (Thuesen et al. 2009; Wernick and Muntener 2010)
Ceftazidime	50–100 mg/kg IM, IV q4–8h (Flammer 2002)	Carnivores: 25–30 mg/kg IV, IM q8–12h (Plumb 2015) Rabbits: 100 mg/kg IM q12h	20 mg/kg IM, IV q72h (Mader 2006; Mitchell and Tully 2009)
Ceftiofur crystalline-free acid (Excede®)	10 mg/kg IM q72h (Sadar et al. 2014) 20 mg/kg IM q96h (Hope et al. 2012)	VOPs: 2 mg/kg IM q24h q7–10 days Ruminants: 6.6 mg/kg SQ once, IM q4d Carnivores: 7 mg/kg SQ (Travis 2007; Jankowski et al. 2012)	Snakes: 15 mg/kg IM (Adkesson et al. 2011)
Cephalexin	50–100 mg/kg PO q4–8h (Bush et al. 1981, Samour 2000)	DO NOT USE in rabbits and certain species of rodents. OK in rats, mice, bats, squirrels, raccoons, opossums, wild felids and canids: 22–60 mg/kg PO q6–12h (Barnard 2009; Plumb 2015)	20–40 mg/kg PO q12h (Funk and Diethelm 2006)
Clindamycin	Most species: 50–100 mg/kg PO q12–24h (Harrison et al. 2006; Lenarduzzi et al. 2011)	DO NOT USE in rabbits/rodents/ruminants (Quesenberry and Carpenter 2004; Mitchell and Tully 2009) Carnivores: 15–30 mg/kg PO q12h Felids only: 11–33 mg/kg PO q24h (Plumb 2015)	5 mg/kg PO, IM q24h (Mader 2006; Mitchell and Tully 2009; Plumb 2015)
Doxycycline	Most species: 25–50 mg/kg PO q 12–24h	Carnivores: 5–10 mg/kg PO q12h (Plumb 2015) Rabbits, rodents: 2.5–5 mg/kg PO q12h (Quesenberry and Carpenter 2004)	Chelonians: 10 mg/kg PO q24h × 10–45 days for mycoplasmosis (Wright 1997; Mitchell and Tully 2009) Amphibians: 5–10 mg/kg PO q12h, q24h 10–50 mg/kg PO q24h (Wright and Whitaker 2001)
Enrofloxacin: injectable may cause tissue necrosis; in general, more than 1 IM injection not advised; appears stable when compounded (Petritz et al. 2013); dilute 1:10 to reduce irritation	Most species: 20–30 mg/kg PO, SQ, q24h (pulse dosing; if giving SQ, may dilute with saline 1:1) (Waxman et al. 2013) 15 mg/kg PO, IV q12–24h; may be given in food items (Wack et al. 2012) IV administration in owls may result in weakness, tachycardia, vasoconstriction; no detected effect on cartilage in day-old chicks	Canids: 5–20 mg/kg PO, IM, IV q24h (Plumb 2015) Felids: 5 mg/kg PO q24h (Plumb 2015) (contraindicated in young, growing canids and felids) Rabbits, rodents: 5–10 mg/kg PO, IM q12h (Donnelly 2004)	Chelonians: 5–10 mg/kg PO, IM q24–48h (James et al. 2003) Snakes: 10 mg/kg IM then 5–10 mg/kg IM, PO q48h (Young et al. 1997) Amphibians: 10 mg/kg q24h applied topically 5–10 mg/kg PO, SQ, IM q24h (Wright and Whitaker 2001)

(Continued)

	Birds	Mammals	Reptiles and Amphibians
Gentamicin: potential for nephrotoxicity high	Diluted to 5 mg/mL with sterile saline and used as sinus flush or for nebulization	Rodents: 1.5–2.5 mg/kg SQ, IM, IV q12h (Adamcak and Otten 2000)	Most reptiles: 2.5 mg/kg loading dose, then 1.5 mg/kg q96h; Amphibians: 8 µg/mL in 0.5% saline as 24 h bath × 5 days made fresh daily; 2–4 mg/kg IM q72h × 4 (Jacobson 1999)
Metronidazole	Most species: 25–50 mg/kg PO q12–24h	Rodents: 10–40 mg/kg PO q24h (Quesenberry and Carpenter 2004); Felids: 10–15 mg/kg PO q12h (Plumb 2015)	Amphibians: 50 mg/kg PO q24h × 3 days; 50 mg/L bath for up to 24 h (Wright and Whitaker 2001)
Penicillin G procaine	Not used routinely	DO NOT USE in rabbits/rodents; Carnivores: 20 000–40 000 IU/kg IV q6h; SQ, IM q12h (Plumb 2015); Cervids: 44 000–66 000 IU/kg IM, SQ q24h (Plumb 2015)	10 000–20 000 IU/kg SQ, IM, IV q8–12h
Piperacillin/tazobactam (Zosyn®, Wyeth)	100 mg/kg IV, IM q 6–12h (Nemetz and Lennox 2004)	Canids: 50 mg/kg IV q8h (Kuehn 2015)	Reptiles: 100 mg/kg IM, SQ q48h (dose extrapolated from PK study on piperacillin in pythons); Amphibians: 100 mg/kg IM, SQ q24h (based on piperacillin dose) (Wright 1997)
Trimethoprim/sulfadiazine (Tribrissen, Schering-Plough)	30–48 mg/kg PO q12h (Flammer 2002)	Rabbits, rodents: 30–48 mg/kg PO q12h (Adamcak and Otten 2000; Jenkins 2004); Carnivores: 15–30 mg/kg PO q12h; Bats: 15–30 mg/kg PO q12h (Barnard 2009)	Reptiles: 30 mg/kg PO q24h × 2d; then q48h (Jacobson 1999); Amphibians: 15 mg/kg PO q24h up to 21 days (Wright and Whitaker 2001)
Tylosin (Tylan®): injectable may cause tissue necrosis	Finch mycoplasmosis: 1 mg/mL of drinking water; give as only water source for 21 days; change water daily; make new solution q2 days (Mashima et al. 1997)	Carnivores: 10–40 mg/kg PO q12h (Plumb 2015); Rabbits: 10 mg/kg PO q12–24h (Quesenberry and Carpenter 2004); Not recommended for use in rodents; Cervids: 5–10 mg/kg IM or slow IV q24h not to exceed 5d (Plumb 2015)	Chelonians: mycoplasmosis 5 mg/kg IM once daily × 10d (Gauvin 1993)

Antifungals

	Birds	Mammals	Reptiles and Amphibians
Amphotericin B: efficacy against aspergillosis may be low; MIC indicated (Silvanose et al. 2011) Internal mycoses: study in leopard frogs naturally infected with *Batrachochytrichium dendrobatidis* showed reduction of infection but not complete fungal clearance	1.5 mg/kg IV q8h × 3–7 days (Flammer 1993) 1–1.5 mg/kg IT or intralesional via endoscope (dilute with sterile water if larger volume needed) (Jenkins 1991; Beynon et al. 1996) 7 mg/mL sterile water nebulization × 15 min q12h	Carnivores: 0.25 mg/kg IV 3 r/w. Total dose 8 mg/kg; 4 mg/kg if used with an azole (Oglesbee 2011b) Rabbits, rodents: 1 mg/kg IV q24h (Sanati et al. 1997)	Reptiles: 0.1 mg/kg intrapulmonary or intralesional q24h × 4w (Hernandez-Divers 2001) Amphibians: 1 mg/kg ICe q24h; 15 µg/mL continuous immersion bath (Wright and Whitaker, 2001; Holden et al. 2014)
Griseofulvin: administer with fatty meal; may cause bone marrow depression; monitor CBC during treatment	Dermatophytosis: 10 mg/kg PO q12h × 21d (Beynon et al. 1996)	Carnivores: dermatophytosis: 25 mg/kg PO q12h or 50 mg/kg PO q24h. Continue therapy 2 weeks beyond clinical resolution (Oglesbee 2011a) Rabbits, rodents: dermatophytosis: 25 mg/kg PO q24h × 28d (Hillyer 1997; Adamcak and Otten 2000)	Not routinely used
Itraconazole: give w/meal for most effective absorption; monitor liver function (Itrafungol® may be used) Chytridiomycosis, topical route best, do not use with larvae	Aspergillosis prophylaxis: 5–10 mg/kg PO q12h × 5–7d, then q24h × 14d, then q48h Aspergillosis treatment: 6–10 mg/kg PO q12–24h (Lumeij et al. 1995; Jones et al. 2000)	Carnivores: 5–10 mg/kg PO q24h (Plumb 2015) Rabbits: 5–10 mg/kg PO q24h for dermatophytosis (Hess 2004) Rodents: 5–10 mg/kg q12–24h (Lightfoot 2000)	Snakes and lizards: 5–10 mg/kg PO q24–48h; blood levels may persist for up to 14d after cessation (Gibbons 2014) Chelonians: 5 mg/kg PO q24h or 15 mg/kg PO q72h (Manire et al. 2003) Amphibians: 10 mg/kg PO q24h; 0.01% in 0.6% salt solution as 5 min bath buffered with sodium bicarbonate q24h × 11d; 0.0025% itraconazole bath × 5 min/day × 6 days (Georoff et al. 2013) Oral and enteric yeast infections: 100 000 units/kg topically and PO q24h (Mader 2006)
Nystatin 100 000 IU/mL suspension: apply topically to oral lesions	Oral candidiasis: 100 000–300 000 IU/kg topically or PO q12h × 7–14d (Dahlhausen 2006)	Carnivores: oral candidiasis: 50 000–150 000 IU topically or PO q6–8h (Plumb 2015) Marsupials: 5000 IU/kg PO q8–12h (Ness and Johnson-Delaney 2012) Rodents: 60 000–100 000 units topically or PO q 8h (Mans and Donnelly 2012)	

(Continued)

	Birds	Mammals	Reptiles and Amphibians
Terbinafine	Raptors: 22 mg/kg PO q24h (Bechert et al. 2010) Questionable efficacy against aspergillosis; may be more effective when used in combination with itraconazole	Carnivores: dermatophytosis: 10–20 mg/kg PO q24h. Can do pulse therapy (7 d on, 21 d off) (Plumb 2015) Rabbits: 8–20 mg/kg PO q24h (Hess 2004) Rodents: 10–40 mg/kg PO q24h (Oglesbee 2011a)	Reptiles: 10 mg/kg PO q24h (Klaphake 2005a) Amphibians: 0.01% bath 15 min q24h (Wright 2014) 0.005–0.01% bath × 5 min × 5d. Dilute in ethanol (Bowerman et al. 2010)
Voriconazole	Raptors: 12.5 mg/kg PO q12h × 3 days then q12–24 h for 44–100 days (di Somma et al. 2007)	Canids: 4 mg/kg PO q12h (Plumb 2015) Not recommended in felids due to significant side effects	10 mg/kg PO q24h (Waeyenberghe et al. 2010)

Antiparasitics

	Birds	Mammals	Reptiles and Amphibians
Carbaryl powder 5% (Sevin® dust)	For ectoparasites, dust over feathers (Samour 2000)	Most species: for ectoparasites, dust lightly q7d (Morrisey and Carpenter 2004)	No data
Nitenpyram (Capstar®): Capstar wound flush: one 11.4 mg tablet crushed and mixed with 30 mL sterile 0.9% NaCl	Topical flush	Carnivores: fleas, myiasis: 11.4 mg (1 tablet) PO for animals weighing 0.9–11.36 kg (Plumb 2015) Rodents: myiasis: 1 mg/kg PO once *Can halve and quarter tablets for smaller wildlife patients	Reptiles: for maggots (extra-label): crush one 11.4 mg tablet into powder and give PO, as an enema, or on wound one time (Klaphake 2005a)
Fenbendazole (Panacur®): toxicosis reported in vultures, storks (Bonar et al. 2003); pigeons, doves (Howard et al. 2002); porcupines (Weber et al. 2006); rabbits (Graham et al. 2014)	May cause feather abnormalities if used during molt. Mortality reported in cormorants with *Cyathostoma* sp within 24 h of deworming. (Barron, pers. commun. 2016)	Canids, felids (Plumb 2015): ascarids, hookworms, whipworms, *Taenia*: 50 mg/kg PO q24h × 3–5d *Paragoninus*:25–50 mg/kg PO q12h × 10–14d *Giardia*: 50 mg/kg PO q24h × 3–7d Ursids: 10 mg/kg PO q24h × 3d Rabbits: 10–20 mg/kg PO q24h × 5d; repeat q14d Prairie dogs and other rodents: 10–25 mg/kg PO q24h × 5d (Lightfoot 2000) Ruminants: 15 mg/kg PO q24h × 3d Marsupials: *Capillaria*: 25 mg/kg PO q24h × 5d	Reptiles*: 25–50 mg/kg PO q24h × 4 treatments (Diaz-Figueroa and Mitchell 2006) Amphibians*: 50 mg/kg PO q24h × 3–5d. Repeat in 14–21d. (Wright and Whitaker 2001) 25–50 mg/kg PO q24h × 3d. Repeat in 14d (Wright 2014)
***Leukopenia may occur with prolonged treatment or overdosage (Neiffer et al. 2005; Wright 2014)**	25–50 mg/kg PO q24h × 5d; repeat in two weeks (Huckabee 2000)		
Fipronil	Topical light spray 1× (Redig 2003)	Most species; do NOT use in rabbits (Cooper and Penaliggon 1997; Plumb 2015)	No data
Imidacloprid/Moxidectin	0.2 mg/kg topically PRN (BSAVA)	Most species: 0.2 mg/kg topically PRN (Wagner and Wendlberger 2000)	No data
Ivermectin Intravenous lipid emulsion has been successfully used to treat ivermectin toxicosis in mammals (Kidwell et al. 2014)	Most species: *Knemidokoptes, Dermanyssus*, ascarids, *Capillaria*, gapeworm: 0.2–0.4 mg/kg PO, SQ, topical once q7–14d Intramuscular administration may result in propylene glycol (PG) toxicosis, particularly in smaller birds. Can dilute solution further with PG if needed for smaller animals if giving PO or topically	Canids: Sarcoptes: 0.3–0.4 mg/kg PO, SQ q7d for weeks Endoparasites (*Capillaria, Oslerus, Eucoleus, Pneumonyssoides*): 0.2–0.4 mg/kg SQ once Felids: *Aelurostrongylus*: 0.4 mg/kg SQ once Rabbits, rodents: *Sarcoptes*, fur mites, ear mites: 0.3–0.4 mg/kg SQ q10–14d (Quesenberry and Carpenter 2004) Bats: toxicosis reported; use not recommended	Reptiles: DO NOT USE IN CHELONIANS, SKINKS, INDIGO SNAKES Nematodes, mites: 0.2 mg/kg PO, SQ, IM, topical q14d (Diaz-Figueroa and Mitchell 2006) Amphibians: 0.2–0.4 mg/kg PO once; 0.2–0.4 mg/kg PO or IM q14d (Wright 1996)

(Continued)

	Birds	Mammals	Reptiles and Amphibians
Metronidazole	Most species: 25–50 mg/kg PO q12–24h (Cybulski et al. 1996)	Carnivores: *Giardia*: 15–25 mg/kg PO q12h × 5–7d (Plumb 2015) Rabbits: anaerobic infections: 20 mg/kg PO q12h or 40 mg/kg PO q24h × 3–5d (Ivey and Morrisey 2000) Rodents: 10–40 mg/kg PO q24h (Brown and Donnelly 2012)	Reptiles: 20 mg/kg PO q24h or 40 mg/kg q48h (Kolmstetter et al. 1998; Bodri et al. 2001) Amphibians: 10 mg/kg PO once; 10 mg/kg PO q24h 5–10d; 50 mg/kg PO q24h for 3–5d; 50 mg/L bath for up to 24h (Poynton and Whitaker 1994; Wright 1996)
Mefloquine	Raptors: *Plasmodium*: 30 mg/kg PO at time 0h, 12h, 24h, 48h (Tavernier et al. 2005)	Not applicable	Not applicable
Praziquantel (Droncit®)	Cestodes, trematodes: 10 mg/kg PO repeat in 7–14 days; higher doses needed to treat schistosomes (Blankespoor et al. 2001)	Carnivores: cestodes: 5–10 mg/kg PO, SQ Trematodes: 20–25 mg/kg PO q24h × 3–10d (Plumb 2015) Rabbits, rodents: cestodes, trematodes: 5–10 mg/kg PO, SQ, IM; repeat in 10d (Jenkins 2004)	Reptiles: cestodes, trematodes: 8 mg/kg PO, SQ, IM; repeat in 14d (Diaz-Figueroa and Mitchell 2006) Amphibians: 10 mg/L bath up to 3h q7–21d; 8–24 mg/kg PO, SQ, ICe or topically q7–21d (Wright 1996)
Pyrantel pamoate	4.5–25 mg/kg PO once; can repeat in 2 weeks (Samour 2000)	Carnivores, rabbits: 5–10 mg/kg PO after meal q2–3weeks (Ivey and Morrisey 2000; Plumb 2015) Rodents: 50 mg/kg PO once (Adamcak and Otten 2000)	5 mg/kg PO q14d
Quinacrine	Hemoparasites: 5–10 mg/kg PO q24h × 7d	Rodents; antiprotozoal: 75 mg/kg PO q8h (Adamcak and Otten 2000)	Hemoparasites: 20–100 mg/kg PO q48h × 2–3w
Selamectin (Revolution®)	6 mg/kg topical spray for lice (anecdotal reports)	All species: 6–12 mg/kg topically once, repeat 10–14d for mites or q30d for fleas (Oglesbee 2011a)	Not recommended for chelonians
Sulfadimethoxine (Albon®)	25–50 mg/kg PO q12–24h × 3–7d	Carnivores: coccidiosis: 55 mg/kg PO, then 25 mg/kg PO q24h × 10–20d Ruminants: coccidiosis: 55 mg/kg PO, then 25 mg/kg PO q24h >4d or until clinical signs resolve Rabbits (Gentz et al. 1995): coccidiosis: 50 mg/kg PO once. Then 25 mg/kg PO q24h × 21d Rodents: coccidiosis: 50 mg/kg PO, then 25 mg/kg PO q24h × 10–20d	50 mg/kg PO q24h × 5d then q48h PRN (Diaz-Figueroa and Mitchell 2006)

Fluids and Emergency Drugs

	Birds	Mammals	Reptiles and Amphibians
Activated charcoal	2–8 g/kg PO PRN (Samour 2000)	Carnivores: 1–4 g/kg with 5–10 mL of water per g of charcoal PO q4–6h (Plumb 2015) Rabbits, rodents: 2–3 g/kg PO (Idid and Lee 1996)	No data
Atropine (0.54 mg/mL) **QUICK DOSE FOR CARNIVORE** **CPCR: 0.5 mL/10lb (or 5 kg) IV;** **1 mL/10lb (or 5 kg) intratracheal** **QUICK DOSE FOR AVIAN CPCR:** **0.1 mL/100 g IM, IV, IO, IT**	Bradycardia: 0.2 mg/kg IM, IV, IO CPCR: 0.5 mg/kg IM, IV, IO, IT (O'Malley 2011) Organophosphate toxicity: 0.2 mg/kg IM q3–4h PRN (Harrison et al. 2006)	Carnivores: bradycardia: 0.02–0.04 mg/kg IM, IV (Plumb 2015) CPCR: 0.04 mg/kg IV, IO; repeat q3–5 min PRN for maximum of 3 doses OR 0.08–0.1 mg/kg intratracheal; dilute with 5–10 mL sterile water before administration (Plumb 2015) Organophosphate toxicity: 0.2–0.5 mg/kg; give ¼ dose IV and remainder IM, SQ (Plumb 2015) Rodents: organophosphate toxicity: 10 mg/kg SQ q20min (Ivey and Morrisey 2000) Preanesthetic: 0.05 mg/kg IM, SQ (Heard 2004) Rabbits: many have serum atropinase and need higher doses: 0.8–1 mg/kg IM, SQ (Olson et al. 1994)	Organophosphate toxicity: 0.1–0.2 mg/kg SQ, IM (Gauvin 1993; Wright and Whitaker 2001)
Crystalloid bolus volume for shock	10–15 ml/kg IV, IO over 5–10 minutes	90 mL/kg – administer ¼ of total dose over 15 min, then reassess heart rate, blood pressure, mucous membranes	No data
Diazepam **QUICK DOSE FOR CARNIVORE** **STATUS EPILEPTICUS: 0.5 mL/10lb** **IV; 1 mL/10lb rectally**	Seizures: 0.5–1 mg/kg IM, IV, IO, PRN (Samour 2000)	Carnivores: status epilepticus or cluster seizures: 0.5–1 mg/kg IV, intranasally, rectally. Repeat twice PRN (Plumb 2015) Rabbits, rodents: 1–3 mg/kg IM, IV, IO (Oglesbee 2011a)	Seizures: 0.5 mg/kg, IM (Hernandez-Divers 2003)
Dexamethasone sodium phosphate; **methylprednisolone sodium succinate**	Steroid use generally not recommended in birds (Rosenthal 2004), but the exception may be a single dose of Dex SP in cases of acute retinal trauma (Korbel, pers. commun.)	High-dose (e.g. 30 mg/kg IV), fast-acting corticosteroids are no longer recommended for use in shock or CNS trauma (still controversial); recent studies have not demonstrated significant benefit and it actually may cause increased deleterious effects (Plumb 2015)	Currently not recommended
Dextrose 50%	Hypoglycemia: 50–100 mg/kg IV slow bolus; can dilute with fluids (Ritchie 1990)	Hypoglycemia: 0.5 g/kg IV bolus (dilute by half to make a 25% solution), follow up with CRI of 5% dextrose in a balanced electrolyte solution (Plumb 2015) Small mammal CPR: 0.25 mL/kg, 50% dextrose diluted 50% w/saline (Lichtenberger 2012)	Hypoglycemia: 0.5 g/kg IV slow bolus (Funk and Diethelm 2006)
Edetate calcium disodium (CaEDTA) Nephrotoxic; consider administration of fluids during treatment to maintain hydration	35 mg/kg IM, IV q12h × 5d. Recheck lead levels after 5 days of treatment; if still elevated, allow 3-day rest period before restarting treatment (Harrison et al. 2006)	Most species: 25 mg/kg SQ q6–12h × 5d. Recheck lead levels after 5 days of treatment; if still elevated, allow 5–7-day rest period before restarting treatment. (Lightfoot 2000; Deeb and Carpenter 2004; Plumb 2015)	Chelonians: 35 mg/kg IM q24h (Chitty 2003)

(Continued)

	Birds	Mammals	Reptiles and Amphibians
Epinephrine 1:1000 (1 mg/mL) **Large mammal cheat dose: 0.5–1 mL per 10 lbs (or 5 kg) IV, IO, IT** **Small mammal/avian/reptile cheat dose: 0.01 mL per 100 g IV, IO, IT**	0.1 mg/kg IV, IO, IT (Harris 2003)	Most species: use of low-dose (0.01 mg/kg IV/IO) epinephrine administered every 3–5 min early in CPR is recommended, but high-dose (0.1 mg/kg IV/IO) epinephrine may be considered after prolonged CPR: 0.1–0.2 mg/kg IV, IO, IT; dilute in 5–10 mL sterile water or saline for IT administration (Ramer et al. 1999; Lichtenberger 2012; Plumb 2015)	0.1 mg/kg IV, intracardiac (Funk and Diethelm 2006)
Furosemide	Pulmonary edema, ascites: 0.15–2 mg/kg/day IM, PO (Pees et al. 2006)	Carnivores: pulmonary edema, ascites: 2–4 mg/kg IM, IV q1–2h until respiration improves (Plumb 2015) Rabbits: pulmonary edema: 1–4 mg/kg IM, IV q4–12h (Huston 2004)	Pulmonary edema, ascites: 2–5 mg/kg q12–24h PO, IM, IV (Gauvin 1993)
Hetastarch	10–15 mL/kg IV, IO bolus over 15 min q8h for up to 4 treatments (Joseph 1998); maximum of 20 mL/kg/day	Canids: 10–20 mL/kg IV bolus 15–30 min 1–2 mL/kg/h IV CRI; do not exceed 25 mL/kg/day Felids: 5–10 mL/kg IV bolus over 15–30 min 1–2 mL/kg/h IV CRI; do not exceed 10 mL/kg/day (Plumb 2015) Rabbits: 20 mL/kg IV (Mitchell and Tully 2009)	Reptiles: 3–5 mL/kg IV, IO bolus over several minutes; do not exceed 10 mL/kg/day (author experience) Amphibians: Hetastarch 6% in 0.9% saline; bath not to exceed 1h without reassessment (Wright 2014)
Hypertonic saline (HTS) 7.5%	Hypovolemic shock, head trauma: 3 mL/kg IV, IO; consider using with a colloid to prolong effect (1 part HTS:5 parts HES; max bolus volume 15 mL/kg) (author experience)	Head trauma, pulmonary contusions: 4–6 mL/kg slow bolus; consider using with a colloid to prolong effect (Plumb 2015)	No data
Maintenance fluid rate	70–120 mL/kg/day	Carnivores: 40–60 mL/kg/day OR $(140 \times BW)^{0.73}$/day Rabbits, rodents: 75–100 mL/kg/day	25–30 mL/kg/day Reptile lactated Ringer's solution (LRS): 1 part LRS + 1 part 5% dextrose +1 part 0.9% NaCl OR 1 part LRS + 2 parts 2.5% dextrose in 0.45% NaCl Amphibian LRS: 6.6 g NaCl, 0.15 g KCL, 0.15 g $CaCl_2$, 0.2 g $NHCO_3$, in 1 L H_2O for treating hydrocoelom and SQ edema (soak 24h or until stable)
Mannitol	0.2–2 mg/kg IV over 10–20 min q24h (Joseph 1998)	Carnivores: most species: traumatic brain injury: 0.5–1.5 g/kg IV over 10–20 min. Repeat q6–8h PRN for maximum of three boluses and only if patient is showing response (Plumb 2015)	No data
Pralidoxime (2-PAM)	10–20 mg/kg IM q8–12h (Jones 2007) 10–100 mg/kg IM q24–48h (Samour 2000)	Carnivores: 20 mg/kg IM, SQ or IV (slowly) q6–12h until nicotinic signs are present	

Nutritional Supplements and Miscellaneous

	Birds	Mammals	Reptiles and Amphibians
Acetylcysteine: OK in refrigerator for 6 months; do not freeze	Nebulize 50 mg as a 2% solution diluted with saline over 15–30 min for mucoid nasal discharge. Monitor respiration (author experience)	Most species: nebulize 50 mg as a 2% solution diluted with saline (Oglesbee 2011a, b; Plumb 2015)	Tortoises: nebulize 50 mg as a 2% solution diluted with saline over 30–60 min for mucoid nasal discharge (author experience)
Calcium gluconate: dilute the 23% solution 1:1 with saline or sterile water for IV or IM administration	Hypocalcemic tetany, dystocia: 50–100 mg/kg IV slowly to effect (can be given IM if venous access is unavailable)	Most species hypocalcemia: 94–140 mg/kg IV slowly to effect; monitor respiration and cardiac rhythm during administration. Halt administration if arrhythmias occur (Plumb 2015) Hyperkalemic cardiotoxicity (serum K+ >8 mEq/L): 50–100 mg/kg IV over 10–20 min; monitor ECG (Plumb 2015)	Reptiles: Hypocalcemic tetany, dystocia: 100 mg/kg SQ, IM, ICe q6–24h (Funk and Diethelm 2006) Amphibians: 2–5% daily baths with 2 IU vitamin D3 per 10–100 mL of water (Wright 2006)
Cimetidine	10–25 mg/kg PO, IM, IV q12h (Guinotte et al. 1993; Tully 1996)	Most species: 5–10 mg/kg IM, IV, PO, SQ q6–12h (Ivey and Morrisey 2000; Plumb 2015)	Reptiles: 4 mg/kg IM, PO q8–12h (Gauvin 1993)
Diphenhydramine	2–4 mg/kg IM, IV, PO q12h (Ritchie and Harrison 1997)	Most species: 2–5 mg/kg PO, SQ, IM, IV (Barnard 2009; Plumb 2015)	No data
Famotidine	Not effective in chickens, even at high doses (Guinotte et al. 1993)	Most species: 0.5 mg/kg IM, IV, PO, SQ q6–12h (Oglesbee 2011a, b; Plumb 2015)	No data
Iron dextran	10 mg/kg IM q7d (Samour 2008)	Carnivores: 10–20 mg/kg IM followed by oral therapy (Plumb 2015) Rabbits: 4–6 mg/kg IM once (Quesenberry and Carpenter 2004)	Reptiles: 12 mg/kg IM 1–2×/week (Mader 2006; Mitchell and Tully 2009)
Isoxsuprine	Raptors: 5–10 mg/kg PO q24h (Redig 2003)	Canids: 1 mg/kg PO q24h (Plumb 2015)	No data
Lactulose	0.2–1 mL/kg PO q8–12h (Samour 2000)	Carnivores: 0.25–0.5 mL/kg PO q6–8h until stools are loose (Plumb 2015)	Reptiles: 0.3–0.5 mL/kg PO q12–24h (Stahl 1999; author experience)
Loperamide	No data	Most species: 0.1 mg/kg PO q8h × 3d. Then q24h × 2d. Give in 1 mL water (Ivey and Morrisey 2000; Oglesbee 2011a, b)	No data
Maropitant	No data	Carnivores: 0.5–1 mg/kg SQ or IV slow q24h OR 2–4 mg/kg PO q24h up to 5 consecutive days (Oglesbee 2011a, b; Plumb 2015)	No data

(Continued)

	Birds	Mammals	Reptiles and Amphibians
Meclizine	No data	Most species: 2–12 mg/kg PO q12–24h (Ivey and Morrisey 2000; Oglesbee 2011a, b; Plumb 2015)	No data
Metoclopramide	Raptors, waterfowl: 0.5–2 mg/kg IV, IM, PO q8–12h PRN (Samour 2000; author experience)	Carnivores: 0.2–0.4 mg/kg PO, SQ q6–8h Rabbits: 0.2–1.0 mg/kg IM, PO, SQ q12h (Oglesbee 2011a, b)	Reptiles: 0.06 mg/kg PO q24h × 7d (Divers 1996) Chelonians: 1–10 mg/kg PO q24h
Omeprazole	10–100 mg/kg PO q24h (author uses 20 mg/kg PO q24h) × 3d. Feed only soft foods as increase in gut pH limits ability to digest bones, etc. (Guinotte et al. 1993; Hinrichsen et al. 1997)	Carnivores: 0.5–1 mg/kg PO q24h (Plumb 2015)	No data
Oxytocin	3–5 IU/kg IM. May repeat q30m × 3 if ureterovaginal sphincter dilated (Samour 2000) Alternatively, use PGE2A gel topically if ureterovaginal sphincter not dilated (Bowles 2006)	Most species: 0.2–3 IU/kg IM, IV, SQ	Reptiles: 5–20 IU/kg. Repeat in 20–60 min if required. Better in turtles than snakes/lizards. Efficacy increased if used with PGF2A (Feldman, pers. commun.)
Simethicone (66 mg/mL)	No data	Most species (adult or infant): 60 mg/kg PO q8–12h or at every feeding for infants (Oglesbee 2011a, b). Also consider burping nursing neonates after every feeding	No data
Succimer (DMSA)	20–40 mg/kg PO q12h		
Sucralfate	25 mg/kg PO q12h	Most species: 25–125 mg/kg PO q8h; give 30–60 min after histamine-2 blockers	
Vitamin B complex (dose based on thiamine/B1)	10–30 mg/kg IM q7d (Samour 2008)	Carnivores: 10–20 mg/kg IM, SQ q8–12h PRN (Plumb 2015) Ruminants: 10 mg/kg IV, then 10 mg/kg IM q12h for 2–3d (Plumb 2015) Rodents: 2–20 mg/kg SQ, IM (Quesenberry and Carpenter 2004; Mitchell and Tully 2009)	Reptiles: 5–10 mg/kg SQ, IM (Mader 2006)
Vitamin E-selenium (Bo-Se 1 mg/mL; Mu-Se 5 mg/mL)	Prevention of capture myopathy in ratites, other long-legged species: 0.06 mg/kg IM once Raptors: vitamin E only: 15 mg/kg IM, PO (Mainka et al. 1994)	Ruminants: 0.3 mL/10 lbs SQ, IM (Plumb 2015)	Reptiles: no data Amphibians: 100 IU/kg PO q7d (Wright 2014)

To reduce nasal congestion (author's experience; we put in insulin syringe, cut the needle off at hub and then use to put drop up nose)

No data

Most species:
hypertonic saline (dilute to 2% with normal saline) 3–4 drops each nostril 3–4×/day

Cerenia (reduces substance P, the primary inflammatory cytokine involved in nasal inflammation): dilute 1:10 with normal saline and put 1 drop in each nostril 1–2×/day

Phenylephrine hydrochloride:
1 drop each nostril 1–2×/day for no more than 3 days to try to avoid rebound effect
Oxymetazoline HCL 0.05%
(OR xylometazoline 0.05%):1 drop each nostril 1–2×/day for no more than 3 days to try to avoid rebound effect

Tortoises:
hypertonic saline (dilute to 2% with normal saline) 3–4 drops each nostril 3–4×/day

"Carnivores" may include wild North American felids, canids, procyonids, ursids, and mustelids.

"Rodents" may include wild North American flying, tree, and ground squirrels; rats, mice, beaver, prairie dogs, ground hogs, and porcupines

NOTE: Many species of wildlife are hunted for human consumption. Drugs prohibited for use in food animals should not be administered to these species if they will be released to the wild and/or consumed by humans. See www.farad.org for list of drugs prohibited from use in food animals.

CBC, complete blood count; CNS, central nervous system; CPCR, cardiopulmonary cerebral resuscitation; CRI, constant rate infusion; ECe, epicoelomic; ECG, electrocardiogram; ICe, intracoelomic; IM, intramuscular; IN, intranasal; IO, intraosseous; IP, intraperitoneal; IT, intratracheal; IU, international unit; IV, intravenous; MIC, minimum inhibitory concentration; SQ, subcutaneous; NSAID, nonsteroidal antiinflammatory drug; OTM, orotransmucosal; PO, orally; PRN, as needed; SQ, subcutaneous.

References

Adamcak, A. and Otten, B. (2000). Rodent therapeutics. *Vet. Clin. North Am. Exotic Anim. Pract.* 3 (1): 221–240.

Adkesson, M., Fernandez-Varon, E., Cox, S. et al. (2011). Pharmacokinetics of a long-acting ceftiofur formulation (ceftiofur crystalline free acid) in the ball python (*Python regius*). *J. Zoo Wildl. Med.* 42 (3): 444–450.

Baker, B.B., Sladky, K.K., and Johnson, S.M. (2011). Evaluation of the analgesic effects of oral and subcutaneous tramadol administration in red-eared slider turtles. *J. Am. Vet. Med. Assoc.* 238: 220–227.

Barnard, S.M. (ed.) (2009). *Bats in Captivity: Volume 1– Biological and Medical Aspects*, 494–558. Washington, DC: Logos Press.

Bechert, U., Christensen, J.M., Poppenga, R. et al. (2010). Pharmacokinetics of terbinafine after single oral dose administration in Red-Tailed Hawks (*Buteo jamaicensis*). *J. Avian Med. Surg.* 24 (2): 122–130.

Beynon, P.H., Forbes, N.A., and Harcourt-Brown, N.H. (1996). *Manual of Pigeons, Raptors, and Waterfowl.* Ames, IA: Iowa State University Press.

Black, P.A., Cox, S.K., Macek, M. et al. (2010). Pharmacokinetics of tramadol hydrochloride and its metabolite O-desmethyltramadol in peafowl (Pavo cristatus). *J. Zoo Wildl. Med.* 41: 671–676.

Blankespoor, C.L., Reimink, R.L., and Blankespoort, H.D. (2001). Efficacy of praziquantel in treating natural schistosome infections in common mergansers. *J. Parasitol.* 87: 424–426.

Bloomfield, R.B., Brooks, D., and Vulliet, R. (1997). The pharmacokinetics of a single intramuscular dose of amikacin in red-tailed hawks (Buteo jamaicensis). *J. Zoo Wildl. Med.* 28: 55–61.

Bodri, M.S., Rambo, T.M., Wagner, R.A. et al. (2006). Pharmacokinetics of metronidazole administered as a single oral bolus to corn snakes, Elaphe guttata. *J Herpetol Med Surg* 16 (1): 15–19.

Bonar, C.J., Lewandowski, A.H., and Schaul, J. (2003). Suspected fenbendazole toxicity in 2 vulture species (*Gyps africanus, Torgos tracheliotus*) and Marabou storks (*Leptotilus crumeniferus*). *J. Avian Med. Surg.* 17 (1): 16–19.

Bowerman, J., Rombough, C., Weinstock, S. et al. (2010). Terbinafine hydrochloride in ethanol effectively clears Batrachochytrium dendrobatidis in amphibians. *J. Herpetol. Med. Surg.* 20 (1): 24–28.

Bowles, H.L. (2006). Evaluating and treating the reproductive system. In: *Clinical Avian Medicine* (ed. G.J. Harrison and T.L. Lightfoot), 528. Palm Beach, FL: Spix Publishing.

Brown, C. and Donnelly, T.M. (2012). Disease problems of small rodents. In: *Ferrets, Rabbits, and Rodents: Clinical Medicine and Surgery*, 3e (ed. K.E. Quesenberry and J.W. Carpenter), 354–372. St Louis, MO: Elsevier Saunders.

Bush, M., Locke, D., Neal, L.A., and Carpenter, J.W. (1981). Pharmacokinetics of cephalothin and cephalexin in selected avian species. *Am. J. Vet. Res.* 42 (6): 1014–1017.

Caligiuri, R., Kollias, G.V., Jacobson, E. et al. (1990). The effects of ambient temperature on amikacin pharmacokinetics in gopher tortoises. *J. Vet. Pharmacol. Ther.* 13 (3): 287–291.

Carpenter, J.W., Olsen, J.H., Hunter, R.P. et al. (2005). Pharmacokinetics of azithromycin in the blue and gold macaw. *J Zoo Wildl Med* 36 (4): 606–609.

Catbagan, D.L., Quimby, J.M., Mama, K.R. et al. (2011). Comparison of the efficacy and adverse effects of sustained-release buprenorphine hydrochloride following subcutaneous administration and buprenorphine hydrochloride following oral transmucosal administration in cats undergoing ovariohysterectomy. *Am. J. Vet. Res.* 72 (4): 461–466.

Ceulemans, S.M., Guzman, D.S., Olsen, G.H. et al. (2014). Evaluation of thermal antinociceptive effects after intramuscular administration of buprenorphine hydrochloride to American kestrels (Falco sparverius). *Am. J. Vet. Res.* 75: 705–710.

Chitty JR. (2003). Lead toxicosis in a Greek tortoise. Proceedings of the Association of Reptilian and Amphibian Veterinarians: p. 101.

Coke, R.L., Hunter, R.P., Isaza, R. et al. (2003). Pharmacokinetics and tissue concentrations of azithromycin in ball pythons (Python regius). *Am. J. Vet. Res.* 64 (2): 225–228.

Cole, G.A., Paul-Murphy, J., Krugner-Higby, L. et al. (2009). Analgesic effects of intramuscular administration of meloxicam in Hispaniolan parrots (Amazona ventralis) with experimentally induced arthritis. *Am. J. Vet. Res.* 70: 1471–1476.

Cooper, P.E. and Penaliggon, J. (1997). Use of frontline spray on rabbits. *Vet. Rec.* 140 (20): 535–536.

Cybulski, W., Larrson, P., Tjalve, H. et al. (1996). Disposition of metronidazole in hens (Gallus gallus) and quail (Coturnix coturnix japonica): pharmacokinetics and whole-body autoradiography. *J. Vet. Pharmacol. Ther.* 19: 352–358.

Dahlhausen, R.D. (2006). Implications of mycoses in clinical disorders. In: *Clinical Avian Medicine* (ed. G.J. Harrison and T.L. Lightfoot), 701. Palm Beach, FL: Spix Publishing.

Deeb, B.J. and Carpenter, J.W. (2004). Neurologic and musculoskeletal diseases. In: *Ferrets, Rabbits, and Rodents: Clinical Medicine and Surgery*, 2e (ed. K.E. Quesenberry and J.W. Carpenter), 209. St Louis, MO: Saunders.

de la Navarre B. (2011). Common parasitic diseases of reptiles and amphibians. Proceedings of the Western Veterinarians Conference.

Delk, K.W., Carpenter, J.W., Kukanich, B. et al. (2014). Pharmacokinetics of meloxicam administered orally to rabbits (Oryctolagus cuniculus) for 29 days. *Am. J. Vet. Res.* 75: 195–199.

DeMarco, J.H., Heard, D.J., Fleming, G.J. et al. (2002). Ivermectin toxicosis after topical administration in dog-faced fruit bats (Cynopterus brachyotis). *J. Zoo Wildl. Med.* 33 (2): 147–150.

Desmarchelier, M., Troncy, E., Fitzgerald, G. et al. (2012). Analgesic effects of meloxicam administration on postoperative orthopedic pain in domestic pigeons (Columba livia). *Am. J. Vet. Res.* 73: 361–367.

Di Somma, A. et al. (2007). The use of Voriconazole for the treatment of Aspergillosis in Falcons (*Falco* Species). *J. Avian Med. Surg.* 21 (4): 307–316.

Diaz-Figueroa, O. and Mitchell, M.A. (2006). Gastrointestinal anatomy and physiology. In: *Reptile Medicine and Surgery*, 2e (ed. D.R. Mader), 155. St Louis, MO: Saunders Elsevier.

Divers SJ. (1996). Constipation in snakes with particular reference to surgical correction in a Burmese python (Python molurus bivittatus). Proceedings of the Association of Reptilian and Amphibian Veterinarians: pp. 119–123.

Donnelly, T.M. (2004). Disease problems of small rodents. In: *Ferrets, Rabbits, and Rodents: Clinical Medicine and Surgery*, 2e (ed. K.E. Quesenberry and J.W. Carpenter), 305–306. St Louis, MO: Saunders.

Fernández-Varón, E., Carceles, C., Espuny, A. et al. (2004). Pharmacokinetics of a combination preparation of ampicillin and sulbactam in turkeys. *Am. J. Vet. Res.* 65: 1658–1663.

Fernández-Varón, E., Carceles, C., Espuny, A. et al. (2006). Short communication: pharmacokinetics of an Ampicillin–Sulbactam (2:1) combination after intravenous and intramuscular administration to chickens. *Vet. Res. Commun.* 30: 285–291.

Flammer K.(1993). An overview of antifungal therapy in birds. Proceedings of the Association of Avian Veterinarians: pp. 1–4.

Flammer K. (2002). Treatment of bacterial and mycotic diseases of the avian gastrointestinal tract. Proceedings of the North American Veterinarians Conference: pp. 851–852.

Flammer K, Massey JG, Roudybush T, Meek C. (2011). Doxycycline-medicated pelleted diet in cockatiels. Proceedings of the Annual Conference of the Association of Avian Veterinarian: p. 15.

Flecknell, P.A. (2001). Analgesia of small mammals. *Vet. Clin. North Am. Exot Anim. Pract.* 4: 47–56.

Flecknell, P.A., Orr, H.E., Roughan, J.V. et al. (1999). Comparison of the effects of oral or subcutaneous carprofen or ketoprofen in rats undergoing laparotomy. *Vet. Rec.* 144: 65–67.

Fleming, G.J. and Robertson, S.A. (2012). Assessments of thermal antinociceptive effects of butorphanol and human observer effect on quantitative evaluation of analgesia in green iguanas (Iguana iguana). *Am. J. Vet. Res.* 73: 1507–1511.

Foley, P.L., Liang, H., and Crichlow, A.R. (2011). Evaluation of a sustained-release formulation of buprenorphine for analgesia in rats. *J. Am. Assoc. Lab. Anim. Sci.* 50: 198–204.

Funk, R.S. and Diethelm, G. (2006). Reptile formulary. In: *Reptile Medicine and Surgery*, 2e (ed. D.R. Mader), 1120. St Louis, MO: Saunders Elsevier.

Gades, N.M., Danneman, P.J., Wixson, S.K. et al. (2000). The magnitude and duration of the analgesic effect of morphine, butorphanol, and buprenorphine in rats and mice. *Contemp. Top. Lab. Anim. Sci.* 39: 8–13.

Gamble, K.C. (2008). Plasma fentanyl concentrations achieved after Transdermal fentanyl patch application in prehensile-tailed skinks, Corucia zebrata. *J. Herpetol. Med. Surg.* 18: 81–85.

Gauvin, J. (1993). Drug therapy in reptiles. *Sem. Avian Exotic Pet. Med.* 2 (1): 48–59.

Gentz, E.J., Harrenstein, L.A., and Carpenter, J.W. (1995). Dealing with gastrointestinal, genitourinary, and musculoskeletal problems in rabbits. *Vet. Med.* 90 (4): 365–372.

Georoff, T.A., Moore, R.P., Rodriguez, C. et al. (2013). Efficacy of treatment and long-term follow-up of Batrachochytrium dendrobatidis PCR-positive anurans following itraconazole bath treatment. *J. Zoo Wildl. Med.* 44 (2): 395–403.

Gibbons, P.M. (2014). Therapeutics. In: *Current Therapy in Reptile Medicine and Surgery*, 3e (ed. D.R. Mader and S.J. Divers), 57–69. St Louis, MO: Elsevier.

Giorgi, M., de Vito, V., Owen, H. et al. (2014). PK/PD evaluations of the novel atypical opioid tapentadol in red-eared slider turtles. *Medycyna Weterynaryjna* 70: 530–535.

Giorgi, M., Lee, H.-K., Rota, S. et al. (2015). Pharmacokinetic and pharmacodynamic assessments of tapentadol in yellow-bellied slider turtles(Trachemys scripta scripta) after a single intramuscular injection. *J. Exotic Pet. Med.* 24: 317–325.

Graham, J., Garner, M.M., and Reavill, D.R. (2014). Benzimidazole toxicosis in rabbits: 13 cases (2003 to 2011). *J. Exotic. Pet. Med.* 23 (2): 188–195.

Greenacre, C., Paul-Murphy, J., Sladky, K.K. et al. (2005). Reptile and amphibian analgesia. *J. Herpetol. Med. Surg.* 15: 24–30.

Greenacre, C., Schumacher, J., and Talke, G. (2006). Comparative anti-nociception of morphine, butorphanol, and buprenorphine versus saline in green iguanas, Iguana iguana, using electro-stimulation. *J. Herpetol. Med. Surg.* 16: 2006.

Griggs, R.B., Bardo, M.T., and Taylor, B.K. (2015). Gabapentin alleviates affective pain after traumatic nerve injury. *Neuroreport* 26: 522–527.

Guinotte, F., Gautron, J., Soumarmon, A. et al. (1993 Oct). Gastric acid secretion in the chicken: effect of histamine H2 antagonists and H+/K(+)-ATPase inhibitors on gastro-intestinal pH and of sexual maturity calcium carbonate level and particle size on proventricular H+/K+ ATPase activity. *Comp. Biochem. Physiol. Comp. Physiol.* 106 (2): 319–327.

Guzman, D.S., Flammer, K., Paul-Murphy, J.R. et al. (2011). Pharmacokinetics of butorphanol after intravenous, intramuscular, and oral administration in Hispaniolan Amazon parrots (Amazona ventralis). *J. Avian. Med. Surg.* 25: 185–191.

Harris D.(2003). Emergency management of acute illness and trauma in avian patients. Proceedings of the Atlantic Coast Veterinarians Conference.

Harrison, G.J., Lightfoot, T.L., and Flinchum, G.B. (2006). Emergency and critical care. In: *Clinical Avian Medicine* (ed. G.J. Harrison and T.L. Lightfoot), 228. Palm Beach, FL: Spix Publishing.

Hawkins, M.G. and Pascoe, P.J. (2007). Cagebirds. In: *Zoo Animal and Wildlife Immobilzation and Anesthesia* (ed. G. West, D. Heard and N. Caulkett), 285. Ames, IA: Blackwell.

Hawkins, M.G. and Pascoe, P.J. (2012). Anesthesia, analgesia, and sedation of small mammals. In: *Ferrets, Rabbits, and Rodents: Clinical Medicine and Surgery*, 3e (ed. K.E. Quesenberry and J.W. Carpenter), 429–451. St Louis, MO: Elsevier Saunders.

Hawkins, M.G., Wright, B.D., Pascoe, P.J. et al. (2003). Pharmacokinetics and anesthetic and cardiopulmonary effects of propofol in red-tailed hawks (Buteo jamaicensis) and great horned owls (Bubo virginianus). *Am. J. Vet. Res.* 64: 677–683.

Heard, D.J. (2004). Anesthesia, analgesia, and sedation of small mammals. In: *Ferrets, Rabbits, and Rodents*, 2e (ed. K. Quesenberry and J. Carpenter), 356–369. St Louis, MO: Saunders.

Heard, D.J. (2007). Rodents. In: *Zoo Animal & Wildlife Immobilization and Anesthesia* (ed. G. West, D. Heard and N. Caulkett), 655–663. Ames, IA: Wiley Blackwell.

Hernandez-Divers, S.J. (2001). Pulmonary candidiasis caused by Candida albicans in a Greek tortoise (Testudo graeca) and treatment with intrapulmonary amphotericin B. *J. Zoo Wildl. Med.* 32 (3): 352–359.

Hernandez-Divers, S. (2003). Reptile critical care. *Exotic DVM* 5: 81–87.

Hess, L. (2004). Dermatologic diseases. In: *Ferrets, Rabbits, and Rodents: Clinical Medicine and Surgery*, 2e (ed. K.E. Quesenberry and J.W. Carpenter), 199. St Louis, MO: Saunders.

Hilf, M., Swanson, D., and Wagner, R. (1991). A new dosing schedule for gentamicin in blood pythons (Python curtus): a pharmacokinetic study. *Res. Vet. Sci.* 50: 127–130.

Hillyer, E.V. (1997). Dermatologic diseases. In: *Ferrets, Rabbits, and Rodents: Clinical Medicine and Surgery* (ed. E.V. Hillyer and K.E. Quesenberry), 212–219. St Louis, MO: Saunders.

Hinrichsen, J.P., Neira, M., Lopez, C. et al. (1997 Jul). Omeprazole, a specific gastric secretion inhibitor on oxynticopeptic cells, reduces gizzard erosion in broiler chicks fed with toxic fish meals. *Comp. Biochem. Physiol. C: Pharmacol. Toxicol. Endocrinol.* 117 (3): 267–273.

Holden, W.M., Ebert, A.R., Canning, P.F., and Rollins-Smith, L.A. (2014). Evaluation of amphotericin B and chloramphenicol as alternative drugs for treatment of chytridiomycosis and their impacts on innate skin defenses. *Appl Environ Microbiol.* 80 (13): 4034–4041.

Hope, K.L., Tell, L.A., Byrne, B.A. et al. (2012). Pharmacokinetics of a single intramuscular injection of ceftiofur crystalline-free acid in American black ducks (*Anas rubripes*). *Am. J. Vet. Res.* 73: 620–627.

Howard, L.L., Papendick, R., Stalis, I.H. et al. (2002). Fenbendazole and albendazole toxicity in pigeons and doves. *J. Avian Med. Surg.* 16 (3): 203–210.

Huckabee, J.R. (2000). Raptor therapeutics. *Vet. Clin. North Am. Exot. Anim. Pract.* 3 (1): 91–116.

Huston, S.H. (2004). Cardiovascular diseases. In: *Ferrets, Rabbits, and Rodents: Clinical Medicine and Surgery*, 2e (ed. K.E. Quesenberry and J.W. Carpenter), 213. St Louis, MO: Saunders.

Idid, S.Z. and Lee, C.Y. (1996). Effects of Fuller's earth and activated charcoal on oral absorption of paraquat in rabbits. *Clin. Exp. Pharmacol. Physiol.* 23: 697–681.

Ivey, E.S. and Morrisey, J.K. (2000). Therapeutics for rabbits. *Vet. Clin. North Am. Exot. Anim. Pract.* 3 (1): 183–220.

Jacobson ER. (1999). Bacterial infections and antimicrobial treatment in reptiles. Proceedings of the North American Veterinarians Conference.

James, S.B., Calle, P.P., Raphael, B.L. et al. (2003). Comparison of injectable versus oral enrofloxacin pharmacokinetics in red-eared slider turtles, Trachemys scripta elegans. *J. Herpetol. Med. Surg.* 13 (1): 5–10.

Jankowski, G., Adkesson, M., Langan, J. et al. (2012). Cystic endometrial hyperplasia and pyometra in three captive African hunting dogs (*Lycaeon pictus*). *J. Zoo Wildl. Med.* 43 (1): 99–100.

Jenkins JR. (1991). Aspergillosis. Proceedings of the Association of Avian Veterinarians: pp. 328–330.

Jenkins, J.R. (2004). Gastrointestinal diseases. In: *Ferrets, Rabbits, and Rodents: Clinical Medicine and Surgery*, 2e (ed. K.E. Quesenberry and J.W. Carpenter), 169. St Louis, MO: Saunders Elsevier.

Johnson JD. (2002). Medical management of ill chelonians. Proceedings of the Western Veterinarians Conference.

Jones, M. (2007). Avian toxicology. Proceedings of the Western Veterinarians Conference.

Jones, M.P., Orosz, S.E., Cox, S.K., and Frazier, D.L. (2000). Pharmacokinetic disposition of itraconazole in red-tailed hawks (Buteo jamaicensis). *J. Avian Med. Surg.* 14 (1): 15–22.

Joseph, V. (1998). Emergency care of raptors. *Vet. Clin. North Am. Exotic Anim. Pract.* 1 (1): 77–98.

Kidwell, J.H., Buckley, G., Allen, A. et al. (2014). Use of IV lipid emulsion for treatment of ivermectin toxicosis in a cat. *J. Am. Anim. Hosp. Assoc.* 50 (1): 59–61.

Klaphake, E. (2005a). Sneezing turtles and wheezing snakes. Proceedings of the Western Veterinarians Conference.

Klaphake E. (2005b). Reptilian parasites. Proceedings of the Western Veterinarians Conference.

Kolmstetter, C.M., Frazier, D., Cox, S., and Ramsay, E.R. (1998). Pharmacokinetics of metronidazole in the green iguana. *Iguana iguana. Bull Assoc Reptilian Amphibian Vet.* 8: 4–7.

Kuehn, N. (2015). *North American Companion Animal Formulary: A Comprehensive Guide for Drug Usage in Dogs and Cats*, 11e. Port Huron, MI: North American Compendiums, Inc.

Lenarduzzi, T., Langston, C., and Ross, M.K. (2011). Pharmacokinetics of clindamycin administered orally to pigeons. *J. Avian Med. Surg.* 25: 259–265.

Letcher J, Papich M. (1994). Pharmacokinetics of intramuscular administration of three antibiotics in bullfrogs (Rana beiana). Proceedings of the Association of Reptilian and Amphibian Veterinarians/American Asociation of Zoo Veterinarians: pp. 79–93.

Lichtenberger, M. (2012). Emergency and critical care of small mammals. In: *Ferrets, Rabbits, and Rodents: Clinical Medicine and Surgery*, 3e (ed. K.E. Quesenberry and J.W. Carpenter), 532–544. St Louis, MO: Elsevier Saunders.

Lightfoot, T.L. (2000). Therapeutics of African pygmy hedgehogs and prairie dogs. *Vet. Clin. North Am. Exot. Anim. Pract.* 3 (1): 155–172.

Lumeij, J.T., Gorgevska, D., and Woestenborghs, R. (1995). Plasma and tissue concentrations of itraconazole in racing pigeons (Columba livia domestica). *J. Avian Med. Surg.* 9 (1): 32–35.

Mader, D. (ed.) (2006). *Reptile Medicine and Surgery*, 2e. St Louis, MO: Saunders.

Mainka, S.A., Dierenfeld, E.S., Cooper, R.M., and Black, S.R. (1994). Circulating alpha-tocopherol following intramuscular or oral vitamin E administration in Sawinson's hawks. *J. Zoo Wildl. Med.* 25 (2): 229–232.

Manire, C., Rhinehart, H., Pennick, G. et al. (2003). Steady-state plasma concentrations of itraconazole after oral administration in Kemp's ridley sea turtles, *Lepidochelys kempi. J. Zoo Wildl. Med.* 34 (2): 171–178.

Mans, C. and Donnelly, T.M. (2012). Disease problems of chinchillas. In: *Ferrets, Rabbits, and Rodents: Clinical Medicine and Surgery*, 3e (ed. K.E. Quesenberry and J.W. Carpenter), 311–325. St Louis, MO: Elsevier Saunders.

Mans, C., Lahner, L.L., Baker, B.B. et al. (2012). Antinociceptive efficacy of buprenorphine and hydromorphone in red-eared slider turtles (Trachemys scripta elegans). *J. Zoo Wildl. Med.* 43: 662–665.

Mashima, T.Y., Ley, D.H., Stoskopf, M.K. et al. (1997). Evaluation of treatment of conjunctivitis associated with mycoplasma gallisepticum in house finches (Carpodacus mexicanus). *J. Avian Med. Surg.* 11 (1): 20–24.

Mitchell, M. and Tully, T. Jr. (eds.) (2009). *Manual of Exotic Pet Practice.* St Louis, MO: Saunders Elsevier.

Morrisey, J.K. and Carpenter, J.W. (2004). Formulary. In: *Ferrets, Rabbits, and Rodents: Clinical Medicine and Surgery*, 2e (ed. K.E. Quesenberry and J.W. Carpenter), 439. St Louis, MO: Saunders.

Neiffer, D.L., Lydick, D., Burks, K., and Doherty, D. (2005). Hematologic and plasma biochemical changes associated with fenbendazole administration in Hermann's tortoises (testudo hermanni). *J. Zoo Wildl. Med.* 36 (4): 661–672.

Nemetz LP, Lennox AM. (2004). Zosyn: a replacement for pipracil in the avian patient. Proceedings of the Association of Avian Veterinarians.

Ness, R.D. and Johnson-Delaney, C.A. (2012). Sugar gliders. In: *Ferrets, Rabbits, and Rodents: Clinical Medicine and Surgery*, 3e (ed. K.E. Quesenberry and J.W. Carpenter), 393–410. St Louis, MO: Elsevier Saunders.

Oglesbee, B.L. (2011a). Guinea pigs. In: *Blackwell's Five-Minute Veterinary Consult: Small Mammal*, 2e (ed. B.L. Oglesbee), 226–341. Ames, IA: Wiley Blackwell.

Oglesbee, B.L. (2011b). Ferrets. In: *Blackwell's Five-Minute Veterinary Consult: Small Mammal*, 2e (ed. B.L. Oglesbee), 46–224. Ames, IA: Wiley Blackwell.

Olson, M.E., Vizzutti, D., Marck, D.W., and Cox, A.K. (1994). The parasympatholytic effects of atropine sulfate and glycopyrrolate in rats and rabbits. *Can. J. Vet. Res.* 58: 254–258.

O'Malley, B. (2011). Avian emergencies. World Small Animal Veterinary Association World Congress Proceedings.

Pees, M., Krautwald-Junghanns, M.E., and Straub, J. (2006). Cardiovascular system. In: *Avian Clinical Medicine* (ed. G.J. Harrison and T.L. Lightfoot), 388. Palm Beach, FL: Spix Publishing.

Petritz, O.A., Guzman, D.S., Wiebe, V.J. et al. (2013). Stability of three commonly compounded extemporaneous enrofloxacin suspensions for oral administration to exotic animals. *J. Am. Vet. Med. Assoc.* 243: 85–90.

Plumb, D.C. (2015). *Plumb's Veterinary Drug Handbook*, 8e. Ames, IA: Wiley Blackwell.

Poynton, S.L. and Whitaker, B.R. (1994). Protozoa in poison dart frogs (Dendro-batidae): clinical assessment and identification. *J Zoo Wildl Med.* 25: 29–39.

Quesenberry, K. and Carpenter, J. (eds.) (2004). *Ferrets, Rabbits, and Rodents: Clinical Medicine and Surgery*, 2e. St Louis, MO: Saunders.

Ramer, J.C., Paul-Murphy, J., and Benson, K.G. (1999). Evaluating and stabilizing critically ill rabbits – part I. *Comp. Cont. Ed. Pract. Vet.* 21 (1): 30–40.

Redig, P.T. (2003). Falconiformes. In: *Zoo and Wild Animal Medicine*, 5e (ed. M.E. Fowler and R.E. Miller), 150–161. St Louis, MO: Saunders.

Ritchie, B. (1990). Fluid therapy in the avian patient. *Vet Med Rep.* 2: 316–319.

Ritchie, B.W. and Harrison, G.J. (1997). Formulary. In: *Avian Medicine: Principles and Application* (ed. B.W. Ritchie, G.J. Harrison and L.R. Harrison), 454–478. Lake Worth, FL: Wingers Publishing.

Rosenthal, K.L. (2004). Therapeutic contraindications in exotic pets. *Sem. Avian Exotic Pet. Med.* 13 (1): 44–48.

Sadar MJ, Hawkins MG, Drzenovich T, et al. (2014). Pharmacokinetic-pharmacodynamic integration of an extended-release ceftiofur formulation administered to red-tailed hawks (*Buteo jamaicensis*). Proceedings of the Annual Conference of the Association of Avian Veterinarians: p.11.

Samour, J. (2000). Pharmaceutics commonly used in avian medicine. In: *Avian Medicine* (ed. J. Samour), 388–418. St. Louis, MO: Mosby.

Samour, J. (ed.) (2008). *Avian Medicine*, 2e. Philadelphia, PA: Mosby Elsevier.

Sanati, H., Ramos, C.F., Bayer, A.S., and Ghannoum, M.A. (1997). Combination therapy with Amphotericin B and fluconazole against invasive candidiasis in neutropenic-mouse and infective-endocarditis rabbit models. *Antimicrob. Agents Chemother.* 41: 1345–1348.

Schott R. (2015). Triaging the wildlife patient. Proceedings of the SAVMA Symposium.

Schumacher, J. (2011). Respiratory medicine of reptiles. *Vet. Clin. Exot. Anim.* 14: 207–224.

Scott, D. (2010). Formulary. In: *Raptor Medicine, Surgery and Rehabiliation*, 30. Boston: CABI.

Silvanose, C., Bailey, T., and di Somma, A. (2011). In vitro sensitivity of Aspergillus species isolated from respiratory tract of falcons. *Vet. Scan.* 6 (2): 95.

Stahl SJ. (1999). Medical management of bearded dragons. Proceedings of the North American Veterinarians Conference: 789–792.

Tavernier, P., Saggese, M., van Wettere, A., and Redig, P. (2005). Malaria in an eastern screech owl (Otus asio). *Avian Dis.* 49 (3): 433–435.

Thuesen, L. et al. (2009). Selected pharmacokinetic parameters for Cefovecin in hens and green iguanas. *J. Vet. Pharmacol. Ther.* 32 (6): 613–617.

Travis, E. (2007). Ileocecocolic strictures in two captive cheetahs (Acinonyx jubatus jubatus). *J. Zoo Wildl. Med.* 38 (4): 574–578.

Tully, T.N. (1996). Therapeutics. In: *Ratite Management, Medicine, and Surgery* (ed. T.N. Tully and S.M. Shane), 155–163. Malabar, FL: Krieger.

Vennen, K.M. and Mitchell, M.A. (2009). Rabbits. In: *Manual of Exotic Pet Practice* (ed. M.A. Mitchell and T.N. Tully), 392. St Louis, MO: Saunders Elsevier.

Wack, A.N., KuKanich, B., Bronson, E. et al. (2012). Pharmacokinetics of enrofloxacin after single dose oral and intravenous administration in the African penguin (Spheniscus demersus). *J. Zoo Wildl. Med.* 43: 309–316.

Waeyenberghe, L. et al. (2010). Voriconazole, a safe alternative for treating infections caused by the *Chrysosporium* anamorph of *Nannizziopsis vriesii* in bearded dragons (*Pogona vitticeps*). *Med. Mycol.* 48 (6): 880–885.

Wagner, R. and Wendlberger, U. (2000). Field efficacy of moxidectin in dogs and rabbits naturally infested with Sarcoptes spp., Demodex spp. and Psoroptes spp. mites. *Vet. Parasitol.* 93 (2): 149–158.

Waxman, S., Prados, A.P., de Lucas, J. et al. (2013). Pharmacokinetic and pharmacodynamic properties of enrofloxacin in Southern crested caracaras (*Caracara plancus*). *J. Avian Med. Surg.* 27: 180–186.

Weber, M.A., Miller, M.A., Neiffer, D.L., and Terrell, S.P. (2006). Presumptive fenbendazole toxicosis in North American porcupines. *J. Am. Vet. Med. Assoc.* 228 (8): 1240–1242.

Wernick, M. and Muntener, C.R. (2010). Cefovecin: a new long-acting cephalosporin. *J. Exotic Pet. Med.* 19 (4): 317–322.

Wright, K.M. (1996). Amphibian husbandry and medicine. In: *Reptile Medicine and Surgery* (ed. D.R. Mader), 436–459. Philadelphia: W.B. Saunders.

Wright KM. (1997). Common medical problems of tortoises. Proceedings of the North American Veterinarians Conference.

Wright, K.M. (2006). Amphibian formulary. In: *Reptile Medicine and Surgery*, 2e (ed. D.R. Mader), 1140–1146. St Louis, MO: Saunders Elsevier.

Wright, K. (2014). Amphibian therapy. In: *Current Therapy in Reptile Medicine & Surgery* (ed. D. Mader and S. Divers), 281–288. St. Louis, MO: Elsevier Saunders.

Wright, K.M. and Whitaker, B.R. (2001). Pharmacotherapeutics. In: *Amphibian Medicine and Captive Husbandry* (ed. K.M. Wright and B.R. Whitaker), 309–330. Malabar, FL: Krieger Publishing.

Yarto-Jaramillo, E. (2015). Rodentia. In: *Fowler's Zoo and Wild Animal Medicine*, vol. 8 (ed. R.E. Miller and M.E. Fowler), 384–422. St Louis, MO: Elsevier Saunders.

Young, L.A., Schumacher, J., Papich, M. et al. (1997). Disposition of enrofloxacin and its metabolite ciprofloxacin after intramuscular injection in juvenile Burmese pythons (Python molurus bivittatus). *J. Zoo. Wildl. Med.* 28 (1): 71–79.

Index

Numbers in *italics* refer to figures; numbers in **bold** refer to tables.

Medical Management of Wildlife Species: A Guide for Practitioners, First Edition. Edited by Sonia M. Hernandez,
Heather W. Barron, Erica A. Miller, Roberto F. Aguilar and Michael J. Yabsley.
© 2020 John Wiley & Sons, Inc. Published 2020 by John Wiley & Sons, Inc.